Exercise and Physical Activity During Pregnancy and Postpartum

Rita Santos-Rocha
Editor

Exercise and Physical Activity During Pregnancy and Postpartum

Evidence-Based Guidelines

Second Edition

Springer

Editor
Rita Santos-Rocha
Sport Sciences School of Rio Maior - ESDRM
Polytechnic Institute of Santarém
Rio Maior, Portugal

ISBN 978-3-031-06136-3 ISBN 978-3-031-06137-0 (eBook)
https://doi.org/10.1007/978-3-031-06137-0

Previous editions published with Springer International Publishing

This Springer imprint is published by the registered company Springer Nature Switzerland AG
The registered company address is: Gewerbestrasse 11, 6330 Cham, Switzerland

Foreword

Exercise and a healthy lifestyle during pregnancy are key to preventing chronic disease risk in both mother and her developing fetus [1]. Maternal benefits of exercise include improved fitness [2], prevention of excessive pregnancy weight gain [3], weight retention and potential obesity [4], gestational diabetes [5], hypertension [6], maternal depression [7], and reduction in cesarean section rates [8]. Maternal exercise has also been linked to appropriate birth weight [9] and prevention of chronic disease development in the offspring [1]. When these benefits are considered, it is surprising that many healthcare providers do not advocate a healthy lifestyle for pregnant individuals. The second edition of this well-rounded book provides updated information in each chapter plus the inclusion of the insights into the early postpartum period. The first two chapters present information regarding education of healthcare providers and fitness professionals of the importance of health promotion during pregnancy (Chap. 1) and the importance of psychological and behavioral support necessary for women to be successful in beginning or maintaining physical activity during pregnancy (Chap. 2). Lack of information and social support are two reasons why pregnant women may not be engaged in physical activity. Knowledge of benefits of prenatal exercise may lead to a more favorable attitude towards exercise among participants, healthcare providers, and exercise professionals from an international perspective as Chap. 7 presents evidence-based guidelines for exercising during pregnancy that are practice-oriented. Guidelines for exercise testing and prescription for pregnant individuals are presented in Chap. 8, followed by suggestions for programming exercise classes that includes steps for planning and conducting classes, and monitoring pregnant individuals and providing exercise adaptations during pregnancy for safe physical activity (Chap. 9).

Pregnancy affects every system of the body, and it is important to understand the physiological changes (Chap. 3), body composition alterations (Chap. 4), and the biomechanical adaptations (Chap. 5) to pregnancy and the implications for physical activity. In addition, pregnancy alterations to the musculoskeletal system (including the pelvic floor, pelvic girdle, and lower back) may increase risk factors for musculoskeletal disorders (such as diastasis recti), impairments (such as urinary incontinence), and pain in the lower back and pelvic girdle (Chap. 6). Recommendations for treatment and guidance for recovery of functional capacity related to potential impairment and disorders of the musculoskeletal system are also important features of Chap. 6. Prenatal exercise can also be used as a therapy for musculoskeletal health of the pregnant exerciser and athlete to improve and restore physical function (Chap. 12).

Nutritional and energy requirements of the pregnant individual who exercises including the athlete are outlined in Chap. 13 with the dietary recommendations for these individuals bridging the gap between science and practice with a summary of main dietary recommendations found in Chap. 14. Dietary intake before, during, and after maternal exercise is important to monitor to maintain adequate energy availability while avoiding unhealthy behaviors such as alcohol or drug use. New to this edition is Chap. 10 with a focus on exercise prescription and adaptations in the early postpartum, considered the "fourth trimester" with emphasis on planning, conducting, and monitoring exercise classes to assist in transitioning back to exercise and physical activity after giving birth, followed by Chap. 11 which discusses strengthening the competences of future healthcare professionals in promoting physical activity during pregnancy and the postpartum period using educational strategies and digital health.

The second edition provides chapters written by experts in their respective fields with a summary of revised and up-to-date evidence-based literature and presented in a comprehensive format that can be used by healthcare providers and fitness professionals to assist and engage individuals who wish to be physically active and follow a healthy lifestyle throughout pregnancy and into the "fourth trimester."

References

1. Nagpal TS, Mottola MF. Physical activity throughout pregnancy is key to preventing chronic disease. Reproduction. 2020;160:R111–8.
2. Ruchat SM, Davenport MH, Giroux I, Hillier M, Batada A, Hammond JA, Sopper MM, Mottola MF. Walking program of low or vigorous intensity during pregnancy confers an aerobic benefit. Int J Sports Med. 2012;33:661–6.
3. Ruchat SM, Mottola MF, Skow RJ, Nagpal TS, Meah VL, James M, Riske L, Sobierajski F, Kathol AJ, Marchand AA, Nuspl M, Weeks A, Gray CE, Poitras VJ, Jaramillo Garcia A, Barrowman N, Slater LG, Adamo KB, Davies GA, Barakat R, Davenport MH. Effectiveness of exercise interventions in the prevention of excessive gestational weight gain and postpartum weight retention: a systematic review and meta-analysis. Br J Sports Med. 2018;52(21):1347–56.
4. Mottola MF. Pregnancy, physical activity and weight control to prevent obesity and future chronic disease risk in both mother and child. Curr Women's Health Rev. 2015;11(1):31–40.
5. Davenport MH, Ruchat SM, Poitras VJ, Jaramillo Garcia A, Gray CE, Barrowman N, Skow RJ, Meah VL, Riske L, Sobierajski F, James M, Kathol AJ, Nuspl M, Marchand AA, Nagpal TS, Slater LG, Weeks A, Adamo KB, Davies GA, Barakat R, Mottola MF. Prenatal exercise for the prevention of gestational diabetes mellitus and hypertensive disorders of pregnancy: a systematic review and meta-analysis. Br J Sports Med. 2018;52(21):1367–75.
6. Barakat R, Pelaez M, Cordero Y, Perales M, Lopez C, Mottola MF. Exercise initiated in early pregnancy protects against hypertension, excessive weight gain and macrosomia: randomized control trial. Am J Obstet Gynecol. 2016;214(5):649.e1–8.
7. Vargas-Terrones M, Nagpal TS, Perales M, Prapavessis P, Mottola MF, Barakat R. Physical activity and prenatal depression: going beyond statistical significance by assessing the impact of reliable and clinical significant change. Psychol Med. 2021;51(4):688–93.

8. Shojaei B, Loripoor M, Sheikhfathollahi M, Aminzadeh F. The effect of walking during late pregnancy on the outcomes of labor and delivery: a randomized clinical trial. J Educ Health Promot. 2021;10:277–85.
9. Wiebe HW, Boule N, Chari R, Davenport MH. The effect of supervised prenatal exercise on fetal growth. A meta-analysis. Obstet Gynecol. 2015;125:1185–94.

Michelle F. Mottola

R. Samuel McLaughlin Foundation—Exercise and Pregnancy Laboratory, School of Kinesiology, Faculty of Health Sciences, Department of Anatomy and Cell Biology, Schulich School of Medicine and Dentistry, Children's Health Research Institute
mmottola@uwo.ca https://www.uwo.ca/fhs/EPL/
The University of Western Ontario
London, ON, Canada

Preface

For several years I had the opportunity to work as exercise professional in the health and fitness context with populations of all ages, including pregnant and postpartum women. I do believe in exercise, and I have always been enthusiastic about working with pregnant women in the roles of exercise professional, and later, also as a mother (of Guilherme, Sofia, and Leonor). As a professor and researcher, I have devoted my efforts to the field of exercise and sporting activity during pregnancy and the postpartum period, by means of lectures, workshops, conferences, thesis supervision, and publications.

The current evidence leaves no room for doubt that physical activity and exercise should be part of a healthy lifestyle during pregnancy and the postpartum period. Moreover, physical activity and exercise are beneficial for the health and fitness of both mother and fetus. However, too many pregnant and postpartum women give up or limit their exercise due to undue fear of losing a child or complications during pregnancy and childbirth. On the other hand, sometimes neither the women nor the professionals know what types of exercises are the best, the safest, and the most effective.

Sport, exercise, and physical activity during pregnancy and postpartum is a quite demanding field of knowledge and practice. Exercise professionals must be aware of the many physiological, biomechanical, and psychosocial adaptations caused by pregnancy, as well as the pregnancy-related health conditions, symptoms, and discomforts, bearing in mind the proper pre-exercise and basic fitness evaluations, individualized exercise prescription, exercise selection, adaptation, and safety, while conducting pre- and postnatal exercise programs. Healthcare professionals must develop appropriate health screening, ongoing medical monitoring, and specific treatment as necessary, as well as monitor potential contraindications for exercise, having in mind the quite prevalent health conditions (such as excessive weight gain, gestational diabetes, low back and pelvic girdle pain, urinary incontinence, and diastasis recti). They must also be active agents in the health promotion process by providing counseling on the benefits of physical activity, recreational exercise, sports, and therapeutic exercise, and other aspects of health, such as nutrition, sleep, and behaviors to be avoided. Thus, a multidisciplinary team approach is of particular importance, and communication between exercising or sporting women, medical doctors (obstetricians, gynecologists, general practitioners, or other), midwives, exercise professionals (exercise specialists, coaches, and exercise physiologists), physical therapists, nutritionists, psychologists, among others, is fundamental.

My personal goals were to gather international researchers and practitioners focused on the field of physical activity, exercise, and sports during pregnancy and postpartum, to provide practical and evidence-based knowledge on the topic. This book is intended to fill the gap between evidence-based knowledge on the benefits of physical activity in pregnancy and postpartum, and practice in the implementation of exercise programs, bridging the gap between science and practice, between researchers, health, and exercise professionals, and between women and exercise. The ultimate goal is to help both exercise professionals and healthcare professionals to provide better care to pregnant and postpartum women by means of physical activity, exercise, and sports.

I want to thank from the bottom of my heart all the authors that shared their knowledge and devoted some of their busy schedules to the first and the second editions of the present publication, as well as to all models and photographers.

These authors have different academic and practice backgrounds in gynecology, physiotherapy, nursing, nutrition, psychology, and sports and exercise sciences, and come from countries such as Argentina, Australia, Canada, England, Germany, Lithuania, Norway, Poland, Portugal, Spain, Switzerland, and the Netherlands. The first edition of this book was the first time that authors from different countries have decided to present a collective release of their scientific or practical experience in this topic. The second edition represents an update and reinforcement of this international cooperation.

The second edition is a comprehensive and multidisciplinary volume structured in 14 chapters. The book combines research and exercise/clinical applications and provides a real standard reference in this specific field for medical, health, sports, and exercise professionals, as well as students and researchers.

Chapter 1 will give an overview regarding the concepts of physical activity and exercise and health promotion aspects for the pregnant exerciser. Chapter 2 addresses the current evidence surrounding the psychosocial aspects of an active pregnancy and provides recommendations for providing psychological and behavioral support to women to become or remain active throughout their pregnancy. Chapters 3, 4, and 5 address, respectively, the physiological, body composition, and biomechanical changes during pregnancy, the main forms of assessing these parameters, and their implications for physical activity and exercise. Chapter 6 addresses the most prevalent musculoskeletal impairments during pregnancy and postpartum, such as urinary incontinence, diastasis recti abdominis, pregnancy-related low back pain and/or pelvic girdle pain, and provides recommendations on how to recover functional capacity. Chapter 7 updates the review of the current evidence-based and practice-oriented guidelines for exercising during pregnancy in different countries, regarding the contents related to prenatal exercise programs. Chapter 8 focuses on the components of pre-exercise evaluation, exercise testing, and exercise prescription for pregnant exercisers. Chapter 9 is practice-oriented regarding exercise selection and adaptations during pregnancy. Chapter 10 focuses on the components of pre-exercise evaluation and exercise prescription and is practice-oriented regarding the selection of exercises during the early postpartum period. Chapter 11 focuses on educational strategies and digital health to empower future healthcare professionals in the promotion of physical activity during the perinatal period. Chapter 12 is also practice-oriented to the therapeutic exercise regarding the musculoskeletal health of the pregnant exerciser. Chapter 13 addresses the nutritional requirements for the pregnant exerciser and athlete, and the unhealthy habits to avoid. Finally, Chap. 14 aims to fill the gap between evidence-based knowledge on the impact of dietary habits during pregnancy and particularly the pregnant exerciser and athlete and provides diet recommendations.

The following features of the book should be highlighted:

1. Multidisciplinary volume
2. Combines research and exercise/clinical applications
3. Practice-oriented with increased number of figures and links to videos
4. Updated and extended second edition of the first international collective, evidence-based book on exercise in pregnancy and postpartum.

Hopefully, this book will attract health professionals, exercise and sports professionals, researchers, and students and will increase the recognition of the importance, effectiveness, and safety of the broad area of physical activity, exercise, and sport during pregnancy and postpartum.

This book is dedicated to the memory of Elisa Geranio, editor at Springer, whom I had the pleasure to meet in Vienna, in July 2016, during the Congress of the European College of Sport Science. Elisa Geranio challenged me to this editorial project and provided support until the first edition was submitted.

Rio Maior, Portugal — Rita Santos-Rocha

Contents

Editors and Contributors

About the Editor

Rita Santos-Rocha (Lisbon, 1971) is associate professor at the Sport Sciences School of Rio Maior (ESDRM—Escola Superior de Desporto de Rio Maior)—Polytechnic Institute of Santarém, Portugal, that she supervised as director between 2011 and 2015. She was the president of the scientific board between 2018 and 2022. She is the program director of the master's degree in Physical Activity and Health, and Professor of the bachelor's degrees in Sport, Fitness and Health, in Exercise Testing and Prescription, Public Health and Physical Activity, and Research Methods.

Professor Santos-Rocha is a researcher of the Neuromechanics of Human Movement Group of the Interdisciplinary Centre for the Study of Human Performance (CIPER)—Faculty of Human Kinetics (FMH)—University of Lisbon. Her research interests are mainly focused on the impact of physical activity and exercise programs and gait biomechanics, on pregnant and postpartum women, and other special populations.

She was the leader of the EuropeActive's Educational Standards for the Pregnancy and Postnatal Exercise Specialist published in 2016, which refers to the European Qualification Framework. Professor Santos-Rocha has been collaborating with the Professional Standards Committee of EuropeActive (former European Health & Fitness Association) since 2010, and holds a seat on the scientific board of the Gymnastics Federation of Portugal between 2006 and 2020. She is a founder member of the Portuguese Association of Exercise Physiologists (APFE).

In the past, she worked as a fitness instructor, gymnastics and physical education teacher, and exercise physiologist, with people from 2 to 92 years old, including pregnant and postpartum women. She continues to work in the fitness industry as a training provider and supervisor of exercise professionals and students.

She holds a BSc in Sports Sciences (1996), an MSc in Exercise and Health (2000), and a PhD in Human Movement—Health and Fitness (2006).

Contributors

Liliana Aguiar, PhD Laboratory of Biomechanics and Functional Morphology, Interdisciplinary Centre for the Study of Human Performance - CIPER, Faculty of Human Kinetics – FMH, University of Lisbon, Cruz Quebrada-Dafundo, Portugal

European University (Universidade Europeia), Lisbon, Portugal

School of Health Technology – ESTeSL, Polytechnic Institute of Lisbon, Lisbon, Portugal

Ana-Luisa Alvarez-Falcón, MSc Dietetics Unit, University Hospital of Gran Canaria, Dr. Negrin, Las Palmas de Gran Canaria, Spain

Lou Atkinson, PhD School of Psychology, Aston University, Birmingham, UK

Applied Health Research Group, College of Health & Life Sciences, Aston University, Birmingham, UK

Ruben Barakat, PhD Faculty of Physical Activity and Sport Sciences – INEF, Technical University of Madrid, Madrid, Spain

Kari Bø, PhD Department of Sports Medicine, Norwegian School of Sport Sciences, Oslo, Norway

Department of Obstetrics and Gynecology, Akershus University Hospital, Lørenskog, Norway

Marco Branco, PhD Sport Sciences School of Rio Maior - ESDRM, Polytechnic Institute of Santarém, Rio Maior, Portugal

Laboratory of Biomechanics and Functional Morphology, Interdisciplinary Centre for the Study of Human Performance - CIPER, Faculty of Human Kinetics – FMH, University of Lisbon, Cruz Quebrada-Dafundo, Portugal

Isabel Corrales Gutiérrez, PhD Fetal Medicine Unit, Department of Surgery, University Hospital Virgen Macarena, University of Seville, Seville, Spain

Hélia Dias, PhD Health School of Santarém - ESSS, Polytechnic Institute of Santarém, Santarém, Portugal

Center for Health Technology and Services Research (NursID Group – Innovation & Development in Nursing), University of Porto, Porto, Portugal

Coral Falco, PhD Department of Sport, Food and Natural Sciences, Faculty of Education, Arts and Sports, Western Norway University of Applied Sciences, Bergen, Norway

Inês Ferreira, MSc Directorate General of Health, Ministry of Health, Lisbon, Portugal

Frøydis Hausmann, PhD Department of Sport, Food and Natural Sciences, Faculty of Education, Arts and Sports, Western Norway University of Applied Sciences, Bergen, Norway

Gunvor Hilde, PhD Department of Physiotherapy, OsloMet-Oslo Metropolitan University (former: Oslo and Akershus University College of Applied Sciences), Oslo, Norway

Mathilde Hyvärinen, MSc School of Health Sciences – HESAV, University of Applied Sciences and Arts Western Switzerland - HES-SO, Lausanne, Switzerland

Rui Jorge, PhD Agrarian School of Santarém - ESAS, Polytechnic Institute of Santarém, Santarém, Portugal

Sport Sciences School of Rio Maior - ESDRM, Polytechnic Institute of Santarém, Rio Maior, Portugal

School of Health Sciences - ESSLei, Polytechnic Institute of Leiria, Leiria, Portugal

Claire De Labrusse, PhD School of Health Sciences – HESAV, University of Applied Sciences and Arts Western Switzerland - HES-SO, Lausanne, Switzerland

Patrícia Mota, PhD H&TRC-Health and Technology Research Center, ESTeSL-Lisbon School of Health Technology, Polytechnic Institute of Lisbon, Lisbon, Portugal

Laboratory of Biomechanics and Functional Morphology, Faculty of Human Kinetics, Interdisciplinary Centre for the Study of Human Performance, University of Lisbon, Cruz Quebrada-Dafundo, Portugal

Taniya Singh Nagpal, PhD Faculty of Applied Health Sciences, Brock University, St. Catharines, ON, Canada

Miguel Ángel Oviedo-Caro, PhD Department of Physical Education and Sport, University of Seville, Seville, Spain

Katrine Mari Owe, PhD Norwegian Research Centre for Women's Health, Oslo University Hospital, Oslo, Norway

Simona Pajaujiene, PhD Lithuanian Sports University, Kaunas, Lithuania

Augusto Gil Pascoal, PhD Laboratory of Biomechanics and Functional Morphology, Faculty of Human Kinetics, Interdisciplinary Centre for the Study of Human Performance, University of Lisbon, Cruz Quebrada-Dafundo, Portugal

María Perales, PhD University Camilo José Cela, Madrid, Spain

Research Institute Hospital 12 de Octubre ('i + 12'), Madrid, Spain

Nuno M. Pimenta, PhD Sport Sciences School of Rio Maior – ESDRM, Polytechnic Institute of Santarém, Rio Maior, Portugal

Healthy Weight Laboratory, Interdisciplinary Centre for the Study of Human Performance - CIPER, Faculty of Human Kinetics – FMH, University of Lisbon, Cruz Quebrada-Dafundo, Portugal

Mireille van Poppel, PhD Institute of Human Movement Science, Sport and Health, University of Graz, Graz, Austria

Belén Rodriguez, PhD Tu Gestor de Salud for Nutrition and Sport, Madrid, Spain

Spanish Paralympic Committee, Madrid, Spain

Rita Santos-Rocha, PhD Sport Sciences School of Rio Maior - ESDRM, Polytechnic Institute of Santarém, Rio Maior, Portugal

Laboratory of Biomechanics and Functional Morphology, Interdisciplinary Centre for the Study of Human Performance - CIPER, Faculty of Human Kinetics - FMH, University of Lisbon, Lisbon, Portugal

Franziska Schläppy, BSc Department of Midwifery, School of Health Sciences – HESAV, University of Applied Sciences and Arts Western Switzerland - HES-SO, Lausanne, Switzerland

Maria-Raquel G. Silva, PhD FP-I3ID, FP-BHS and Faculty of Health Sciences, University Fernando Pessoa, Porto, Portugal

CIAS-Research Centre for Anthropology and Health - Human Biology, Health and Society, University of Coimbra, Coimbra, Portugal

CHRC-Comprehensive Health Research Centre - Sleep, Chronobiology and Sleep Disorders, Nova Medical School, Nova University of Lisbon, Lisbon, Portugal

Britt Stuge, PhD Division of Orthopaedic Surgery, Oslo University Hospital, Oslo, Norway

Anna Szumilewicz, PhD Gdansk University of Physical Education and Sport, Gdańsk, Poland

Diana Teixeira, PhD NOVA Medical School - FCM, NOVA University of Lisbon, Lisbon, Portugal

Comprehensive Health Research Centre - CHRC, NOVA Medical School - FCM, NOVA University of Lisbon, Lisbon, Portugal

Megan Teychenne, PhD Deakin University, Geelong, VIC, Australia

Institute for Physical Activity and Nutrition (IPAN), School of Exercise and Nutrition Sciences, Burwood, VIC, Australia

António Prieto Veloso, PhD Laboratory of Biomechanics and Functional Morphology, Interdisciplinary Centre for the Study of Human Performance - CIPER, Faculty of Human Kinetics – FMH, University of Lisbon, Cruz Quebrada-Dafundo, Portugal

Filomena Vieira, PhD Laboratory of Biomechanics and Functional Morphology, Interdisciplinary Centre for the Study of Human Performance - CIPER, Faculty of Human Kinetics – FMH, University of Lisbon, Cruz Quebrada-Dafundo, Portugal

Jennifer Wegrzyk, PhD School of Health Sciences – HESAV, University of Applied Sciences and Arts Western Switzerland - HES-SO, Lausanne, Switzerland

Aneta Worska, MSc Gdansk University of Physical Education and Sport, Gdańsk, Poland

Physical Activity, Exercise, and Health Promotion for the Pregnant Exerciser

1

Mireille van Poppel, Katrine Mari Owe, Rita Santos-Rocha, Hélia Dias, and Miguel Ángel Oviedo-Caro

Abstract

Currently, there is consensus that maintaining light to moderate physical activity during an uncomplicated pregnancy has several benefits for the health of the woman and the fetus. Pregnancy provides good opportunities for promoting women's health and an active lifestyle. The purpose of this chapter is to provide exercise and healthcare professionals with a basic understanding of the importance of an active lifestyle, health promotion, and education during the different stages of pregnancy, by emphasizing the benefits, correlates, and patterns of physical activity during

M. van Poppel (✉)
Institute of Human Movement Science, Sport and Health, University of Graz, Graz, Austria
e-mail: Mireille.van-poppel@uni-graz.at

K. M. Owe
Norwegian Research Centre for Women's Health, Oslo University Hospital, Oslo, Norway
e-mail: Katrine.Mari.Owe@fhi.no

R. Santos-Rocha
Sport Sciences School of Rio Maior - ESDRM, Polytechnic Institute of Santarém, Rio Maior, Portugal

Laboratory of Biomechanics and Functional Morphology, Interdisciplinary Centre for the Study of Human Performance - CIPER, Faculty of Human Kinetics - FMH, University of Lisbon, Lisbon, Portugal
e-mail: ritasantosrocha@esdrm.ipsantarem.pt

H. Dias
Health School of Santarém - ESSS, Polytechnic Institute of Santarém, Santarém, Portugal

Center for Health Technology and Services Research (NursID Group – Innovation & Development in Nursing), University of Porto, Porto, Portugal
e-mail: helia.dias@essaude.ipsantarem.pt

M. Á. Oviedo-Caro
Department of Physical Education and Sport, University of Seville, Seville, Spain

R. Santos-Rocha (ed.), *Exercise and Physical Activity During Pregnancy and Postpartum*, https://doi.org/10.1007/978-3-031-06137-0_1

pregnancy. We highlight the importance of healthcare professionals in promoting the benefits of physical activity and advising women on a healthy and active lifestyle during pregnancy, referring them to a prenatal exercise specialist.

Keywords

Pregnancy · Postpartum · Health promotion · Education for health · Physical activity · Exercise

1.1 Introduction

Currently, there is consensus that maintaining light to moderate physical activity during an uncomplicated pregnancy has several benefits for the health of the woman and the fetus [1–5]. In the last three decades, scientific evidence has clearly supported the importance of physical activity and exercise during pregnancy [6–11]. In the first place, one should clarify the meaning of these terms, because sometimes the terms physical activity and exercise are used interchangeably, and there is no clear consensus on the definitions of fitness or exercise prescription [5].

Physical activity is defined as any bodily movement produced by the contraction of skeletal muscles that results in a substantial increase in caloric requirements over resting energy expenditure [5, 12]. *Exercise* is a type of physical activity consisting of planned, structured, and repetitive bodily movement done to improve and/or maintain one or more components of physical fitness [12] and/or prolong life [13]. In other words, exercise is a subcategory of physical activity. Although energy expenditure is increased during physical activity, it does not always reflect exercise and should not be confused with fitness [14]. Thus, physical activity can be categorized either in different contexts, such as leisure-time, exercise, sports, occupational, household, and transportation activities, or by intensity, i.e., light (less than 3 METs—metabolic equivalents[1]), moderate (between 3 and 5.9 METs), and vigorous (6 METs or more) [14]. The World Health Organization (WHO) guidelines recommend adults to do 150–300 min of intentional physical activity of moderate to vigorous intensity per week for good health and reduction of several diseases [15].

On the contrary, *sedentary behavior* involves activities that less than 1.5 METs [5], and *physical inactivity* is a behavioral state of not achieving on a regular basis, a certain minimum standard of physical activity [14], i.e., fail to meet the WHO recommended level of physical activity required for good health. Physical inactivity is the fourth leading cause of death worldwide [16] and considered the biggest public health problem of the twenty-first century [17].

Physical inactivity during pregnancy may be a significant public health[2] issue due to its prevalence and associates with adverse pregnancy and birth outcomes, as

---

[1] MET = Multiple of resting metabolic rate, used as a measure of exercise intensity [5].

[2] Public health is a field that encompasses many disciplines in an effort to promote and protect health and prevent disease and disability in defined populations and communities [16]. In other words, the science and art of promoting health, preventing disease, and prolonging life through the organized effects of society [17].

well as the short- and long-term risk for several chronic diseases for mother and child. Both exercise and health professional organizations have discipline-specific and endorsed guidelines for physical activity during pregnancy. However, whether interventions exist that translate health evidence of regular physical activity in pregnant women into practice remains unknown.

The purpose of this chapter is to provide exercise and healthcare professionals with a basic understanding of the importance of an active lifestyle, health promotion,[3] and education[4] during the different stages of pregnancy, by emphasizing the benefits, the correlates, and the patterns of physical activity during pregnancy.

1.2 Education for Health and Lifestyle During Pregnancy

1.2.1 Pregnancy as an Opportunity to Promote Health

Assuming the importance of professional health intervention aiming at low-risk pregnancy surveillance, the main components are defined as prenatal care, health education, and preparation for childbirth and parenting [20]. Learning and information sharing must be integrated and permeate all pregnancy care from a health education perspective. Health education is understood as "all intentional activities conducive to learning related to health and disease [...]; can facilitate the acquisition of skills; may also lead to changes in behavior and lifestyles" [21]. In other words, health education can be defined as the processes through which people learn about personal health concepts and behaviors [16]. It is necessary here to identify the indicators of differentiation in adulthood that fit the perspective of adult education. Those indicators should be considered in the operationalization of the different components of pregnancy surveillance, in order to support self-development and learning. This perspective is supported by the principles that guide learning within the andragogic model that Knowles defined in the 1970s: The need to know, the concept of self, the role of experience, the willingness to learn, the orientation of learning, and motivation [22, 23]. Adults are only inclined to start and develop a learning process as long as they recognize its applicability, that is, a process that guides them to solving problems and tasks that they encounter in their life. Since pregnancy is a period of profound physical and psychological changes in a woman's life, it is an opportune moment to change lifestyles and improve health behaviors, based on a philosophy of "woman-centered care" [24, 25].

Thus, for health education during pregnancy and in the postpartum period, the goal of health professionals should be to: increase health literacy and develop parental skills; make learning and information sharing components of each prenatal and postnatal surveillance visit with the pregnant woman/couple and family; establish a relationship of trust that facilitates the expression of expectations, fantasies, beliefs,

[3] Health promotion is the process of enabling people to increase control over the determinants of health and thereby improve their health [18].

[4] Health education can be defined as the processes through which people learn about personal health concepts and behaviors [19].

myths, feelings (positive or negative) and competencies related to pregnancy, birth and parenthood; and promote the right to adequate information for a free and informed decision.

Moreover, a routine health promotion program, encompassing education, advice, and general health assessment in the prepregnancy period can be developed for improving pregnancy outcomes by encouraging behavioral change, or allowing early identification of potentially modifiable risk factors, such as smoking, alcohol intake, poor nutrition [26], poor sleep, as well as physical inactivity.

1.2.2 Preparing for Childbirth and Parenting

The preparation for childbirth and the operationalized parenting in formal courses is an important part of health promotion in maternal, obstetric, and gynecological health [27]. These courses allow women and their partners to experience pregnancy, and from their needs, share, express, and clarify fears, doubts, and anxieties, in a group environment and mutual support, in order to enable them to the tasks that pregnancy and parenting require. The courses often include a theoretical component and a practical component. According to Recommendation 2/2012 of the Board of the College of Maternal and Obstetrical Health Nursing Specialty [28], the theoretical component includes the following topics: labor, labor analgesia, breastfeeding, puerperium, childbirth, among others. The following practical components are worth highlighting: exercises to promote the attachment of the pregnant woman/companion/baby during pregnancy; comfort techniques during labor; the role of the companion to promote the comfort of the parturient, placements during labor and delivery, and the pelvic floor toning exercises. It should be noted that this descriptive statement also refers to the creation and use of opportunities in the preconception, pregnancy, and puerperium periods to promote healthy lifestyles, which reinforces the importance of a care centered on the needs of each woman and structured based on the philosophy of the andragogic model.

1.2.3 Health and Lifestyle Promotion

There is growing evidence that regular physical activity during pregnancy contributes positively to physical and psychological health. Moreover, physical activity significantly affects public health as it reduces the risk of chronic diseases (such as cardiometabolic diseases) and provides numerous protective factors related to psychologic (e.g., mood, self-esteem, etc.) and musculoskeletal parameters (e.g., urinary incontinence, low back pain, etc.), during and after pregnancy. Adverse consequences of inactivity may be an important problem especially among pregnant women.

Pregnancy is a period *par excellence* to identify, modify, and adopt habits and behaviors for healthy lifestyles. The pregnant woman is often motivated to learn when she understands the advantages and benefits of learning. The health professional should seek the congruence between the adult's learning process, its particularity, and the need for personal development within the life cycle. Moreover, the promotion of physical activity may represent an important prevention strategy for public health, and it implies an interaction among several professionals from health and wellbeing settings [29].

We stress the importance of healthcare professionals in promoting the benefits of physical activity, and advising women on a healthy and active lifestyle during pregnancy, referring them to a prenatal exercise specialist. It is also necessary to show that exercise specialist and instructors are well informed regarding the implementation of tailored exercise programs or the inclusion of pregnant women in regular group fitness classes. The best service is for sure provided by multidisciplinary professional groups, including exercise professionals, midwives, physiotherapists, and doctors, who can coach pregnant women to exercise properly.

However, a review by Nascimento et al. [30] reported that most pregnant women are not receiving physical activity and exercise guidance from healthcare providers, during prenatal care meetings, and some pregnant women were told to stop exercise [31]. The latter particularly applies to women pregnant with twins or triplets, who are often classified as contraindicated to physical activity and advised bed rest [32]. Several barriers experienced by healthcare providers have been identified to explain this lack of promotion of physical activity, such as a lack of time and resources and insufficient skills [33]. Nascimento et al. [30] provide suggestions to improve the quality of exercise guidance for pregnant women including the participation of a multidisciplinary team in providing educational strategies, support groups, and education about exercise benefits and safety for both pregnant women and medical professionals involved in prenatal care.

Exercise guidance and recommendations given to pregnant women in prenatal care is a particular issue in health and lifestyle promotion, since women who received some counseling were three times more likely to exercise than those who received no guidance [32, 34]. Indeed, Krans et al. [35] found that the probability that a woman exercised during pregnancy was increased if her obstetrician encouraged her to exercise.

1.3 Public Health and Physical Activity During Pregnancy

1.3.1 Impact of Maternal Physical Activity on Chronic Disease Risk

The recommendations for physical activity in pregnancy are mostly based on the evidence that maternal physical activity reduces the risk of pregnancy and birth complications. Sufficient physical activity in pregnancy may reduce the risk of the great obstetric complications (i.e., preeclampsia, gestational diabetes mellitus, hypertension, preterm, large for gestational age (LGA), small for gestational age (SGA), and other (e.g., varicose veins, deep vein thrombosis, fatigue, stress, anxiety, and depression)) [1, 3, 4, 7, 10, 11, 36].

However, for public health, not only pregnancy and birth outcomes are of relevance, but also the long-term health of both mother and offspring. Although physical activity has beneficial effects for some pregnancy outcomes, in this part the focus will be on four health parameters that are highly relevant for public health: weight status, glucose metabolism, cardiovascular health, and quality of life. The first three are influenced by both pregnancy and physical activity. Quality of life is related to the other health parameters and therefore indirectly influenced.

Pregnancy is obviously associated with weight gain. Gestational weight gain (GWG) is comprised of the accretion of water, protein (fat-free mass), and fat mass in the fetus as well as the placenta, uterus, and amniotic fluid, and expansion of maternal blood volume, mammary gland, and maternal adipose tissue [37]. How much weight women gain and are recommended to gain is dependent on their prepregnancy body mass index (BMI = weight (kg)/height $(m)^2$) [38]. However, many women gain more than the recommended weight, especially overweight and obese women [37]. Excessive GWG in pregnancy is associated with a reduced risk for preterm birth, but increases the risk for cesarean section, large for gestational age, and macrosomia [39]. Furthermore, excessive GWG is related to a higher risk of obesity in the offspring [40]. The prevention of excessive GWG is therefore relevant for both mother and child. There is a high level of evidence that a higher level of physical activity in pregnancy is related to a lower risk of excessive GWG [41–43].

From a public health perspective, it is especially worrying that excessive GWG is also associated with more weight retention postpartum. Weight retention is the difference between prepregnancy and postpartum weight. Women with excess GWG retain the most weight postpartum, and the excess weight gained in pregnancy is still retained up until 20 years later [44]. Therefore, limiting GWG in pregnancy has a long-lasting effect on the weight development of women and reduces the risk of becoming overweight or obese [45]. Since physical activity in pregnancy reduces the risk of excessive GWG, it seems logical to assume it will also reduce postpartum weight retention. However, currently, there is no convincing evidence that physical activity interventions alone in pregnancy are effective in reducing weight retention, with some studies finding reduced weight retention after antenatal intervention [46, 47] and others finding no reduction [48, 49]. However, there are relatively few studies that evaluated physical activity interventions that were initiated in pregnancy for the effect on postpartum weight retention. In contrast, there is good evidence that physical activity interventions initiated postpartum are effective in reducing weight retention [50].

Insulin sensitivity is highly influenced by pregnancy (see Chap. 3 [51], "Physiological Changes"). When women cannot "cope" with the increased insulin resistance in pregnancy with a sufficient increase in insulin secretion, they develop gestational diabetes (GDM). Women who start pregnancy with increased insulin resistance (e.g., due to obesity), or those with compromised insulin secretion, are at higher risk of developing GDM [52]. Pregnancy is therefore considered a metabolic "stress test." Women with GDM during pregnancy have an elevated risk of developing type 2 diabetes postpartum [53].

Many studies on the prevention of gestational diabetes have been conducted in recent years, most of them evaluating an intervention that included a physical activity component. Systematic reviews and meta-analyses of these studies generally conclude that physical activity interventions in pregnancy are effective in reducing the risk of gestational diabetes [43, 54]. However, there are some indications that interventions initiated in the first trimester are effective, but those initiated in the second trimester or later are not [55]. Prevention of GDM does not automatically mean that the women will not develop type 2 diabetes later in life, but that they will have a reduced risk of type 2 diabetes if they maintain their increased physical activity levels. Therefore, continued support and counseling on physical activity after a pregnancy complicated by GDM are needed. Unfortunately, this is not routinely implemented in clinical care and the most effective strategy is unclear yet. A review reported inconsistent findings of the 12 studies that addressed the effectiveness of postpartum interventions for the prevention of type 2 diabetes among women with a history of GDM [56].

Also for the cardiovascular system, pregnancy is a stress test. Gestational hypertensive disorders, including gestational hypertension and preeclampsia, are one of the leading causes of maternal morbidity and mortality [57]. Women who develop preeclampsia are at increased risk for chronic hypertension and cardiovascular disease in later life [58]. There is evidence that physical activity interventions in pregnancy reduce the risk of hypertension in pregnancy [42, 59], but have no effect on the risk of preeclampsia [59]. In contrast, observational studies show that physical activity before or in early pregnancy might be related to a lower risk of preeclampsia [60].

Given the evidence of beneficial effects of physical activity in pregnancy on maternal health, it is not surprising that it also has a positive effect on quality of life of the women during pregnancy. Physical activity has been reported to have a positive effect on quality of life, mainly with regards to physical and pain components [61–63], and maternal perception of health status [64]. Whether physical activity in pregnancy also influences the quality of life later in life is unknown, since no information on the long-term consequences for maternal quality of life is available.

1.3.2 Impact of Maternal Physical Activity on Offspring Health

Also in this part, the focus is mostly on the long-term consequences of maternal physical activity on offspring health, since this has the most implications for public health. Important neonatal outcomes, related to health outcomes in later life, are preterm birth (e.g., [65, 66]), and small- or large-for-gestational age (SGA and LGA, respectively) [67, 68], and body composition [69].

Physical activity in pregnancy is related to a reduced risk of preterm birth [42, 70–72]. Physical activity might also be related to birth weight, although results might depend on the physical intensity level, on which measure of birth weight are used as the outcome and study design. A recent meta-analysis found a small increase in mean birth weight for moderate levels of maternal physical activity and a reduction in birth weight in high maternal levels of physical activity compared to lower levels [73]. Structured exercise interventions showed small reductions in mean birth weight, and reduced the risk of LGA, without influencing the risk of SGA newborns [74].

No conclusive evidence is available for an effect of PA on neonatal body composition, mostly because it is studied relatively little [73]. Observational studies indicate that maternal physical activity might reduce neonatal body fat mass at birth [75–78]. However, one intervention study with high compliance with the exercise intervention did not find a change in offspring fat mass but a reduced lean mass in the intervention group [79]. A systematic review of lifestyle interventions in overweight or obese women reported no effect on neonatal adiposity, but only four studies were included in the review [80].

Long-term relationship of maternal physical activity in pregnancy with offspring obesity [81, 82], or fat percentage [76] has been reported. Other long-term health effects of maternal physical activity are plausible, for instance, through epigenetic changes in the offspring; however, such effects have not been demonstrated in humans yet.

1.4 Correlates of Physical Activity Among Pregnant Women

Given its numerous health benefits for both pregnant women and their children, national and international guidelines have recommended regular PA for all healthy pregnant women since the 1980s [83]. However, only a small proportion of women achieve the recommended levels of PA during pregnancy [33, 84]. In addition, longitudinal studies have shown a decline in PA levels as pregnancy progresses and PA levels are also lower in pregnant women compared to their nonpregnant counterparts [85, 86].

Therefore, identifying and understanding the factors that explain why some women are regularly physically active during pregnancy while others are not is of utmost importance to public health research. Physical activity is a complex behavior determined by the interaction of a large number of personal, social, and environmental factors specific to populations, setting, and type of physical activity. Furthering the understanding of the factors that influence physical activity behavior in specific populations such as pregnant women will aid the development of effective, tailored intervention strategies aimed at increasing the prevalence of physical activity among the pregnant population.

The terms *correlates* and *determinant* are often used synonymously in the literature. *Correlates* are factors statistically associated with or predictive of physical activity but do not imply a causal relationship. Determinants are defined as causal factors and derived from experimental or longitudinal studies [87, 88]. Most studies including pregnant women have only assessed the impact of individual correlates (i.e., psychological and biological) on physical activity during pregnancy [89]. Information on interpersonal, societal, environmental, policy, and global factors have barely been studied in pregnant populations.

Correlates and determinants of physical activity may change as pregnancy progresses due to massive bodily changes associated with pregnancy. If we assume that most women reduce their physical activity levels toward the end of their pregnancy, we may also expect correlates of PA to change. It seems that pregnant women shift from high-intensity exercise (i.e., running, ball games, and fitness training) to moderate and low-intensity exercise such as swimming and bicycling.

1.4.1 Identifying Physically Active Pregnant Women

Women who are regularly physically active before pregnancy are much more likely to continue to be regularly physically active during pregnancy [89–94]. Physically active pregnant women also tend to be older, primiparous, and have higher education [92, 93, 95–99], compared to those not meeting the recommended levels of physical activity or who are inactive during pregnancy. In addition, overweight or obesity status before pregnant and pregnancy-related weight gain are shown to be independently associated with regular exercise during pregnancy [91, 92, 98].

In nonpregnant populations, a negative association between age and physical activity has repeatedly been documented [87]. Depending on the outcome of interest, studies including pregnant women have reported both positive and negative associations with maternal age and physical activity [95, 100, 101].

1.4.2 Identifying Physically Inactive Women

Pregnancy-related factors such as gestational length, multiple pregnancies, pelvic girdle pain, nausea with or without vomiting, assisted reproduction, sub fecundity, sick leave, and other musculoskeletal pain are found to be associated with less likelihood of regular physical activity during pregnancy [92, 94, 97].

Correlates of sedentary behavior among pregnant women overlap but are not the same as for physical activity: smoking [102], having a sitting job, fewer children less than 5 years of age in the household [103], and younger age [102, 103] were related to more sedentary behavior during pregnancy.

1.5 Physical Activity Patterns Among Pregnant Women

There is a lack of information on the specific guidelines and real strategies of adaptation of several recreational and sports activities that might be adapted to healthy pregnant women. These issues are further addressed in Chaps. 7, 8, and 9 [104–106]. However, we believe that in order to better develop safe and effective exercise programs, it is necessary to understand, among other variables: the physical activity patterns of pregnant women; the motivations for exercise during pregnancy; and the characteristics of proper exercise. This information will be useful to develop recommendations for pregnancy-specific exercise programs.

Some studies report the prevalence of physical activity during pregnancy, but little references in the literature report the pattern of exercise and leisure-time physical activity using well-validated measures [84, 86, 89, 92, 96, 107–116]. Although there are international guidelines for physical activity during pregnancy recommending regular physical activity for healthy pregnant women, either sedentary or previously active, the results of such studies conducted in different countries are not favorable. A deep review of these studies is out of the scope of this chapter but the respective analysis, in general, allow to formulate key ideas, as follows.

Regarding the prevalence of physical activity, a high percentage of pregnant women are sedentary; few pregnant women are meeting the international guidelines for physical activity during pregnancy (i.e., completing the minimum of 150 min of aerobic exercise per week); and there is an increasing decline of exercise, leisure time, and work-related physical activities across pregnancy, in comparison with the prepregnancy period, especially in the first and third trimesters. Considering that the prevalence of PA is lower in the first and the third trimesters, and higher in the second trimester, only few women remain active throughout pregnancy, in accordance with the latest review on the topic, by Nascimento et al. [117]. Tavares et al. [118] and Lynch et al. [119] reported that women tend to replace moderate-intensity activities with light-intensity or sedentary activities during pregnancy. Furthermore, the reduction in physical activity level occurred not only in the level of exercise but also in daily activities, such as housework, childcare, transportation, and occupational activities [43]. According to Gaston and Vamos [32], results indicate that promoting physical activity during pregnancy should remain a public health priority.

Regarding the pattern of physical activity and exercise during pregnancy, walking is the most commonly reported form of exercise, followed by water exercise, swimming, and aerobics. Nevertheless, other types of exercise are also reported, such as dancing, cycling, jogging, resistance training, Pilates, yoga, stretching, and pelvic floor exercises. Although there is insufficient data in the literature to assess the specific effects of these types of exercise, there seems to be a consensus that they are safe, effective, and allow a broad span of intensity and complexity to be adapted to pregnant women. Further development of this topic is provided in Chaps. 7, 8, and 9 [104–106].

1.6 Measuring Physical Activity, Sedentary Behavior, and Sleep Pattern

When analyzing physical activity patterns with the aim to investigate its relationship with health, we should take into account that physical activity is part of the activity behaviors that integrate the daily activity of a person. During years, research has mainly studied the potential effect that some activity behavior in isolation, such as physical activity or sedentary activity, has for heath. For instance, scientific evidence has shown how physical activity have potential benefits to reduce the risk of developing hypertension, obesity, or adverse psychological and neonatal outcomes [3, 120–122]; or how sedentary behaviors have potential negative effects on glucose tolerance, mental distress, and pregnancy outcomes [123–126].

Scientific evidence highlights that each activity behavior has unique potential effect on health and also that one activity behavior could influence the other behaviors [126], what supposes the need of a global assessment of all behaviors rather than the assessment of them in isolation. Consequently, it has been required the introduction, for first time, of advice for sedentary behaviors in the update of the World Health Organization guidelines on physical activity [15]; or the integration of physical activity, sedentary behavior, and sleep in the update of the Canadian guidelines [127]. This perspective is related with the concept of healthy lifestyle, which is defined by the American Psychological Association's Thesaurus of Psychological Index Terms as "a pattern of behavior involving lifestyle which ensures optimum health" [128].

To reach a global conclusion when analyzing the effect of activity behavior on health, it is necessary to take into account all activity behaviors. For instance, a pregnant woman could be categorized as physically active, by meeting physical activity recommendations, but also spent a higher amount of time on sedentary activities [129]. If we only focus on the assessment of one behavior in isolation, a possible lack of information could avoid us to lead a conclusion about the influence on health that activity behaviors have.

Additionally, the finite nature of the day, 24 h, makes activity behaviors exhaustive and mutually exclusive components of a person's 24-h day [130]. This nature implies that the time spent in one behavior necessarily has to be displaced from another behavior within the 24-h day. So when analyzing the health effect of an activity behavior, the rest of activity behaviors must not be ignored because they are an influence of the studied behavior and as aforementioned a unique effect on health.

The design of the assessment procedure is very important to guarantee that it fulfills the research objective and do not lead us to misleading results. At first, it is essential to establish the dimensions of the activity behaviors that we want to analyze and to select the most appropriate instruments to obtain the activity behavior's data. In this sense, the research could focus on activity intensity (sleep, sedentary activity, light, moderate, and vigorous physical activity), activity type (walking, working, leisure, etc.), or the posture (reclining, sitting, and standing). Objective instruments such as accelerometry-based devices obtain a measurement of pregnant women's activity intensity [131, 132], while inclinometer-based devices obtain a measure of pregnant women's posture [133]. Subjective instruments such as diaries and questionnaires allow obtaining a measure of the type of activity developed by pregnant women [134–137].

Subsequently, the selection of the most appropriate statistical approach based on the characteristics of the data obtained is also very important. Traditional linear regression models, which allow analyze the relationship between a set of explanatory variables and an outcome, or traditional isotemporal substitution, which allows analyze the theoretical effect of displaced a fixed time between behaviors, show some inconvenient that impossibilities to properly analyze all activity behaviors together, i.e., multicollinearity[5] [138]. To overcome the multicollinearity problem derived from the codependent nature of activity behaviors, compositional log-ratio transformation techniques[6] have been proposed [138]. For instance, the compositional isometric log-ratio transformation allows expressing the time spent in one behavior relative to the time spent in the rest of behaviors [130], which solve the codependency problem when the research applies compositional linear regression and compositional isotemporal substitution models [139]. However, the analysis of the collinearity is still required to ensure that there is an absence of collinearity in the linear regression model [137]. The multivariate pattern analysis, which describes the pattern of associations for the descriptors with the outcome accounting for the correlated structure of the data, is another technique that allows overcoming collinearity problems [140]. However, there is a limitation in the interpretation of the results because it does not allow quantifying time exchange between descriptors or adjusting the regression models [137].

Researchers have to deeply analyze what is the best procedure to answer the research question and reach this objective. The selection of most suitable instruments and statistical approach is required to properly interpret the results and get global conclusions when analyzing the effects of activity behaviors on health.

1.7 Further Research

Although beneficial effects of physical activity in pregnancy on maternal and offspring health are established, some open questions remain. First and foremost, no consensus is reached on the type and intensity of physical activity required, especially for women who start pregnancy obese or with a low fitness level. Second, there is some evidence that the timing of physical activity (intervention) is relevant, with better outcomes for early physical activity (intervention). However, this needs to be studied more systematically. Furthermore, most studies in this field are from developed countries, and voluntary physical activity might have different effects on pregnancy outcomes than nonvoluntary physical activity (e.g., at work or for transport). Reducing physical activity levels according to developing pregnancy and possible pregnancy complaints is not always an option for women in from low-to-middle income (LMIC) countries. Whether this type of physical activity in pregnancy has the same beneficial effect on maternal and offspring outcomes is grossly understudied.

---

[5] Multicollinearity occurs when independent variables in a regression model are correlated, which is a problem when the degree of correlation between variables is high enough because it can cause problems when fitting the model and interpreting the results.

[6] Log-ratio transformation techniques allow to transfer compositional data from the constrained simplex space to the unconstrained real space, where traditional multivariate statistics may be applied.

Although there are international guidelines for physical activity during pregnancy recommending regular physical activity for healthy pregnant women, little is known about the pattern of exercise and physical activity of pregnant women worldwide. Hence, national surveillance studies of physical activity in the population should include pregnant women. Well-designed longitudinal investigations reporting pregnancy-related changes in physical activity by trimester of pregnancy would also help to fill this gap. Not only the various designs but also the various instruments used in the studies limit comparisons of studies on the practice of exercise during pregnancy. It would be of particular importance that researchers would use same precise, reliable, acculturated, and validated instruments for physical activity and exercise measurement whenever applicable, in what concerns to quantity and quality.

Moreover, results indicate a need for more information and motivation for moderate exercise before and throughout pregnancy. Pregnant women is a heterogeneous group, which implies that different women need different approaches. Promoting physical activity remains a priority in public health policy, and pregnant women or those planning a pregnancy should be encouraged to maintain an active lifestyle or to adopt a tailored exercise routine during pregnancy in order to avoid sedentary- and obesity-associated risks.

Research on better and more effective physical activity and exercise interventions that improve long-term compliance to a physically active lifestyle during and after pregnancy is needed. The methods of increasing physical activity in this special population must be developed, implemented, and evaluated.

References

1. Mottola MF, Davenport MH, Ruchat SM, et al. 2019 Canadian guideline for physical activity throughout pregnancy. Br J Sports Med. 2018;52:1339–46.
2. ACNM - American College of Nurse-Midwives. Exercise in pregnancy. J Midwif Women's Health. 2014;59:473–4.
3. ACOG - American College of Obstetricians and Gynecologists. ACOG Committee Opinion No. 804: Physical activity and exercise during pregnancy and the postpartum period. Obstet Gynecol. 2020;135(4):e178–e88.
4. SMA - Sport Medicine Australia. SMA statement the benefits and risks of exercise during pregnancy. Sydney Olympic Park, NSW: SMA; 2016. http://sma.org.au/publications-media/sma-position-statements/. Accessed 31 Dec 2017.
5. ACSM - American College of Sports Medicine. ACSM's guidelines for exercise testing and prescription. 11th ed. Baltimore, MD: Wolters Kluwer; 2021.
6. Kramer MS. Aerobic exercise for women during pregnancy. Cochrane Database Syst Rev. 2002;2:CD000180.
7. Brown W. The benefits of physical activity during pregnancy. J Sci Med Sport. 2002;5(1):37–45.
8. Downs DS, Chasan-Taber L, Evenson KR, Leiferman J, Yeo S. Physical activity and pregnancy: past and present evidence and future recommendations. Res Q Exerc Sport. 2012;83(4):485–502.
9. Kader M, Naim-Shuchana S. Physical activity and exercise during pregnancy. Eur J Physiother. 2014;16(1):2–9.

10. Perales M, Santos-Lozano A, Ruiz JR, Lucia A, Barakat R. Benefits of aerobic or resistance training during pregnancy on maternal health and perinatal outcomes: a systematic review. Early Hum Dev. 2016;94:43–8.
11. Díaz-Burrueco JR, Cano-Ibáñez N, Martín-Peláez S, Khan KS, Amezcua-Prieto C. Effects on the maternal-fetal health outcomes of various physical activity types in healthy pregnant women. A systematic review and meta-analysis. Eur J Obstet Gynecol Reprod Biol. 2021;262:203–15.
12. Caspersen CJ, Powell KE, Christenson GM. Physical activity, exercise, and physical fitness: definitions and distinctions for health-related research. Public Health Rep. 1985;100(2):126–31.
13. Boome T. Regular exercise and disease prevention. ASEP's exercise medicine text for exercise physiologists. Sharjah: Bentham Science Publishers; 2016. p. 3–31. Chapter 1.
14. ACSM - American College of Sports Medicine. ACSM's resources for the exercise physiologist. 2nd ed. Alphen aan den Rijn: Wolters Kluwer; 2018.
15. Bull FC, Al-Ansari SS, Biddle S, Borodulin K, Buman MP, Cardon G, et al. World Health Organization 2020 guidelines on physical activity and sedentary behaviour. Br J Sports Med. 2020;54(24):1451–62.
16. Kohl HW III, Craig CL, Lambert EV, Inoue S, Alkandari JR, Leetongin G, Kahlmeier S, Lancet Physical Activity Series Working Group. The pandemic of physical inactivity: global action for public health. Lancet. 2012;380(9838):294–305.
17. Blair SN. Physical inactivity: the biggest public health problem of the 21st century. Br J Sports Med. 2009;43:1–2.
18. Kohl HW III, Murray TD. Foundations of physical activity and public health. Champaign, IL: Human Kinetics; 2012.
19. Davies M, Macdowall W, editors. Health promotion theory. London: Open University Press; 2006.
20. da Saúde DG. Programa nacional para a vigilância da gravidez de baixo risco (National program for low-risk pregnancy vigilance). Lisboa: DGS; 2015. [Portuguese].
21. Tones K, Tilford S. Health education. Effectiveness, efficiency and equity. 2nd ed. London: Chapman & Hall; 1994.
22. Canário R. Educação de adultos: Um campo e uma problemática (adult education: a field and a problematic). Lisboa: Educa; 1999. [Portuguese].
23. Quintas H. Educação de adultos: vida no currículo e currículo na vida. Perspectivas e reflexões [Adult education: life in a curriculum and curriculum in life]. 1st ed. Lisboa: Agência Nacional para a Qualificação, I.P; 2008. [Portuguese].
24. Barradas A, et al. Livro de bolso: Enfermeiras especialistas em saúde materna e obstétrica/parteiras (pocket book: Midwives). Lisboa: Ordem dos Enfermeiros; 2015. [Portuguese]. http://www.ordemenfermeiros.pt/publicacoes/Documents/LivroBolso_EESMO.pdf. Accessed 30 Dec 2017.
25. Bowden J, Manning V. Health promotion in midwifery: principles and practice. 3rd ed. Boca Raton, FL: CRC Press; 2016.
26. Whitworth M, Dowswell T. Routine pre-pregnancy health promotion for improving pregnancy outcomes. Cochrane Database Syst Rev. 2009;7(4):CD007536.
27. dos Enfermeiros O. Regulamento dos padrões de qualidade dos cuidados especializados em enfermagem de saúde materna, obstétrica e ginecológica (Regulation on quality pattern of nurse care in obstetrics and gynecologics woman health). Lisboa: Ordem dos Enfermeiros; 2011. [Portuguese]. https://membros.ordemenfermeiros.pt/AssembleiasGerais/Documents/AG2011/Ponto10_Reg%20PQCEE%20SMOG.pdf. Accessed Oct 2017.
28. dos Enfermeiros O. Recomendação nº 2/2012: Recomendações para a preparação para o nascimento [Recommendations for birth preparation]. Lisboa: Ordem dos Enfermeiros; 2012. [Portuguese]. http://www.ordemenfermeiros.pt/colegios/Documents/Recomendacao_2-2012.pdf. Accessed Oct 2017.
29. Liguori G, Gallé F, Valeriani F, Romano Spica V. The role of the hygienist in prevention and health promotion through physical activity: the contribute of the Working Group "Movement Sciences for Health" of the Italian Society of Hygiene. Ann Ig. 2015;27(1):11–5.

30. Nascimento SL, Surita FG, Godoy AC, Kasawara KT, Morais SS. Physical activity patterns and factors related to exercise during pregnancy: a cross sectional study. PLoS One. 2015;10(6):e0128953.
31. Meah VL, Davies GA, Davenport MH. Why can't I exercise during pregnancy? Time to revisit medical 'absolute' and 'relative' contraindications: systematic review of evidence of harm and a call to action. Br J Sports Med. 2020;54(23):1395–404.
32. Gaston A, Vamos CA. Leisure-time physical activity patterns and correlates among pregnant women in Ontario, Canada. Matern Child Health J. 2013;17(3):477–84.
33. McParlin C, Bell R, Robson SC, Muirhead C, Araújo-Soares V. What helps or hinders midwives to implement physical activity guidelines for obese pregnant women? A questionnaire survey using the Theoretical Domains Framework. Midwifery. 2017;49:110–6.
34. Whitaker KM, Baruth M, Schlaff RA, Talbot H, Connolly CP, Liu J, Wilcox S. Provider advice on physical activity and nutrition in twin pregnancies: a cross-sectional electronic survey. BMC Pregnan Childb. 2019;19(1):418.
35. Krans EE, Gearhart JG, Dubbert PM, Klar PM, Miller AL, Replogle WH. Pregnant women's beliefs and influences regarding exercise during pregnancy. J Miss State Med Assoc. 2005;46(3):67–73.
36. Pivarnik JM, Chambliss H, Clapp J III, et al. Impact of physical activity during pregnancy and postpartum on chronic disease risk. Med Sci Sports Exerc. 2006;38(5):989–1006.
37. Gilmore LA, Klempel-Donchenko M, Redman LM. Pregnancy as a window to future health: excessive gestational weight gain and obesity. Semin Perinatol. 2015;39(4):296–303.
38. Institute of Medicine. Weight Gain During pregnancy: reexamining the guidelines. Washington, DC: The National Academies Press; 2009.
39. Goldstein RF, Abell SK, Ranasinha S, Misso M, Boyle JA, Black MH, Li N, Hu G, Corrado F, Rode L, Kim YJ, Haugen M, Song WO, Kim MH, Bogaerts A, Devlieger R, Chung JH, Teede HJ. Association of Gestational Weight Gain With Maternal and Infant Outcomes: a systematic review and meta-analysis. JAMA. 2017;317(21):2207–25.
40. Lau EY, Liu J, Archer E, McDonald SM, Liu J. Maternal weight gain in pregnancy and risk of obesity among offspring: a systematic review. J Obes. 2014;2014:524939.
41. Elliott-Sale KJ, Barnett CT, Sale C. Exercise interventions for weight management during pregnancy and up to 1 year postpartum among normal weight, overweight and obese women: a systematic review and meta-analysis. Br J Sports Med. 2015;49(20):1336–42.
42. Muktabhant B, Lawrie TA, Lumbiganon P, Laopaiboon M. Diet or exercise, or both, for preventing excessive weight gain in pregnancy. Cochrane Database Syst Rev. 2015;15(6):CD007145.
43. da Silva SG, Ricardo LI, Evenson KR, Hallal PC. Leisure-time physical activity in pregnancy and maternal-child health: a systematic review and meta-analysis of randomized controlled trials and cohort studies. Sports Med. 2017;47(2):295–317.
44. Nehring I, Schmoll S, Beyerlein A, Hauner H, von Kries R. Gestational weight gain and long-term postpartum weight retention: a meta-analysis. Am J Clin Nutr. 2011;94(5):1225–31.
45. Fraser A, Tilling K, Macdonald-Wallis C, Hughes R, Sattar N, Nelson SM, et al. Associations of gestational weight gain with maternal body mass index, waist circumference, and blood pressure measured 16 y after pregnancy: the Avon Longitudinal Study of Parents and Children (ALSPAC). Am J Clin Nutr. 2011;93:1285–92.
46. Ronnberg A, Hanson U, Ostlund I, Nilsson K. Effects on postpartum weight retention after antenatal lifestyle intervention - a secondary analysis of a randomized controlled trial. Acta Obstet Gynecol Scand. 2016;95(9):999–1007.
47. Phelan S, Phipps MG, Abrams B, Darroch F, Grantham K, Schaffner A, et al. Does behavioral intervention in pregnancy reduce postpartum weight retention? Twelve-month outcomes of the Fit for Delivery randomized trial. Am J Clin Nutr. 2014;99:302–11.
48. Althuizen E, van der Wijden CL, van Mechelen W, Seidell JC, van Poppel MN. The effect of a counselling intervention on weight changes during and after pregnancy: a randomised trial. BJOG. 2013;120(1):92–9.

49. Rauh K, Günther J, Kunath J, Stecher J, Hauner H. Lifestyle intervention to prevent excessive maternal weight gain: mother and infant follow-up at 12 months postpartum. BMC Pregnan Childb. 2015;15:265.
50. Dalrymple KV, Flynn AC, Relph SA, O'Keeffe M, Poston L. Lifestyle Interventions in overweight and obese pregnant or postpartum women for postpartum weight management: a systematic review of the literature. Nutrients. 2018;10:1704.
51. Perales M, Nagpal TS, Barakat R. Physiological changes during pregnancy. Main adaptations and discomforts and implications for physical activity and exercise. In: Santos-Rocha R, editor. Exercise and physical activity during pregnancy and postpartum. Evidence-based guidelines. 2nd ed. Cham: Springer International Publishing; 2022. Chapter 3.
52. Catalano PM, Tyzbir ED, Roman NM, Amini SB, Sims EA. Longitudinal changes in insulin release and insulin resistance in nonobese pregnant women. Am J Obstet Gynecol. 1991;165:1667–72.
53. Bellamy L, Casas JP, Hingorani AD, Williams D. Type 2 diabetes mellitus after gestational diabetes: a systematic review and meta-analysis. Lancet. 2009;373:1773–9.
54. Sanabria-Martínez G, García-Hermoso A, Poyatos-León R, Álvarez-Bueno C, Sánchez-López M, Martínez-Vizcaíno V. Effectiveness of physical activity interventions on preventing gestational diabetes mellitus and excessive maternal weight gain: a meta-analysis. BJOG. 2015;122(9):1167–74.
55. Song C, Li J, Leng J, Ma RC, Yang X. Lifestyle intervention can reduce the risk of gestational diabetes: a meta-analysis of randomized controlled trials. Obes Rev. 2016;17(10):960–9.
56. Guo J, Chen JL, Whittemore R, Whitaker E. Postpartum lifestyle interventions to prevent type 2 diabetes among women with history of gestational diabetes: a systematic review of randomized clinical trials. J Women's Health (Larchmt). 2016;25(1):38–49.
57. Lo JO, Mission JF, Caughey AB. Hypertensive disease of pregnancy and maternal mortality. Curr Opin Obstet Gynecol. 2013;25(2):124–32.
58. Brown MC, Best KE, Pearce MS, Waugh J, Robson SC, Bell R. Cardiovascular disease risk in women with pre-eclampsia: systematic review and meta-analysis. Eur J Epidemiol. 2013;28(1):1–19.
59. Magro-Malosso ER, Saccone G, Di Tommaso M, Roman A, Berghella V. Exercise during pregnancy and risk of gestational hypertensive disorders: a systematic review and meta-analysis. Acta Obstet Gynecol Scand. 2017;96(8):921–31.
60. Aune D, Saugstad OD, Henriksen T, Tonstad S. Physical activity and the risk of preeclampsia: a systematic review and meta-analysis. Epidemiology. 2014;25(3):331–43.
61. Haakstad LA, Bø K. Effect of regular exercise on prevention of excessive weight gain in pregnancy: a randomised controlled trial. Eur J Contracept Reprod Healthc. 2011;16:116–25.
62. Vallim AL, Osis MJ, Cecatti JG, et al. Water exercises and quality of life during pregnancy. Reprod Health. 2011;8:14.
63. Montoya Arizabaleta AV, Orozco Buitrago L, Aguilar de Plata AC, et al. Aerobic exercise during pregnancy improves health-related quality of life: a randomised trial. J Physiother. 2010;56:253–8.
64. Barakat R, Pelaez M, Montejo R, et al. Exercise during pregnancy improves maternal health perception: a randomized controlled trial. Am J Obstet Gynecol. 2011;204:402.e1–7, 19.
65. Bolton CE, Bush A, Hurst JR, Kotecha S, McGarvey L. Lung consequences in adults born prematurely. Postgrad Med J. 2015;91(1082):712–8.
66. Pyhälä R, Wolford E, Kautiainen H, Andersson S, Bartmann P, Baumann N, Brubakk AM, Evensen KAI, Hovi P, Kajantie E, Lahti M, Van Lieshout RJ, Saigal S, Schmidt LA, Indredavik MS, Wolke D, Räikkönen K. Self-reported mental health problems among adults born preterm: a meta-analysis. Pediatrics. 2017;139(4):e20162690.
67. Hammami M, Walters JC, Hockman EM, et al. Disproportionate alterations in body composition of large for gestational age neonates. J Pediatr. 2001;138:817–21.
68. Rogers IS, Ness AR, Steer CD, et al. Associations of birth size and dual-energy X-ray absorptiometry measures of lean and fat mass at 9 to 10 y of age. Am J Clin Nutr. 2006;84:739–47.

69. Simpson J, Smith AD, Fraser A, et al. Programming of adiposity in childhood and adolescence: associations with birth weight and cord blood adipokines. J Clin Endocrinol Metab. 2017;102:499–506.
70. Magro-Malosso ER, Saccone G, Di Mascio D, Di Tommaso M, Berghella V. Exercise during pregnancy and risk of preterm birth in overweight and obese women: a systematic review and meta-analysis of randomized controlled trials. Acta Obstet Gynecol Scand. 2017;96(3):263–73.
71. Vamos CA, Flory S, Sun H, DeBate R, Bleck J, Thompson E, Merrell L. Do physical activity patterns across the lifecourse impact birth outcomes? Matern Child Health J. 2015;19(8):1775–82.
72. Di Mascio D, Magro-Malosso ER, Saccone G, Marhefka GD, Berghella V. Exercise during pregnancy in normal-weight women and risk of preterm birth: a systematic review and meta-analysis of randomized controlled trials. Am J Obstet Gynecol. 2016;215(5):561–71.
73. Bisson M, Lavoie-Guénette J, Tremblay A, Marc I. Physical activity volumes during pregnancy: a systematic review and meta-analysis of observational studies assessing the association with infant's birth weight. AJP Rep. 2016;6(2):e170–97.
74. Wiebe HW, Boulé NG, Chari R, Davenport MH. The effect of supervised prenatal exercise on fetal growth: a meta-analysis. Obstet Gynecol. 2015;125(5):1185–94.
75. Clapp JF III, Capeless EL. Neonatal morphometrics after endurance exercise during pregnancy. Am J Obstet Gynecol. 1990;163(6 Pt 1):1805–11.
76. Clapp JF III. Morphometric and neurodevelopmental outcome at age five years of the offspring of women who continued to exercise regularly throughout pregnancy. J Pediatr. 1996;129:856–63.
77. Harrod CS, Chasan-Taber L, Reynolds RM, et al. Physical activity in pregnancy and neonatal body composition: the Healthy Start study. Obstet Gynecol. 2014;124(2 Pt 1):257–64.
78. Bisson M, Tremblay F, St-Onge O, Robitaille J, Pronovost E, Simonyan D, Marc I. Influence of maternal physical activity on infant's body composition. Pediatr Obes. 2017;12(Suppl 1):38–46.
79. Hopkins SA, Baldi JC, Cutfield WS, McCowan L, Hofman Hoplins PL. Exercise training in pregnancy reduces offspring size without changes in maternal insulin sensitivity. J Clin Endocrinol Metab. 2010;95:2080–8.
80. Baroni NF, Baldoni NR, Alves GCS, Crivellenti LC, Braga GC, Sartorelli DS. Do lifestyle interventions in pregnant women with overweight or obesity have an effect on neonatal adiposity? A systematic review with meta-analysis. Nutrients. 2021;13(6):1903.
81. Mourtakos SP, Tambalis KD, Panagiotakos DB, Antonogeorgos G, Arnaoutis G, Karteroliotis K, Sidossis LS. Maternal lifestyle characteristics during pregnancy, and the risk of obesity in the offspring: a study of 5,125 children. BMC Pregnan Childb. 2015;15:66.
82. Mudd LM, Pivarnik J, Holzman CB, Paneth N, Pfeiffer K, Chung H. Leisure-time physical activity in pregnancy and the birth weight distribution: where is the effect? J Phys Act Health. 2012;9(8):1168–77.
83. Evenson KR, Barakat R, Brown WJ, Dargent-Molina P, Haruna M, Mikkelsen EM, Mottola MF, Owe KM, Rousham EK, Yeo S. Guidelines for physical activity during pregnancy: comparisons from around the world. Am J Lifestyle Med. 2014;8(2):102–21.
84. Evenson KR, Savitz DA, Huston SL. Lesure-time physical activity among pregnat women in the US. Paediat Perinat Epidemol. 2004;18:400–7.
85. Rousham EK, Clarke PE, Gross H. Significant changes in physical activity among pregnant women in the UK as assessed by accelerometry and self-reported activity. Eur J Clin Nutr. 2006;60(3):393–400.
86. Borodulin KM, Evenson KR, Wen F, Herring AH, Benson AM. Physical activity patterns during pregnancy. Med Sci Sports Exerc. 2008;40(11):1901–8.
87. Bauman AE, Reis RS, Sallis JF, Wells JC, Loos RJ, Martin BW. Correlates of physical activity: why are some people physically active and others not? Lancet. 2012;380(9838):258–71.
88. Bauman AE, Sallis JF, Dzewaltowski DA, Owen N. Toward a better understanding of the influences on physical activity: the role of determinants, correlates, causal variables, mediators, moderators, and confounders. Am J Prev Med. 2002;23(2 Suppl):5–14.

89. Gaston A, Cramp A. Exercise during pregnancy: a review of patterns and determinants. J Sci Med Sport. 2011;14:299–305.
90. Chasan-Taber L, Schmidt MD, Pekow P, Sternfeld B, Manson J, Markenson G. Correlates of physical activity in pregnancy among Latina women. Matern Child Health J. 2007;11(4):353–63.
91. Haakstad LA, Voldner N, Henriksen T, Bø K. Why do pregnant women stop exercising in the third trimester? Acta Obstet Gynecol Scand. 2009;88(11):1267–75.
92. Owe KM, Nystad W, Bø K. Correlates of regular exercise during pregnancy: the Norwegian mother and child cohort study. Scand J Med Sci Sports. 2009;19(5):637–45.
93. Zhang Y, Dong S, Zuo J, Hu X, Zhang H, Zhao Y. Physical activity level of urban pregnant women in Tianjin, China: a cross-sectional study. PLoS One. 2014;9(10):e109624.
94. Broberg L, Ersboll AS, Backhausen MG, Damm P, Tabor A, Hegaard HK. Compliance with national recommendations for exercise during early pregnancy in a Danish cohort. BMC Pregnan Childb. 2015;15:317.
95. Petersen AM, Leet TL, Brownson RC. Correlates of physical activity among pregnant women in the United States. Med Sci Sports Exerc. 2005;37(10):1748–53.
96. Schmidt MD, Pekow P, Freedson PS, Markenson G, Chasan-Taber L. Physical activity patterns during pregnancy in a diverse population of women. J Women's Health. 2006;15(8):909–18.
97. Juhl M, Madsen M, Andersen AM, Andersen PK, Olsen J. Distribution and predictors of exercise habits among pregnant women in the Danish National Birth Cohort. Scand J Med Sci Sports. 2012;22(1):128–38.
98. Jukic AMZ, Evenson KR, Herring AH, Wilcox AJ, Hartmann KE, Daniels JL. Correlates of physical activity at two time points during pregnancy. J Phys Act Health. 2012;9(3):325–35.
99. Gjestland K, Bø K, Owe KM, Eberhard-Gran M. Do pregnant women follow exercise guidelines? Prevalence data among 3482 women, and prediction of low-back pain, pelvic girdle pain and depression. Br J Sports Med. 2013;47(8):515–20.
100. Hinton PS, Olson CM. Predictors of pregnancy-associated change in physical activity in a rural white population. Matern Child Health J. 2001;5(1):7–14.
101. Liu J, Blair SN, Teng Y, Ness AR, Lawlor DA, Riddoch C. Physical activity during pregnancy in a prospective cohort of British women: results from the Avon longitudinal study of parents and children. Eur J Epidemiol. 2011;26(3):237–47.
102. Evenson KR, Wen F. Prevalence and correlates of objectively measured physical activity and sedentary behavior among US pregnant women. Prev Med. 2011;53(1–2):39–43.
103. Jones MA, Whitaker K, Wallace M, Barone Gibbs B. Demographic, socioeconomic, and health-related predictors of objectively measured sedentary time and physical activity during pregnancy. J Phys Act Health. 2021;18:1–8.
104. Szumilewicz A, Worska A, Santos-Rocha R, Oviedo-Caro MA. Evidence-based and practice-oriented guidelines for exercising during pregnancy. In: Santos-Rocha R, editor. Exercise and physical activity during pregnancy and postpartum. Evidence-based guidelines. 2nd ed. Cham: Springer International Publishing; 2022. Chapter 7.
105. Santos-Rocha R, Corrales-Gutierrez I, Szumilewicz A, Pajaujiene S. Exercise testing and prescription during pregnancy. In: Santos-Rocha R, editor. Exercise and physical activity during pregnancy and postpartum. Evidence-based guidelines. 2nd ed. Cham: Springer International Publishing; 2022. Chapter 8.
106. Szumilewicz A, Santos-Rocha R. Exercise selection during pregnancy. In: Santos-Rocha R, editor. Exercise and physical activity during pregnancy and postpartum. Evidence-based guidelines. 2nd ed. Cham: Springer International Publishing; 2022. Chapter 9.
107. Zhang J, Savitz DA. Exercise during pregnancy among US women. Ann Epidemiol. 1996;6(1):53–9.
108. Symons Downs D, Hausenblas HA. Women's exercise beliefs and behaviors during their pregnancy and postpartum. J Midwif Womens Health. 2004;49(2):138–44.
109. Clarke PE, Rousham EK, Gross H, Halligan AW, Bosio P. Activity patterns and time allocation during pregnancy: a longitudinal study of British women. Ann Hum Biol. 2005;32(3):247–58.

110. Poudevigne MS, O'Connor PJ. A review of physical activity patterns in pregnant women and their relationship to psychological health. Sports Med. 2006;36(1):19–38.
111. Domingues MR, Barros AJD. Leisure-time physical activity during pregnancy in the 2004 Pelotas Birth Cohort Study. Rev Saude Publica. 2007;41(2):173–80.
112. Tendais I, Figueiredo B, Mota J. Actividade física e qualidade de vida na gravidez. Aná Psicológica. 2007;25(3):489–501. [Portuguese].
113. Gouveia R, Martins S, Sandes AR, Nascimento C, Figueira J, Valente S, Correia S, Rocha E, Silva LJ. Gravidez e exercício – mitos, evidências e recomendações. Acta Medica Port. 2007;20:209–14. [Portuguese].
114. Hegaard HK, Damm P, Hedegaard M, Henriksen TB, Ottesen B, Dykes A, Kjaergaard H. Sports and leisure time physical activity during pregnancy in nulliparous women. Matern Child Health J. 2011;15:806–13.
115. Ribeiro CP, Milanez H. Knowledge, attitude and practice of women in Campinas, São Paulo, Brazil with respect to physical exercise in pregnancy: a descriptive study. Reprod Health. 2011;8:31.
116. Walsh JM, McGowan C, Byrne J, McAuliffe FM. Prevalence of physical activity among healthy pregnant women in Ireland. Int J Gynaecol Obstet. 2011;114(2):154–5.
117. Nascimento SL, Surita FG, Cecatti JG. Physical exercise during pregnancy: a systematic review. Curr Opin Obstet Gynecol. 2012;24(6):387–94.
118. Tavares JS, Melo ASO, Amorim MMR, Barros VO, Takito MY, Benício MHD, Cardoso MAA. Padrão de atividade física entre gestantes atendidas pela estratégia saúde da família de Campina Grande–PB. Rev Bras Epidemiol. 2009;12(1):10–9. [Portuguese].
119. Lynch KE, Landsbaugh JR, Whitcomb BW, Pekow P, Markenson G, Chasan-Taber L. Physical activity of pregnant hispanic women. Am J Prev Med. 2012;43(4):434–9.
120. Davenport MH, Meah VL, Ruchat S-M, Davies GA, Skow RJ, Barrowman N, et al. Impact of prenatal exercise on neonatal and childhood outcomes: a systematic review and meta-analysis. Br J Sports Med. 2018;52(21):1386–96.
121. Davenport MH, McCurdy AP, Mottola MF, Skow RJ, Meah VL, Poitras VJ, et al. Impact of prenatal exercise on both prenatal and postnatal anxiety and depressive symptoms: a systematic review and meta-analysis. Br J Sports Med. 2018;52:1376–85.
122. Fazzi C, Saunders DH, Linton K, Norman JE, Reynolds RM. Sedentary behaviours during pregnancy: a systematic review. Int J Behav Nutr Phys Act. 2017;14(1):32.
123. van Poppel MNM, Simmons D, Devlieger R, van Assche FA, Jans G, Galjaard S, et al. A reduction in sedentary behaviour in obese women during pregnancy reduces neonatal adiposity: the DALI randomised controlled trial. Diabetologia. 2019;62(6):915–25.
124. Dieberger AM, Desoye G, Stolz E, Hill DJ, Corcoy R, Simmons D, et al. Less sedentary time is associated with a more favourable glucose-insulin axis in obese pregnant women-a secondary analysis of the DALI study. Int J Obes. 2021;45(2):296–307.
125. Xiang M, Zhang Z, Liang H. Sedentary behavior relates to mental distress of pregnant women differently across trimesters: an observational study in China. J Affect Disord. 2020;260:187–93.
126. Whitaker KM, Zhang D, Kline CE, Catov J, Barone Gibbs B. Associations of Sleep with sedentary behavior and physical activity patterns across pregnancy trimesters. Womens Health Issues. 2021;31:366.
127. Ross R, Chaput J-P, Giangregorio LM, Janssen I, Saunders TJ, Kho ME, et al. Canadian 24-hour movement guidelines for adults aged 18-64 years and adults aged 65 years or older: an integration of physical activity, sedentary behaviour, and sleep. Appl Physiol Nutr Metab. 2020;45(10 Suppl. 2):S57–102.
128. Tuleya L. Thesaurus of psychological index terms, 11 Washington, DC: American Psychological Association; 2007. xxvi, 463.
129. Di Fabio DR, Blomme CK, Smith KM, Welk GJ, Campbell CG. Adherence to physical activity guidelines in mid-pregnancy does not reduce sedentary time: an observational study. Int J Behav Nutr Phys Act. 2015;12:27.

130. Dumuid D, Pedišić Ž, Stanford TE, Martín-Fernández JA, Hron K, Maher CA, et al. The compositional isotemporal substitution model: a method for estimating changes in a health outcome for reallocation of time between sleep, physical activity and sedentary behaviour. Stat Methods Med Res. 2017;28:346.
131. Smith KM, Lanningham-Foster LM, Welk GJ, Campbell CG. Validity of the SenseWear armband to predict energy expenditure in pregnant women. Med Sci Sports Exerc. 2012;44(10):2001–8.
132. Ehrlich SF, Casteel AJ, Crouter SE, Hibbing PR, Hedderson MM, Brown SD, et al. Alternative wear-time estimation methods compared to traditional diary logs for wrist-Worn ActiGraph accelerometers in pregnant women. J Measur Phys Behav. 2020;3(2):110–7.
133. Barone Gibbs B, Paley JL, Jones MA, Whitaker KM, Connolly CP, Catov JM. Validity of self-reported and objectively measured sedentary behavior in pregnancy. BMC Pregnan Childb. 2020;20(1):99.
134. Chasan-Taber L, Schmidt MD, Roberts DE, Hosmer D, Markenson G, Freedson PS. Development and validation of a pregnancy physical activity questionnaire. Med Sci Sports Exerc. 2004;36(10):1750–60.
135. Oviedo-Caro MA, Bueno-Antequera J, Munguía-Izquierdo D. Measuring sedentary behavior during pregnancy: comparison between self-reported and objective measures. Matern Child Health J. 2018;22(7):968–77.
136. Herring SJ, Foster GD, Pien GW, Massa K, Nelson DB, Gehrman PR, et al. Do pregnant women accurately report sleep time? A comparison between self-reported and objective measures of sleep duration in pregnancy among a sample of urban mothers. Sleep Breath. 2013;17(4):1323–7.
137. Migueles JH, Aadland E, Andersen LB, Brønd JC, Chastin SF, Hansen BH, et al. GRANADA consensus on analytical approaches to assess associations with accelerometer-determined physical behaviours (physical activity, sedentary behaviour and sleep) in epidemiological studies. Br J Sports Med. 2021;56:376.
138. Chastin SFM, Palarea-Albaladejo J, Dontje ML, Skelton DA. Combined effects of time spent in physical activity, sedentary behaviors and sleep on obesity and cardio-metabolic health markers: a novel compositional data analysis approach. PLoS One. 2015;10(10):e0139984.
139. Oviedo-Caro MA, Bueno-Antequera J, Munguia-Izquierdo D. Associations of 24-hours activity composition with adiposity and cardiorespiratory fitness: the PregnActive project. Scand J Med Sci Sports. 2020;30(2):295–302.
140. Aadland E, Andersen LB, Migueles JH, Ortega FB, Kvalheim OM. Interpretation of associations between the accelerometry physical activity spectrum and cardiometabolic health and locomotor skills in two cohorts of children using raw, normalized, log-transformed, or compositional data. J Sports Sci. 2020;38(23):2708–19.

Psychological, Social and Behavioural Changes During Pregnancy: Implications for Physical Activity and Exercise

2

Lou Atkinson and Megan Teychenne

Abstract

Pregnancy is often cited as a time in a woman's life when motivation towards having a healthy lifestyle increases, including a desire to pursue physical activities and improve physical fitness. There is also a growing body of evidence which demonstrates the potential for physical activity to positively influence psychological well-being during pregnancy. However, pregnancy is also a period of intense physical and psychological changes. Alongside the many established social and cultural beliefs associated with pregnancy, these changes contribute significant complexities to women's adoption and maintenance of exercise during this time. In this chapter, we will examine the current evidence surrounding the psychosocial aspects of an active pregnancy and provide recommendations for providing psychological and behavioural support to women to become or remain active throughout their pregnancy.

Keywords

Pregnancy · Physical activity · Exercise · Psychosocial factors · Behaviour change

---

L. Atkinson (✉)
Applied Health Research Group, College of Health & Life Sciences, Aston University, Birmingham, UK

School of Psychology, Aston University, Birmingham, UK
e-mail: l.atkinson1@aston.ac.uk

M. Teychenne
Deakin University, Geelong, VIC, Australia

Institute for Physical Activity and Nutrition (IPAN), School of Exercise and Nutrition Sciences, Burwood, VIC, Australia
e-mail: megan.teychenne@deakin.edu.au

R. Santos-Rocha (ed.), *Exercise and Physical Activity During Pregnancy and Postpartum*, https://doi.org/10.1007/978-3-031-06137-0_2

2.1 Psychological and Social Changes During Pregnancy

Pregnancy is undoubtedly a unique period in a woman's life. As with the physical changes to a woman's body, pregnancy induces a number of non-physical changes, which may be temporary or endure long after the pregnancy is completed.

2.1.1 Identity

A woman's first experience of pregnancy often causes significant shifts in self-identity [1]; however, every pregnancy can be associated with either temporary or permanent changes in perceived roles and identity. During pregnancy, women often describe transitioning to a new mothering identity, which in turn disrupts or diminishes existing identities. For example, there may be a change to the woman's perception of her role as a working professional, or as a sexually attractive partner [2]. Whilst some women welcome or adapt easily to this new identity, others may have more difficulty accepting these changes or balancing their new role alongside existing ones [3]. These shifting identities have the potential to both positively and negatively influence a woman's engagement with physical activity during her pregnancy. For example, if a woman feels that being sexually attractive is less important to her during pregnancy, she may feel reduced motivation to exercise to maintain a healthy weight or toned physique. Women have reported that pregnancy is a time when they feel 'excused' from striving for the socially constructed ideal aesthetic of the female body [2, 4]. Alternatively, women's behaviour can be driven by a desire to retain elements of their prepregnancy self-identity [5]. Hence women who were active pre-pregnancy may wish to continue to exercise if this is important to their sense of self. The new mothering identity may also positively influence women's engagement with an active lifestyle. For example, the desire to protect and nurture their unborn child, as well as an awareness of parents as role models to their offspring, can increase a woman's intentions towards exercise during pregnancy [6] Women may also experience, consciously or unconsciously, social pressure to outwardly demonstrate their commitment to their unborn child by restructuring their lifestyle, such as eating healthily and reducing alcohol consumption, and generally taking care of their bodies [7]. However, these internal drivers and societal expectations towards doing the best for baby can also reduce motivation towards being active. For example, concerns over the safety of physical activity and beliefs about the need to rest during pregnancy are often cited as reasons for reducing or ceasing exercise [8].

Case Study: Yolanda

I've been active all my life and I knew all the benefits of exercising when you're pregnant so I really wanted to continue with my running and teaching my indoor cycling classes, for as long as I was healthy and felt able to. As soon as my bump started showing some of the people in my classes said to me, "Should you still be doing this?" I was a bit shocked that they would say that to someone they didn't really know very well, but even though I knew I wasn't doing anything wrong and my baby was safe, it still made me question myself. And then I thought, if that makes me question if I should be doing those activities—a qualified fitness instructor, who has done all the research and had expert advice about exercising during pregnancy—how would an 'ordinary' woman without that knowledge respond to comments like that? It's no wonder so many women just give up!

2.1.2 Loss of Control

Although women have reported being in awe of the functional adaptations made by their body during pregnancy [2, 9], many women also describe a sense of losing control over their bodies [10] or of their bodies becoming autonomous; automatically and independently doing what is required to create and support a new life [9]. Both the lack of familiarity with their body and the feeling that their body knows best can reduce women's confidence to be physically active. They may no longer be certain how their body will respond to exercise, or may interpret the physical sensations they experience during pregnancy as indicating that some activities are not safe or appropriate [5]. Additionally, women may embrace the opportunity to relinquish control over their bodies, viewing pregnancy as a time when it is socially acceptable to reduce their usual self-restraint and to allow nature to take its course [11], for example reducing exercise and gaining weight. Conversely, some women who have lost or controlled their weight pre-pregnancy report finding the inevitable weight gain associated with pregnancy distressing, expressing feelings of guilt and disappointment at losing their pre-pregnancy shape [12].

Whilst some women describe feeling that their body has 'taken over', research also suggests that some women feel that they are fully responsible for the outcome of their pregnancy, and should anything go wrong this will be as a result of their choices and actions [9]. This sense of personal responsibility is often heightened when achieving pregnancy has not been straightforward, resulting in the woman making significant efforts to seek information and make deliberate behavioural choices aimed at maximising the chances of a successful outcome [5]. This pressure to exert control over their pregnancy can both increase and decrease motivation towards being physically active, depending on whether a woman perceives exercise and activity to be beneficial or risky to her pregnancy.

2.1.3 Cognitive Function

Many women report experiencing some form of cognitive deterioration during pregnancy. For example, women describe being more forgetful or experiencing difficulties in concentrating on a task or performing their usual work-related activities. Although systematic reviews [13] and prospective studies [14] have concluded that there is only limited evidence for impairment of memory or other cognitive functioning during pregnancy, this research does provide some corroboration of women's accounts of 'baby brain'. Several potential causes of these perceived changes in cognitive function have been proposed, including biochemical changes, lifestyle factors and cultural stereotypes [13]; however, more research is needed to identify both cause and effect. Regardless of whether the reported effects can be measured objectively, the perceived changes in a woman's mental capacity can be distressing and add to the sense of being less 'herself' since becoming pregnant. This in turn can contribute to changes in a woman's motivation and perceived capability for regular exercise.

2.1.4 Behavioural Changes

Women may seek to adopt or change many behaviours once they become pregnant. Based on local guidelines, antenatal healthcare professionals will advise women on a variety of areas including nutritional supplements, alcohol consumption, smoking and diet. Women may also seek or receive lay advice from friends, family, or online communities, as well as information or guidance from websites, books, magazines and other media [15]. In fact, many pregnant women report 'information overload', especially in early pregnancy. Due to the cognitive demands of attempting multiple behaviour changes, it is likely that some changes will be more successful than others and research suggests that women may view physical activity as low priority [16]. As such, even when motivation to be active during pregnancy is high, women may find pursuing this to be challenging whilst dealing with so many other changes.

Key Points

- The experience of pregnancy can involve significant psychological, social and behavioural change, which can influence a woman's engagement with physical activities.
- Women may experience social pressure to adopt lifestyle changes which are viewed as nurturing or protective. Beliefs about the relative benefits and risks to the pregnancy of physical activity will influence exercise behaviour.
- A sense of losing control over her body, or experiencing the natural changes to her body can be disconcerting for women and may reduce confidence to pursue pre-pregnancy activities.

2.2 The Influence of Physical Activity and Exercise on Psychological Well-Being During Pregnancy

The benefits of physical activity on mental health and well-being for the general population have been well documented [17, 18]. For men and women of various ages and life stages, physical activity has been shown to be beneficial for reducing depressive symptoms [18, 19], anxiety symptoms [20] as well as improving sleep [21] and overall well-being [22]. But what about during pregnancy? Do the same psychological benefits of exercise exist? Let us look at the current level of evidence that has investigated the relationship between physical activity and the aforementioned psychological factors (e.g. depressive and anxiety symptoms, sleep and overall well-being).

2.2.1 Depressive Symptoms

Pregnancy is a time in which women may be at high risk of experiencing depression and/or depressive symptoms [23]. Considering antenatal depression can lead to premature labour, higher infant stress hormone levels and reduced attachment and mother–child bonding [24], it is important to identify strategies to prevent and/or manage depressive symptoms during pregnancy. Pregnant women are sometimes reluctant to use or be prescribed antidepressant medication during pregnancy due to concerns about potential side effects [25], and therefore seek out alternative therapies to alleviate depressive symptoms, which may include physical activity.

Unlike that of the general population, there is currently limited evidence which investigates the link between physical activity during pregnancy and risk of depression (either antenatal or postnatal depression). A 2015 systematic review of intervention studies [26] identified just six studies that have investigated the effectiveness of exercise trials on antenatal depression, and concluded a small to moderate effect of physical activity on reducing depressive symptoms during pregnancy, which has been since confirmed from in a 2018 meta-analysis of 21 RCTs [27]. Further, a previous narrative review identified six observational studies that investigated the association between physical activity during pregnancy and depression [28], with most of those studies demonstrating an inverse association between physical activity during pregnancy and depressive symptoms (i.e. physical activity was linked to lower risk of depressive symptoms during pregnancy). Moreover, another systematic review suggested that there is a small body of evidence that shows leisure-time physical activity during pregnancy may be linked to lower risk of depression in the postpartum period [29]. Although this finding was not consistent with the findings of a meta-analysis of seven RCTs [27], that meta-analysis did suggest studies were low quality, with a serious risk of bias and therefore further high-quality evidence is needed.

Although further research investigating the link between physical activity and depression in pregnancy is required, it is noteworthy to mention that of the studies reviewed to date, no studies suggested that physical activity during pregnancy would increase the risk of depression. Rather, both reviews suggested that whilst there is some evidence to suggest that physical activity during pregnancy may be linked to lower risk of depressive symptoms for the mother, clear cut conclusions regarding the overall effectiveness of physical activity for preventing and/or treating depression could not be made due to the limited number of studies, as well as the relatively low to moderate quality of existing studies.

2.2.2 Anxiety Symptoms

Anxiety disorders are particularly common during pregnancy [30] and have been shown to be linked to preterm birth and poor neurodevelopmental outcomes (e.g. learning, motor development and behaviour) of children [31]. Like that of depression, anxiety during pregnancy can be managed through medication, counselling and psychotherapy. Yet, physical activity/exercise has been suggested as a possible alternative to these treatments. So how effective is physical activity for preventing and/or managing anxiety during pregnancy? Whilst there is some evidence to suggest physical activity is linked to lower levels of anxiety symptoms in the general population [20], a much smaller body of research exists for the impact of physical activity during pregnancy on anxiety. Although a 2011 narrative review of observational studies suggested there is some evidence (i.e. two studies) to show that physical activity during pregnancy may be linked to lower risk of anxiety/anxiety symptoms [28], a more recent meta-analysis [27] suggested that of the three existing RCTs examining the impact of pre-natal physical activity on anxiety, there was no association. However, this was based on low-quality evidence, highlighting the need for more high-quality research in this area. Given that physical activity may benefit mental health through psychological pathways such as **distraction** from negative thoughts and **mastery** of skills and goals [32], it is certainly plausible that physical activity during pregnancy would help to prevent and manage anxiety symptoms. However, further research is needed in order to make clear cut conclusions.

Case Study: Alana

When I fell pregnant, I was going through an extremely stressful time in my life. I was working full-time in a demanding job, in the process of moving house and had other personal issues I was working through. I had always been an active person and so I used exercise as a way to reduce my stress and anxiety during this time. Before work each morning I would go for a half hour walk around a park which was surrounded by bushland and wildlife. Prior to pregnancy I would run 4–5 times per week, however, I felt quite uncomfortable running when I was pregnant and so "took up" brisk walking instead. As my belly grew, my pace certainly slowed down (particularly up the steep hills!), but I always felt a sense of calm, happiness, and satisfaction after completing my walks. I'm not sure if it was the fresh air, natural environment, music tunes I was listening to, or the physical activity itself, but I feel that walking is what kept my mental health in-check when I was pregnant.

2.2.3 Sleep

Sleep disturbances are often experienced by women during pregnancy, potentially due to hormonal and physiological changes (e.g. discomfort, more frequent urination) [33] as well pregnant women being predisposed to certain sleep disorders (e.g.

insomnia, restless leg syndrome) [34]. As an alternative to sleeping pills, which often lead to dependence and other negative effects, physical activity has been proposed as a safer method to improve sleep quality in the general population [35]. Although some studies suggest that vigorous-intensity exercise is linked to better sleep [36], other studies have shown that physical activity undertaken at light to moderate intensity, such as walking, was linked to improved sleep [21, 37], with bouts of activity of 1 h or more linked to longer sleep duration [21].

Amongst pregnant women, the link between physical activity and sleep quality and/or duration has largely not been studied and evidence is still inconclusive. Cross-sectional studies have shown weak to no evidence of an association [38, 39], whilst one prospective study has shown that exercise during early pregnancy was linked to greater continuity of sleep [40]. Very few intervention studies have examined the effects of physical activity on sleep during pregnancy, yet of those studies, results have shown that aerobic exercise [41] and yoga [42] were beneficial in improving sleep quality (e.g. reducing insomnia symptoms, increasing continuity of sleep). Whilst a recent meta-analysis which included seven RCTs concluded that exercise had a positive impact on the sleep quality of pregnant women, but did not improve insomnia symptoms [43]. It is clear that further studies are needed to enable evidence-based conclusions regarding physical activity and sleep in pregnancy to be made. However, given that those with the strongest study design (i.e. experimental studies) have shown positive results on the effect of physical activity and sleep quality in pregnancy, physical activity could be a promising method for improving sleep in pregnant women.

2.2.4 Summary

Although evidence is somewhat promising regarding the potential of physical activity for the prevention/treatment of mental health problems and sleep disorders during pregnancy, further research is required to make clear cut conclusions in this population group. In particular, research is needed to investigate the specific dose (e.g. duration, intensity) and domain (e.g. leisure time, domestic, work, travel) of physical activity for preventing and/or managing symptoms of depression, anxiety and sleep problems during pregnancy, in order to provide guidance on recommendations during the antenatal period.

Key Points

- Much evidence in the general population suggests leisure-time physical activity is beneficial for mental health (i.e. depression and anxiety) and sleep quality
- Although some evidence of positive effect of physical activity on antenatal depressive and anxiety symptoms, very little research has investigated the link between physical activity and depressive and anxiety symptoms during pregnancy

- Only a handful of studies have investigated the link between physical activity and sleep in pregnant women, with conflicting findings
- However, no detrimental effects of physical activity on mental health or sleep have been observed within the current body of evidence.

2.3 Psychosocial Barriers and Facilitators to Being Active During Pregnancy

In the general population, adults report a large number of factors that influence their physical activity levels. These factors can be modifiable (i.e. we can change or influence these as health practitioners) or non-modifiable (i.e. we cannot change/influence these as health practitioners, e.g. demographic factors such as age, education, income), and are often categorised as individual, social, physical environmental and policy factors, according to the ecological model of behaviour change [44]. Some pregnant women may report a lot of barriers to being active, whilst others may just report one or two. So let us look at some of the most commonly reported 'modifiable' influences (either barriers or facilitators) on being active during pregnancy.

2.3.1 Individual Factors

Individual factors have been shown to be the most commonly cited barriers to physical activity amongst pregnant women [8, 45]. Physical symptoms of pregnancy, lack of time and misinformation (about health-related outcomes of antenatal exercise) are amongst the list of key individual factors that influence participation in physical activity during pregnancy.

2.3.2 Physical Symptoms

2.3.2.1 Fatigue

We have already discussed how physical activity may affect sleep. On the flip side of the coin, lack of sleep and fatigue have been cited as barriers to being physically active during pregnancy [45, 46], with one study suggesting that pregnant women rated sleep as more important than being physically active [45]. Another qualitative study showed that 'feeling tired' either due to work or the physical changes experienced in pregnancy was the second most commonly cited barrier to being active during pregnancy [8].

2.3.2.2 Nausea

Experiencing nausea, most commonly as 'morning sickness', has been cited as a key barrier to being physically active during pregnancy [8, 46]. During severe morning sickness, women may not be physically capable of being active. However, some researchers have suggested that being active during pregnancy may potentially help alleviate symptoms of morning sickness [47]. Since the direction of the relationship between morning sickness/nausea and exercise is still unclear, further studies are required to determine the causal pathways.

2.3.2.3 Discomfort, Physical Limitations and High-Risk Pregnancies

The physical demands of pregnancy lead to most women experiencing some level of physical discomfort as their pregnancy progresses. Symptoms such as shortness of breath, musculoskeletal pain or soreness and feeling awkward as weight increases are commonly cited as barriers to being physically active [45, 48]. Whilst these symptoms are normal in healthy pregnancy and may not be considered contraindications to physical activity by exercise professionals, they certainly provide a significant psychological barrier. It should also be noted that a proportion of pregnant women may experience pregnancy-related physical limitations such as severe pelvic and back pain, or may be classified as having a 'high-risk' pregnancy (e.g. previous foetal death, reproductive tract abnormalities [49]) which are likely to prevent them from being as physically active as pregnant women without physical limitations or complications [8]. These are important factors to consider when designing physical activity programs for pregnant women, as a 'one size fits all approach' will never be appropriate (see Chap. 8 for guidance on contraindications and modifications to exercise during pregnancy).

2.3.2.4 Lack of Time

Like that of the general population, having a lack of time to be active is a commonly cited barrier amongst pregnant women [8, 46]. This is often explained by pregnant women having family, childcare and/or work commitments [8, 46] that tend to be prioritised over their own health and well-being. The perceived lack of time during pregnancy may also be linked to the tiredness mentioned above, as women have described having 'shorter days' to fit everything in during pregnancy, due to the increased need for sleep [45].

2.3.2.5 Motivation

Having a lack of motivation to be active is often cited by pregnant women as a barrier to exercise [8, 45]. It may be that the fatigue from the pregnancy and lack of time contribute to lowering motivation levels of pregnant women. Women also appear to defer motivation for physical activity to the postnatal period, as they feel that they will be keen to lose weight after the baby is born, and exercise would contribute to this [45, 50].

On the other hand, some pregnant mothers are motivated to be active in order to protect and nurture their baby [51] or because they perceive labour will be easier if they are fit/physically active [52]. General maternal health and well-being, decreasing stress, improving fitness and improving appearance have also been cited by women as motivating factors for physical activity during pregnancy [48].

2.3.2.6 Attitudes and Beliefs

A comprehensive systematic review of attitudes, barriers and enablers to physical activity during pregnancy concluded from 11 quantitative and 13 qualitative studies that women generally held positive attitudes towards physical activity during their pregnancy, indicating that it was important, beneficial and safe [48]. However, the same review also concluded that fears about safety were a barrier to physical activity. This corroborates previous studies which indicated that lack of knowledge about how much and how to exercise safely in pregnancy, and concerns about harming their unborn child are common barriers to antenatal physical activity [8, 45, 46]. Providing clear, evidence-based information to women about the benefits and 'dispelling myths' [46] of physical activity during pregnancy may be imperative for antenatal health.

2.3.3 Social Factors

Social factors such as social support from friends, family and GPs have been shown in the general population to be important for influencing physical activity. When examining the social factors that may predict physical activity during pregnancy, findings are relatively similar, with perhaps a little more emphasis on healthcare professionals and social norms.

2.3.3.1 Social Norms

Social norms refer to behaviour that is seen as socially 'acceptable'. Often pressure is placed on pregnant women by others to ensure they are 'rested' and 'not overdoing it', or they simply follow what their family and friends have done in their pregnancies [52]. Similarly, women may form perceptions of the type and amount of exercise that is 'good for pregnancy' by observing others' behaviour long before experiencing their own pregnancy [5]. Social norms related to antenatal physical activity can vary amongst cultural groups [46] and therefore information and interventions may need to be tailored to the cultural background of women.

2.3.3.2 Healthcare Professional Advice

Pregnant women often suggest that being provided with a lack of (or even misinformation) from their antenatal healthcare provider has prevented them from being active during their pregnancy [8, 46]. One qualitative study found that women without any health or pregnancy-related complications were told by their doctor to limit or even discontinue physical activity whilst they were pregnant [25]. Further, research in South Africa has shown that most (83%) medical practitioners were unaware of what the physical activity recommendations during pregnancy were, and very few practitioners (19%) provided women with informational brochures on physical activity during pregnancy [53]. This finding is of concern, given that healthcare professionals are a trusted source of information and are seen as the best mode of providing health-related information to women during pregnancy [54].

2.3.3.3 Social Support

Social support is increasingly recognised as an important determinant of antenatal physical activity [55]. Studies suggest that having emotional (e.g. working out together) or informational (e.g. being told by friends that exercise is good during pregnancy) support from friends and/or family acts as a facilitator to antenatal physical activity [52]. On the contrary, a lack of emotional (e.g. no one to exercise with) and of informational social support has been suggested to be a barrier to physical activity during pregnancy [35, 45]. Having a partner who is active has been shown to be associated with higher physical activity levels for the pregnant woman [56] suggesting that it may be important to encourage and support physical activity in both parties.

> **Case Study: Estelle**
> When I was pregnant, I was well aware of the physical activity guidelines for pregnant women. I was a PE teacher, with a keen interest in sports and exercise, and kept up to date with research in the area. However, when I attended the antenatal education classes run at the hospital, I was told that pregnant women were not to be as active as other women, and rather just exercise at a low intensity a couple of times per week. I was quite shocked by the misinformation nurses were providing to women.

2.3.4 Physical Environmental Factors

Environmental factors that are linked to physical activity during pregnancy have not been as widely cited, nor studied, as individual or social factors [8]. However, physical environmental determinants such as access to transport and facilities, as well as non-modifiable determinants such as the weather [45, 52], have been suggested to influence physical activity amongst pregnant women.

2.3.4.1 Transport

Having a lack of transport (e.g. not owning a car) has been linked to increased physical activity in pregnant women, as they are required to walk or cycle from place to place [45], and some women choose to walk rather than drive as a means of staying active [52]. Therefore, promoting active transport may be a particularly useful strategy for pregnant women, given that they often cite a lack of time to be active in leisure time. Having said that, women also find a lack of transportation to be a barrier [45], as they are reliant on partners or friends to drive them to facilities (see below). Weather has also been shown to be an influencing factor [52] suggesting that active travel may be a less appealing option during cold and wet seasons.

2.3.4.2 Access to Facilities

Access to facilities that are safe, aesthetically pleasing and inexpensive has been suggested by pregnant women to be an important factor in being physically active [45, 52]. As with the general population, many pregnant women perceive the costs of attending exercise classes or facilities to be unaffordable [57]. Provision of free to use facilities such as pleasant walking trails or subsidised access to gyms/leisure centres may be effective methods of supporting women to be active during their pregnancy [52].

2.3.5 Summary

There are a broad range of factors that influence physical activity during pregnancy, which encompass the individual, social and physical environmental constructs of the ecological model for behaviour change. Targeting these constructs, and in particular, focussing on the key barriers/facilitators to antenatal physical activity is important when designing programs and interventions to enhance physical activity in pregnant women.

Key Points
- Pregnant women report a range of individual, social and environmental influences on physical activity
- These include factors such as: Lack of time, physical symptoms of pregnancy, misinformation (from friends, family and health professionals) and social norms
- Targeting these factors in the design of antenatal physical activity programs/interventions will increase the chance of changing physical activity behaviours

2.4 Behaviour Change Strategies

As this chapter has detailed, there are unique and significant challenges to achieving an active lifestyle during pregnancy. However, the psychological and physical benefits (see Chap. 3) provide substantial incentives for women to strive for an active pregnancy, and for health and exercise professionals to support those efforts. The following section outlines the evidence from a variety of behaviour change interventions aimed at promoting and supporting physical activity during pregnancy. The following section combines this evidence with theoretically derived behaviour change strategies to suggest a number of practical techniques which could be implemented to support women to achieve their personal physical activity goals.

2.4.1 Systematic Reviews

A small number of systematic reviews have been conducted to examine the effectiveness of behaviour change interventions aimed at maintaining or increasing physical activity during pregnancy [58–60]. The earliest of these reviews [58] took the stance that physical activity usually declines during pregnancy, hence increasing physical activity or preventing declines in physical activity levels were both considered 'desirable' outcomes. This review found that eight of the ten interventions reporting changes in physical activity showed a desirable difference between participants in the intervention and those in the control group. In regard to the format of successful physical activity interventions during pregnancy, it was observed that most ($n = 5$) involved regular face-to-face meetings, half ($n = 4$) focused solely on physical activity (as opposed to an intervention aimed at changing multiple behaviours) and only three were offered over a long time period (i.e. 20 weeks or more). With regard to specific behaviour change techniques employed, all five of the interventions that used 'Goals and Planning' demonstrated desirable physical activity outcomes. Results were more mixed for other behaviour change techniques (e.g. 'Repetition of desired behaviours and Substitution of unwanted behaviours' and 'Comparison of outcomes/Pros and Cons'), whilst two interventions did not use any recognised behaviour change techniques but still demonstrated favourable physical activity outcomes through education alone.

In a later review [59], five of the 15 RCTs examined reported a statistically significant difference in physical activity between the intervention and control groups, in favour of the intervention group. Analysis of intervention delivery methods identified that seven trials employed individual interviews, three trials employed group interviews, two trials used multimedia and one trial used a brochure. Analysis of behaviour change strategies identified that goal setting techniques were most frequently used ($n = 11$), with problem solving ($n = 9$), instruction ($n = 9$), self-monitoring ($n = 8$), feedback ($n = 4$) and modelling ($n = 1$) techniques also used.

A further review focused only on interventions to increase physical activity in pregnant women with overweight or obesity [60]. Meta-analyses conducted on data from 13 studies indicated that interventions in this population were effective in increasing physical activity, but cautioned that the included studies were highly heterogeneous. In fact, the authors of all of these reviews concluded that the highly varied methods and intervention strategies used to date, and an overall lack of high quality intervention studies hampered the ability to draw conclusions about intervention effectiveness [58–60]. However, by examining the evidence from intervention studies conducted to date, we can gain some insight into potential strategies to support women to remain active during pregnancy.

2.4.2 Walking Interventions

Walking is one of the most commonly reported forms of exercise amongst pregnant women and is recommended as a low-intensity, safe exercise during pregnancy that almost all women should be able to perform. As a natural movement that most women undertake in their everyday activities, many of the psychological barriers to exercise often do not relate to walking, such as concerns about injury, uncertainty about how to perform it or social pressure to avoid over exertion. Walking also requires no specialist equipment or facilities and can be more easily incorporated into a busy lifestyle than attending sessions at a fixed time and location, thereby reducing the pragmatic and financial barriers to exercise.

It is therefore surprising that only a few behavioural interventions have focused on walking as the primary exercise modality. Two short-term (8–10 weeks) trials of unsupervised walking programs resulted in good adherence to the recommendation to walk for 30 min, three times per week [61, 62]. A trial of a more structured and intensive walking program (40 min, five times per week) resulted in higher daily steps at 28 weeks gestation after 10 weeks of intervention; however, the effect was no longer significant at 36 weeks [63], suggesting that women found it difficult to maintain recommended levels of walking in late pregnancy. In another trial, women who were overweight or obese, and had low activity levels, were advised to walk 30 min on most days of the week for 20 weeks, starting at between 12 and 15 weeks gestation [64]. Although women were advised to perform the walking in any setting, they were also provided with treadmills for unsupervised home use. Although results showed some positive outcomes, such as higher frequency and duration of walks in late pregnancy in the intervention group, overall total step counts were not higher in the intervention group compared to controls. The impact of being provided with a treadmill at home is unknown and the lack of difference in overall step counts between intervention and control may indicate that if women were using the treadmill at home they may have reduced other forms of walking.

These combined results suggest that provision of a relatively simple exercise program that can be performed in or around the home, with or without specialist equipment, may be beneficial in supporting women to maintain an active pregnancy.

2.4.3 Supervised Individual or Group Exercise

As previously mentioned, many women are uncertain about how to exercise safely during pregnancy, and concerns about harming the baby are often cited as reasons for reducing or ceasing activity. It is perhaps therefore unsurprising that interventions which provide closely supervised exercise sessions are some of the most successful at increasing and maintaining activity levels during pregnancy. Several trials of have shown significant increases in physical activity at completion of the intervention, and significantly higher physical activity levels than control groups. These have included:

- Walking sessions three times per week for sedentary women. Sessions were supervised by physical education professionals and medical and physiotherapy students, and women wore heart rate monitors throughout [65].
- One 60-min group exercise session per week delivered by a physiotherapist, comprising low-impact aerobics, body weight-based strength exercises and abdominal and pelvic floor exercises, plus a structured home exercise programme of endurance training, strength and balance exercises [66].
- A weekly group exercise session in a community venue, delivered by licensed fitness trainers, comprising aerobics, stretching and strength exercises, plus a recommended home-based exercise program and instruction video designed by an exercise physiologist [67].
- Twice weekly 60-min exercise classes at a local gym, delivered by trained instructors [68].

- Supervised stationary cycling sessions three times per week for women with overweight and obesity, including both steady state and interval training [69].
- Two 70-min moderate-intensity exercise sessions per week, delivered by a certified fitness instructor and with a nurse present, plus educational and motivational support [70].

It is likely that these types of intervention are successful because the level of supervision and monitoring reduces women's fears and anxieties around the safety of exercise for her baby. When performed in groups with other pregnant women, participants may also be receiving social support and encouragement from similar others. Additionally, participating in a trial may simply have provided an opportunity to attend a pregnancy-specific exercise session that may not otherwise have been available. It is interesting to note the success of these face-to-face interventions given the previously mentioned findings that lack of time to exercise is a common barrier to being active during pregnancy. These results suggest that whilst finding the time to attend a supervised exercise session may be challenging, women who do attend may be more successful at remaining active through their pregnancy than those who attempt to be active on their own.

2.4.4 Information and Behavioural Counselling

Some of the successful interventions which have focused on delivering advice about the benefits of being active during pregnancy have also employed behavioural counselling techniques, aimed at facilitating changes to some of the psychosocial determinants of physical activity and exercise behaviour. For example, Jackson et al. [71] successfully used a behavioural assessment, a 'Video Doctor' computer program and an educational worksheet to deliver tailored nutrition, diet and weight gain education using principles from Motivational Interviewing. However, Smith et al. [72] tested found no effect on overall light physical activity or total MET-minutes of exposure to a web-based behavioural intervention based on Social Cognitive Theory [73] on women with low pre-pregnancy activity levels. The intervention included modules on goal setting and action planning, an exercise tracker and a community forum, and was compared to exposure to a website which only provided general diet and physical activity guidelines. These mixed results suggest that a digital intervention may have the potential to support women to achieve an active pregnancy, but further research and development are needed.

Other brief interventions include a leaflet [74] or slideshow [75] based on Protection Motivation Theory (PMT). Both were intended to increase participants' perceived vulnerability to and severity of negative outcomes associated with low physical activity during pregnancy, by presenting factual information regarding these risks. The leaflet and slideshow also included information regarding the benefits of exercise, and practical exercise suggestions, to increase participants' response efficacy (their perception of how effective being physically active will be at reducing the risk of negative outcomes) and self-efficacy (their perception of their own ability to do the required amount of physical activity), respectively. A goal setting section aimed to facilitate participants' implementation of their intentions, and the slideshow also included planning activities. Results of both trials demonstrated a significant effect on physical activity levels and showed that the interventions had been effective at manipulating most of the PMT constructs. These results indicate that relatively brief interventions which target some of the health beliefs around exercise in pregnancy, and providing tools to help women plan and overcome barriers, may be successful at both increasing and maintaining activity levels during pregnancy.

In contrast, more complex and longer duration interventions have shown mixed results. In a trial of a comprehensive lifestyle advice programme for women with overweight or obesity [76], those in the intervention group received information and advice on diet and physical activity, and were encouraged to use goal setting, identification of barriers, problem solving and self-monitoring as behavioural strategies, over multiple 121 sessions between 20 and 36 weeks gestation. Some women were also given access to supervised walking sessions. The trial results demonstrated that women in the intervention group had significantly increased their total physical activity, compared with women in the control group. The authors noted that the increase represented an additional 15–20 min brisk walking on most days of the week. However, this was largely comprised of overall increase in household activity, and access to the supervised walking sessions appeared to have no effect on overall physical activity. In a similar trial comprising both dietary and physical activity elements, women in the intervention group were again encouraged to use goal setting, self-monitoring, problem solving and identification of barriers, during a series of eight weekly group sessions, and were also provided with tools such as a pedometer, log book and DVD of a pregnancy-specific exercise regime [77]. The results of this trial showed no increase in physical activity in either the intervention or control groups [78]. Thus, in women who have excess weight during pregnancy, alternative strategies may be needed to encourage participation in sport or exercise.

2.4.5 Combined Interventions

A few trials have combined a significant element of behavioural counselling with detailed exercise programs. Ko et al. [79] tested an intervention which included gym-based exercise sessions with an instructor, a structured home-based exercise programme and a number of behaviour change techniques delivered both face to face and through the mail. At the end of the trial, women in the intervention group showed a slower decline in activity levels as pregnancy progressed, higher MET-hours per week and a smaller percentage reported no physical activity, compared to those in the control group. Simmons et al. [80] trialled a behavioural coaching intervention for women with obesity which included face-to-face, telephone, and email coaching sessions based on motivational interviewing, a detailed exercise prescription and provision of pedometers and exercise bands. Results showed significantly higher moderate- to vigorous-intensity physical activity in women in the intervention group. Similar results were demonstrated in another intervention which combined free access to a fitness centre, supervised group exercise sessions and coaching by a physiotherapist to help women to integrate physical activity into their daily lives [81].

2.4.6 Summary

In summary, the evidence from interventions to date is far from conclusive and demonstrates that a range of support options may be beneficial, as women are likely to have different experiences, needs and characteristics. Additionally, most trials have focused on women who were inactive or had overweight or obesity prior to becoming pregnant. Therefore, evidence regarding interventions to support active women to maintain their pre-pregnancy activity levels is lacking. However, the research evidence does give some indication that the most successful strategies involve face-to-face support, over a relatively extended time period, and includes behavioural counselling, detailed exercise prescription, and provision of specialised equipment or training sessions.

Key Points

- Some women may need and/or want support to adopt or maintain positive physical activity/exercise behaviours during their pregnancy.
- Support strategies should be tailored for the individual woman's preferences and needs. Detailed information and instruction on how to perform safe exercises, ongoing monitoring and feedback from healthcare and/or exercise professionals, and access to specialised exercise sessions and/or equipment are likely to be beneficial.
- Interventions may be more successful if they are provided face to face, and over the duration of the pregnancy.

2.5 Using Theory to Support Physical Activity in Pregnancy

In this chapter so far, we have seen that pregnancy as a life stage can induce unique sets of both motivating factors, and barriers for physical activity. Hence whilst pregnant women may be keen to participate in physical activities for their own wellbeing and their baby's health, they may struggle to carry out those good intentions. These women may benefit from additional support from their healthcare or exercise professional, or even from friends and family. By utilising behaviour change theory, we can identify strategies and tools that are likely to both increase women's motivation and ability to get or stay active during their pregnancy.

2.5.1 The COM-B Model

The COM-B model [82] (Fig. 2.1) is a simplified model of behaviour, based on the Theoretical Domains Framework (TDF) [83] which itself was derived from a large number of established theories of behaviour change, with the intention of simplifying and improving the use of theory in informing behaviour change services and programs. As such, the COM-B provides a simple method of understanding the factors which influence the behaviour, and identifying specific behaviour change techniques (BCTs) which can affect these factors to increase the likelihood that the desired behaviour will be performed.

The model posits that, in order for a behaviour to occur, an individual must have:

- The capability to do it—this includes both the physical ability and the psychological ability such as knowledge and the ability to work out how to perform the behaviour.
- The opportunity to do it—this includes having physical resources such as time, money, facilities, etc. and the right social environment, e.g. the behaviour is perceived as acceptable or beneficial amongst the individual's social circle.
- The motivation to do it—this motivation may be reflective, based on reasoned assessment of relative value of doing the behaviour compared to not doing it or doing something else, or it may be less conscious more automatic motivation such as internal desires, impulses or reflex reactions.

As shown in the diagram above, perceptions about capability and opportunity can also influence motivation levels. Additionally, an individual's past experience and current behaviour also influence motivation and perceptions of capability and opportunity, which in turn influence the likelihood of undertaking the behaviour in the future. For example, if a pregnant woman learns that exercising is good for her and her baby she may have increased motivation for being active. However, if she was not good at sports in school and has avoided sport and exercise ever since, her motivation to get active will likely be reduced because she is worried that she will not be good at it. Although the combination of these factors will be unique to every individual woman, we can use the evidence outlined above for the most common barriers and facilitators for physical activity in pregnancy to identify which of these factors will be important, and to identify appropriate methods to support women who may otherwise struggle to maintain activity levels through their pregnancy (Table 2.1).

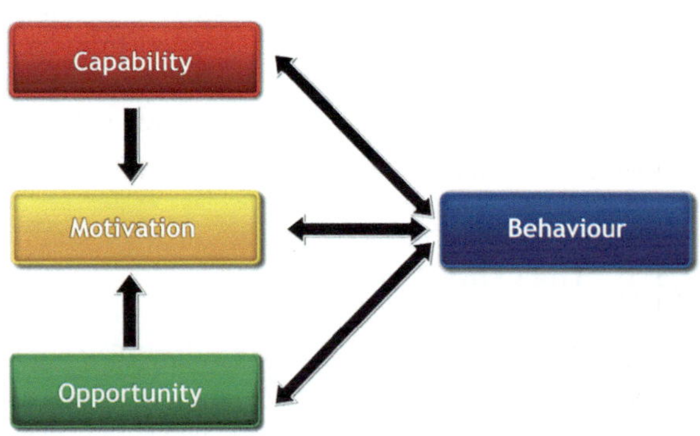

Fig. 2.1 The COM-B model

Table 2.1 Common barriers to physical activity during pregnancy and cognitive behavioural strategies to overcome these based on the COM-B constructs

COM-B construct	Common issues	Strategies
Physical capability	Aches and pains, increased weight and other physical symptoms of pregnancy can restrict the types of activities women can participate in	Understand what restrictions (actual or perceived) the woman is facing and:
		• Suggest alternative exercises or activities
		• Provide information regarding which exercises and activities are safe (or not) for her personal situation
	Fatigue, breathlessness and sleep problems can reduce energy levels leaving women feeling less able to exercise	Ask the woman what types of activities she feels able to undertake and:
		• Suggest low-intensity activities and activities which can be done in small bouts
		• Suggest the woman starts with small amounts of low intensity and slowly increases duration, frequency and/or intensity each week
Psychological capability	Lack of knowledge about safe and/or beneficial exercises can reduce women's confidence to be active	Understand the woman's current knowledge and provide:
		• Detailed instructions on frequency, intensity, time and type of physical activity. Where possible, include diagrams, videos or demonstrations
		• Easy to understand information about recommendations for an active pregnancy, and the benefits to mum and baby
	The combination of tiredness, mood changes and general cognitive overload can decrease the ability to work through the mental processes needed to carry out physical activity, e.g. making plans, or even simply remembering to do it	Reassure the woman that it is normal to experience these physical and/or mental symptoms, and provide:
		• Planning tools to enable the woman to make specific plans for her physical activity. Encourage her to include as much detail as possible, e.g. when, where, with whom, for how long, etc. Self-monitoring tools like an exercise diary, pedometer or a wearable or smartphone fitness tracker may also be helpful
		• Suggestions to 'prompt' the woman to be active, for example reminders in her calendar/on her phone, arranging for a friend or relative to remind/ask her about exercise, etc.
Physical opportunity	Lack of accessible facilities or pregnancy-specific activities	Reassure the woman that almost all types of physical activity are safe and beneficial, and can be accumulated throughout the day in small bouts.
		• Help the woman to identify opportunities within her daily routine to be active, such as walking to work, playing games with her children, doing squats whilst waiting for a pot to boil, etc
		• Provide home-based activities/workouts, which require no specialist equipment and minimum space
	Lack of time and/or money	Where possible:
		• Provide vouchers or subsidised access to local classes or facilities
		• Provide classes or activities at times when women are not working or too tired, with childcare facilities

(continued)

Table 2.1 (continued)

COM-B construct	Common issues	Strategies
Social opportunity	Social norms are to rest and/or avoid activity during pregnancy	Reassure the woman that being active is recommended for her during pregnancy, and:
		• Help her to identify a friend, family member or colleague who is willing to exercise/be active with her—encourage her to make arrangements for regular activity sessions together
		• Encourage her to attend groups/sessions specifically for pregnant women, and/or arrange to meet with other pregnant women in an active way, e.g. walk, swim, take children to the park
		• Encourage providers of activities to promote these to pregnant women
		• Provide role models who are similar or aspirational, who were active in their pregnancies
Reflective motivation	Inaccurate information or beliefs about exercise during pregnancy	Provide information about the benefits of being active during pregnancy, and the increased risks of being inactive. This should be:
		• Proactively provided, as many women will not ask for it
		• From a credible source
		• Easy to understand, consistent and non-judgmental
		• Focused on all types of physical activity, not just sport or exercise
		• Not just aimed at pregnant women—e.g. provided pre-conception or between pregnancies
Automatic motivation	Women follow the same behaviour of their previous pregnancies, or retain their low activity pre-pregnancy lifestyle, through habit	Encourage the woman to think of this pregnancy as an opportunity for change:
		• Suggest making a list of the Pros and Cons of being active during this pregnancy
		• Suggest keeping an exercise diary or using an activity monitor to raise awareness of current activity levels
	Women unconsciously replicate the activity levels/behaviour of their mothers, aunts, sisters and friends	Assure the woman that every pregnancy is unique.
		• Encourage her to try an activity and make a note of how she feels afterwards
		• Suggest the woman arranges a reward for herself for achieving her exercise goals

2.6 Conclusion

In this chapter, we have examined both the influence of psychosocial factors on women's physical activity during pregnancy and the effect of physical activity on a woman's psychological well-being during her pregnancy. This highlights the complexities of achieving and maintaining an active pregnancy, but also the significant benefits. Subsequently, we examined the evidence for successful strategies to support women's behavioural goals and suggested techniques to remove barriers and increase a woman's ability to stay active during her pregnancy. As every woman is unique, it is vital that interventions and support strategies are tailored to a woman's individual needs. However, an understanding of the multiple psychosocial factors at play is clearly imperative in enabling healthcare and exercise professionals to provide women with appropriate care and advice throughout their pregnancy.

References

1. Bailey L. Refracted selves? A study of changes in self-identity in the transition to motherhood. Sociology. 1999;33(2):335–52. https://doi.org/10.1177/S0038038599000206.
2. Hodgkinson EL, Smith DM, Wittkowski A. Women's experiences of their pregnancy and postpartum body image: a systematic review and meta-synthesis. BMC Pregnan Childb. 2014;14(1):330. https://doi.org/10.1186/1471-2393-14-330.
3. Smith JA. Identity development during the transition to motherhood: an interpretative phenomenological analysis. J Reproduct Infant Psychol. 1999;17(3):281–99. https://doi.org/10.1080/02646839908404595.
4. Olander EK, Atkinson L, Edmunds JK, French DP. The views of pre- and post-natal women and health professionals regarding gestational weight gain: an exploratory study. Sex Reprod Healthc. 2011;2(1):43–8. https://doi.org/10.1016/j.srhc.2010.10.004.
5. Atkinson L, Shaw RL, French DP. Is pregnancy a teachable moment for diet and physical activity behaviour change? An interpretative phenomenological analysis of the experiences of women during their first pregnancy. Br J Health Psychol. 2016;21(4):842–58. https://doi.org/10.1111/bjhp.12200.
6. Clissold TL, Hopkins WG, Seddon RJ. Lifestyle behaviours during pregnancy. N Z Med J. 1991;104(908):111–2.
7. Ogle JP, Tyner KE, Schofield-Tomschin S. Watching over baby: expectant parenthood and the duty to be well. Sociol Inq. 2011;81(3):285–309. https://doi.org/10.1111/j.1475-682X.2011.00377.x.
8. Connelly M, Brown H, van der Pligt P, Teychenne M. Modifiable barriers to leisure-time physical activity during pregnancy: a qualitative study investigating first time mother's views and experiences. BMC Pregnan Childb. 2015;15(1):100. https://doi.org/10.1186/s12884-015-0529-9.
9. Carter SK. Beyond control: body and self in women's childbearing narratives. Sociol Health Ill. 2010;32(7):993–1009. https://doi.org/10.1111/j.1467-9566.2010.01261.x.
10. Neiterman E, Fox B. Controlling the unruly maternal body: losing and gaining control over the body during pregnancy and the postpartum period. Soc Sci Med. 2017;174:142–8. https://doi.org/10.1016/j.socscimed.2016.12.029.
11. Clark A, Skouteris H, Wertheim EH, Paxton SJ, Milgrom J. My baby body: a qualitative insight into women's body-related experiences and mood during pregnancy

and the postpartum. J Reproduct Infant Psychol. 2009;27(4):330–45. https://doi.org/10.1080/02646830903190904.
12. Nash M. Weighty matters: negotiating 'fatness' and 'in-betweenness' in early pregnancy. Fem Psychol. 2012;22(3):307–23. https://doi.org/10.1177/0959353512445361.
13. Henry JD, Rendell PG. A review of the impact of pregnancy on memory function. J Clin Exp Neuropsychol. 2007;29(8):793–803. https://doi.org/10.1080/13803390701612209.
14. Christensen H, Leach LS, Mackinnon A. Cognition in pregnancy and motherhood: prospective cohort study. Br J Psychiatry. 2010;196(2):126–32. https://doi.org/10.1192/bjp.bp.109.068635.
15. Beckham AJ, Urrutia RP, Sahadeo L, Corbie-Smith G, Nicholson W. "We know but we don't really know": diet, physical activity and cardiovascular disease prevention knowledge and beliefs among underserved pregnant women. Matern Child Health J. 2015;19(8):1791–801. https://doi.org/10.1007/s10995-015-1693-2.
16. Atkinson L, Jackson B, Hodges K. Results of an online survey of UK women's views and experiences of physical activity information sources during pregnancy - final report. Coventry: Tommys; 2014.
17. Bauman AE. Updating the evidence that physical activity is good for health: an epidemiological review 2000-2003. J Sci Med Sport. 2004;7(1 Suppl):6–19.
18. Teychenne M, Ball K, Salmon J. Physical activity and likelihood of depression in adults: a review. Prev Med. 2008;46(5):397–411. https://doi.org/10.1016/j.ypmed.2008.01.009.
19. Schuch FB, Vancampfort D, Richards J, Rosenbaum S, Ward PB, Stubbs B. Exercise as a treatment for depression: a meta-analysis adjusting for publication bias. J Psychiatr Res. 2016;77:42–51. https://doi.org/10.1016/j.jpsychires.2016.02.023.
20. Strohle A. Physical activity, exercise, depression and anxiety disorders. J Neural Transm (Vienna). 2009;116(6):777–84. https://doi.org/10.1007/s00702-008-0092-x.
21. Youngstedt SD. Effects of exercise on sleep. Clin Sports Med. 2005;24(2):355–65. https://doi.org/10.1016/j.csm.2004.12.003.
22. Da Costa D, Rippen N, Drista M, Ring A. Self-reported leisure-time physical activity during pregnancy and relationship to psychological well-being. J Psychosom Obstet Gynecol. 2003;24:111–9.
23. Marcus SM. Depression during pregnancy: rates, risks and consequences. Can J Clin Pharmacol. 2009;16(1):15–22.
24. Bonari L, Pinto N, Ahn E, Einarson A, Steiner M, Koren G. Perinatal risks of untreated depression during pregnancy. Can J Psychiatr. 2004;49(11):726–35.
25. Einarson A, Choi J, Einarson TR, Koren G. Adverse effects of antidepressant use in pregnancy: an evaluation of fetal growth and preterm birth. Depress Anxiety. 2010;27(1):35–8. https://doi.org/10.1002/da.20598.
26. Daley AJ, Foster L, Long G, Palmer C, Robinson O, Walmsley H, Ward R. The effectiveness of exercise for the prevention and treatment of antenatal depression: systematic review with meta-analysis. BJOG. 2015;122(1):57–62. https://doi.org/10.1111/1471-0528.12909.
27. Davenport MH, McCurdy AP, Mottola MF, Skow RJ, Meah VL, Poitras VJ, Jaramillo Garcia A, Gray CE, Barrowman N, Riske L, Sobierajski F, James M, Nagpal T, Marchand AA, Nuspl M, Slater LG, Barakat R, Adamo KB, Davies GA, Ruchat SM. Impact of prenatal exercise on both prenatal and postnatal anxiety and depressive symptoms: a systematic review and meta-analysis. Br J Sports Med. 2018;52(21):1376–85. https://doi.org/10.1136/bjsports-2018-099697.
28. Shivakumar G, Brandon AR, Snell PG, Santiago-Munoz P, Johnson NL, Trivedi MH, Freeman MP. Antenatal depression: a rationale for studying exercise. Depress Anxiety. 2011;28(3):234–42. https://doi.org/10.1002/da.20777.
29. Teychenne M, York R. Physical activity, sedentary behavior, and postnatal depressive symptoms: a review. Am J Prev Med. 2013;45(2):217–27. https://doi.org/10.1016/j.amepre.2013.04.004.
30. Ross LE, McLean LM. Anxiety disorders during pregnancy and the postpartum period: a systematic review. J Clin Psychiatry. 2006;67(8):1285–98.

31. Schetter CD, Tanner L. Anxiety, depression and stress in pregnancy: implications for mothers, children, research, and practice. Curr Opin Psychiatry. 2012;25(2):141.
32. Paluska SA, Schwenk TL. Physical activity and mental health: current concepts. Sports Med. 2000;29(3):167–80.
33. Lee KA. Alterations in sleep during pregnancy and postpartum: a review of 30 years of research. Sleep Med Rev. 1998;2(4):231–42.
34. Sahota PK, Jain SS, Dhand R. Sleep disorders in pregnancy. Curr Opin Pulm Med. 2003;9(6):477–83.
35. Fox KR. The influence of physical activity on mental well-being. Public Health Nutr. 1999;2(3a):411–8.
36. Quan SF, O'Connor GT, Quan JS, Redline S, Resnick HE, Shahar E, Siscovick D, Sherrill DL. Association of physical activity with sleep-disordered breathing. Sleep Breath. 2007;11(3):149–57. https://doi.org/10.1007/s11325-006-0095-5.
37. Sherrill DL, Kotchou K, Quan SF. Association of physical activity and human sleep disorders. Arch Intern Med. 1998;158(17):1894–8. https://doi.org/10.1001/archinte.158.17.1894.
38. Borodulin K, Evenson KR, Monda K, Wen F, Herring AH, Dole N. Physical activity and sleep among pregnant women. Paediatr Perinat Epidemiol. 2010;24(1):45–52.
39. Loprinzi PD, Loprinzi KL, Cardinal BJ. The relationship between physical activity and sleep among pregnant women. Ment Health Phys Act. 2012;5(1):22–7. https://doi.org/10.1016/j.mhpa.2011.12.002.
40. Baker JH, Rothenberger SD, Kline CE, Okun ML. Exercise during early pregnancy is associated with greater sleep continuity. Behav Sleep Med. 2016;16:1–14. https://doi.org/10.1080/15402002.2016.1228649.
41. Tella B, Sokunbi O, Akinlami O, Afolabi B. Effects of aerobic exercises on the level of insomnia and fatigue in pregnant women. Int J Gynecol Obstet. 2011;15(1):1.
42. Beddoe AE, Lee KA, Weiss SJ, Powell Kennedy H, Yang C-PP. Effects of mindful yoga on sleep in pregnant women: a pilot study. Biol Res Nurs. 2010;11(4):363–70.
43. Yang SY, Lan SJ, Yen YY, Hsieh YP, Kung PT, Lan SH. Effects of exercise on sleep quality in pregnant women: a systematic review and meta-analysis of randomized controlled trials. Asian Nurs Res. 2020;14(1):1–10. https://doi.org/10.1016/j.anr.2020.01.003.
44. Sallis JF, Owen N, Fisher EB. Ecological models of health behavior. In: Health behavior and health education: theory, research, and practice, vol. 4. San Francisco, CA: Jossey-Bass; 2008. p. 465–86.
45. Evenson KR, Moos M-K, Carrier K, Siega-Riz AM. Perceived barriers to physical activity among pregnant women. Matern Child Health J. 2009;13(3):364.
46. Downs DS, Chasan-Taber L, Evenson KR, Leiferman J, Yeo S. Physical activity and pregnancy. Res Q Exerc Sport. 2012;83(4):485–502. https://doi.org/10.1080/02701367.2012.10599138.
47. Foxcroft KF, Rowlands IJ, Byrne NM, McIntyre HD, Callaway LK. Exercise in obese pregnant women: the role of social factors, lifestyle and pregnancy symptoms. BMC Pregnan Childb. 2011;11(1):4.
48. Harrison AL, Taylor NF, Shields N, Frawley HC. Attitudes, barriers and enablers to physical activity in pregnant women: a systematic review. J Physiother. 2018;64(1):24–32. https://doi.org/10.1016/j.jphys.2017.11.012.
49. Aubry RH, Pennington JC. Identification and evaluation of high-risk pregnancy: the perinatal concept. Clin Obstet Gynecol. 1973;16(1):3–27.
50. Weir Z, Bush J, Robson SC, McParlin C, Rankin J, Bell R. Physical activity in pregnancy: a qualitative study of the beliefs of overweight and obese pregnant women. BMC Pregnan Childb. 2010;10:18. https://doi.org/10.1186/1471-2393-10-18.
51. Cioffi J, Schmied V, Dahlen H, Mills A, Thornton C, Duff M, Cummings J, Kolt GS. Physical activity in pregnancy: women's perceptions, practices, and influencing factors. J Midwif Women's Health. 2010;55(5):455–61.
52. Leiferman J, Swibas T, Koiness K, Marshall JA, Dunn AL. My baby, my move: examination of perceived barriers and motivating factors related to antenatal physical activity. J Midwif Women's Health. 2011;56(1):33–40. https://doi.org/10.1111/j.1542-2011.2010.00004.x.

53. Watson ED, Oddie B, Constantinou D. Exercise during pregnancy: knowledge and beliefs of medical practitioners in South Africa: a survey study. BMC Pregnan Childb. 2015;15(1):245.
54. van der Pligt P, Campbell K, Willcox J, Opie J, Denney-Wilson E. Opportunities for primary and secondary prevention of excess gestational weight gain: general practitioners' perspectives. BMC Fam Pract. 2011;12(1):124.
55. Coll CV, Domingues MR, Goncalves H, Bertoldi AD. Perceived barriers to leisure-time physical activity during pregnancy: a literature review of quantitative and qualitative evidence. J Sci Med Sport. 2017;20(1):17–25. https://doi.org/10.1016/j.jsams.2016.06.007.
56. Leppänen M, Aittasalo M, Raitanen J, Kinnunen TI, Kujala UM, Luoto R. Physical activity during pregnancy: predictors of change, perceived support and barriers among women at increased risk of gestational diabetes. Matern Child Health J. 2014;18(9):2158–66. https://doi.org/10.1007/s10995-014-1464-5.
57. Reichert F, Barros AJD, Domingues M, Hallal P. The role of perceived personal barriers to engagement in leisure-time physical activity. Am J Public Health. 2007;97:515. https://doi.org/10.2105/AJPH.2005.070144.
58. Currie S, Sinclair M, Murphy MH, Madden E, Dunwoody L, Liddle D. Reducing the decline in physical activity during pregnancy: a systematic review of behaviour change interventions. PLoS One. 2013;8(6):e0066385. https://doi.org/10.1371/journal.pone.0066385.
59. James P, Morgant R, Merviel P, Saraux A, Giroux-Metges MA, Guillodo Y, Dupré PF, Muller M. How to promote physical activity during pregnancy: a systematic review. J Gynecol Obstet Hum Reprod. 2020;49(9):101864. https://doi.org/10.1016/j.jogoh.2020.101864.
60. Flannery C, Fredrix M, Olander EK, McAuliffe FM, Byrne M, Kearney PM. Effectiveness of physical activity interventions for overweight and obesity during pregnancy: a systematic review of the content of behaviour change interventions. Int J Behav Nutr Phys Act. 2019;16(1):97. https://doi.org/10.1186/s12966-019-0859-5.
61. Taniguchi C, Sato C. Home-based walking during pregnancy affects mood and birth outcomes among sedentary women: a randomized controlled trial. Int J Nurs Pract. 2016;22(5):420–6. https://doi.org/10.1111/ijn.12453.
62. Zarezadeh T, Nemati N. Effects of 8 week regular walking on the neonate in nulliparous women. Koomesh. 2016;17(2):403–10.
63. Yeo S, Davidge S, Ronis DL, Antonakos CL, Hayashi R, O'Leary S. A comparison of walking versus stretching exercises to reduce the incidence of preeclampsia: a randomized clinical trial. Hypertens Pregnan. 2008;27(2):113–30. https://doi.org/10.1080/10641950701826778.
64. Kong KL, Campbell CG, Foster RC, Peterson AD, Lanningham-Foster L. A pilot walking program promotes moderate-intensity physical activity during pregnancy. Med Sci Sports Exerc. 2014;46(3):462–71. https://doi.org/10.1249/MSS.0000000000000141.
65. De Oliveria Melo AS, Silva JLP, Tavares JS, Barros VO, Leite DFB, Amorim MMR. Effect of a physical exercise program during pregnancy on uteroplacental and fetal blood flow and fetal growth: a randomized controlled trial. Obstet Gynecol. 2012;120(2 Part 1):302–10. https://doi.org/10.1097/AOG.0b013e31825de592.
66. Stafne SN, Salvesen KÅ, Romundstad PR, Torjusen IH, Mørkved S. Does regular exercise including pelvic floor muscle training prevent urinary and anal incontinence during pregnancy? A randomised controlled trial. BJOG. 2012;119(10):1270–9. https://doi.org/10.1111/j.1471-0528.2012.03426.x.
67. Hui A, Back L, Ludwig S, Gardiner P, Sevenhuysen G, Dean H, Sellers E, McGavock J, Morris M, Bruce S, Murray R, Shen GX. Lifestyle intervention on diet and exercise reduced excessive gestational weight gain in pregnant women under a randomised controlled trial. BJOG. 2012;119(1):70–7. https://doi.org/10.1111/j.1471-0528.2011.03184.x.
68. Sagedal LR, Sanda B, Overby NC, Bere E, Torstveit MK, Lohne-Seiler H, Hillesund ER, Pripp AH, Henriksen T, Vistad I. The effect of prenatal lifestyle intervention on weight retention 12 months postpartum: results of the Norwegian Fit for Delivery randomised controlled trial. BJOG. 2017;124(1):111–21. https://doi.org/10.1111/1471-0528.13863.
69. Wang C, Wei Y, Zhang X, Zhang Y, Xu Q, Sun Y, Su S, Zhang L, Liu C, Feng Y, Shou C, Guelfi KJ, Newnham JP, Yang H. A randomized clinical trial of exercise during pregnancy to prevent gestational diabetes mellitus and improve pregnancy outcome in overweight and

obese pregnant women. Am J Obstet Gynecol. 2017;216(4):340–51. https://doi.org/10.1016/j.ajog.2017.01.037.
70. Symons Downs D, DiNallo JM, Birch LL, Paul IM, Ulbrecht JS. Randomized Face-to-face vs. Home exercise interventions in pregnant women with gestational diabetes. Psychol Sport Exerc. 2017;30:73–81. https://doi.org/10.1016/j.psychsport.2017.02.003.
71. Jackson RA, Stotland NE, Caughey AB, Gerbert B. Improving diet and exercise in pregnancy with Video Doctor counseling: a randomized trial. Patient Educ Couns. 2011;83(2):203–9. https://doi.org/10.1016/j.pec.2010.05.019.
72. Smith K, Lanningham-Foster L, Welch A, Campbell C. Web-based behavioral intervention increases maternal exercise but does not prevent excessive gestational weight gain in previously sedentary women. J Phys Act Health. 2016;13(6):587–93. https://doi.org/10.1123/jpah.2015-0219.
73. Albert B. Social foundations of thought and action: a social cognitive theory. New York, NY: Prentice-Hall; 1986.
74. Gaston A, Prapavessis H. Maternal-fetal disease information as a source of exercise motivation during pregnancy. Health Psychol. 2009;28(6):726–33. https://doi.org/10.1037/a0016702.
75. Gaston A, Prapavessis H. Using a combined protection motivation theory and health action process approach intervention to promote exercise during pregnancy. J Behav Med. 2014;37(2):173–84. https://doi.org/10.1007/s10865-012-9477-2.
76. Dodd JM, Cramp C, Zhixian S, Yelland LN, Deussen AR, Grivell RM, Moran LJ, Crowther CA, Turnbull D, McPhee AJ, Wittert G, Owens JA, Robinson JS, For the LRTG. The effects of antenatal dietary and lifestyle advice for women who are overweight or obese on maternal diet and physical activity: the LIMIT randomised trial. BMC Med. 2014;12(1):161–79. https://doi.org/10.1186/s12916-014-0161-y.
77. Poston L, Briley AL, Barr S, Bell R, Croker H, Coxon K, Essex HN, Hunt C, Hayes L, Howard LM, Khazaezadeh N, Kinnunen T, Nelson SM, Oteng-Ntim E, Robson SC, Sattar N, Seed PT, Wardle J, Sanders TAB, Sandall J. Developing a complex intervention for diet and activity behaviour change in obese pregnant women (the UPBEAT trial); Assessment of behavioural change and process evaluation in a pilot randomised controlled trial. BMC Pregnan Childb. 2013;13:148. https://doi.org/10.1186/1471-2393-13-148.
78. Hayes L, Bell R, Robson S, Poston L. Association between physical activity in obese pregnant women and pregnancy outcomes: the UPBEAT pilot study. Ann Nutr Metab. 2014;64(3–4):239–46. https://doi.org/10.1159/000365027.
79. Ko CW, Napolitano PG, Lee SP, Schulte SD, Ciol MA, Beresford SA. Physical activity, maternal metabolic measures, and the incidence of gallbladder sludge or stones during pregnancy: a randomized trial. Am J Perinatol. 2014;31(1):39–48. https://doi.org/10.1055/s-0033-1334455.
80. Simmons D, Devlieger R, Van Assche A, Jans G, Galjaard S, Corcoy R, Adelantado JM, Dunne F, Desoye G, Harreiter J, Kautzky-Willer A, Damm P, Mathiesen ER, Jensen DM, Andersen L, Lapolla A, Dalfra MG, Bertolotto A, Wender-Ozegowska E, Zawiejska A, Hill D, Snoek FJ, Jelsma JGM, Van Poppel MNM. Effect of physical activity and/or healthy eating on GDM risk: the DALI lifestyle study. J Clin Endocrinol Metab. 2017;102(3):903–13. https://doi.org/10.1210/jc.2016-3455.
81. Vinter CA, Jensen DM, Ovesen P, Beck-Nielsen H, Jørgensen JS. The LiP (Lifestyle in Pregnancy) study: a randomized controlled trial of lifestyle intervention in 360 obese pregnant women. Diabetes Care. 2011;34:2502. https://doi.org/10.2337/dc11-1150.
82. Michie S, van Stralen MM, West R. The behaviour change wheel: a new method for characterising and designing behaviour change interventions. Implement Sci. 2011;6:42. https://doi.org/10.1186/1748-5908-6-42.
83. Cane J, O'Connor D, Michie S. Validation of the theoretical domains framework for use in behaviour change and implementation research. Implement Sci. 2012;7(1):37.

3

Physiological Changes During Pregnancy: Main Adaptations, Discomforts, and Implications for Physical Activity and Exercise

María Perales, Taniya Singh Nagpal, and Ruben Barakat

Abstract

Almost the entire female body naturally modifies and changes during pregnancy, and in many cases, these modifications occur normally; however, there may be imbalances that occur that can cause complications or pathologies.

In fact, pregnancy is known as the most changing period in a human life as there is no other time that produces the same quantity and quality of bodily modifications. Due to the varied changes the body experiences, pregnancy and childbirth can determine the future well-being of the mother and her child.

The pregnant body must work for 40 weeks to achieve adequate fetal growth and development and this causes a constant effort to maintain balance in all organs and systems. In summary, due to the many modifications that occur during pregnancy, exercise during pregnancy should be given unique and special considerations when compared to nonpregnant populations. However, from a scientific point of view, none of these modifications contradicts exercise in healthy pregnant women without obstetric contraindications.

M. Perales (✉)
University Camilo José Cela, Madrid, Spain

Research Institute Hospital 12 de Octubre ('i + 12'), Madrid, Spain
e-mail: mperales@ucjc.edu

T. S. Nagpal
Faculty of Applied Health Sciences, Brock University, St. Catharines, ON, Canada
e-mail: tnagpal@brocku.ca

R. Barakat
Faculty of Physical Activity and Sport Sciences – INEF, Technical University of Madrid, Madrid, Spain
e-mail: rubenomar.barakat@upm.es

R. Santos-Rocha (ed.), *Exercise and Physical Activity During Pregnancy and Postpartum*, https://doi.org/10.1007/978-3-031-06137-0_3

Keywords

Pregnancy · Physiology · Cardiovascular · Hematologic · Metabolic · Physical activity · Exercise

3.1 Cardiovascular Changes

The human body during pregnancy changes day by day to continuously adapt its functions to ensure the development of an independent individual [1]. It is essential to optimize maternal health during this period.

The fetus is completely dependent on the mother. In a normal pregnancy, the maternal cardiovascular system undergoes essential changes in its structure and function which are necessary to support fetal demands and this leads to a considerable amount of stress on the maternal heart [2]. These changes (see Table 3.1) begin around the fifth week of pregnancy and continue until 1 year after delivery [3, 4].

General hemodynamic changes include an increase in maternal heart rate (30%) [5, 6] and blood volume (40–45%) [7]. Red blood cells also increase during pregnancy but less than blood volume (18–25%) [8], and this produces a decrease in hematocrit known as physiological anemia of pregnancy [5].

Table 3.1 Main cardiovascular changes during pregnancy

			Trimester		
	Change	Magnitude	First T	Second T	Third T
Hemodynamic changes					
Vascular resistance	↓	30%	↓	↓	↑
Blood volume	↑	40–45%	↑	↑	–
Cardiac output	↑	30–50%	↑	↑	NC
Heart rate	↑	15–30%	↑	↑	↑
Stroke volume	↑	20–30%	↑	↑	NC
Systolic blood pressure	–	–	–	–	–
Diastolic blood pressure	↓	10 mmHg	↓	↓/=	↑
Structural changes					
Aorta artery elasticity	↑	30%	↑	–	–
Heart size	↑	30%	↑	↑	↑
Left atrial	↑	16–40%	↑	↑	↑
Left ventricular					
Left ventricular diastolic dimension	↑	20%	↑	–	–
Left ventricular systolic dimension	↑	10%	↑	↑	↑
Left ventricular wall thickness	↑	15–25%	↑	↑	↑
Left ventricular stress	↑	17%	↑	–	↓
Left ventricular mass	↑	50%	↑	↑	↑
Systolic function	NC				
Diastolic function	↓		↑	↑	↓

NC no consensus

Hemodynamic alterations continue to occur throughout pregnancy with different changes taking place in each trimester. Total maternal vascular resistance decreases around 30% up to 28 weeks of pregnancy and then there is a considerable increase until term [6, 9]. This change leads to a reduction in maternal blood pressure (specifically diastolic blood pressure) during the first and second trimesters, and a normal increase during the third trimester [10, 11].

There is a general consensus that maternal cardiac output and stroke volume increase by 30–50% and 20–30%, respectively, in the first and second trimesters. However, previous literature has been inconsistent on what occurs during the third trimester as some authors report a decrease in cardiac output and stroke volume [5, 6], while there is also research supporting an increase [11, 12] or no variation at all [13–15]. Furthermore, it is important to note that most of these hemodynamic changes depend on maternal parity, age, and body mass index (BMI; [16, 17]).

Hemodynamic modifications on the maternal heart persist for a longer time than other hemodynamic and functional changes that occur during pregnancy. The increase in stroke volume is attributed to an increase in blood volume and preload, as demonstrated by the increase in left atrial and left ventricular end-diastolic dimensions and consequently the size of the heart gradually increases by approximately 30% [5, 18]. A slight increase in the left ventricular systolic dimension is also observed in a normal pregnancy [19].

To minimize stress on the heart, the walls of the heart increase in thickness beginning in the first weeks of gestation [2]. This response leads to a change in geometric left ventricular patterning usually toward eccentric hypertrophy and this is typically associated with an exercise stimulus and pregnancy. Abnormal structural adaptations may also lead to concentric remodeling or concentric hypertrophy and this may cause health complications during and after pregnancy [20].

Additional structural modifications include the aorta artery which increases in its flexibility by approximately 30% [21], in response to the normal reduction in total maternal vascular resistance [2].

In regards to maternal heart function, literature has been inconsistent on what potential changes occur with some research suggesting an improvement in systolic function [19] However, there are also reports of impaired systolic function [22] or no change taking place [6, 9]. As pregnancy progresses, the heart's capacity to relax increases which implies an enhancement in diastolic function up to the beginning of the third trimester. Following this, a normal decline in diastolic function until labor has been observed [11, 15].

3.1.1 Implications of Exercise During Pregnancy on the Maternal Heart

The changes that occur in the maternal heart during pregnancy are reversible in healthy women, but it is estimated that approximately 1% of pregnancies are complicated by heart disease in Europe [23]. There are some risk factors associated with an unhealthy lifestyle during pregnancy that may compromise maternal and fetal health.

A growing body of evidence supports that adopting or continuing a sedentary lifestyle during pregnancy increases the risk for developing gestational hypertension or diabetes and gaining excessive weight, and these are considered the risk factors for heart failure and cardiovascular dysfunction [24]. During labor, physically inactive women show limitations in the intensity and duration of pushes which lead to greater stress on the maternal heart and this may increase the risk of developing cardiovascular disease later in life [25].

Maintaining or starting to exercise during pregnancy may have great physiological benefits for the mother and the newborn. However, it is important to keep in mind some exercise considerations to accommodate for the naturally occurring maternal cardiovascular response to pregnancy and in order to avoid any additional stress on the maternal heart.

3.1.1.1 Maternal Cardiovascular Response to Exercise

During aerobic exercise, vascular resistance is reduced and this produces an increase in cardiac output, stroke volume, and heart rate [26]. This hemodynamic response depends on the gestational age, intensity, modality, and fitness level [27].

Importantly, maximal maternal heart rate is lower in pregnant women compared to nonpregnant women during submaximal exercise [28]. The physiological increase in maternal heart rate at rest and the maximal heart rate reduction produce a decrease in maternal heart rate reserve [29]. Exercise programs for pregnant women should control the intensity of the activity not only by a heart rate monitor but also by using the Borg Scale of Perceived Exertion [30] to ensure the safety of the woman.

Maternal position during exercise also plays an essential role in the cardiovascular response. Aortocaval compression occurs when the gravid uterus compresses the maternal abdominal aorta and inferior vena cava. This impedes venous return which decreases cardiac output and stroke volume and may reduce uteroplacental perfusion resulting in fetal acidosis [31]. This phenomenon occurs in 90% of pregnant women when they adopt a supine position or are lying on their right side [31].

3.1.1.2 Maternal Cardiovascular Adaptations to Exercise

There is limited evidence on the cardiovascular adaptations that occur in response to exercise during pregnancy [32, 33]. Findings from both studies were consistent, especially in the third trimester where results showed that the effects of exercise are hidden by the physiological pregnancy adaptations. No significant improvement in hemodynamic, functional, or structural results was observed; however, authors clarify that moderate regular exercise from late first trimester to term does not produce an additional change or adverse impact on the maternal heart [32, 33].

A nonsignificant trend was found in regards to maternal heart structure. Sedentary women tend to increase the proportion of abnormal left ventricular patterning, particularly concentric remodeling, which was not observed in active women [33]. This result is potentially relevant because cardiac remodeling during pregnancy is associated with a higher risk for maternal and fetal complications such as preeclampsia, hypertension, and preterm delivery [20].

Regular moderate exercise has also shown to be effective for the prevention of important cardiovascular risks during pregnancy such as antenatal depression and excessive gestational weight gain [33].

Further studies related to cardiovascular adaptations during pregnancy in response to exercise are necessary to clarify the most effective dose of exercise required based on maternal characteristics for the most physiological benefit overall.

3.2 Hematological Changes

Hematological modifications occur in response to pregnancy to meet the bodily requirements for both the mother and growing fetus such as nutrient transport to maintain fetal well-being [34].

Blood volume increases by 45% (1800 mL), and this includes an increase in blood volume or plasma (around 1500 mL) and cythemia (around 350 mL). This "hemodilution" will maintain adequate uteroplacental flow [35].

An additional gr of iron (daily) is required during pregnancy due to the increase in red blood cells (citemia) and fetal–placental iron requirements. This need is more essential from the second half of gestation (extra caution is recommended when engaging in strenuous physical activity) [36].

During pregnancy, hemoglobin concentration below 11 g/100 mL is considered anemia. Normal pregnancy in a woman with a deficit of iron reserves can lead to iron deficiency anemia [36].

During pregnancy, there is a decrease in folates, which are essential for fetal development. It is advisable for a woman who is trying to conceive to take a certain amount of folic acid a few months before pregnancy [37].

There is also a state of hypercoagulability (increased fibrinogen and other factors of coagulation). These changes are required for coagulation at the time of delivery. An increase of plasma fibrinogen justifies the elevation for the rate of globular sedimentation. A mild leukocytosis is established in 20% of pregnant women. Lymphocytes decrease in number and in absolute percentage, especially at the beginning of pregnancy, and continue throughout [36].

3.3 Respiratory Changes

The physiological requirements and normal modifications that occur during pregnancy include a relevant interaction between cardiovascular and respiratory functions. During exercise, this interaction also exists [34].

Oxygen and carbon dioxide are transported in both directions between the atmosphere and maternal and fetal cells. This is a complex process with challenges and anatomical and physiological implications that occur due to pregnancy [35].

The changes in the respiratory system cause alterations in anatomical and functional structures. These changes occur in early pregnancy due to hormonal influence and small volumetric alterations. These modifications include variations in lung dimension and capacity and respiratory mechanisms [35, 38].

The upper respiratory tract is (in some cases) affected by changes in the mucosa of the nasopharynx, for example, hyperemia, edema, and excessive secretion. This generates obstructive symptoms for normal breathing functions [36].

Furthermore, as a result of the expansion of the uterus, the average diaphragmatic position when the pregnant woman is standing is elevated by 4 cm [39].

As pregnancy progresses, the growing uterus significantly increases intra-abdominal pressure and this causes the ribs to become more horizontal. However, the ribs compensate for this by increasing the anteroposterior and transverse diameters of the rib cage by approximately 2 cm. The substernal angle is also increased by about 70° in the first trimester and 105° in the final stage of gestation and the circumference of the thoracic cage increases by about 5–7 cm [39].

At the beginning of pregnancy, the woman breathes more deeply but not more frequently, primarily due to an increase in progesterone. The consequence of this is that alveolar ventilation increases above pregestational values. As there is a higher tidal volume, the volume of expiratory reserve decreases, but vital capacity is maintained by a slight increase in inspiratory capacity [36].

Another characteristic of pregnancy at the respiratory level is the increase of oxygen consumption by 10–20% and a reduction in PCO2. This increases the tidal volume while decreasing the residual volume and functional residual capacity. The combination of reduced residual functional capacity and increased oxygen consumption results in reduced oxygen reserves. There is also an increase in oxygen uptake when breathing due to an increase in diaphragmatic work [36].

The ventilation/minute also increases, resulting in respiratory alkalosis, again in this case due to progesterone and additionally by the increase in estrogen. Despite this respiratory alkalosis, the acid–base state is maintained by compensatory metabolic acidosis. The arterial pH remains at 7.44 as a result of primary respiratory alkalosis and compensatory acidosis. The main purpose of these maternal respiratory mechanisms is to reduce arterial PCO2 and thus generate a mild maternal alkalosis that ensures placental gas exchange and prevents fetal acidosis [36, 40].

3.4 Metabolic Changes

The body's goal during pregnancy is to ensure fetal growth and development and this generates continuous adjustments in the maternal metabolic system throughout the 40 weeks of gestation. From a general point of view, normal metabolic processes are altered during pregnancy to adapt to the exact needs of the developing fetus [34, 35, 41].

During pregnancy, the protein content in body tissue is increased. Carbohydrates accumulate in the liver, muscles, and placenta. Under the skin, fat deposits increase, especially in the chest and buttocks area. The concentration of both types of cholesterol and blood fat is also increased. The pregnant body accumulates salts of various minerals essential for the normal development of the fetus, including calcium, phosphorus, potassium, and iron. In addition, hormonal changes favor the retention of water in tissues [35].

Weight gain is the most obvious change during pregnancy. Traditionally, total maternal weight gain of 10–13 kg was considered adequate (with many individual variations). However, currently the recommendations are based on maternal prepregnancy BMI [34, 42] (Table 3.2).

Many parameters influence maternal weight gain during pregnancy (Table 3.3), including the interstitial fluid and the increase of fatty tissue (deposit).

Maternal weight gain determined by the increase in fat reserves has significant variability. When the total weight gain is 11 kg, the average fat deposit at the end of pregnancy is 1800 g, but it can be much higher (3–4 kg or even more), it can be null, or even negative; this means that the pregnant woman's body consumes the reserve fat that she had previously accumulated [40, 43].

In healthy pregnant women during the first half of gestation (anabolic phase), the weight gain depends mostly on the accumulation of fatty deposits and normal changes in the maternal body in response to pregnancy. In this phase, the contribution that fetal weight has on total maternal weight gain is not significant. As pregnancy progresses, weight gain is primarily due to fetal growth and less due to maternal bodily changes [40].

Fat reserves accumulated in the first half of gestation are used during the third trimester, mainly in the last 4 weeks when the fetus has a rapid increase in body fat percentage. From the biological point of view, maternal weight gain during pregnancy should be lower when prepregnancy BMI is higher; that is, when a woman's

Table 3.2 Institute of medicine weight gain recommendations for pregnancy

Prepregnancy body mass index category	Recommended intervals of total weight gain (kg)
<18.5	12.5–18
18.5–24.9	11.5–16
25–29.9	7–11.5
≥30	5–9

Table 3.3 Analysis of maternal weight gain during pregnancy [40]

	Weight gain in grams			
	Week 10	Week 20	Week 30	Week 40
Fetus	5	300	1500	3400
Placenta	20	170	430	650
Amniotic fluid	30	350	750	800
Uterus	140	320	600	970
Mamas	45	180	360	405
Blood	100	600	1300	1250
Interstitial liquid	0	30	80	1680
Fat deposits	310	2050	3480	3345
Total weight gain	650	4000	8500	12,500

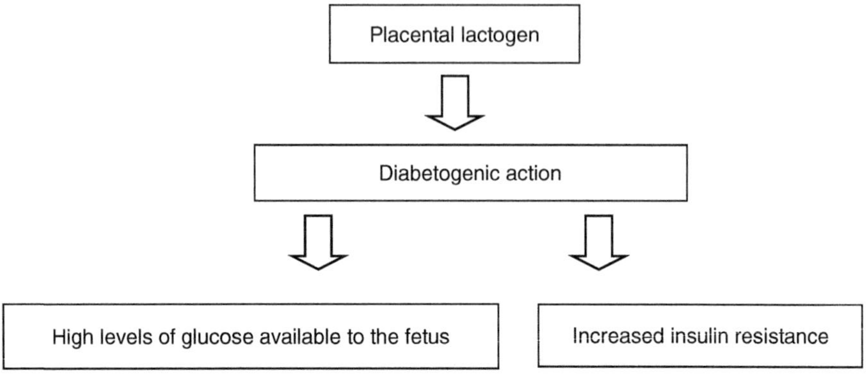

Fig. 3.1 Metabolism of carbohydrates in the second half of pregnancy [40]

fat deposit is higher before pregnancy, her BMI will be greater, and therefore less weight gain is recommended during pregnancy [34].

Metabolism of carbohydrates: In nondiabetic women, pregnancy is associated with profound metabolic changes, which can be studied in both fasting and postprandial situations (after the first intake) [40].

After an overnight fast, glucose levels are lower in pregnant women than nonpregnant women, especially in the second and third trimesters. The decrease in glucose decreases the level of insulin and this exaggerates ketosis by starvation. Therefore, after fasting during pregnancy, the levels of beta-hydroxybutyric acid and acetoacetic acid are higher than in nonpregnant women [40]

When pregnant women are fasting, there is an increase in the likelihood of hypoglycemia (very important), hypoinsulinemia, and hyperketonemia. This is due to facilitated diffusion of glucose from the mother to the fetus as a basic mechanism, and the existence of a greater volume of maternal distribution for glucose.

Thus, in the postprandial state, the maternal response is characterized by hyperinsulinemia, hyperglycemia, hypertriglyceridemia, and decreased sensitivity to insulin (insulin resistance) [40]. Pregnancy is, therefore, a diabetogenic experience. The factors responsible for this diabetogenic effect are placental hormones (placental lactogen), especially in the second half of pregnancy (Fig. 3.1) [34, 35, 40].

Metabolism of fats: Plasma lipids increase in the second half of pregnancy. This increase affects total lipids, cholesterol, phospholipids, and free fatty acids [40].

3.5 Locomotor Changes

Changes in the locomotor system are responsible for many common symptoms during pregnancy. Paresthesia and pain in the upper extremities occur as a consequence of an accentuated cervical lordosis and collapse of the scapular belt. These complications occur more frequently in the third trimester [34, 35, 44].

Traditionally, hyperlordosis has been considered a complication or even a pathology that occurs during pregnancy [34].

Currently, it is considered that this hyperlordosis is only apparent because the pregnant woman compensates for the deviation of her center of gravity, not by means of hyperlordosis but by displacing the entire craniocaudal axis backward. This new position can cause low back pain, especially if there is poor postural hygiene. Occasionally, a lumbosciatica originates due to compression of the sciatic nerve, and this may cause an increase in pain and functional disability (Fig. 3.2) [40].

Carpal tunnel syndrome is caused by the compression of the median nerve as it passes through the carpal tunnel on the anterior side of the wrist. It is characterized by pain and paresthesia usually experienced at night in the territory that is innervated by the median nerve and after delivery this reverts back to its normal state [40].

The rectus abdominis muscles are occasionally separated from the midline, creating a diastasis of the recti of variable extension. Sometimes, the uterus is only covered by a thin layer of peritoneum, fascia, and skin [34].

The mobility of the sacroiliac joints increases during pregnancy due to hormonal action, especially due to an increase in relaxin. The increase in joint relaxation can potentially diffuse pain. At the end of pregnancy, paresthesia may occur in the lower extremities (thigh and back of the leg), as a consequence of compressive changes (edema of the sheaths, pressure of the fetal head). In fact, this may contribute to the amount and quality of physical activity that a pregnant woman can perform in the final stage of pregnancy [45].

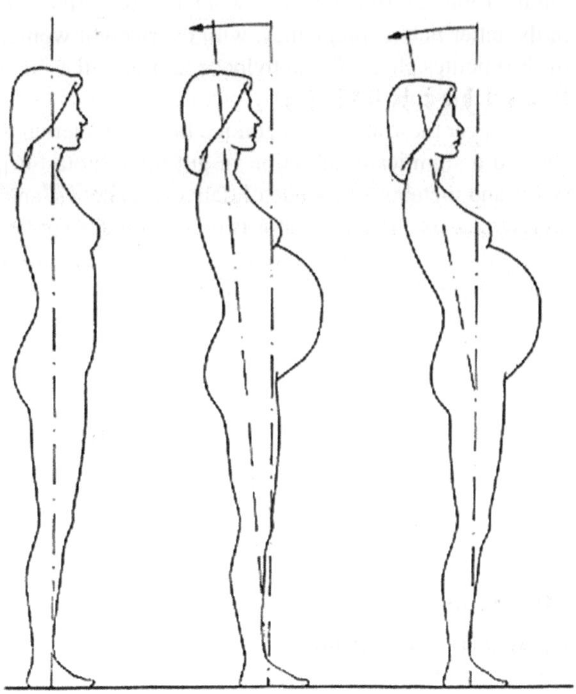

Fig. 3.2 Displacement of the center of gravity [40]

3.6 Microbiome Changes During Pregnancy

The human body has particular microbial population, including bacteria, archaea, fungi, and viruses. It is an important health factor due to mothers share their microbes and microbiome metabolites with the fetus in utero, during delivery and during lactation. This factor is also essential because it that is influenced and influences in maternal physiological changes during gestation with a high impact in maternal and fetus health from the beginning of life by altering pregnancy outcomes [46].

The womb is not sterile and microbial exposure may begin in utero. The placenta and amniotic fluid have been reported to serve as potential sources of intrauterine microbial transmission from the mother to the developing fetus. In healthy pregnant women, microbiota change dramatically, not only in bacterial load but also in its composition, from the first to the third trimester. Notably, this change is a key to promote a healthy pregnancy and normal fetal development [46]. Microbiota changes during pregnancy are characterized by increased abundance of members of the Actinobacteria and Proteobacteria phyla, as well as a reduction in individual richness [47]. These changes include placenta, gut, vaginal, and oral microbiota and are affected by gestational age.

Interestingly, microbiota during pregnancy is affected by such important factors as diet and physical exercise, not only during pregnancy but also prior it. Factor such as women body mass index prior to pregnancy correlated to neonatal gut microbiota composition in vaginally delivered, but not C-section [48]. The maternal gut microbiota differs between women with normal weight and obesity particularly in the latter half of pregnancy, with overweight women demonstrating increases in the Firmicutes phylum (Staphylococcus) as well as increases in some Proteobacteria (Escherichia coli) [49].

However these are not the unique factors, maternal weight gain during pregnancy showed a significant alteration in gut microbiota [46], as well as maternal health status and metabolism, mode of delivery, genetics, and use of antibiotics [50].

Exercise as a modify factor is recommended for healthy pregnancy with a great impact on intestinal microbiota. The scope of exercise biology extends well beyond energy expenditure and has emerged as an effective tool in the prevention and treatment of common diseases. Most studies to understand the impact of exercise on microbiota were performed by animal model. However, the anti-inflammatory effect of regular exercise, particular a combination of aerobic and resistance exercise, has been reported by much high-quality studies [51]. Exercise prescription is increasingly recognized as a safe and effective treatment for many diseases by adding further support for the potential influence of exercise on the brain-gut-microbiome axis [51].

Keeping in mind that microbiota can be "trained" even during pregnancy with a great effect in the present and future health generation [51], pregnancy, and also the postnatal period, are critical windows of opportunity for the prevention of metabolic diseases in the next generation.

References

1. Ezcurdia GM. Ejercicio físico y deportes durante el embarazo. In: Fabre Gonzalez E, editor. Manual de asistencia al embarazo normal. Madrid: Grupo de trabajo sobre asistencia al embarazo normal. Sección de Medicina Perinatal. Sociedad Española de Ginecología y Obstetricia; 2001. Chapter 11.
2. Melchiorre K, Sharma R, Thilaganathan B. Cardiac structure and function in normal pregnancy. Curr Opin Obstet Gynecol. 2012;24(6):413–21.
3. Duvekot JJ, Cheriex EC, Pieters FA, Menheere PP, Peeters LH. Early pregnancy changes in hemodynamics and volume homeostasis are consecutive adjustments triggered by a primary fall in systemic vascular tone. Am J Obstet Gynecol. 1993;169(6):1382–92.
4. Clapp JF III, Capeless E. Cardiovascular function before, during, and after the first and subsequent pregnancies. Am J Cardiol. 1997;80(11):1469–73.
5. Kametas NA, McAuliffe F, Cook B, Nicolaides KH, Chambers J. Maternal left ventricular transverse and long-axis systolic function during pregnancy. Ultrasound Obstet Gynecol. 2001;18(5):467–74.
6. Geva T, Mauer MB, Striker L, Kirshon B, Pivarnik JM. Effects of physiologic load of pregnancy on left ventricular contractility and remodeling. Am Heart J. 1997;133(1):53–9.
7. Thornburg KL, Jacobson SL, Giraud GD, Morton MJ. Hemodynamic changes in pregnancy. Semin Perinatol. 2000;24(1):11–4.
8. Hytten F. Blood volume changes in normal pregnancy. Clin Haematol. 1985;14(3):601–12.
9. Gilson GJ, Samaan S, Crawford MH, Qualls CR, Curet LB. Changes in hemodynamics, ventricular remodeling, and ventricular contractility during normal pregnancy: a longitudinal study. Obstet Gynecol. 1997;89(6):957–62.
10. Atkins AF, Watt JM, Milan P, Davies P, Crawford JS. A longitudinal study of cardiovascular dynamic changes throughout pregnancy. Eur J Obstet Gynecol Reprod Biol. 1981;12(4):215–24.
11. Mesa A, Jessurun C, Hernandez A, et al. Left ventricular diastolic function in normal human pregnancy. Circulation. 1999;99(4):511–7.
12. Mabie WC, DiSessa TG, Crocker LG, Sibai BM, Arheart KL. A longitudinal study of cardiac output in normal human pregnancy. Am J Obstet Gynecol. 1994;170(3):849–56.
13. Mashini IS, Albazzaz SJ, Fadel HE, et al. Serial noninvasive evaluation of cardiovascular hemodynamics during pregnancy. Am J Obstet Gynecol. 1987;156(5):1208–13.
14. Robson SC, Hunter S, Boys RJ, Dunlop W. Serial study of factors influencing changes in cardiac output during human pregnancy. Am J Phys. 1989;256(4 Pt 2):H1060–5.
15. Valensise H, Novelli GP, Vasapollo B, et al. Maternal cardiac systolic and diastolic function: relationship with uteroplacental resistances. A Doppler and echocardiographic longitudinal study. Ultrasound Obstet Gynecol. 2000;15(6):487–97.
16. Turan OM, De Paco C, Kametas N, Khaw A, Nicolaides KH. Effect of parity on maternal cardiac function during the first trimester of pregnancy. Ultrasound Obstet Gynecol. 2008;32(7):849–54.
17. Dagher FJ, Lyons JH, Finlayson DC, Shamsai J, Moore FD. Blood volume measurement: a critical study prediction of normal values: controlled measurement of sequential changes: choice of a bedside method. Adv Surg. 1965;1:69–109.
18. Sociedad Europea de cardiologia (ESC). Guía de práctica clínica de la ESC para el tratamiento de las enfermedades cardiovasculares durante el embarazo. Rev Esp Cardiol. 2012;65(2):171.e1–e44.
19. Savu O, Jurcut R, Giusca S, et al. Morphological and functional adaptation of the maternal heart during pregnancy. Circ Cardiovasc Imaging. 2012;5(3):289–97.
20. Novelli GP, Valensise H, Vasapollo B, et al. Left ventricular concentric geometry as a risk factor in gestational hypertension. Hypertension. 2003;41(3):469–75.
21. Hall ME, George EM, Granger JP. The heart during pregnancy. Rev Esp Cardiol. 2011;64(11):1045–50.

22. Schannwell CM, Zimmermann T, Schneppenheim M, Plehn G, Marx R, Strauer BE. Left ventricular hypertrophy and diastolic dysfunction in healthy pregnant women. Cardiology. 2002;97(2):73–8.
23. Roos-Hesselink JW, Duvekot JJ, Thorne SA. Pregnancy in high risk cardiac conditions. Heart. 2009;95(8):680–6.
24. Wolfe LA, Weissgerber TL. Clinical physiology of exercise in pregnancy: a literature review. J Obstet Gynaecol Can. 2003;25(6):473–83.
25. Sohnchen N, Melzer K, Tejada BM, et al. Maternal heart rate changes during labour. Eur J Obstet Gynecol Reprod Biol. 2011;158(2):173–8.
26. Artal R, Platt LD, Sperling M, Kammula RK, Jilek J, Nakamura R. I. Maternal cardiovascular and metabolic responses in normal pregnancy. Am J Obstet Gynecol. 1981;140(2):123–7.
27. Pivarnik JM. Cardiovascular responses to aerobic exercise during pregnancy and postpartum. Semin Perinatol. 1996;20(4):242–9.
28. Soultanakis HN, Artal R, Wiswell RA. Prolonged exercise in pregnancy: glucose homeostasis, ventilatory and cardiovascular responses. Semin Perinatol. 1996;20(4):315–27.
29. Wolfe LA, Mottola MF. Aerobic exercise in pregnancy: an update. Can J Appl Physiol. 1993;18(2):119–47.
30. Borg GA. Psychophysical bases of perceived exertion. Med Sci Sports Exerc. 1982;14(5):377–81.
31. Lee SW, Khaw KS, Ngan Kee WD, Leung TY, Critchley LA. Haemodynamic effects from aortocaval compression at different angles of lateral tilt in non-labouring term pregnant women. Br J Anaesth. 2012;109(6):950–6.
32. Wolfe LA, Preston RJ, Burggraf GW, McGrath MJ. Effects of pregnancy and chronic exercise on maternal cardiac structure and function. Can J Physiol Pharmacol. 1999;77(11):909–17.
33. Perales M, Santos-Lozano A, Sanchis-Gomar F, Luaces M, Pareja-Galeano H, Garatachea N, Barakat R, Lucia A. Maternal cardiac adaptation to a physical exercise program during pregnancy. Med Sci Sports Exerc. 2016;48(5):896–906.
34. Barakat R. El ejercicio físico durante el embarazo. Madrid: Pearson Alhambra; 2006.
35. Artal R, Wiswell R, Drinkwater B. Exercise in pregnancy. 2nd ed. Baltimore, MD: Williams and Wilkins; 1991.
36. Fernandez V, Rodriguez Melcon Y, Baron V. Modificaciones de la sangre en el embarazo. Cambios circulatorios y respiratorios. Alteraciones de los sistemas digestivos y urinarios. Sistema óseo y dientes. Cambios en la piel. Otras modificaciones. In: Tratado de Ginecología, Obstetricia y Medicina de la Reproducción, vol. 1. Madrid: Sociedad Española de Ginecología y Obstetricia. Panamericana; 2003.
37. Cunningham FG, Leveno KJ, Bloom SL, Hauth JC, Rouse DJ, Spong CY. Hematological changes. In: Cunningham FG, Leveno KJ, Bloom SL, Hauth JC, Rouse DJ, Spong CY, editors. Williams obstetrics. 23rd ed. New York, NY: McGraw-Hill; 2010. p. 114.
38. Alaily AB, Carrol KB. Pulmonary ventilation in pregnancy. Br J Obstet Gynecol. 1978;85:518–24.
39. Cunningham FG, Leveno KJ, Bloom SL, Hauth JC, Rouse DJ, Spong CY. Respiratory tract. In: Cunningham FG, Leveno KJ, Bloom SL, Hauth JC, Rouse DJ, Spong CY, editors. Williams obstetrics. 23rd ed. New York, NY: McGraw-Hill; 2010. p. 121.
40. De Migue LJ, Sánchez M. Cambios fisiológicos y adaptación materna durante el embarazo. In: Fabre Gonzalez E, editor. Manual de asistencia al embarazo normal. 2nd ed. Grupo de trabajo sobre asistencia al embarazo normal. Sección de Medicina Perinatal. Sociedad Española de Ginecología y Obstetricia Madrid; 2001. Chapter 4.
41. Barakat R, Perales M, Garatachea N, Ruiz JR, Lucia A. Exercise during pregnancy. A narrative review asking: what do we know? Br J Sports Med. 2015;49(21):1377–81.
42. Rasmussen KM, Yaktine AL, Institute of Medicine (Committee to Reexamine IOM Pregnancy Weight Guidelines, Food and Nutrition Board and Board on Children, Youth, and Families). Weight gain during pregnancy: reexamining the guidelines. Washington, DC: National Academic Press; 2009. Provides new guidelines for weight gain during pregnancy that are

based on minimizing the risks of inadequate or excessive gains to mothers as well as their infants.
43. Cerqueira M. Metabolismo en el embarazo. Modificaciones endocrinas. Modificaciones psíquicas. In: Tratado de Ginecología, Obstetricia y Medicina de la Reproducción, vol. 1. Madrid: Sociedad Española de Ginecología y Obstetricia. Ed. Panamericana; 2003.
44. Barakat R, Perales M. Resistance exercise in pregnancy and outcome. Clin Obstet Gynecol. 2016;59(3):591–9.
45. Cunningham FG, Leveno KJ, Bloom SL, Hauth JC, Rouse DJ, Spong CY. Other system. musculoskeletal system. In: Cunningham FG, Leveno KJ, Bloom SL, Hauth JC, Rouse DJ, Spong CY, editors. Williams obstetrics. 23rd ed. New York, NY: McGraw-Hill; 2010. p. 129.
46. Nuriel-Ohayon M, Neuman H, Koren O. Microbial changes during pregnancy, birth, and infancy. Front Microbiol. 2016;7:1031.
47. Koren O, Goodrich JK, Cullender TC, Spor A, Laitinen K, Bäckhed HK, Gonzalez A, Werner JJ, Angenent LT, Knight R, Bäckhed F, Isolauri E, Salminen S, Ley RE. Host remodeling of the gut microbiome and metabolic changes during pregnancy. Cell. 2012;150(3):470–80.
48. Mueller NT, Shin H, Pizoni A, Werlang IC, Matte U, Goldani MZ, Goldani HA, Dominguez-Bello MG. Birth mode-dependent association between pre-pregnancy maternal weight status and the neonatal intestinal microbiome. Sci Rep. 2016;6:23133.
49. Santacruz A, Collado MC, García-Valdés L, Segura MT, Martín-Lagos JA, Anjos T, Martí-Romero M, Lopez RM, Florido J, Campoy C, Sanz Y. Gut microbiota composition is associated with body weight, weight gain and biochemical parameters in pregnant women. Br J Nutr. 2010;104(1):83–92.
50. Soderborg TK, Borengasser SJ, Barbour LA, Friedman JE. Microbial transmission from mothers with obesity or diabetes to infants: an innovative opportunity to interrupt a vicious cycle. Diabetologia. 2016;59(5):895–906.
51. O'Sullivan O, Cronin O, Clarke SF, Murphy EF, Molloy MG, Shanahan F, Cotter PD. Exerc Microbiota Gut Microb. 2015;6(2):131–6.

Body Composition Changes During Pregnancy and Effects of Physical Exercise

4

Nuno M. Pimenta, Frøydis Hausmann, Coral Falco, and Mireille van Poppel

Abstract

The study of body composition is a fascinating branch of the biological sciences where research and clinical practice stimulate and complement each other. A strong theoretical background is needed to support the assessment and interpretation of body composition measurements, in order to have an impact and usefulness in the clinical setting, and clinical practice underscores the usefulness and makes sense of research. Body composition is a key component of health-related fitness with physical, morphological, and particularly important health-related implications during pregnancy. Pregnancy poses a major challenge for the study of body composition, as several techniques and overall methods and related assumptions are often not applicable, and pregnancy therefore requires specific assessment approaches. In the present chapter, we present a look into body composition fundamentals, how body composition can be assessed during pregnancy, and what adaptations should be taken into consideration in the assessment and

N. M. Pimenta (✉)
Sport Sciences School of Rio Maior – ESDRM, Polytechnic Institute of Santarém, Rio Maior, Portugal

Healthy Weight Laboratory, Interdisciplinary Centre for the Study of Human Performance - CIPER, Faculty of Human Kinetics – FMH, University of Lisbon, Cruz Quebrada-Dafundo, Portugal
e-mail: npimenta@esdrm.ipsantarem.pt

F. Hausmann · C. Falco
Department of Sport, Food and Natural Sciences, Faculty of Education, Arts and Sports, Western Norway University of Applied Sciences, Bergen, Norway
e-mail: froydis.hausmann@hvl.no; Coral.Falco@hvl.no

M. van Poppel
Institute of Human Movement Science, Sport and Health, University of Graz, Graz, Austria
e-mail: Mireille.van-poppel@uni-graz.at

R. Santos-Rocha (ed.), *Exercise and Physical Activity During Pregnancy and Postpartum*, https://doi.org/10.1007/978-3-031-06137-0_4

interpretation of body composition data. In the final section of the present chapter, a focus will be put on the effect of exercise on body composition during pregnancy.

Keywords

Pregnancy · Body composition · Assessment · Physical activity · Exercise

4.1 Introduction

The study of body composition is strongly associated to, and sometimes confused for, the study of obesity; however, body composition includes the study of body components far beyond body mass index and fat mass alone. The present chapter will focus on the challenge of assessing different body composition components in pregnant women, particularly on those components that have been found to show a wide variation during pregnancy and that are associated with health outcomes both during and after pregnancy, for either the mother or the newborn. This includes, of course, not only body fat (BF), including its content and distribution, but also total body water (TBW) and other fat-free mass (FFM) components.

Body composition is considered to be a component of health-related fitness and has physical, morphological and particularly important health-related implications for the overall, apparently healthy, population [1, 2] including women during and after pregnancy [3–8]. In the final section of the present chapter, we will focus on the effect of exercise and its prescription components (Frequency, Intensity, Time and Type plus Volume and Progression: FITT_VP) on body composition during pregnancy and its body composition-related consequences.

4.2 Body Composition Overview

The field of body composition research can be organized in three interconnecting areas: (1) body composition levels and their organizational rules; (2) body composition methodology; and (3) body composition biological effects [9, 10]. The present chapter focuses on two of these areas: on one hand, this chapter focuses on methodology and aims to highlight the challenge of body composition assessment in pregnancy; on the other hand, this chapter also focuses on the biological effects meaning that it aims to detail the effects of pregnancy and of exercise during pregnancy on body composition and also the effects of variations in body composition on different health outcomes for the pregnant and post-pregnant women and the newborn.

4.2.1 Body Composition Levels

Over the years, a wide variation could be observed in the terminology and methodology used in the study of body composition. The terminology and the five-level model suggested by Wang and colleagues [9] (see Fig. 4.1) was a critical milestone in the field of body composition research and is still fairly consensual and up-to-date, despite the advances in technology that occurred since. In the five-level model, it is assumed that each component within each level is mutually exclusive and the sum of all components in the same level is equivalent to whole-body mass [9].

The **atomic level** includes 11 major components, including oxygen, hydrogen, carbon, and nitrogen which altogether account for more than 96% of whole-body mass [10]. At the atomic level, the quantification of total body potassium has been widely used in the assessment of body composition in pregnancy [8]. The atoms considered in the mentioned atomic level are the constituents of molecules including water, carbohydrates, proteins, lipids, bone minerals, and soft tissue minerals, which are the six major components at the **molecular level** [10]. This is probably one of the most considered levels in body composition analysis. At the molecular level, it is possible to use multicomponent models for body composition analysis, but the assumptions used in several estimation methods at this level of body composition analysis may prove invalid when used in pregnancy [11], as discussed further in this chapter. The **cellular level** includes three components: extracellular solids, extracellular fluids, and cells, which include all body cell mass (including adipocytes). Total body cell mass is often assessed using total body potassium count, as potassium is nearly all intracellular and the estimation of body cell mass can be done from this assumption. The **tissue-organ level** results from the differentiation of cells into tissues and organs, including adipose tissue, skeletal muscle, visceral organs, and bone. To assess body composition at tissue-organ level, image methods

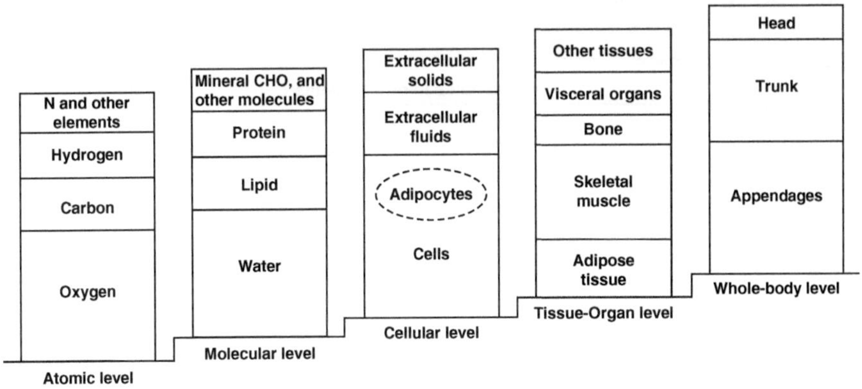

Fig. 4.1 The five-level model in body composition suggested by Wang and colleagues (adapted from Shen and colleagues [10], p. 4). *N* nitrogen, *CHO* carbohydrates

are required such as ultrasound or magnetic resonance imaging (MRI). The fifth level, the **whole-body level**, can be assessed using simple measures of weight or height, and can also be divided into regions such as the head, limbs, and trunk, which can be assessed with various anthropometric techniques, such as circumferences, skinfolds, and lengths, which are particularly useful in clinical settings.

The five-level model, as proposed by Wang and colleagues [9], present a clear, consensually accepted framework for the human body composition field (research/analysis/intervention). The biological rationale, criteria, assumptions, and terminology present in the five-level model are assumed as valid for all humans (pregnant and non-pregnant). This is the theoretical framework that is used throughout the present chapter.

4.2.2 Fat and Adipose Tissue

Body fat is a common concern when analyzing human body composition. When one refers to lipids, considered at the molecular level, it is important to acknowledge this refers to all of such molecules in the body, including essential non-fat lipids (lipids that are not in the form of triglycerides; e.g., phospholipids), both in adipose and other tissues; lipids in the form of triglycerides stored within the adipose tissue; and lipids in the form of triglycerides stored in other tissues. The commonly used word "fat" may be used interchangeably with BF but is distinguished from adipose tissue. The latter, assessed at the cellular level, refers to the adipocytes, which are cells that comprise BF and non-fat lipids, such as phospholipids, but include also other components essential to the survival and function of these cells (about 80% of adipose tissue is fat and the remainder 20% are water, proteins, and minerals) [12]. In this case, BF refers to triglycerides, which are the molecular form in which lipids are stored in the body. BF can be stored in the adipose tissue and in other tissues as well (see Fig. 4.2) [10].

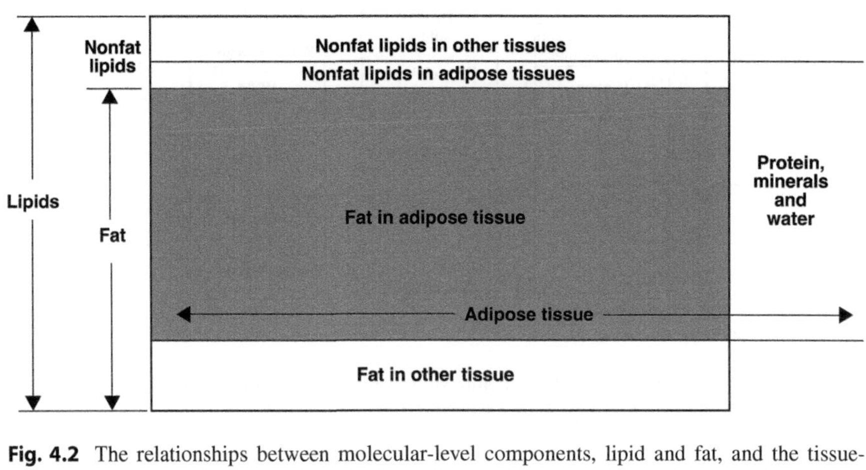

Fig. 4.2 The relationships between molecular-level components, lipid and fat, and the tissue-organ-level component, adipose tissue. (Adapted from Shen and colleagues [10], p. 12)

This terminology seems valid in pregnancy and gives a clear approach to the analysis of these specific components of body composition. This is the biological and terminological framework assumed in the present chapter and considered throughout.

4.2.3 Fat Depots and Adipose Tissue location

BF distribution analysis started with the study of body shape [13]. At the beginning of the twentieth century, after World War II, insurance companies identified a higher risk of mortality related to certain BF distribution phenotypes [14]. In the conviction that BF accumulation in different regions of the body could have different predictive values for adverse health outcomes, classifications of BF distribution were developed, such as Vague's classification [15, 16] that distinguished central BF accumulation (android) from peripheral, preferentially lower, BF accumulation (gynoid). BF distribution has long been shown to be related with other adverse outcomes, including diabetes, CVD, some forms of cancer, besides mortality [14]. BF distribution markers have been suggested to be more consistent and strong predictors of cardiometabolic risk in healthy non-pregnant women, as compared to whole-body markers of generalized adiposity [17], and the potential usefulness of such BF distribution markers for public health has been recognized [18] including in pregnancy [19–22].

Image methods have been assumed as a criterion in the study of BF distribution, yet image methods, often used as reference methods to quantify adipose tissue [23, 24], most often can only assess adipose tissue (as well as other tissues) but not BF [12]. Furthermore, some established image methods, such as DEXA, are prevented from usage during pregnancy due to potentially hazardous radiation exposure [8, 25]. Body composition assessment during pregnancy will be discussed in detail in the next subsection.

Shen and colleagues [12] presented a classification of adipose tissue location, based on image methods, to give coherence to the wide terminology that was being used. In general, adipose tissue is divided into subcutaneous and internal adipose tissues. Significant differences in the biologic behavior of such BF depots have been identified in pregnant as compared with non-pregnant women [26]. Subcutaneous adiposity may be divided into superficial and deep subcutaneous adipose tissue. It has also been given some importance to this division of subcutaneous adipose tissue [27]. Internal adipose tissue can also be further divided into visceral and non-visceral, and these can subsequently be divided into many other specific BF depots, all according to their specific location [12]. Sometimes BF may be stored in the visceral region, outside of adipocytes, near the organs. This is called ectopic fat and seems to have important health implications [28–30]. This terminology was developed using image methods and some specific adipose tissue locations may prove difficult to assess using other methods (particularly internal adipose tissue), whereas subcutaneous adipose tissue seams fairly accessible for clinical assessment using anthropometric techniques or other.

Along with robust laboratory methods for human body composition assessment, many clinical markers of BF content and distribution have been suggested, including simple anthropometric measurements and resulting calculated body indexes, as discussed ahead in the present chapter. These anthropometric variables and indexes assess body composition at a whole-body level to evaluate body dimensions and morphology, and often are used as BF content and distribution surrogates.

4.3 Body Composition During Pregnancy

The study of overweight and obesity has been overwhelming in the field of human body composition research, maybe because of both the pandemic dimension of its prevalence in developed countries [31, 32] and the associated health implications of such widespread condition [14, 33, 34]. The study of body composition in specific subpopulations, such as pregnancy, is not as overwhelming as in the general population or in other specific subpopulations but is still quite enlightening [8]. From the biochemical point of view, pregnancy is, above all, a challenge of body composition in which a being, the mother, is converting a set of nutrients into a new being, the child. The mother is therefore conceiving the first body composition with which her child is going to born with. In order to do that the mother also has to build an adequate milieu in which the fetus can have a healthy development. This includes building up the placenta and increasing body fluid, including amniotic fluid and extra blood volume to support the fetus, increasing energy reserves to support the gradual growth and development of the fetus and to support future lactation. All these expansions observed in specific body components during pregnancy have a significant impact on maternal body mass, or weight, and on body composition.

4.3.1 Pregnancy and Obesity

Obesity has been defined as an excess of adipose tissue [1]; however, adipose tissue is difficult to assess, requiring expensive and limited access imaging methods such as computed tomography (which use is prevented during pregnancy due to hazardous radiation exposure) or magnetic resonance imaging [12]. Obesity has also been referred to as an excess of BF [27, 35], which should be easier to estimate than adipose tissue. However, the most widely used definition of obesity is "a state of excessive weight" mostly because of the simple and inexpensive marker recommended by most prominent organizations [2, 36–39]: the body mass index (BMI = weight [kg]/height [m]^2). There are no specific BMI cutoffs for the diagnosis of obesity in pregnant women. Obesity must be assessed using pre-pregnancy BMI. During pregnancy, for monitoring healthy gestational weight gain, the weight in kilograms is preferred and recommended, instead of BMI. Pre-pregnancy BMI is usually difficult to assess because most women only attend maternal care after getting pregnant and not before. Pre-pregnancy BMI is, however, determinant for defining individual weight gain goals [40]. Individualization for obese women is less specific because healthy gestational weight gain recommendations for each class of pre-pregnancy obesity are lacking [41].

Obesity is linked to many diseases and morbidities and ultimately, to higher mortality rates in the non-pregnant [11, 42], and has also been related with hazardous health outcomes during and after pregnancy, both for the mother and the offspring [43]. Pregnancy in women who are obese, as assessed by pre-pregnancy BMI, is associated with higher risk of gestational diabetes, pregnancy-induced hypertension (including eclampsia and preeclampsia) [44, 45] and hyperemesis gravidarum [46]. Pre-pregnant obese mothers are also more likely to have fetal deaths [47], stillbirths [48, 49], preterm births [50], neonatal and perinatal death [47], large for age neonates [51] and also increased risk of infant death [47], obesity during childhood [52], and congenital heart defects [53] in their offspring. Maternal obesity is also associated with a phenomenon that has been called "developmental overnutrition" of the fetus which is associated with increased fetal skeletal growth and BF accumulation, which may explain the large-for-age neonates and future offspring increased obesity and adiposity levels and, possibly other adiposity-related cardiometabolic imbalances [54]. It has recently been reported that type 1 diabetes is 20% more common, and strikes at younger ages, in children of mothers that were obese as compared to controls, regardless of GWG [55].

Taken together, obesity is a risk factor for women who want to have children as it imposes high risks for both the mother and the offspring both during pregnancy and throughout the lifespan. This underlies the recommendation of the IOM for overweight and obese women to lose weight before getting pregnant to ensure better health outcomes [40]. The potential for prevention of common diseases in future generations by reducing maternal obesity and excessive weight gain during pregnancy definitely needs to be explored. Nevertheless, surplus fat and enlarged adipocytes seem to be the key for altered metabolism and related metabolic impairments in obesity [27, 56, 57], rather than just an excess of body weight alone [58].

4.3.2 Pregnancy and Weight Gain

Weight gain during pregnancy, most often called gestational weight gain (GWG), is expected and important for a healthy pregnancy and pregnancy outcome. Nevertheless, GWG should occur within healthy boundaries. A great deal of importance has been given to GWG, and recommendations exist (Table 4.1) aiming to optimize maternal and offspring health outcomes, as has been re-examined by the Institute of Medicine (IOM) from their original guidelines for weight gain during pregnancy [40]. The importance of having a controlled weight gain during pregnancy has gained increased significance particularly in the current context of obesity epidemic, mainly because it is recognized that the prevalence of overweight and obesity has increased among women in reproductive age, as has overall BMI and GWG of pregnant women, since the publication of the original guidelines from the IOM in 1990 [59], as acknowledge in their latest review [40], leading to increased

Table 4.1 Recommendation for total and rate of weight gain during pregnancy of singleton fetuses, according to initial BMI [Adapted from the Institute of Medicine [40]]

Pre-pregnancy BMI	Total GWG	GWG in the first trimester	Average rate of GWG in the second and third trimesters	Range rate of GWG in the second and third trimesters
Underweight (BMI < 18.5 kg/m^2)	12.5–28.0 kg	0.5–2.0 kg	0.51 kg/week	0.44–0.58 kg/week
Normal weight (BMI = [18.5; 24.9] kg/m^2)	11.5–16.0 kg	0.5–2.0 kg	0.42 kg/week	0.35–0.50 kg/week
Overweight (BMI = [25.0; 29.9] kg/m^2)	7.0–11.5 kg	0.5–2.0 kg	0.28 kg/week	0.23–0.33 kg/week
Obese (BMI ≥ 30.0 kg/m^2)	5.0–9.0 kg	0.5–2.0 kg	0.22 kg/week	0.17–0.27 kg/week

BMI body mass index, *GWG* gestational weight gain

risk of adverse pregnancy-related outcomes. It is also recognized that healthy gestational weight gain recommendations for different classes of obesity are lacking [41].

Accordingly, guidelines for GWG were published (Table 4.1) presenting recommended GWG ranges and rate, fitted to mother's initial (pre-pregnant) BMI [40]. Two aspects immediately stand out from IOM guidelines: mothers' pre-pregnancy BMI is inversely related to recommended GWG, meaning that women with lower pre-pregnancy BMI may gain more weight during pregnancy than women with higher BMIs and be within GWG guidelines for healthy pregnancies and outcomes; recommended GWG rate tends to be rather slow in the first trimester and increases in a nearly linear fashion throughout the second and third trimesters.

Research has shown pre-pregnancy BMI to be inversely associated with GWG, meaning that women with higher pre-pregnancy BMI tend to experience lower GWG [60, 61]. However, conflicting results have been found as well, showing higher GWG (consistently above IOM guidelines) in women with higher pre-pregnancy BMI, as compared to medium or low pre-pregnancy BMI women [62]. Taken together, this highlights the importance of an individualized approach and follow-up of pregnancy, regardless of pre-pregnancy BMI, to keep GWG within a healthy range.

It is important to acknowledge that these guidelines apply only to singleton pregnancies and specific guidelines should be used for women with a multiple pregnancy. Furthermore, alternative guidelines for whole GWG at pregnancy term have been suggested for pregnant women of twins (Table 4.2) but, in this case, healthy recommendations for underweight women, as assessed by pre-pregnant BMI, are not yet known and, therefore, have not been disclosed [40]. These guidelines reflect the GWG observed between the 25th and 75th percentiles of mothers of twins with ≥2.5 kg at term (37–42 weeks of gestation). This means that these guidelines are based on Gaussian normality rather than sound risk-related assessment and healthy outcomes. Furthermore, it has been recognized that the study of overall GWG in multiple pregnancies has been considerably neglected [63].

Table 4.2 Recommendation for total and rate of weight gain during pregnancy of twins, according to initial BMI [Adapted from the Institute of Medicine [40]]

Pre-pregnancy BMI	Total GWG
Underweight (BMI < 18.5 kg/m^2)	12.5–28.0 kg
Normal weight (BMI = [18.5; 24.9] kg/m^2)	17.0–25.0 kg
Overweight (BMI = [25.0; 29.9] kg/m^2)	14.0–23.0 kg
Obese (BMI ≥ 30.0 kg/m^2)	11.0–19.0 kg

BMI body mass index, *GWG* gestational weight gain

According to IOM guidelines, women who fall outside the recommended GWG experience higher risk of maternal and offspring adverse outcomes [40]. Excessive GWG has been shown to be associated with increased risk of undesired outcomes, including gestational diabetes and resulting fetal macrosomia [64], preterm delivery [65, 66], complications during labor, post-partum weight and BF retention and subsequent maternal obesity [62], and increased risk of unsuccessful breastfeeding [25, 40]. High GWG also seems to increase the risk of obesity in offspring during childhood, but high pre-pregnancy BMI has a stronger influence [52]. Insulin resistance tends to be higher in pregnant women due to changes in pregnancy-related hormones [67]. This seems to result from a normal adaptation caused by the increase of production of placenta growth hormones that have an insulin resistance effect on the mother [68], possibly to ensure that glucose is available for the fetus and is not all accounted for by the mother. The association of GWG with hypertensive pregnancy disorders is not consistent and contradictory results have been published [40]; however, it has recently been shown that GWG in the first two trimesters was independently associated with the development of hypertensive pregnancy disorders [69]. Nevertheless, pre-pregnancy BMI seems to be the strongest correlate with such disorders [69].

It has recently been reported that pregnant women with normal pre-pregnancy BMI who fall outside the GWG Institute of Medicine guidelines (either gaining too much or too little weight) do not present a higher risk of infant mortality in the first year of life as compared to the ones whose GWG fall within guidelines [70]. It is admitted that higher attention has been given to excess GWG; however, low GWG has been shown to be associated with preterm delivery [65]. To this concern, despite the increasing concordant results in diverse populations of pregnant women [66], conflicting results exist, particularly in under and normal weight pregnant women [71].

As mentioned before, IOM's guidelines recommend less GWG in the first trimester and near linearly increases throughout the second and third trimesters [40]. However, not all women follow such a standard pattern within each trimester's recommended GWG and/or GWG rate boundaries and may diverge along part or all of the pregnancy course [72]. Regardless of the total amount of GWG or the GWG rate per specific trimester, less but pertinent attention was given to the pattern of GWG [72]. Because, as elegantly explained by Widen and colleagues [72], two pregnant women can exhibit the exact same amount of total GWG but one may have had a low GWG in early pregnancy and then have a steep increase in GWG later in pregnancy, while others may have had a steady GWG, within IOM's guidelines, throughout the course of pregnancy. Apparently, women who show medium to high rate of GWG in the second trimester and high rate of GWG in the third trimester have associated higher gains in BF, estimated to be within 3–5 kg [72]. Regarding the offspring outcomes, women who showed high GWG in the second trimester tend to have bigger newborns at birth, approximately 1 cm more in length and 350 g in weight [72].

The health risks associated with obesity or overweight or even with GWG, including its amount, rate, or pattern, are often attributed to excess or increasing BF in these women. The study of body composition and the composition of GWG is not well explored in pregnancy [72] mostly because assessment is challenging [11], as will be discussed ahead in the present chapter. The next subsection of this chapter will focus on existing literature regarding the variation and correlates of different body components during pregnancy. Furthermore, the study of the composition of GWG is not well explored in pregnancy and warrants further research [72].

4.3.3 Pregnancy and Body Components

As widely mentioned, GWG is expected and important for healthy pregnancies and healthy pregnancy outcomes for the mother and newborn throughout the lifespan. However, GWG does not occur proportionally in all body components. It has been shown that, on average, FFM tends to increase more than BF through the course of pregnancy (58% vs. 42%, respectively), but FFM weight gain is also more reversible than BF after delivery [62]. Increases in total body water (TBW) and FFM, but not BF, were shown to be highly correlated with the birth weight of offspring [62, 73]. This can be a contributing factor for explaining offspring different birth weights and sizes from mothers with the same pre-pregnancy BMI and/or GWG, but maybe different pregnancy-related body composition changes. The increase in TBW, protein, and FM seem to be linearly correlated with GWG but different patterns can be observed [62]. However, not all body components show an increase during pregnancy. Bone mineral content (BMC) decreases during pregnancy, resulting in lower values post-partum as compared to pre-pregnancy [62]. This seems more evident in lower as compared to higher pre-pregnancy BMI mothers [62]. One could think that pregnant women could recover from this reduction in BMC after delivering, but results show the opposite, BMC tends to continue decreasing after delivery at least up to the 27 weeks postpartum [62]. Furthermore, BMC losses during 9 months of lactation may be fourfold higher than the losses observed during pregnancy [74]. This has been recognized as a significant risk for osteoporosis and morbidity [75]. Regardless of this significant reduction in BMC, it has been shown to be mostly a transient condition and women frequently recover to their initial BMC [76]. Ultimately, these results call for the particular attention given to the pregnancy follow-up, particularly in low BMI women. Women should be advised about the suitable amounts of calcium intake to support the mother and the developing fetus, and also about the proper osteoblastotrophic amount and type of physical exercise [76, 77]. The kinetics of BMC during pregnancy is not available as it is usually assessed by Dual-energy X-ray Absorptiometry (DXA) which use is prevented in pregnant women due to the risk of hazardous exposure to radiation; therefore, it is only used pre-pregnancy and postpartum [62].

As mentioned earlier, GWG tends to be higher in women with lower pre-pregnancy BMI [60, 61]. However, it was shown that higher or excessive GWG is primarily attributable to excessive BF increases and not to FFM changes [62, 78]. This was found more pronounced in women with higher pre-pregnancy BMI, as compared with women with lower pre-pregnancy BMI, but gestational FFM gain showed no differences between different levels of pre-pregnancy BMI [62, 78]. This underlines the importance of close monitoring and follow-up of mothers, particularly those with higher pre-pregnancy BMI, regarding BF. An individualized approach may be key to help mothers keep GWG within healthy range throughout the course of pregnancy. This is particularly important as it was also observed that higher weight and BF retention after delivery was observed in mothers who presented higher GWG and BF increases during pregnancy [62, 79]; FFM and TBW gains during pregnancy were not correlated with weight and BF retention after delivery [60, 62, 80]; Pre-pregnancy BMI was not a determinant of weight and BF retention after delivery [62, 79]; and women who gained weight above IMO guidelines retained more weight and more BF after delivery [62]. This underlines the important public health message of adhering to IOM guidelines, including the beginning of pregnancy at a healthy weight and keeping GWG within the recommended range.

The pathophysiological pathway that links BF and related morbidities is still not completely disclosed. Nevertheless, it seems rather consistent that the altered metabolism associated with excessive BF, rather than body weight alone, plays a key role in obesity [56, 81–84]. The scientific evidence on the association of maternal body composition with different health outcomes during and after pregnancy is fairly less abundant than that relating pre-pregnancy BMI or GWG with the same outcomes [25]. During the course of pregnancy, mostly in late pregnancy, it is commonly observed an increase in insulin resistance, which is a normal physiological adaptation to pregnancy [85] mostly induced by placental hormones [68] apparently to limit maternal glucose uptake allowing adequate nutrient supply to the growing fetus [86]. The increase in adipocyte fat content results in increased size and number of adipocytes [87], leading to adipocyte functional changes that results in deregulated secretion of pro-inflammatory cytokines (adipokines). This adipocyte deregulation may contribute to increase inflammation and further increase insulin resistance (IR) [88, 89], possibly leading to gestational diabetes mellitus (GDM) [67] and other cardiometabolic risk factors and hazardous outcomes [90, 91]. The abnormal adipokine expression associated with increased overall adiposity or BF [27, 57] is also associated with increased risk of adverse maternal hypertensive disorders, including eclampsia and pre-eclampsia [92–97]. Visceral adipose tissue, but not subcutaneous adipose tissue, seems to be an important predictor of hyperemesis gravidarum, which is known to be a condition characterized by severe nausea, vomiting, weight loss, and possibly dehydration [46]. Taken together, this highlights the importance of carefully monitor and manage overall body composition, particularly BF, throughout the course of pregnancy to help diagnose and avoid preventable hazardous risks and enhance pregnancy outcomes.

As noticed BF is not the only body component related with hazardous pregnancy courses and outcomes. Low plasma volume, which can be a consequence of low TBW, may undermine cardiac output, and together this can lead to reduced uterine blood flow and fetal growth restriction [98]. On the other hand, high TBW has been found to be associated with hypertensive pregnancy disorders, including eclampsia and preeclampsia, which may also lead to hazardous outcomes [99]. These findings together underline the importance of keeping TBW within a healthy range throughout the course of pregnancy [31]. The next section focuses on the assessment of body composition during pregnancy.

4.4 Body Composition Assessment in Pregnancy

The assessment of body composition in pregnant women has always been a challenge [11, 32]. This can be attributed to three main reasons [25]: (1) the assumptions and standard references used for non-pregnant often prove to be invalid in pregnant women; (2) available methods for use in pregnancy cannot distinguish mother from fetus body composition; and (3) not all body composition assessment methods/instruments are considered safe to be used in pregnancy.

During pregnancy, women show a differentiated growth of several body regions and components resulting in gestational weight gain. One of such body components showing an important and steeper growth during pregnancy is total body water (TBW) [62]. It was shown that FFM increment by the term of pregnancy was about 57% of total pregnancy weight gain for mothers with low or high pre-pregnancy BMI and 67% for mothers with normal BMI [62]. Increments in TBW represented 85% of total pregnancy FFM gain for mothers with low or normal pre-pregnancy BMI and 83% for mothers with high pre-pregnancy BMI. In non-pregnant women, TBW is assumed to represent 73.2% of FFM. However, during pregnancy, TBW increases to a higher proportion of FFM instead of the assumed 73.2% [33]. Bone mineral content tends to decrease during pregnancy [62], which together with the increase in TBW leads to a drop in body density. These changes observed in body composition during pregnancy prevent the use of general assumptions during pregnancy. Strategies to overcome such limitations in pregnancy body composition assessment will be discussed ahead.

Another basic limitation in body composition assessment is the difficulty to distinguish between the mother's body composition and gestational weight gain and that of the fetus, as well as the placenta and amniotic fluid [11, 25]. This makes it particularly challenging to assess the mother's weight, body composition, and relative changes, independently. Therefore, most assessment methods usually assume

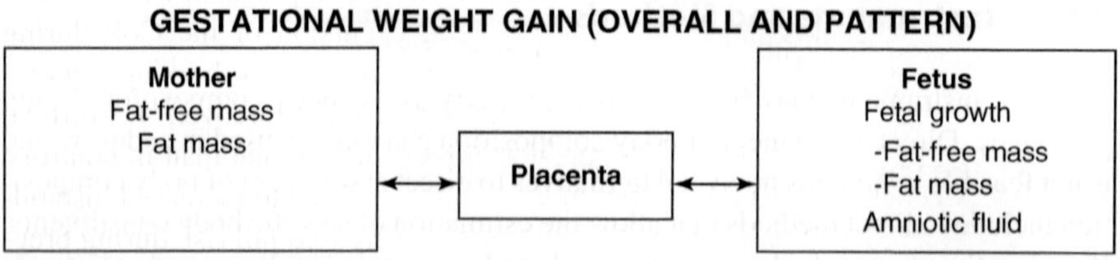

Fig. 4.3 Schematic summary of the components of gestational weight gain. (Adapted from the Institute of Medicine [40])

and assess pregnant women as a whole not distinguishing either the fetus or the placenta mass from that of the mother (Fig. 4.3).

Current methods may help to estimate some components of GWG; particularly up-to-date techniques to estimate fetal mass and body composition based on ultrasound or MRI-based techniques may play an important role to overcome this challenge [34, 100]. However, no significant validation studies have been put out in this field, and the sophistication of such methods, requiring highly specialized professionals and expensive equipment, also limits its broader use [25]. The composition of human placenta has been assessed and it is known to include on average 87% of water, nearly 11% of protein, and less than 1% of fat [101, 102]. Placentas' composition is substantially different from that of non-pregnant whole-body composition, which underlines the first mentioned limitation regarding profound body composition changes during pregnancy and unusable non-pregnant assumptions during this period. Furthermore, placenta molecular composition and mass are hardly assessed during human pregnancy in vivo; it is commonly assessed only at the time of delivery [101, 102]. Current and promising methods will be discussed ahead.

The third reason for body composition assessment to be a challenge during pregnancy lies in the fact that pregnancy is a unique phase of a woman's and new-being's life, characterized by a massive and fast cell replication which needs to occur without adverse interferences such as hazardous radiation or others, associated with any assessment-related procedures, that may expose either the fetus or the mother to any avoidable risk [11, 25]. These include mostly imaging methods such as Dual-energy X-ray Absorptiometry (DXA) or Computed Tomography (CT) scans [8, 25, 42, 103]. Accordingly, the tools for body composition assessment in pregnancy are limited when compared to what is available and used for the assessment of non-pregnant persons. Considering these challenges and limitations, this section will focus on feasible techniques and methods for the assessment of body composition during pregnancy, particularly on those that are easy and practical for use in clinical practice. A description and brief review regarding each body composition marker will be presented. This subsection is therefore divided into two parts: the first part regards the well-established laboratory methods and the second part regards selected body composition clinical markers such as weight, BMI, body circumferences, and skinfolds.

4.4.1 Instruments and Methods

Different instruments may be required to properly assess body composition during pregnancy. Direct assessment of body composition can only be used in cadavers and is not feasible in humans in vivo. Alternatives to direct assessment of body composition include indirect methods that allow the estimation of specific body constituents. Based on the previously detailed five-level model presented by Wang and colleagues [9], body composition is assessed in compartment models. The sum of all compartments, in each level, represents the whole-body mass of a person. For each body composition compartment, specific instruments and methods apply. However, it is important to understand that not all instruments and methods are usable during pregnancy mainly for safety reasons but sometimes also for precision reasons. In this section, we will discuss the different body composition assessment models and methods and which methods are appropriate to be used during pregnancy in each model.

4.4.1.1 Laboratory Body Composition Assessment

The five-level model is a cornerstone in the assessment of body composition and is used as a reference [9, 10] including in pregnancy [8, 11]. Accordingly, the body is divided into several components or compartments [9]. Most often multi-compartment body composition models analyze body composition at the molecular level, dividing the body into BF, TBW, protein, and minerals. This constitutes the common gold standard four-compartment (4-C) model (e.g., BF + TBW + total body protein + minerals) [10]. However, other compartmentalizations can be used under the molecular model: the three-compartment model which usually considerers both protein and minerals together in a component that may be called "dry lean mass" (BF + TBW + dry lean mass); and the most widely used two-compartment model (BF + FFM) which is the most often assessed overall [10] but, due to several assumptions implied, proves invalid when using standard conversion factors in pregnancy [25]. The three and four-compartment models would be better options in terms of precision but are far more difficult and expensive to use and are impractical in clinical settings [8, 25]. These latest multi-compartment models need to be assessed with a combination of laboratory methods [10].

Four-Compartment Model

As mentioned earlier, the four-compartment (4-C) model divides the body into four components: BF, TBW, mineral, and protein. The 4-C model is considered to be the reference approach to be used in the validation of other body composition assessment techniques [10]. For the assessment of body components in a 4-C model, it is mandatory to assess at least three components, and the fourth component can be calculated by exclusion, because the sum of all components is equal to whole-body mass [8]. In a 4-C model, each body component needs to be assessed using robust laboratory methods [10].

The reference method for the assessment of TBW uses the dilution principle with stable radiolabeled tracers, or isotopes, such as deuterium dilution [8, 11, 25]. This method needs the collection of a physiologic baseline sample of body fluid, usually urine or saliva. A fixed amount labeled water (e.g., 100 mg/kg of body weight) is then administered. Spot urine samples are then collected. Two methods have been reported for use in the estimation of TBW based on labeled water: the plateau method, which involves the collection of second body fluid sample after a predetermined period (e.g., 4 h) to ensure equilibrium [25, 104]; and the back-extrapolation method involves several collections of body fluid samples during up to 14 days [25, 33, 62]. Collected samples are analyzed using gas-isotope ratio mass spectrometry [8, 105].

By using a reference method for the assessment of TBW, it is possible to have a considerable amount of confidence that the pregnancy-associated variation in TBW is being controlled and will not introduce significant amounts of error in body composition estimations. However, the assessment of TBW using stable radiolabeled tracers requires highly specialized technicians and expensive laboratory equipment which undermines its feasibility, particularly in clinical settings. Furthermore, pregnant women may not be willing to ingest stable radiolabeled isotopes, which limits the use of this method [25].

Alternative TBW assessment methods have been used during pregnancy, comprising bioelectrical impedance analysis [31, 99, 106] or spectroscopy [107]. However, despite the fact that reference values obtained during pregnancy have been published [31], to our knowledge, validation studies for these techniques against a reference method in pregnant women are lacking [25].

The assessment of body protein in pregnant women is carried out by calculating cell mass from measurements of total body potassium (TBK) [8]. Gamma radiation spontaneously arises from potassium and this may be assessed using a whole-body counter [108, 109]. The assessment of gamma radiation allows the quantification of body potassium and calculations can be done thereafter [8, 110]. Potassium studies do not require administration of exogenous isotopes and do not involve any exposure to exogenous radiation [8, 11] and are therefore considered to be safe and have been used during pregnancy [111]. Whole-body counting requires specific equipment, which is not common and hard to access, and specialized technicians are needed preventing routine usage of this method.

The assessment of body mineral is done using Dual-energy X-ray Absorptiometry (DXA). Because DXA involves exposure to minimal but potentially hazardous radiation, its use is prevented during pregnancy [8, 25, 42, 103]. Therefore, in order to assess the mineral component of the 4-C model, DXA assessments are made before pregnancy or after delivery, in the assumption that it does not change throughout pregnancy [8, 11, 25, 33]. This assumption however excludes fetal and placenta BMC accretion and does not account for the mothers BMC reduction throughout pregnancy [25, 62]. For this reason, the need for further research regarding BMC assessment in pregnancy has been highlighted and, in the event that significant BMC variation throughout pregnancy is acknowledged, correction factors would need to be developed [25].

Body fat mass may be assessed by exclusion of all other three components from whole-body weight [BF = Body weight – (TBW + Protein + mineral)].

Different approaches to the 4-C model have been used in pregnancy [112]. This includes the use of stable isotopes to assess TBW; pre or post pregnancy DXA for mineral and the assessment of body volume to assess body density and BF [113]. Body volume may be assessed using one of two methods: underwater weighing, also known as hidrodensitometry, and air displacement plethysmography (ADP) [25]. Both techniques are well accepted and have been used in pregnancy; however, underwater weighing requires more collaboration from the subject and ADP has been suggested to be preferable for the assessment of body composition during pregnancy [25, 114]. By using this approach, protein can then be calculated by exclusion [Protein = Body weight − (TBW + Mineral + BF)]. This approach avoids the need of a scintillator for whole-body potassium counting, which may not be available in many labs.

Three-Compartment Model

The three-compartment (3-C) model divides the body into three components, usually: BF, TBW, and dry FFM (comprising mineral and protein together) [115]. This model despite being potentially less accurate than the 4-C because it does not account for the ratio between mineral and protein, has the virtue of accounting for variations in TBW which can be the most variable body component during pregnancy [8, 115]. This approach also avoids the need of a scintillator for whole-body potassium counting, which may not be easy to find and use. In this model, TBW is assessed as in the 4-C model [8, 11, 25, 60, 115]. The estimation of BF can be done using body density corrected for TBW (Table 4.3) [116]. Dry FFM is calculated by exclusion of the former two components (TBW and BF) from whole-body mass (Dry FFM = body mass − [TBX + BF]) [11, 25, 115].

Table 4.3 Equations for estimation and monitoring of BF, developed and validated for use in pregnancy [116]

Population	Gestational age	Equations
Pregnant women without edema or with leg edema only	10 weeks	BF [kg] = (Weight [kg]/100) × ((496.4/Db [×10^3 kg/m^3]) − 451.6)
	20 weeks	BF [kg] = (Weight [kg]/100) × ((502.2/Db [×10^3 kg/m^3]) − 458.0)
	30 weeks	BF [kg] = (Weight [kg]/100) × ((510.8/Db [×10^3 kg/m^3]) − 467.5)
	40 weeks	BF [kg] = (Weight [kg]/100) × ((522.5/Db [×10^3 kg/m^3]) − 480.5)
Pregnant women with generalized edema	10 weeks	BF [kg] = (Weight [kg]/100) × ((496.4/Db [×10^3 kg/m^3]) − 451.6)
	20 weeks	BF [kg] = (Weight [kg]/100) × ((504.7/Db [×10^3 kg/m^3]) − 460.8)
	30 weeks	BF [kg] = (Weight [kg]/100) × ((518.1/Db [×10^3 kg/m^3]) − 475.7)
	40 weeks	BF [kg] = (Weight [kg]/100) × ((537.3/Db [×10^3 kg/m^3]) − 497.0)

BF body fat, in kilograms, *Db* body density, in ×10^3 kg/m^3

Other divisions of body components have been used in the 3-C, but usually not in pregnancy, such as that assessed by DXA, which divides the body into the following: BF, mineral and lean soft tissue (comprising TBW and protein, together).

Two-Compartment Model

The two-compartment model divides the body into BF and FFM [10]. Many approaches for the assessment of body composition in a 2-C model use only one instrument to estimate BF and FFM, usually based on the assessment of either: body volume [e.g., assessed by hydrodensitometry or ADP [25]] to calculate body density (Body density = Body weight/body volume) and, from there, estimate BF and FFM based on the assumptions of a fixed density of BF (0.9 g/cm^3) and FFM (1.1 g/cm^3); or TBW estimates [e.g., assessed by stable isotopes dilution [111] or by bioelectric impedance [107]] that will allow to estimate FFM and, by exclusion, BF based on the assumption of a stable hydration of FFM (TBW = 0.73 × FFM) [10]. As mentioned in the previous subsections, several assumptions regarding the relative constancy of FFM composition, used in non-pregnant persons for body composition assessment on a 2-C model, are not valid during pregnancy [115]. The increase in TBW, which is the FFM component with the lowest density (1 g/cm^3), lowers the average overall FFM density. In addition, the decrease in body mineral observed during pregnancy, which is the FFM component with the highest density (about 3.06 g/cm^3), also contributes to a lower average overall FFM density [33, 62]. Taken together, these body composition adaptations to pregnancy limit the use of body density-based methods in a 2-C model. Furthermore, the changes in the proportion of TBW to FFM, which is assumed to be 73% in non-pregnant persons, also make this assumption invalid and therefore not usable during pregnancy, also compromising the use of TBW-based techniques for the assessment of body composition in a 2-C model during pregnancy. Regardless of all the limitations of the 2-C model, it has been reported that, when the estimates of BF are calculated using corrected or gestational age-specific methods, it can produce reliable mean fat estimates for the assessment of larger samples [114, 115]. To account for TBW variation throughout the course of pregnancy, Van Raaij et al. [116] developed a set of gestational age-specific equations to assess FM from assessed body density (Table 4.3). It has recently been recognized that the assessment of BF on a 2-C model using ADP can be reliable in routine assessments also at the individual level [114]. Variations in FFM density have been found to be higher at mid-pregnancy (Week 14) as compared with late pregnancy (Week 32) making 2-C model-based assessments more accurate at later stages [42].

Non-molecular Model Body Composition Assessment

Different approaches may be used in the assessment of body composition during pregnancy that fall outside the molecular model. Assessments at the cellular level using TBW and TBK or bioelectric impedance, either multi-frequency analysis or spectroscopy [107], to assess intra- and extra-cellular water may give estimates of body cell mass [117]. However, to our knowledge, validation studies for the estimation of body cell mass using these techniques during pregnancy are lacking.

Assessments at the tissue-organ level using imaging methods such as magnetic resonance imaging, or spectroscopy, or even computed tomography may give estimates of local adipose tissue, muscle, and bone area [12]. However, it is important to acknowledge that some image methods involve radiation emissions considered to be potentially hazardous during pregnancy (e.g., computed tomography) and therefore cannot be used to assess pregnant women [8, 25, 42, 103]. The use of ultrasound is widespread during pregnancy to assess mainly fetal development [34, 100], yet it has also been used to assess the mother's body composition, including bone mineral density [118], subcutaneous adipose thickness [119], and visceral fat thickness [120], with promising results. MRI is a reference method to assess different depots of visceral adipose tissue [12], yet has been used in pregnancy mainly to assess malformations or other pregnancy-related problems when other assessments raise suspicion and/or are not conclusive [121]. The advantages of using MRI rely mainly on its confirmed excellent tissue contrast. Although there is no evidence that MRI is harmful during pregnancy, to either the mother or fetus, there still seems to be a lack of consensus as to whether any true risk exists [121]. Recommendations have recognized the acceptance and usefulness of MRI during pregnancy when alternative non-ionizing imaging methods are suboptimal, or if the information to be obtained by MRI would require more invasive procedures (e.g., biopsy or amniocentesis) [121]. In accordance, to our knowledge, MRI has not been used as a body composition assessment tool in pregnant women, as non-ionizing alternatives are available. Furthermore, no significant validation studies have been put out in this field and the sophistication of such methods, requiring highly specialized professionals and expensive equipment, also limits its broader use [25, 106] making this approach less feasible and desirable [122].

4.4.1.2 Clinical Markers of Body Composition/Obesity in Pregnancy

This subsection focusses on established and promising clinical markers of body composition including bioelectric impedance, skinfolds thickness, body circumferences, as well as body indexes. A description and review regarding each clinical marker will be presented in the following subsections. To better organize the information, this subsection is divided into four parts: the first part regards the well-established BMI; the second part regards the use of bioelectric impedance in clinical settings; third part focuses on the use of skinfold thickness; and the fourth part reviews selected body circumferences.

Body Mass Index

The body mass index (BMI), calculated as weight, in kg, divided by squared height, in meters (BMI = weight [kg]/height $[m]^2$), is a simple marker of excess body weight, easy to measure, highly precise, and strongly associated with overall fat in non-pregnant people [123]. Accordingly, BMI has been shown to explain 74% and 55% of the variation of whole absolute and relative BF (as assessed by DXA), respectively [124]. Similar results showing a significant relationship between BMI and BF were also found in pregnancy, both in obese [125] and non-obese [126]. The assessment of BMI in pregnancy has, however, been used mostly to assess hazards in pregnancy, related to pre-pregnancy obesity [40]. For this reason, the recommendations for the assessment and classification of BMI in non-pregnant people should be used for the assessment and classification of pre-pregnancy BMI [40]. Gestational follow-up and health care usually only begin after the first weeks of pregnancy, and it is sometimes hard to assess pre-pregnancy BMI. During the course of pregnancy, the progression of body weight, the so-called gestational weight gain has been preferred for follow-up [40] and weight has even been long considered the most feasible and desired measure to use for the monitoring of body composition progression during pregnancy [122].

The endorsement of the use of BMI as a marker for obesity has relied recurrently on same arguments, including: BMI measurement is simple, non-invasive, reliable, and inexpensive [127]; BMI is associated with body composition, particularly to fat [128], and is also related with hazardous health outcomes during and after pregnancy for both the mother and the offspring, as reviewed earlier in the present chapter. It is important to acknowledge that BMI assesses body composition at a whole-body level, considering Wang's five-level model [9], and does not assess any specific body composition component, though having, as mentioned, a significant association not only with generalized fatness [121] but also with different components of lean tissue, such as muscle or bone [21]. Therefore, when assessing obesity, BMI may be deceptive [17]. Even though the usefulness of BMI may be accepted in the assessment of secular trends of the prevalence of obesity at the population level, BMI has been suggested to only provide a crude measurement of total adiposity and does not accurately diagnose obesity, at least at the individual level [125, 129]. The limitations of BMI have been reported extensively [21, 100, 125], and several other markers have been advocated [23, 126, 130], as further detailed.

Bioelectric Impedance

Bioelectric impedance has been used during pregnancy and its usefulness has proven to be encouraging for the assessment of TBW and related impairments [31, 99, 107, 130, 131]. It is important to distinguish between different types of bioelectric impedance devices, despite the fact that all have been used during pregnancy with acceptable results, including single-frequency bioelectric impedance analysis (BIA), which includes the emission of and electric current at a single frequency of 50 kHz [31, 99, 130, 131]; multi-frequency BIA, which includes the emission a several electric currents at different fixed frequencies, usually 5, 50, 100, and 200 kHz [127–129]; and bioelectrical impedance spectroscopy, which uses a spectrum of frequencies usually ranging from 5 kHz to 1 MHz [107]. Bioelectric impedance relies on assumptions and relationships regarding electrical properties of biological tissues and components [25]. It uses a very low amperage electric current that uses the water content of the body as a conductor, to estimate TBW [25]. The bioelectric impedance, or resistance offered to the passage the electrical current through the body tissues allows for estimation of TBW from which estimates of BF and FFM may be derived [25, 116].

Bioelectric impedance has proven to be an inexpensive, simple, non-invasive, reliable, and fast clinical approach method to assess hydration status, which is well tolerated by patients during pregnancy [1–5] and a prediction model specifically developed to be used during pregnancy for the estimation of TWB, using bioelectrical impedance data together with other TBW predictors, was developed based on isotope dilution

$$TBW = 0.7\,A + 0.051\,B - 0.069\,C - 0.029\,D + 0.043\,E + 2.833$$

A = Height2 / Impedance
B = Abdominal circumference
C = Weight
D = Reactance
E = Hematocrit

Fig. 4.4 Multiple-regression equation to predict total body water (TBW) by using bioelectrical impedance, anthropometric, and biochemical measures specifically in pregnant women. (Adapted from Lukaski et al. [131])

technique (Fig. 4.4) [131]. Reference values for bioelectric impedance assessments and resulting indexes have also been published for pregnancy [31]. The assessment of TBW, using BIA may even help to identify, in early gestation, mothers at risk of developing different clinical phenotypes of hypertensive disorders of pregnancy and fetal growth restriction [99, 127]. Estimation of TBW can then be used to assess pregnancy risks (e.g., gestational hypertensive disorders [99] or fetal growth restriction [98]). The use of BIA to directly estimate BF during pregnancy has proven less reliable [114]. In order to assure accurate results and better quality assessments, sound guidelines should be followed for the use of bioelectric impedance [132].

Furthermore, BIA has also shown good accuracy and high predictive capacity for the risk of developing preeclampsia, when done at 17–20 weeks of gestation on women who never gave birth (nulliparous women) [1]. Namely, extracellular water/intracellular water ≤ 0.618, skeletal muscle mass ≥ 25 kg, and body fat percentage $\geq 44\%$, were very strong predictors of preeclampsia, particularly when combined [1]. BIA-derived markers such as body fat percentage and fat mass index (kg/m^2) have also been found to be associated with the incidence of GDM, and the later was suggested to be used as a GDM predictor [1]. Skeletal muscle mass percentage, also assessed using BIA, was found inversely associated with the risk of GDM [1]. Additional markers assessed using BIA, particularly the phase angle, have been used and reported during pregnancy and proven innovative and promising for risk assessment, still, further research in the pregnant/postpartum population was recommended to elucidate any links with perinatal or future health outcomes [1] and, accordingly, underscore its usefulness in this population.

Skinfold Thickness

Skinfold thickness (SFT) has been considered a useful clinical tool for the assessment of body composition during pregnancy, particularly in larger samples or in low resources settings [114]. The use of overall anthropometric methods, including SFT, is considered to be absolutely free from health hazards to the mother and fetus, which is one priority concern, and therefore has been considered to be well accepted by pregnant women [8]. The advantages of SFT have been stated and include being low cost, highly portable, simple to use and teach [8] and has shown to be considerably accurate as a surrogate of BF during pregnancy [114]. Additionally, this technique has the advantage of allowing the monitoring follow-up of local accumulation and distribution of adipose tissue [133]. In spite of all the advantages, the measurement of SFT also has some limitations including the risk of intra- and inter-observer errors, which can occur if extensive measurement training and skill are not assured [25]. Nevertheless, it has been reported that, when proper training was present, the measurement of biceps, triceps, and subscapular skinfolds can be reliably obtained, even in overweight and obese pregnant women, by multiple observers, and is suitable for research settings [134]. Another important drawback of SFT in pregnancy is the kinetics of subcutaneous tissue compressibility throughout the course of pregnancy, which is believed to be modified by changed hydration of adipose tissue [8, 25]. Decreased compressibility of SFT in adolescent pregnancy has been reported, resulting in increases in SFT, in spite of no increase in adipose tissue fat content, causing potential BF overestimation [135]. As pregnancy is associated with increasing TBW [62], these decreases in SFT compressibility may be expected to be observed in pregnant women of different ages, however, to our knowledge, this is not yet confirmed.

Despite all limitations of SFT in pregnancy, several SFT sites have been reported to be used during pregnancy, the most established being that of the triceps; biceps; subscapular; suprailiac [103, 111, 114, 126, 133, 136–145]. In spite of less common SFT sites used in pregnancy, the mid-thigh is also frequently used [103, 140–143, 146]. Several equations, developed in non-pregnant women, for estimation of BF using SFT have been used in pregnancy [136–139], yet equations specifically developed and validated to be used in pregnancy are now available (Table 4.4). Still, available equations are for specific gestational ages and no equations exist to be used throughout all pregnancy

Table 4.4 Equations for estimation and monitoring of BF, developed and validated for use in pregnancy

References	Population	Gestational age	Equations
Paxton et al. [103]	White, black and Hispanic women in New York City, NY, USA	37 weeks	BF [kg] = 0.40 (weight at Week 37 [kg]) + 0.16 (Biceps SFT at Week 37 [mm]) – 0.15 (thigh SFT at Week 37 [mm]) – 0.09 (wrist circumference at Week 39) + 0.10 (pre-pregnancy weight [kg]) – 6.56
		14–37 weeks	BF change [kg] = 0.77 (weight change [kg]) + 0.07 (change in thigh SFT [mm]) – 6.13
		14–37 weeks	BF change [kg] = 0.84 (weight change [kg]) – 6.49
Presley et al. [140]	Predominantly white women in Cleveland, OH, USA	30 weeks	BF (kg) = (weight [kg] × 0.33529) + (triceps SFT [mm] × 0.65664) – (subscapular SFT [mm] × 0.4373) + (suprailiac SFT [mm] × 0.43461) – 13.0538
Kannieappan et al. [134]	Overweight and obese women	Between 10th and 20th week	BF (%) = 12.7 + 0.457 × triceps SFT [mm] + 0.352 × subscapular SFT [mm] + 0.103 × biceps SFT [mm] – 0.057 × height + 0.265 × arm circumference [cm]

BF body fat, *SFT* skinfold thickness

regardless of gestation time. Future studies should focus on establishing sound anthropometric approaches for the estimation of body composition continuously throughout pregnancy and also for the estimation of body composition-related hazards for the mother and the fetus during pregnancy.

Skinfolds tend to increase throughout the course of pregnancy (see Table 4.5). Apparently it is possible to observe increases as soon as early pregnancy, and also from this to late pregnancy [146]. This trend has repeatedly been observed but not consistently, as concurring results have also been observed particularly in the upper limbs [103, 148]. Interestingly, women with abnormal glucose tolerance tend to present consistently higher skinfolds in pre and early pregnancy [146]. The steeper increase in skinfolds' size observed in late-pregnancy, in women who without abnormal glucose tolerance, faded these differences between these two groups [146].

One highly constant of SFT assessment in pregnancy is the high individual variability that can be observed in the literature (see Table 4.5). It should also be acknowledged the terminological/methodological diversity found in the literature. For instance, we have found different names for the same SFT site [e.g., lower-thigh SFT [146] has also been called knee SFT [142] or supra-patellar SFT [140], despite using the same measurement protocol] and also different measurement protocols have been proposed for the same SFT (e.g., supra-iliac crest have been measured using varying anatomical landmarks, including; (1) at the midpoint between the anterior superior iliac spine and the lowest rib [140–142] and (2) just above the iliac crest in the mid-axillary line [111, 114, 148]). This arbitrariness prohibits generalization of skinfold measurement for monitoring pregnancy in clinical settings, and also prevents the determination of skinfold measurement reference cutoffs for the identification of abnormal body composition gestation-related changes and the prediction of hazardous health outcomes for both the mother and the fetus. Research and practice should follow standardized guidelines for anthropometric assessment, also in pregnancy.

Bottom line, SFT seems highly valuable for use in clinical practice and may be used to assess body composition of pregnant women in a 2-C model. The high individual variability of SFT throughout the course of pregnancy advises individualization in the follow-up of whole and depot-specific BF during pregnancy [139]. It has been suggested that the use of SFT measurements themselves can be preferred for the assessment and follow-up of adiposity during pregnancy, instead of using SFT to calculate BF and FFM [25]. We recommend the classical standardized protocols from Lohman and colleagues [149] for the assessment of skinfolds to avoid terminological/methodological randomness.

Body Circumferences

Body circumferences have been shown to be less skill dependent and have lower inter-observer variation, as compared with overall skinfold measurement [150, 151], including in pregnancy [134]. Body circumferences, sometimes called body girths [152], have also been widely used and recommended, for use in clinical settings. Waist circumference measurement has been extensively used

Table 4.5 Skinfold thickness dimensions during singleton pregnancy, expressed as mean ± sd (range) [mm, unless otherwise noted]

References	Population	Pre-pregnancy	<16 weeks	16–28 weeks	>28 weeks
Taggart et al. [111]	Healthy woman from Aberdeen, UK (26.1 ± 3.6 years)	No data	Bic SFT = 7.4 ± 3.1	Bic SFT = 8.7 ± 3.8	Bic SFT = 8.7 ± 3.8
			Tri SFT = 15.7 ± 5.1	Tri SFT = 18.0 ± 6.3	Tri SFT = 18.0 ± 6.3
			Sub SFT = 11.8 ± 4.6	Sub SFT = 14.7 ± 4.2	Sub SFT = 14.7 ± 4.2
			Costal SFT = 11.4 ± 4.7	Costal SFT = 16.6 ± 5.5	Costal SFT = 16.6 ± 5.5
			Thigh SFT = 34.8 ± 10.7	Thigh SFT = 30.7 ± 11.1	Thigh SFT = 30.7 ± 11.1
			SIliac SFT = 7.9 ± 3.1	SIliac SFT = 13.6 ± 5.3	SIliac SFT = 13.6 ± 5.3
			Knee SFT = 11.7 ± 3.8	Knee SFT = 8.7 ± 2.7	Knee SFT = 8.7 ± 2.7
			Sum SFT* = 100.7 ± 30.2		
Pipe et al. [111]	Normal weight woman from London, UK (19–40 years)	Normal weight	Sum SFTβ = 48.6 ± 10.2	Sum SFTβ = 57.7 ± 13.6	Sum SFTβ = 59.6 ± 11.5
Catalano et al. [146]	Healthy lean women from Vermont, US (control group: **normal** glucose tolerance at baseline)	Sum SFT# = 74.0 ± 14.8	Sum SFT# = 89.0 ± 22.4		Sum SFT# = 109.8 ± 19.8
[Control]		BMI = 20.8 ± 2.3 kg/m²			
Catalano et al. [146]	Healthy lean women from Vermont, US (**Abnormal** glucose tolerance during pregnancy at baseline)	Sum SFT# = 88.7 ± 16.8	Sum SFT# = 93.5 ± 18.3		Sum SFT# = 108.9 ± 16.3
[AGT]		BMI = 20.6 ± 1.1 kg/m²			
Paxton et al. [103]	Ethnic diverse women from New York, US (26 ± 4.8 years)	UW = 10.5%;	Bic SFT = 15.6 ± 8.4		Bic SFT = 16.0 ± 8.4
		NW = 61.5%;	Tri SFT = 23.5 ± 8.6		Tri SFT = 24.6 ± 8.5
		OW = 14.5%;	Sub SFT = 24.7 ± 11.8		Sub SFT = 27.7 ± 11.0
		Ob = 13.5%.	Thigh SFT = 38.5 ± 14.7		Thigh SFT = 43.6 ± 13.4
			Torax SFT = 19.3 ± 8.1		Torax SFT = 17.3 ± 6.5
			UIliac SFT = 22.0 ± 9.0		UIliac SFT = 25.7 ± 8.1
			Calf SFT = 23.4 ± 7.1		Calf SFT = 26.0 ± 7.0
			Chest SFT = 13.0 ± 7.1		Chest SFT = 13.9 ± 7.9

(continued)

Table 4.5 (continued)

References	Population	Pre-pregnancy	<16 weeks	16–28 weeks	>28 weeks
Soltani et al. [141]	Women from Sheffield, UK.	(NW) BMI = 22.7 ± 1.3 kg/m²	(NW) Sum SFT∂ = 84.30 ± 25.31		
	NW: 26.44 ± 5.32 years	(OW) BMI = 27.2 ± 1.4 kg/m²	(OW) Sum SFT∂ = 125.02 ± 22.76		
	OW: 26.91 ± 4.50 years Ob: 27.68 ± 3.83 years	(Ob) BMI = 34.5 ± 3.54 kg/m²	(Ob) Sum SFT∂ = 158.74 ± 21.52		
Presley et al. [140]	Two groups of Healthy women from Cleveland, Ohio, US.	Development group:			Development group:
	Development group:	BMI = 25.8 ± 4.2 kg/m²			Bic SFT = 8.6 ± 5.1
	30.3 ± 4.4 years	Validation group:			Tri SFT = 18.8 ± 4.7
	Validation group:	BMI = 27.9 ± 6.2 kg/m²			Sub SFT = 16.2 ± 7.9
	30.4 ± 4.5 years				Costal SFT = 17.6 ± 7.1
					Thigh SFT = 33.4 ± 12.6
					SIliac SFT = 15.3 ± 6.8
					SPatellar SFT = 10.6 ± 5.4
					Validation group:
					Bic SFT = 8.7 ± 3.8
					Tri SFT = 18.0 ± 6.3
					Sub SFT = 14.7 ± 4.2
					Costal SFT = 16.6 ± 5.5
					Thigh SFT = 30.7 ± 11.1
					SIliac SFT = 13.6 ± 5.3
					SPatellar SFT = 8.7 ± 2.7
Stevens-Simon et al. [135]	Ethnic diverse adolescents from Denver, CO, US (13–19 years)	BMI = 21.9 ± 5.1 (15.8–36.8) kg/m²	Bic SFT = 10.7 ± 8.0		Bic SFT = 12.4 ± 6.4
			Tri SFT = 16.2 ± 6.3		Tri SFT = 20.5 ± 8.8
			Sub SFT = 15.7 ± 7.1		Sub SFT = 21.5 ± 8.8
			Thigh SFT = 22.2 ± 8.1		Thigh SFT = 27.4 ± 8.3
			Costal SFT = 11.4 ± 5.6		Costal SFT = 15.7 ± 6.6
			SIliac SFT = 12.3 ± 8.4		SIliac SFT = 17.4 ± 6.9

López et al. [147] [offspring <3 kg]	Urban Women from Argentina (19–49 years), offspring birth weight <3.0 kg	BMI = normal	Bic SFT = 8.3 (7.7–8.9)	Bic SFT = 10.1 (9.4–10.7)	Bic SFT = 11.3 (10.6–11.9)
			Tri SFT = 16.1 (15.0–17.3)	Tri SFT = 18.6 (17.5–19.8)	Tri SFT = 19.9 (18.8–20.9)
			Sub SFT = 16.9 (15.8–17.9)	Sub SFT = 19.9 (18.8–21.0)	Sub SFT = 21.9 (20.9–22.9)
López et al. [147] [offspring >3 kg]	Urban women from Argentina (19–49 years), offspring birth weight >3.0 kg	BMI = normal	Bic SFT = 11.0 (10.5–11.5)	Bic SFT = 12.5 (11.9–12.1)	Bic SFT = 13.5 (12.9–14.1)
			Tri SFT = 20.6 (19.8–21.4)	Tri SFT = 22.8 (22.9–23.6)	Tri SFT = 24.4 (23.6–25.1)
			Sub SFT = 20.7 (19.9–21.5)	Sub SFT = 23.6 (22.7–24.4)	Sub SFT = 25.2 (24.3–26.1)
Kannieappan et al. [134]	Overweight and obese women from Australia (29.7 ± 5.2 years)	BMI = 29.2 (27.6–33.6) kg/m^2	Bic SFT = 13.21 (6.5–21.3)		
			Tri SFT = 24.13 (11.1–38.8)		
			Sub SFT = 25.37 (22.0–47.4)		
Branco et al. [148]	Healthy Caucasian women from Portugal (33.2 ± 1.6 years, range 32–37)	BMI = 22.5 ± 3.1	Bic SFT = 6.8 ± 2.6	Bic SFT = 6.7 ± 3.1	Bic SFT = 7.1 ± 2.9
			Tri SFT = 16.2 ± 3.9	Tri SFT = 17.5 ± 4.2	Tri SFT = 16.3 ± 4.4
			Sub SFT = 11.5 ± 4.4	Sub SFT = 12.6 ± 4.4	Sub SFT = 13.3 ± 4.1
			Thigh SFT = 20.4 ± 7.5	Thigh SFT = 23.4 ± 9.4	Thigh SFT = 23.8 ± 8.1
			Calf SFT = 13.4 ± 5.7	Calf SFT = 14.1 ± 6.5	Costal SFT = 14.3 ± 5.0
			SIliac SFT = 19.1 ± 4.0	SIliac SFT = 20.7 ± 4.9	SIliac SFT = 19.0 ± 5.1
			Sum SFT§ = 124.7 ± 24.5	Sum SFT§ = 131.5 ± 30.5	Sum SFT§ = 130.7 ± 27.7

Sd standard deviation, *Sum SFTβ* sum of four skinfold thickness (biceps, triceps, subscapular, suprailiac), *Sum SFT#* sum of seven skinfold thickness (biceps, triceps, subscapular, costal, suprailiac, mid and lower-thigh), *BMI* body mass index, *Bic SFT* biceps skinfold thickness, *Tri SFT* triceps skinfold thickness, *Sub SFT* subscapular skinfold thickness, *Thigh SFT* thigh skinfold thickness, *Costal SFT* costal or subcostal skinfold thickness, *SIliac SFT* supra-iliac, iliac or iliac crest skinfold thickness, *UIliac SFT* upper-iliac skinfold thickness, *Calf SFT* calf skinfold thickness, *SPatellar* SFT supra-patellar skinfold thickness, *NO* normal-weight, *OW* overweight, *Ob* obese, *(NW) Sum SFT∂* sum of five skinfold thickness (triceps, biceps, subscapular, suprailiac and mid-thigh), *Sum SFT§* sum of six skinfold thickness (biceps, triceps, subscapular, thigh, calf, suprailiac)

*Sum SFT means the sum of all sites, namely: bicep SFT + Tricep SFT + Subscapular SFT + Costal SFT + Thigh SFT + Suprailiac SFT + Knee SFT in different settings and populations and is one of the most studied body circumferences [18, 153–155]; however, its usefulness may be compromised during pregnancy because of the wide morphological and body composition changes in this specific region of the body during pregnancy. Yet, abdominal circumference, as measured horizontally at the level of the navel [149], has been used during pregnancy [99, 131, 145]. Apparently, the abdominal circumference is useful in the prediction of TBW, explaining 27% of TBW variation throughout pregnancy, and therefore it has been proposed to be included in a multivariate prediction model of TBW (Fig. 4.4) [131]. Accordingly, both high abdominal circumference and TBW have also been shown to be associated with hypertensive disorders of pregnancy [99, 127].

The circumference of the upper arm, as measured using Lohman and colleagues guidelines [152], has been recognized as the most relevant circumference measurement to be used in pregnancy [25, 122]. Upper arm circumference has been used for decades in the assessment of malnutrition in diverse populations, including children and overall population in underdeveloped countries population, particularly in emergency settings [156–161] and it has been recommended that it should be used more often in nutritional studies [162, 163]. Upper arm circumference has been widely used during pregnancy [114, 138, 153]. It seems highly associated with gestational weight and may even be used as an alternative to weight in settings where a weight scale is not available [153]. Cutoff values for the diagnosis of increased risk for low offspring birthweight have been proposed for mid-upper arm circumference (Table 4.6) [153].

Paxton and colleagues [103] have proposed wrist circumference at the 39th week of gestation to be useful for the calculation of BF, based on a multivariate model (Fig. 4.4); however, the wrist circumference measurement protocol is not disclosed. In the absence of other protocol to be included in Paxton and colleagues' equation (Fig. 4.4), we recommend the measurement of wrist circumference perpendicular to the long axis of the forearm just distal to the styloid process of the radius and ulna, which are easily palpable, as proposed by Lohman and colleagues [152]. Neck circumference seems to be related to the risk of developing maternal hypertensive disorders [164] and gestational diabetes mellitus [165] and, accordingly, has recently been proposed as a promising clinical marker to monitor obesity throughout pregnancy [166]. Other body circumferences have been sparsely used during pregnancy [151] with no confirmed clinical usefulness to date.

Table 4.6 Recommended mid-upper arm circumference cutoff values for the diagnosis of increased risk for low birth-weight offspring [Adapted from Lopez et al. [153]]

	16 weeks of gestation	28 weeks of gestation	36 weeks of gestation
Mid-upper arm circumference (cm)	24.5	25.5	26.5

4.5 Effect of Exercise on Body Composition in Pregnancy and Postpartum

The importance of a physical active and healthy lifestyle during pregnancy is well documented and highly recommended [167–171]. Maternal exercise during pregnancy has a positive effect on mother and offspring, both the short- and long-term effects. Physical Activity (PA) may also reduce the risk for caesarean birth, gestational hypertensive disorders, and preterm birth [172]. Many hormones which are involved in the regulation of metabolic homeostasis are influenced by our lifestyle factors, and it should be of great interest to minimize sedentary lifestyle [169].

The American College of Obstetricians and Gynaecologists (ACOG) has set the PA recommendations for all healthy women during pregnancy and postpartum, which is 150 min moderate intensity per week [172–174]. However, there is evidence showing that PA decreases during pregnancy and pregnant women rarely meet the recommendations. After delivery, PA tends to increase again, but not to the same level as before the pregnancy [171, 175]. PA may help to keep a good balance between energy intake and expenditure in the gestation, which has several beneficial effects, such as reduced risk of excessive weight gain, improved glucose metabolism, and a positive effect on the reduced risk of gestational diabetes (GDM) [169, 171, 176, 177]. Too much weight gain is associated with increased risk for gestational hypertension, preeclampsia, caesarean delivery, and extended hospital stay [177]. During pregnancy, normal weight women would gain approximately 11.5–16 kg. This could change the traditional BMI category from normal to overweight [168, 169, 178, 179]. However, it seems that the obese women are more likely to have excessive weight gain [176, 180], while women with a healthy BMI are more likely to gain weight below the Institute of Medicine's recommendations (IOM) for gestational weight gain (GWG) [176].

4.5.1 Effect of Exercise on Gestational Weight Gain and Body Composition

Previous studies have analyzed if offering a supervised exercise training during pregnancy would have an effect on GWG in women. There is evidence that supervised exercise women shows lower GWG compared to a control group [180], and that more active women gain less weight during pregnancy and are at lower risk of excess GWG [181]. However, other studies found no associations between PA and GWG [169, 170, 178, 182]. It has been argued that PA interventions alone are not enough to reduce the GWG [183] and that a combined diet and PA-based interventions during pregnancy is more effective [184, 185], and retain less weight postpartum [186–188]. The use of an e-based intervention can be useful in controlling GWG in obese mothers [189]. Different studies [190, 191] have shown a beneficial effect of technology-based PA interventions in pregnant woman, but opposite findings can also be found [192, 193]. Overall, these studies evaluated self-reported outcomes [191], utilized steps from Fitbit manually reported by participants [192] or had a short duration on the intervention [190]. The lack of effect of Moderate to Vigorous Physical Activity (MVPA) on GWG [193] highlights the need to combine smart phone's apps with face-to-face interventions, which has shown stronger effects on GWG for interventions targeting dietary behaviors compared with PA [194].

Behavioral intervention on PA and diet combined has been shown to reduce sum of skinfold thickness in one large RCT [195] but not in another [196]. The association of mid-pregnancy PA with maternal adiposity and GWG, in ethnicities from an economically deprived city in the UK, showed that more than 50% of the women are inactive [170]. In white British women, more mid-pregnancy PA was associated with smaller triceps skinfold thickness. Active white British women were less adipose, had smaller triceps skinfolds, and a smaller mid-upper arm circumference. Moderately active Pakistani-origin women had a larger mid-upper arm circumference compared to inactive Pakistani-origin women [170]. Chiavaroli and colleagues [197] observed that while there was a reduction in adiposity in both groups of mothers, exercisers were also lighter, and leaner compared to pre-pregnancy. Exercise in pregnancy, in mothers who were not previously physically active, may be associated with some subtle adverse consequences to the offspring in childhood like have less weight.

Even though the amount of PA is reduced (metabolic equivalent of task: MET index from 5.0 to 3.0 h/week) throughout pregnancy [178] and the body fat mass (FM) increases [169], there is no conclusive evidence between the association between PA and Body Composition (BC) measurements in either early or late gestation [178, 193]. Pregnant women adhered to an exercise program showed a decrease in body fat (BF), and body fat percentage (BF%), while non-active showed an increase [169]. In overweight and obese pregnant women, the weight gain seems to be more due to free fat mass (FFM) than to FM, and BF% decreased especially among obese women. With poor dietary quality, women showed less FFM [178]. Obese women gained less weight and increased less FM than overweight women. Only women with excess GWG gained FM (and FFM) and the change was significantly different between women with excess and ideal WG. Moreover, BF% decreased significantly less in obese women than in women with ideal GWG [178].

There is evidence that pregnant women have a higher basal metabolic rate (BMR) than of non-pregnant, and that MET values in healthy women, are lower for pregnant than non-pregnant women, mainly explained by the increased BMR during pregnancy [198]. The effect of pregnancy on MET-values may be influenced by the intensity of the activity and BC. Significant relationships between total body fat (TBF) and measured MET for pregnant women were found for activities with high but not for low intensity. For all activities (except running), energy expenditure (kJ/min) of the pregnant was slightly higher than for the non-pregnant but only the values for walking at 5.6 km/h were significantly different. The value for sitting was significantly lower for pregnant.

Maternal leptin levels increase over the course of pregnancy [169]. However, it is evidence that PA during pregnancy remarkably reduces leptin levels (inducing a decrease in food intake and increasing energy expenditure via hypothalamic interactions), which can explain the lower BF content and change in FM for this group of women [169, 199]. MVPA is associated with lower leptin levels and weight change in healthy pregnant women with MVPA above the median than those below, although these differences were not statistically significant [200] which may reflect the concomitant change in FM [169, 199].

Short- and long-term maternal outcomes after exercise throughout pregnancy, show that, on the immediate postpartum period [187, 201], normal-weight and overweight/obese women exposed to PA (included low-intensity exercise) plus diet showed greater weight reduction [186] and retained less weight postpartum [186–188]. Among overweight and obese women, postpartum weight retention (PPWR) was not significantly lower in the exercise group, and both groups returned to their early pregnancy body weight 3 months postpartum [182]. In a 1-year follow-up after birth, the effects of exercise during pregnancy on metabolism and body composition showed no differences in body mass index (BMI) nor BF% between women, who exercised in pregnancy, even though both groups showed a reduction in BF% 2 weeks after delivery. However, at 7 years, women who exercised in pregnancy, showed a significant reduction in weight and BMI, and had lower systolic blood pressure [197].

It seems that women with excess weight gain exhibits a higher daily intake than women with ideal weight gain [178] and that PPWG is the result of increased energy intake after pregnancy rather than decreased energy expenditure [202]. This can explain the fact that training programs to control the GWG is remarkably better in women with overweight and obesity compared with those who are underweight and normal weight [193].

4.5.2 Recommendations of Physical Activity and Exercise During Pregnancy and Postpartum

In this context, terms as PA and exercise will be used. PA is defined as any bodily movement produced by skeletal muscles that results in energy expenditure [203]. Exercise is defined as "planned, structured and repetitive bodily movements done to improve one or more components of physical fitness" [172].

Most pregnant women can perform PA, and for those with medical problems individual exercise programs should be tailored [172]. For women with uncomplicated pregnancies, there is no evidence that regular PA during pregnancy may cause miscarriage, poor fetal growth, musculoskeletal injury, or premature delivery [172, 204–206]. According to the ACOG's recommendations, women with uncomplicated pregnancies should perform both aerobic and strength training regularly before, during, and after pregnancy [172]. They should do at least 150 min of moderate intensity aerobic activity per week during pregnancy and the postpartum period. Women who are used to vigorous-intensity aerobic activity or who were physically active before pregnancy can continue these activities during pregnancy and the postpartum period [172, 207, 208]. Physical activity throughout pregnancy seems to provide many benefits. Regular aerobic exercise during pregnancy has been shown to improve or maintain physical fitness. PA does not only have a positive effect on physical conditions such as decreased incidence of: GDM [209], gestational hypertensive disorders [210], preeclampsia, caesarean birth, premature birth, and decreased postpartum recovery time [171, 182, 211, 212]. The study to Magro-Malosso and colleagues [211] documented a significantly reduced risk of gestational hypertensive disorders, gestational hypertension, and caesarean birth in women who performed aerobic exercise 30–60 min 2–7 times per week. PA may also be an essential factor in psychological conditions such as preventing depressive disorders in the postpartum period [213, 214]. Marin-Jimenez and colleagues [215] found that a greater self-reported overall physical fitness, including cardiorespiratory fitness, in pregnancy was associated with less bodily, lumbar, and sciatic pain.

An exercise program for pregnant women should have a moderate intensity for at least 20–30 min preferably every day [172, 197, 216]. The program should consist of aerobic training, strength training, stretching, body awareness, and pelvic floor muscles and strengthening. Examples of aerobic exercises are walking, stationary cycling [198], dancing, and water aerobics. A strength training program can consist of weight-bearing exercises such as squats, push-ups, diagonal lifts on all fours, oblique abdominal crunches, and pelvic floor muscle exercises, with three sets of 10 repetitions of each exercise separated by 1-min rest between sets. In addition, three sets of the "plank exercise" for 30 s can be added [182]. Another type of exercise program for pregnant women can be twice a week for 60 min with 1 day of moderate-intensity aerobic exercises such as Nordic walking or walking, and the other day of moderate-intensity strength training on different machines targeting major muscle groups in the body [169], and in addition 30 min with body awareness, pelvic floor muscles, and stretching until normal length. Regardless, contact activities with high risk for abdominal trauma or imbalance should be avoided [172].

During the pregnancy period, both anatomical and physiological changes occur, such as weight gain and a shift of the center of gravity, which often results in progressive lordosis. As a result, many women experience low back pain [172, 217]. Strength training for the abdominal and back muscles could be of great importance to minimize the problems [174]. Exercises that increase body awareness are also recommended to cope with the gravity shift. Due to the buoyancy in the water, exercise in water may be a good alternative since the weight load on the spine will be reduced [174]. Blood volume, heart rate, and stroke volume normally increase during pregnancy. A physiologic decrease in pulmonary reserve occurs and the ability to exercise anaerobically is impaired. Oxygen availability for aerobic exercise and increased workload consistently lags [172]. This must be considered when training pregnant women. Especially women who are overweight or obese may have a limited ability to participate in more strenuous physical activities during pregnancy. On the other hand, aerobic training in pregnancy has been shown to increase aerobic capacity in normal weight and overweight pregnant women [172]. It is also demonstrated that 30 min of strenuous exercise is well tolerated by women and fetuses in both active and inactive pregnant women in their second trimester. However, it is not recommended to continue exercising vigorously during the third trimester due to the risk to deliver infants weighing 200–400 g less [172]. If the pregnant women have been sedentary before pregnancy, they should follow a more gradual progression of exercise. It has not been established an upper level of safe exercise intensity, but according to the ACOG's recommendations women who are regular exercisers before pregnancy and who have uncomplicated, healthy pregnancies should be able to engage in high-intensity exercise programs, such as jogging and aerobics, with no adverse effects. Activity restrictions should not be given routinely to reduce for example preterm birth [172]. Maintaining a supine position during exercise after 20 weeks of gestation may result in decreased venous return due to aortocaval compression from the gravid uterus, leading to hypotension. This should be taken in consideration when prescribing exercises in pregnancy [172]. To avoid this problem, it is recommended to perform alternative exercises standing on all fours, instead of a supine position. Pregnant women should stay well hydrated during exercise, wear loose-fitting clothing, and avoid high heat and humidity to protect against heat stress, particularly during the first trimester [172].

For postpartum women, PA should primarily focus on daily exercises for the pelvic floor muscles and they can start exercising immediate postpartum [218]. It is also a great interest to do abdominal strengthening exercises, which should include abdominal crunch exercises and the drawing-in exercise, a maneuver that increases abdominal pressure by pulling in the abdominal wall muscles. Those exercises have shown to decrease the incidence of diastasis recti abdominis and decrease the inter-rectus distance, which is important [172, 219, 220]. We do not recommend running and jumping during the first 6 weeks of postpartum. In general, one should be careful with such activities for the first 6 months. Although PA in pregnancy and postpartum is associated with minimal risks and have been shown to benefit most women, still more research is needed, particularly regarding the optimal type of exercise, frequency, duration, and intensity [172].

4.6 Conclusion

This chapter reviews body composition rules and fundamentals to support why and how body composition should be assessed during pregnancy. Pregnancy is characterized by profound adaptations and alterations in body composition which must be taken into consideration in the assessment and interpretation of body composition data. Body composition is considered a relevant component of health-related fitness and is shown to be predictive of several pregnancy-related risks which underline the importance of carefully monitoring and follow-up fitness component during this exquisite phase of women and newborn's life. Even though research regarding body composition during pregnancy is not as overwhelming as in the overall population, it was possible to find and report specific techniques and methods to use in pregnancy to assess body composition and to show established cutoff values regarding some of these methods. Accordingly, pregnancy has been highlighted as an opportunity to protect or enhance current and future health of the mother and the offspring. This has also been argued to be a cornerstone for the future sustainability of health care systems, whose will have to increasingly focus on prevention to ensure sustainability. From this standpoint, exercise seems critical to promote healthy pregnancies, including assuring healthy body composition trajectories throughout the course of pregnancy, and is a strong candidate for a core component of pregnancy health care.

4.7 Further Research

There are validated methods for the assessment of body composition, which are mainly proposed for specific gestational ages. Further research should focus on providing and strengthen findings regarding assessment tools and reference data that are simple to use in clinical practice and allow for the assessment of body composition throughout the course of all pregnancy. Furthermore, research is also warranted on the cause–effect association and underlying mechanisms between body composition and pregnancy-related pathologies of pregnancy and puerperium. Only with such data can the relationship between maternal body composition and related outcomes in mother and child be studied in depth.

Future research should also focus on collecting and reporting detailed data on women's body composition responses to exercise, particularly on the effect of exercise on specific body components and resulting health outcomes during pregnancy and thereafter, and how this impacts pregnancy, postpartum, and the newborn. This data is cornerstone to reinforce physical activity and exercise guidelines for pregnancy and for pregnant women to benefit the most from this healthy lifestyle component.

References

1. CDC. Physical activity and health: a report of the surgeon general. Atlanta, GA: Department of Health and Human Services, Centers for Disease Control and Prevention, National Center for Chronic Disease Prevention and Health Promotion; 1996.
2. ACSM. ACSM's guidelines for exercise testing and prescription. 10th ed. Philadelphia, PA: Wolters Kluwer; 2017. 480 p. Revised.
3. Vernini JM, Moreli JB, Costa RAA, Negrato CA, Rudge MVC, Calderon IMP. Maternal adipokines and insulin as biomarkers of pregnancies complicated by overweight and obesity. Diabetol Metab Syndr. 2016;8(1):68. http://dmsjournal.biomedcentral.com/articles/10.1186/s13098-016-0184-y. Accessed 25 Oct 2017.
4. Mitanchez D, Jacqueminet S, Nizard J, Tanguy M-L, Ciangura C, Lacorte J-M, et al. Effect of maternal obesity on birthweight and neonatal fat mass: a prospective clinical trial. PLoS One. 2017;12(7):e0181307.
5. Schmitt NM, Nicholson WK, Schmitt J. The association of pregnancy and the development of obesity–results of a systematic review and meta-analysis on the natural history of postpartum weight retention. Int J Obes. 2007;31(11):1642–51.
6. Cedergren MI. Maternal morbid obesity and the risk of adverse pregnancy outcome. Obstet Gynecol. 2004;103(2):219–24.
7. Rooney BL, Schauberger CW. Excess pregnancy weight gain and long-term obesity: one decade later. Obstet Gynecol. 2002;100(2):245–52.

8. McCarthy EA, Strauss BJ, Walker SP, Permezel M. Determination of maternal body composition in pregnancy and its relevance to perinatal outcomes. Obstet Gynecol Surv. 2004;59(10):731–42.
9. Wang Z-M, Pierson RN, Heymsfield SB. The five-level model: a new approach to organizing body-composition research. Am J Clin Nutr. 1992;56(1):19–28.
10. Shen W, St-Onge M, Wang Z, Heymsfield S. Study of body composition: an overview. In: Heymsfield S, Lohman TG, Wang Z, Going S, editors. Human body composition. 2nd ed. Champaign, IL: Human Kinetics; 2005. p. 3–16.
11. Lederman SA. Pregnancy. In: Heymsfield SB, Lohman TG, Wang Z, Going SB, editors. Human body composition. 2nd ed. Champaign, IL: Human Kinetics; 2005. p. 299–312.
12. Shen W, Wang Z, Punyanita M, Lei J, Sinav A, Kral JG, et al. Adipose tissue quantification by imaging methods: a proposed classification. Obes Res. 2003;11(1):5–16.
13. Kissebah AH, Krakower GR. Regional adiposity and morbidity. Physiol Rev. 1994;74(4):761–811.
14. Bray G. Overweight, mortality, and morbidity. In: Bouchard C, editor. Physical activity and obesity. Champaign, IL: Human Kinetics; 2000. p. 31–54.
15. Vague J. [Importance of the measurement of fat distribution in pathology]. Bull Mem Soc Med Hop Paris 1950;66(31–32):1572–4.
16. Vague J. The degree of masculine differentiation of obesities: a factor determining predisposition to diabetes, atherosclerosis, gout, and uric calculous disease. Am J Clin Nutr. 1956;4(1):20–34.
17. Canoy D, Boekholdt SM, Wareham N, Luben R, Welch A, Bingham S, et al. Body fat distribution and risk of coronary heart disease in men and women in the European Prospective Investigation Into Cancer and Nutrition in Norfolk cohort: a population-based prospective study. Circulation. 2007;116(25):2933–43.
18. Nishida C, Ko GT, Kumanyika S. Body fat distribution and noncommunicable diseases in populations: overview of the 2008 WHO Expert Consultation on Waist Circumference and Waist-Hip Ratio. Eur J Clin Nutr. 2010;64(1):2–5.
19. Zhang S, Folsom AR, Flack JM, Liu K. Body fat distribution before pregnancy and gestational diabetes: findings from coronary artery risk development in young adults (CARDIA) study. BMJ. 1995;311(7013):1139.
20. Stevens-Simons C, Thureen P, Barret J, Stamm E. Regional body fat distribution and insulin resistance during adolescent pregnancy. J Am Diet Assoc. 2002;102(4):563–5.
21. Landon MB, Osei K, Platt M, O'dorisio T, Samuels P, Gabbe SG. The differential effects of body fat distribution on insulin and glucose metabolism during pregnancy. Am J Obstet Gynecol. 1994;171(4):875–84.
22. Ozias MK, Li S, Hull HR, Brooks WM, Petroff MG, Carlson SE. Abdominal visceral adiposity influences CD4+ T cell cytokine production in pregnancy. Cytokine. 2015;71(2):405–8.
23. Rossner S, Bo WJ, Hiltbrandt E, Hinson W, Karstaedt N, Santago P, et al. Adipose tissue determinations in cadavers--a comparison between cross-sectional planimetry and computed tomography. Int J Obes. 1990;14(10):893–902.
24. Abate N, Burns D, Peshock RM, Garg A, Grundy SM. Estimation of adipose tissue mass by magnetic resonance imaging: validation against dissection in human cadavers. J Lipid Res. 1994;35(8):1490–6.
25. Widen EM, Gallagher D. Body composition changes in pregnancy: measurement, predictors and outcomes. Eur J Clin Nutr. 2014;68(6):643–52.
26. Mazaki-Tovi S, Vaisbuch E, Tarca AL, Kusanovic JP, Than NG, Chaiworapongsa T, et al. Characterization of visceral and subcutaneous adipose tissue transcriptome and biological pathways in pregnant and non-pregnant women: evidence for pregnancy-related regional-specific differences in adipose tissue. Sanchez-Margalet V, editor. PLoS One. 2015;10(12):e0143779.
27. Tchernof A, Despres JP. Pathophysiology of human visceral obesity: an update. Physiol Rev. 2013;93(1):359–404.
28. Goodpaster BH. Measuring body fat distribution and content in humans. Curr Opin Clin Nutr Metab Care. 2002;5(5):481–7.

29. Sardinha LB, Teixeira PJ. Measuring adiposity and fat distribution in relation to health. In: Heymsfield SB, Lohman TG, Wang Z, Going SB, editors. Human body composition. 2nd ed. Champaign, IL: Human Kinetics; 2005. p. 177–202.
30. Despres JP. Abdominal obesity and cardiovascular disease: is inflammation the missing link? Can J Cardiol. 2012;28(6):642–52.
31. Ghezzi F, Franchi M, Balestreri D, Lischetti B, Mele MC, Alberico S, et al. Bioelectrical impedance analysis during pregnancy and neonatal birth weight. Eur J Obestet Gynecol. 2001;98(2):171–6.
32. Forbes GB. Human body composition - growth, aging, nutrition, and activity. Berlin: Springer; 1987. www.springer.com/cn/book/9781461291008. Accessed 9 Nov 2017.
33. Kopp-Hoolihan LE, Van Loan MD, Wong WW, King JC. Fat mass deposition during pregnancy using a four-component model. J Appl Physiol. 1999;87(1):196–202.
34. Ikenoue S, Waffarn F, Sumiyoshi K, Ohashi M, Ikenoue C, Buss C, et al. Association of ultrasound-based measures of fetal body composition with newborn adiposity: fetal body composition and newborn adiposity. Pediatr Obes. 2017;12:86–93.
35. Frankenfield DC, Rowe WA, Cooney RN, Smith JS, Becker D. Limits of body mass index to detect obesity and predict body composition. Nutrition. 2001;17(1):26–30.
36. WHO. Measuring obesity-classification and description of anthropometric data. Report on a WHO consultation on the epidemiology of obesity. Warsaw: WHO Regional Office for Europe; 1987.
37. WHO. Obesity: preventing and managing the global epidemic - report of a WHO consultation on obesity. Executive summary. Geneva: World Health Organization; 1997.
38. NIH. Clinical guidelines on the identification, evaluation, and treatment of overweight and obesity in adults--the evidence report. National Institutes of Health. Obes Res. 1998;6(Suppl 2):51S–209S.
39. CSEP. Canadian Society for Exercise Physiology-Physical Activity Training for Health (CSEP-PATH). 2nd ed. Ottawa, ON: Canadian Society for Exercise Physiology; 2019.
40. IOM (Institute of Medicine). Weight gain during pregnancy: reexamining the guidelines. Washington, DC: The National Academies Press; 2009. http://www.nap.edu/catalog/12584. Accessed 18 Dec 2017.
41. Rasmussen KM, Abrams B, Bodnar LM, Butte NF, Catalano PM, Maria Siega-Riz A. Recommendations for weight gain during pregnancy in the context of the obesity epidemic. Obstet Gynecol. 2010;116(5):1191–5.
42. Forsum E, Henriksson P, Löf M. The Two-component model for calculating total body fat from body density: an evaluation in healthy women before, during and after pregnancy. Nutrients. 2014;6(12):5888–99.
43. Gaillard R. Maternal obesity during pregnancy and cardiovascular development and disease in the offspring. Eur J Epidemiol. 2015;30(11):1141–52.
44. Athukorala C, Rumbold AR, Willson KJ, Crowther CA. The risk of adverse pregnancy outcomes in women who are overweight or obese. BMC Pregnan Childb. 2010;10(1):56.
45. Höhn N, Junge S. [The relationship of maternal obesity, excessive weight gain in pregnancy and pre-eclampsia]. Geburtshilfe Frauenheilkd 1979;39(12):1079–82.
46. Kosus A, Eser A, Kosus N, Usluogullari B, Hizli D. Hyperemesis gravidarum and its relation with maternal body fat composition. J Obstet Gynaecol. 2016;36(6):822–6.
47. Aune D, Saugstad OD, Henriksen T, Tonstad S. Maternal body mass index and the risk of fetal death, stillbirth, and infant death: a systematic review and meta-analysis. JAMA. 2014;311(15):1536.
48. Chu SY, Kim SY, Lau J, Schmid CH, Dietz PM, Callaghan WM, et al. Maternal obesity and risk of stillbirth: a metaanalysis. Am J Obstet Gynecol. 2007;197(3):223–8.
49. Yao R, Ananth CV, Park BY, Pereira L, Plante LA. Obesity and the risk of stillbirth: a population-based cohort study. Am J Obstet Gynecol. 2014;210(5):457.e1–9.
50. Lee H-J, Ha J-E, Bae K-H. Synergistic effect of maternal obesity and periodontitis on preterm birth in women with pre-eclampsia: a prospective study. J Clin Periodontol. 2016;43(8):646–51.

51. Rasmussen S, Irgens L, Espinoza J. Maternal obesity and excess of fetal growth in preeclampsia. BJOG Int J Obstet Gynaecol. 2014;121(11):1351–8.
52. Leonard SA, Rasmussen KM, King JC, Abrams B. Trajectories of maternal weight from before pregnancy through postpartum and associations with childhood obesity. Am J Clin Nutr. 2017;106:1295.
53. Cai G, Sun X, Zhang L, Hong Q. Association between maternal body mass index and congenital heart defects in offspring: a systematic review. Am J Obstet Gynecol. 2014;211(2):91–117.
54. Lawlor DA. The Society for Social Medicine John Pemberton Lecture 2011. Developmental overnutrition—an old hypothesis with new importance?*. Int J Epidemiol. 2013;42(1):7–29.
55. Lindell N, Carlsson A, Josefsson A, Samuelsson U. Maternal obesity as a risk factor for early childhood type 1 diabetes: a nationwide, prospective, population-based case–control study. Diabetologia. 2018;61(1):130–7.
56. Boden G. Role of fatty acids in the pathogenesis of insulin resistance and NIDDM. Diabetes. 1997;46(1):3–10.
57. Koska J, Stefan N, Permana PA, Weyer C, Sonoda M, Bogardus C, et al. Increased fat accumulation in liver may link insulin resistance with subcutaneous abdominal adipocyte enlargement, visceral adiposity, and hypoadiponectinemia in obese individuals. Am J Clin Nutr. 2008;87(2):295–302.
58. Tanaka S, Togashi K, Rankinen T, Perusse L, Leon AS, Rao DC, et al. Is adiposity at normal body weight relevant for cardiovascular disease risk? Int J Obes Relat Metab Disord. 2002;26(2):176–83.
59. IOM (Institute of Medicine). Nutrition during pregnancy: Part I: Weight gain, Part II: Nutrient supplements. Washington, DC: National Academies Press; 1990. http://www.nap.edu/catalog/1451. Accessed 18 Dec 2017.
60. Lederman SA, Paxton A, Heymsfield SB, Wang J, Thornton J, Pierson RN. Body fat and water changes during pregnancy in women with different body weight and weight gain. Obstet Gynecol. 1997;90(4 Pt 1):483–8.
61. Gunderson EP, Abrams B, Selvin S. Does the pattern of postpartum weight change differ according to pregravid body size? Int J Obes. 2001;25(6):853.
62. Butte NF, Ellis KJ, Wong WW, Hopkinson JM, Smith EO. Composition of gestational weight gain impacts maternal fat retention and infant birth weight. Am J Obstet Gynecol. 2003;189(5):1423–32.
63. Bodnar LM, Pugh SJ, Abrams B, Himes KP, Hutcheon JA. Gestational weight gain in twin pregnancies and maternal and child health: a systematic review. J Perinatol. 2014;34(4):252–63.
64. Mohammadbeigi A, Farhadifar F, Zadeh NS, Mohammadsalehi N, Rezaiee M, Aghaei M. Fetal macrosomia: risk factors, maternal, and perinatal outcome. Ann Med Health Sci Res. 2013;3(4):546.
65. Han Z, Lutsiv O, Mulla S, Rosen A, Beyene J, Mcdonald SD, et al. Low gestational weight gain and the risk of preterm birth and low birthweight: a systematic review and meta-analyses: low gestational weight gain and PTB/LBW. Acta Obstet Gynecol Scand. 2011;90(9):935–54.
66. Huang A, Ji Z, Zhao W, Hu H, Yang Q, Chen D. Rate of gestational weight gain and preterm birth in relation to prepregnancy body mass indices and trimester: a follow-up study in China. Reprod Health. 2016;13:93. https://www.ncbi.nlm.nih.gov/pmc/articles/PMC4983027/. Accessed 12 Aug 2016.
67. Jayabalan N, Nair S, Nuzhat Z, Rice GE, Zuñiga FA, Sobrevia L, et al. Cross talk between adipose tissue and placenta in obese and gestational diabetes mellitus pregnancies via exosomes. Front Endocrinol. 2017;8:239. http://www.frontiersin.org.https.sci-hub.hk/articles/10.3389/fendo.2017.00239/full#B126. Accessed 26 Dec 2017.
68. Barbour LA, Shao J, Qiao L, Pulawa LK, Jensen DR, Bartke A, et al. Human placental growth hormone causes severe insulin resistance in transgenic mice. Am J Obstet Gynecol. 2002;186(3):512–7.
69. Ruhstaller K, Bastek J, Thomas A, Mcelrath T, Parry S, Durnwald C. The effect of early excessive weight gain on the development of hypertension in pregnancy. Am J Perinatol. 2016;33(12):1205–10.

70. Friedmann I, Balayla J. Gestational weight gain and the risk of infant mortality amongst women with normal prepregnancy BMI: the Friedmann-Balayla model. J Matern Fetal Neonatal Med. 2018;31(3):325–32.
71. Sharma AJ, Vesco KK, Bulkley J, Callaghan WM, Bruce FC, Staab J, et al. Associations of Gestational Weight Gain with preterm birth among underweight and normal weight women. Matern Child Health J. 2015;19(9):2066–73.
72. Widen EM, Factor-Litvak PR, Gallagher D, Paxton A, Pierson RN, Heymsfield SB, et al. The pattern of gestational weight gain is associated with changes in maternal body composition and neonatal size. Matern Child Health J. 2015;19(10):2286–94.
73. Wang Y, Mao J, Wang W, Qiou J, Yang L, Chen S. Maternal fat free mass during pregnancy is associated with birth weight. Reprod Health. 2017;14(1):47. http://reproductive-health-journal.biomedcentral.com/articles/10.1186/s12978-017-0308-3. Accessed 9 Nov 2017.
74. Kovacs CS, Kronenberg HM. Maternal-fetal calcium and bone metabolism during pregnancy, puerperium, and lactation. Endocr Rev. 1997;18(6):832–72.
75. O'Sullivan SM, Grey AB, Singh R, Reid IR. Bisphosphonates in pregnancy and lactation-associated osteoporosis. Osteoporos Int. 2006;17(7):1008–12.
76. Kovacs CS, Ralston SH. Presentation and management of osteoporosis presenting in association with pregnancy or lactation. Osteoporos Int. 2015;26(9):2223–41.
77. Medicine AC of S. Exercise testing and prescription for population with other chronic diseases and health conditions. In: ACSM's guidelines for exercise testing and prescription. 10th ed. Philadelphia, PA: Lippincott Williams and Wilkins; 2017. p. 297–376. Revised.
78. Berggren EK, Groh-Wargo S, Presley L, Hauguel-de Mouzon S, Catalano PM. Maternal fat, but not lean, mass is increased among overweight/obese women with excess gestational weight gain. Am J Obstet Gynecol. 2016;214(6):745.e1–5.
79. Gunderson EP, Abrams B. Epidemiology of gestational weight gain and body weight changes after pregnancy. Epidemiol Rev. 1999;21(2):261–75.
80. Bogaerts A, De Baetselier E, Ameye L, Dilles T, Van Rompaey B, Devlieger R. Postpartum weight trajectories in overweight and lean women. Midwifery. 2017;49:134–41.
81. Sobhonslidsuk A, Jongjirasiri S, Thakkinstian A, Wisedopas N, Bunnag P, Puavilai G. Visceral fat and insulin resistance as predictors of non-alcoholic steatohepatitis. World J Gastroenterol. 2007;13(26):3614–8.
82. Brunzell JD, Hokanson JE. Dyslipidemia of central obesity and insulin resistance. Diabetes Care. 1999;22(Suppl 3):C10–3.
83. Goodpaster B, Kelley DE. Obesity and diabetes: body composition determinants of insulin resistance. In: Heymsfield SB, Lohman TG, Wang Z, Going SB, editors. Human body composition. 2nd ed. Champaign, IL: Human Kinetics; 2005. p. 356–76.
84. Akagiri S, Naito Y, Ichikawa H, Mizushima K, Takagi T, Handa O, et al. A mouse model of metabolic syndrome; increase in visceral adipose tissue precedes the development of fatty liver and insulin resistance in high-fat diet-fed male KK/Ta mice. J Clin Biochem Nutr. 2008;42(2):150–7.
85. Sonagra AD. Normal pregnancy- a state of insulin resistance. J Clin Diagn Res. 2014;8:CC01. http://jcdr.net/article_fulltext.asp?issn=0973-709x&year=2014&volume=8&issue=11&page=CC01&issn=0973-709x&id=5081. Accessed 3 Jan 2018.
86. Díaz P, Powell TL, Jansson T. The role of placental nutrient sensing in maternal-fetal resource allocation. Biol Reprod. 2014;91(4):82. https://academic.oup.com/biolreprod/article-lookup/doi/10.1095/biolreprod.114.121798. Accessed 3 Jan 2018.
87. Coppack SW. Adipose tissue changes in obesity. Biochem Soc Trans. 2005;33(5):1049–52.
88. Poulos SP, Hausman DB, Hausman GJ. The development and endocrine functions of adipose tissue. Mol Cell Endocrinol. 2010;323(1):20–34.
89. Challier JC, Basu S, Bintein T, Minium J, Hotmire K, Catalano PM, et al. Obesity in pregnancy stimulates macrophage accumulation and inflammation in the placenta. Placenta. 2008;29(3):274–81.
90. Aleksandrova K, Mozaffarian D, Pischon T. Addressing the perfect storm: biomarkers in obesity and pathophysiology of cardiometabolic risk. Clin Chem. 2018;64(1):142–53.

91. Bakhai A. Adipokines--targeting a root cause of cardiometabolic risk. QJM. 2008;101(10):767–76.
92. Amash A, Holcberg G, Sapir O, Huleihel M. Placental secretion of interleukin-1 and interleukin-1 receptor antagonist in preeclampsia: effect of magnesium sulfate. J Interf Cytokine Res. 2012;32(9):432–41.
93. Leme Galvão LP, Menezes FE, Mendonca C, Barreto I, Alvim-Pereira C, Alvim-Pereira F, et al. Analysis of association of clinical aspects and *IL1B* tagSNPs with severe preeclampsia. Hypertens Pregnan. 2016;35(1):112–22.
94. Kalinderis M, Papanikolaou A, Kalinderi K, Ioannidou E, Giannoulis C, Karagiannis V, et al. Elevated serum levels of interleukin-6, interleukin-1β and human chorionic gonadotropin in pre-eclampsia: IL-6, IL-1β and HCG in pre-eclampsia. Am J Reprod Immunol. 2011;66(6):468–75.
95. Phillips J, McBride CA, Morris E, Crocker AM, Bernstein I. Adiposity, but not obesity, is associated with arterial stiffness in young nulliparous women. Reprod Sci. 2018;25:909.
96. Huda SS, Jordan F, Bray J, Love G, Payne R, Sattar N, et al. Visceral adipose tissue activated macrophage content and inflammatory adipokine secretion is higher in pre-eclampsia than in healthy pregnancys. Clin Sci. 2017;131(13):1529–40.
97. D'anna R, Baviera G, Corrado F, Giordano D, Di Benedetto A, Jasonni VM. Plasma adiponectin concentration in early pregnancy and subsequent risk of hypertensive disorders. Obstet Gynecol. 2005;106(2):340–4.
98. Rosso P, Donoso E, Braun S, Espinoza R, Fernández C, Salas SP. Maternal hemodynamic adjustments in idiopatic fetal growth retardation. Gynecol Obstet Investig. 1993;35:162–5.
99. Piuri G, Ferrazzi E, Bulfoni C, Mastricci L, Di Martino D, Speciani AF. Longitudinal changes and correlations of bioimpedance and anthropometric measurements in pregnancy: simple possible bed-side tools to assess pregnancy evolution. J Matern Fetal Neonatal Med. 2017;30(23):2824–30.
100. Toro-Ramos T, Paley C, Pi-Sunyer FX, Gallagher D. Body composition during fetal development and infancy through the age of 5 years. Eur J Clin Nutr. 2015;69(12):1279–89.
101. Chang S, Lodico L, Williams Z. Nutritional composition and heavy metal content of the human placenta. Placenta. 2017;60:100–2.
102. Pratt JP, Kaucher M, Richards AJ, Williams HH, Macy IC. Composition of the human placenta: I. Proximate composition. Am J Obstet Gynecol. 1946;52(3):402–8.
103. Paxton A, Lederman SA, Heymsfield SB, Wang J, Thornton JC, Pierson RN. Anthropometric equations for studying body fat in pregnant women. Am J Clin Nutr. 1998;67(1):104–10.
104. Denne SC, Patel D, Kalhan SC. Total body water measurement in normal and diabetic pregnancy: evidence for maternal and amniotic fluid equilibrium. Neonatology. 1990;57(5):284–91.
105. Wong WW, Lee LS, Klein PD. Deuterium and oxygen-18 measurements on microliter samples of urine, plasma, saliva, and human milk. Am J Clin Nutr. 1987;45(5):905–13.
106. Larciprete G, Valensise H, Vasapollo B, Altomare F, Sorge R, Casalino B, et al. Body composition during normal pregnancy: reference ranges. Acta Diabetol. 2003;40(S1):s225–32.
107. Lof M, Forsum E. Evaluation of bioimpedance spectroscopy for measurements of body water distribution in healthy women before, during, and after pregnancy. J Appl Physiol. 2004;96(3):967–73.
108. Anderson EC, Schuch RL, Fisher WR, Langham W. Radioactivity of people and foods. Science. 1957;125(3261):1273–8.
109. Smith T, Cronquist A. A versatile and economic whole-body counter based on liquid scintillation detector modules. Br J Radiol. 1977;50:332–9.
110. Ellis KJ. Whole-body counting and neutron activation analysis. In: Human body composition. 2nd ed. Champaign, IL: Human Kinetics Publishers; 2005. p. 51–62. Revised.
111. Pipe NGJ, Smith T, Halliday D, Edmonds CJ, Williams C, Coltart TM. Changes in fat, fat-free mass and body water in human normal pregnancy. BJOG Int J Obstet Gynaecol. 1979;86(12):929–40.

112. Gilmore LA, Butte NF, Ravussin E, Han H, Burton JH, Redman LM. Energy intake and energy expenditure for determining excess weight gain in pregnant women. Obstet Gynecol. 2016;127(5):884–92.
113. Fuller NJ, Jebb SA, Laskey MA, Coward WA, Elia M. Four-component model for the assessment of body composition in humans: comparison with alternative methods, and evaluation of the density and hydration of fat-free mass. Clin Sci. 1992;82(6):687–93.
114. Marshall NE, Murphy EJ, King JC, Haas EK, Lim JY, Wiedrick J, et al. Comparison of multiple methods to measure maternal fat mass in late gestation. Am J Clin Nutr. 2016;103(4):1055–63.
115. Hopkinson JM, Butte NF, Ellis KJ, Wong WW, Puyau MR, Smith EO. Body fat estimation in late pregnancy and early postpartum: comparison of two-, three-, and four-component models. Am J Clin Nutr. 1997;65(2):432–8.
116. Van Raaij JM, Peek ME, Vermaat-Miedema SH, Schonk CM, Hautvast JG. New equations for estimating body fat mass in pregnancy from body density or total body water. Am J Clin Nutr. 1988;48(1):24–9.
117. De Lorenzo A, Andreoli A, Matthie J, Withers P. Predicting body cell mass with bioimpedance by using theoretical methods: a technological review. J Appl Physiol. 1997;82(5):1542–58.
118. To WWK, Wong MWN. Changes in bone mineral density of the os calcis as measured by quantitative ultrasound during pregnancy and 24 months after delivery: bone mineral density changes after pregnancy. Aust N Z J Obstet Gynaecol. 2011;51(2):166–71.
119. Kennedy N, Peek M, Quinton A, Lanzarone V, Martin A, Benzie R, et al. Maternal abdominal subcutaneous fat thickness as a predictor for adverse pregnancy outcome: a longitudinal cohort study. BJOG Int J Obstet Gynaecol. 2016;123(2):225–32.
120. Bartha JL, Marín-Segura P, González-González NL, Wagner F, Aguilar-Diosdado M, Hervias-Vivancos B. Ultrasound evaluation of visceral fat and metabolic risk factors during early pregnancy. Obesity. 2007;15(9):2233–9.
121. Tocchio S, Kline-Fath B, Kanal E, Schmithorst VJ, Panigrahy A. MRI evaluation and safety in the developing brain. Semin Perinatol. 2015;39(2):73–104.
122. Norgan NG. Maternal body composition: methods for measuring short-term changes. J Biosoc Sci. 1992;24(3):367–77.
123. Keys A, Fidanza F, Karvonen MJ, Kimura N, Taylor HL. Indices of relative weight and obesity. J Chronic Dis. 1972;25(6):329–43.
124. Craig P, Samaras K, Freund J, Culton N, Halavatau V, Campbell L. BMI inaccurately reflects total body and abdominal fat in Tongans. Acta Diabetol. 2003;40(Suppl 1):S282–5.
125. Sewell MF, Huston-Presley L, Amini SB, Catalano PM. Body mass index: a true indicator of body fat in obese gravidas. J Reprod Med. 2007;52(10):907–11.
126. Lindsay CA, Huston L, Amini SB, Catalano PM. Longitudinal changes in the relationship between body mass index and percent body fat in pregnancy. Obstet Gynecol. 1997;89(3):377–82.
127. Gernand AD, Christian P, Schulze KJ, Shaikh S, Labrique AB, Shamim AA, et al. Maternal nutritional status in early pregnancy is associated with body water and plasma volume changes in a pregnancy cohort in rural Bangladesh. J Nutr. 2012;142(6):1109–15.
128. Contreras Campos ME, Rodríguez-Cervantes N, Reza-López S, Ávila-Esparza M, Chávez-Corral DV, Levario-Carrillo M. Body composition and newborn birthweight in pregnancies of adolescent and mature women: body composition in pregnant adolescents. Matern Child Nutr. 2015;11(2):164–72.
129. Dittmar M, Reber H. Validation of different bioimpedance analyzers for predicting cell mass against whole-body counting of potassium (40K) as a reference method. Am J Hum Biol. 2004;16(6):697–703.
130. Berlit S, Tuschy B, Stojakowits M, Weiss C, Leweling H, Suetterlin M, et al. Bioelectrical impedance analysis in pregnancy: reference ranges. In Vivo. 2013;27(6):851–4.
131. Lukaski HC, Siders WA, Nielsen EJ, Hall CB. Total body water in pregnancy: assessment by using bioelectrical impedance. Am J Clin Nutr. 1994;59(3):578–85.

132. Obuchowska A, Standyło A, Kimber-Trojnar Ż, Leszczyńska-Gorzelak B. The possibility of using bioelectrical impedance analysis in pregnant and postpartum women. Diagnostics. 2021;11(8):1370.
133. Kyle UG, Bosaeus I, De Lorenzo AD, Deurenberg P, Elia M, Manuel Gómez J, et al. Bioelectrical impedance analysis—part II: utilization in clinical practice. Clin Nutr. 2004;23(6):1430–53.
134. Trindade CR, Torloni MR, Mattar R, Sun SY. Good performance of bioimpedance in early pregnancy to predict preeclampsia. Pregnan Hypertens. 2021;26:24–30.
135. Liu Y, Liu J, Gao Y, Zheng D, Pan W, Nie M, et al. The body composition in early pregnancy is associated with the risk of development of gestational diabetes mellitus late during the second trimester. Diabetes Metab Syndr Obes Targets Ther. 2020;13:2367–74.
136. Bijlholt M, Maslin K, Ameye L, Shawe J, Bogaerts A, Devlieger R. Phase angle and bio-impedance values during the first year after delivery in women with previous excessive gestational weight gain: innovative data from the Belgian INTER-ACT study. Int J Environ Res Public Health. 2021;18(14):7482.
137. Lopez LB, Calvo EB, Poy MS, del Valle Balmaceda Y, Camera K. Changes in skinfolds and mid-upper arm circumference during pregnancy in Argentine women. Matern Child Nutr. 2011;7(3):253–62.
138. Kannieapan LM, Deussen AR, Grivell RM, Yelland L, Dodd JM. Developing a tool for obtaining maternal skinfold thickness measurements and assessing inter-observer variability among pregnant women who are overweight and obese. BMC Pregnan Childb. 2013;13(42):1–6.
139. Stevens-Simon C, Thureen P, Barrett J, Stamm E. Skinfold caliper and ultrasound assessments of change in the distribution of subcutaneous fat during adolescent pregnancy. Int J Obes Relat Metab Disord. 2001;25(9):1340.
140. Durnin J, Grant S, McKillop FM, Fitzgerald G. Energy requirements of pregnancy in Scotland. Lancet. 1987;330(8564):897–900.
141. Durnin J. Energy requirements of pregnancy: an integrated study in five countries: background and methods. Lancet. 1987;330(8564):895–6.
142. Durnin JVGA. Energy requirements of pregnancy. Diabetes. 1991;40(S2):152–6.
143. Sohlström A, Forsum E. Changes in total body fat during the human reproductive cycle as assessed by magnetic resonance imaging, body water dilution, and skinfold thickness: a comparison of methods. Am J Clin Nutr. 1997;66(6):1315–22.
144. Presley LH, Wong WW, Roman NM, Amini SB, Catalano PM. Anthropometric estimation of maternal body composition in late gestation. Obstet Gynecol. 2000;96(1):33–7.
145. Soltani H, Fraser RB. A longitudinal study of maternal anthropometric changes in normal weight, overweight and obese women during pregnancy and postpartum. Br J Nutr. 2000;84(01):95.
146. Taggart NR, Holliday RM, Billewicz WZ, Hytten FE, Thomson AM. Changes in skinfolds during pregnancy. Br J Nutr. 1967;21(02):439.
147. Ehrenberg HM, Huston-Presley L, Catalano PM. The influence of obesity and gestational diabetes mellitus on accretion and the distribution of adipose tissue in pregnancy. Am J Obstet Gynecol. 2003;189(4):944–8.
148. Villar J, Cogswell M, Kestler E, Castillo P, Menendez R, Repke JT. Effect of fat and fat-free mass deposition during pregnancy on birth weight. Am J Obstet Gynecol. 1992;167(5):1344–52.
149. Tuazon MAG, Van Raaij JMA, Hautvast JGA, Barba CVC. Energy requirements of pregnancy in the Philippines. Lancet. 1987;330(8568):1129–31.
150. Catalano PM, Roman-Drago NM, Amini SB, Sims EA. Longitudinal changes in body composition and energy balance in lean women with normal and abnormal glucose tolerance during pregnancy. Am J Obstet Gynecol. 1998;179(1):156–65.
151. Branco M, Santos-Rocha R, Vieira F, Silva M-R, Aguiar L, Veloso AP. Influence of body composition on gait kinetics throughout pregnancy and postpartum period. Scientifica. 2016;2016:1–12.

152. Lohman TG, Roche AF, Martorell R. Anthropometric standardization reference manual. Champaign, IL: Human Kinetics; 1988.
153. López LB, Calvo EB, Poy MS, del Valle Balmaceda Y, Cámera K. Changes in skinfolds and mid-upper arm circumference during pregnancy in Argentine women: skinfolds and MUAC changes in pregnant Argentine women. Matern Child Nutr. 2011;7(3):253–62.
154. Heyward V, Wagner DR. Applied body composition assessment. Champaign, IL: Human Kinetics; 2004.
155. Stewart A, Marfell-Jones M, Olds T, de Ridder H. International standards for anthropometric assessment. Lower Hutt: ISAK; 2011.
156. Bern C, Nathanail L. Is mid-upper-arm circumference a useful tool for screening in emergency settings? Lancet. 1995;345(8950):631–3.
157. Vijayaraghavan K, Sastry JG. The efficacy of arm circumference as a substitute for weight in assessment of protein-calorie malnutrition. Ann Hum Biol. 1976;3(3):229–33.
158. Lindtjorn B. Measuring acute malnutrition: a need to redefine cut-off points for arm circumference? Lancet. 1985;2(8466):1229–30.
159. Carter EP. Comparison of weight:height ratio and arm circumference in assessment of acute malnutrition. Arch Child. 1987;62(8):833–5.
160. Hall G, Chowdhury S, Bloem M. Use of mid-upper-arm circumference Z scores in nutritional assessment. Lancet. 1993;341(8858):1481.
161. Demanet JC, Rorive G, Samii K, Van Cauwenberge H, Smets P. Effect of weight on prevalence of hypertension, and its interaction with the arm circumference: Belgian Hypertension Committee epidemiological study. Clin Sci Mol Med Suppl. 1976;3:665s–7s.
162. Harries AD, Jones LA, Heatley RV, Newcombe RG, Rhodes J. Precision of anthropometric measurements: the value of mid-arm circumference. Clin Nutr. 1984;2(3-4):193–6. PubMed PMID: 16829433.
163. Olukoya AA. Identification of underweight women by measurement of the arm circumference. International journal of gynaecology and obstetrics: the official organ of the International Federation of Gynaecology and Obstetrics. 1990;31(3):231–5. PubMed PMID: 1969363.
164. Shao J-T, Yu J, Qi J-Q, Liu X-D. The relationship between neck circumference and pregnancy-induced hypertension in the third trimester pregnant women. Hypertens Pregnan. 2014;33(3):291–8.
165. He F, He H, Liu W, Lin J, Chen B, Lin Y, et al. Neck circumference might predict gestational diabetes mellitus in Han Chinese women: a nested case-control study. J Diabetes Investig. 2017;8(2):168–73.
166. Anglim B, O'Higgins A, Daly N, Farren M, Turner MJ. Maternal obesity and neck circumference. Ir Med J. 2015;108(6):179–80.
167. Clapp JF, Capeless EL. Neonatal morphometrics after endurance exercise during pregnancy. Am J Obstet Gynecol. 1990;163(6 Pt 1):1805–11.
168. Bisson M, Tremblay F, St-Onge O, Robitaille J, Pronovost E, Simonyan D, et al. Influence of maternal physical activity on infant's body composition: maternal activity and neonatal adiposity. Pediatr Obes. 2017;12:38–46.
169. Ferrari N, Bae-Gartz I, Bauer C, Janoschek R, Koxholt I, Mahabir E, et al. Exercise during pregnancy and its impact on mothers and offspring in humans and mice. J Dev Orig Health Dis. 2018;9(1):63–76.
170. Collings PJ, Farrar D, Gibson J, West J, Barber SE, Wright J. Associations of Pregnancy Physical Activity with Maternal Cardiometabolic Health, Neonatal delivery outcomes and body composition in a biethnic cohort of 7305 mother–child Pairs: the born in Bradford study. Sports Med. 2020;50(3):615–28.
171. Leppänen MH, Raitanen J, Husu P, Kujala UM, Tuominen PP, Vähä-Ypyä H, et al. Physical activity and body composition in children and their mothers according to mother's gestational diabetes risk: a seven-year follow-up study. Medicina. 2019;55(10):635.
172. ACOG. Physical activity and exercise during pregnancy and the postpartum period. Obstet Gynecol. 2020;135(4):e178–85.

173. Mottola MF, Davenport MH, Ruchat S-M, Davies GA, Poitras VJ, Gray CE, et al. 2019 Canadian guideline for physical activity throughout pregnancy. Br J Sports Med. 2018;52(21):1339–46.
174. Smith R, Reid H, Matthews A, Calderwood C, Knight M, Foster C. Infographic: physical activity for pregnant women. Br J Sports Med. 2018;52(8):532–3.
175. Gaston A, Cramp A. Exercise during pregnancy: a review of patterns and determinants. J Sci Med Sport. 2011;14(4):299–305.
176. Rogozińska E, Zamora J, Marlin N, Betrán AP, Astrup A, Bogaerts A, et al. Gestational weight gain outside the Institute of Medicine recommendations and adverse pregnancy outcomes: analysis using individual participant data from randomised trials. BMC Pregnan Childb. 2019;19(1):322.
177. Rasmussen KM, Yaktine AL, Institute of Medicine (U.S.). Weight gain during pregnancy: reexamining the guidelines. Washington, DC: National Academies Press; 2009. 854 p.
178. Pellonperä O, Koivuniemi E, Vahlberg T, Mokkala K, Tertti K, Rönnemaa T, et al. Body composition measurement by air displacement plethysmography in pregnancy: comparison of predicted versus measured thoracic gas volume. Nutrition. 2019;60:227–9.
179. Wasenius NS, Simonen M, Penttinen L, Salonen MK, Sandboge S, Eriksson JG. Effect of maternal weight during pregnancy on offspring muscle strength response to resistance training in late adulthood. Adv Med Sci. 2018;63(2):353–8.
180. Muhammad HFL, Pramono A, Rahman MN. The safety and efficacy of supervised exercise on pregnant women with overweight/obesity: a systematic review and meta-analysis of randomized controlled trials. Clin Obes. 2021;11(2):e12428. https://onlinelibrary.wiley.com/doi/10.1111/cob.12428. Accessed 20 Sep 2021.
181. da Silva SG, Ricardo LI, Evenson KR, Hallal PC. Leisure-time physical activity in pregnancy and maternal-child health: a systematic review and meta-analysis of randomized controlled trials and cohort studies. Sports Med. 2017;47(2):295–317.
182. Garnæs KK, Mørkved S, Salvesen KÅ, Salvesen Ø, Moholdt T. Exercise training during pregnancy reduces circulating insulin levels in overweight/obese women postpartum: secondary analysis of a randomised controlled trial (the ETIP trial). BMC Pregnan Childb. 2018;18(1):18. https://bmcpregnancychildbirth.biomedcentral.com/articles/10.1186/s12884-017-1653-5. Accessed 12 Jan 2018.
183. Thangaratinam S, Rogozinska E, Jolly K, Glinkowski S, Roseboom T, Tomlinson JW, et al. Effects of interventions in pregnancy on maternal weight and obstetric outcomes: meta-analysis of randomised evidence. BMJ. 2012;344(4):e2088.
184. The International Weight Management in Pregnancy (i-WIP) Collaborative Group. Effect of diet and physical activity based interventions in pregnancy on gestational weight gain and pregnancy outcomes: meta-analysis of individual participant data from randomised trials. BMJ. 2017;358:j3119.
185. Thangaratinam S, Rogozińska E, Jolly K, Glinkowski S, Duda W, Borowiack E, et al. Interventions to reduce or prevent obesity in pregnant women: a systematic review. Health Technol Assess. 2012;16(31):iii. https://www.journalslibrary.nihr.ac.uk/hta/hta16310/. Accessed 20 Sep 2021.
186. Choi J, Fukuoka Y, Lee JH. The effects of physical activity and physical activity plus diet interventions on body weight in overweight or obese women who are pregnant or in postpartum: a systematic review and meta-analysis of randomized controlled trials. Prev Med. 2013;56(6):351–64.
187. Phelan S, Phipps MG, Abrams B, Darroch F, Grantham K, Schaffner A, et al. Does behavioral intervention in pregnancy reduce postpartum weight retention? Twelve-month outcomes of the Fit for Delivery randomized trial. Am J Clin Nutr. 2014;99(2):302–11.
188. Sagedal L, Sanda B, Øverby N, Bere E, Torstveit M, Lohne-Seiler H, et al. The effect of prenatal lifestyle intervention on weight retention 12 months postpartum: results of the Norwegian Fit for Delivery randomised controlled trial. BJOG Int J Obstet Gynaecol. 2017;124(1):111–21.

189. Huberty JL, Buman MP, Leiferman JA, Bushar J, Hekler EB, Adams MA. Dose and timing of text messages for increasing physical activity among pregnant women: a randomized controlled trial. Transl Behav Med. 2017;7(2):212–23.
190. Hayman M, Reaburn P, Browne M, Vandelanotte C, Alley S, Short CE. Feasibility, acceptability and efficacy of a web-based computer-tailored physical activity intervention for pregnant women - the Fit4Two randomised controlled trial. BMC Pregnan Childb. 2017;17(1):96.
191. Willcox J, Wilkinson S, Lappas M, Ball K, Crawford D, McCarthy E, et al. A mobile health intervention promoting healthy gestational weight gain for women entering pregnancy at a high body mass index: the txt4two pilot randomised controlled trial. BJOG Int J Obstet Gynaecol. 2017;124(11):1718–28.
192. Choi J, Hyeon LJ, Vittinghoff E, Fukuoka Y. mHealth physical activity intervention: a randomized pilot study in physically inactive pregnant women. Matern Child Health J. 2016;20(5):1091–101.
193. Sandborg J, Söderström E, Henriksson P, Bendtsen M, Henström M, Leppänen MH, et al. Effectiveness of a smartphone app to promote healthy weight gain, diet, and physical activity during pregnancy (HealthyMoms): randomized controlled trial. JMIR MHealth UHealth. 2021;9(3):e26091.
194. Walker R, Bennett C, Blumfield M, Gwini S, Ma J, Wang F, et al. Attenuating pregnancy weight gain—what works and why: a systematic review and meta-analysis. Nutrients. 2018;10(7):944.
195. Tanner-Smith EE, Steinka-Fry KT, Gesell SB. Comparative effectiveness of group and individual prenatal care on gestational weight gain. Matern Child Health J. 2014;18(7):1711–20.
196. Agha M, Agha RA, Sandell J. Interventions to reduce and prevent obesity in pre-conceptual and pregnant women: a systematic review and meta-analysis. PLoS One. 2014;9(5):e95132. https://www.ncbi.nlm.nih.gov/pmc/articles/PMC4020754/. Accessed 14 May 2014.
197. Chiavaroli V, Hopkins SA, Derraik JGB, Biggs JB, Rodrigues RO, Brennan CH, et al. Exercise in pregnancy: 1-year and 7-year follow-ups of mothers and offspring after a randomized controlled trial. Sci Rep. 2018;8(1):12915.
198. Forsum E, Janerot-Sjöberg B, Löf M. MET-values of standardised activities in relation to body fat: studies in pregnant and non-pregnant women. Nutr Metab. 2018;15(1):45.
199. Clapp JF III, Kiess W. Effects of pregnancy and exercise on concentrations of the metabolic markers tumor necrosis factor α and leptin. Am J Obstet Gynecol. 2000;182(2):300–6.
200. van der Wijden CL, Delemarre-van de Waal HA, van Mechelen W, van Poppel MNM. The relationship between moderate-to-vigorous intensity physical activity and insulin resistance, insulin-like growth factor (IGF-1)-system 1, leptin and weight change in healthy women during pregnancy and after delivery. Clin Endocrinol. 2015;82(1):68–75.
201. Haas JS, Jackson RA, Fuentes-Afflick E, Stewart AL, Dean ML, Brawarsky P, et al. Changes in the health status of women during and after pregnancy. J Gen Intern Med. 2005;20(1):45–51.
202. Most J, Altazan AD, St. Amant M, Beyl RA, Ravussin E, Redman LM. Increased energy intake after pregnancy determines postpartum weight retention in women with obesity. J Clin Endocrinol Metab. 2020;105(4):e1601–11.
203. Caspersen CJ, Powell KE, Christenson GM. Physical activity, exercise, and physical fitness: definitions and distinctions for health-related research. Public Health Rep. 1985;100(2):126–31.
204. de Oliveria Melo AS, Silva JLP, Tavares JS, Barros VO, Leite DFB, Amorim MMR. Effect of a physical exercise program during pregnancy on uteroplacental and fetal blood flow and fetal growth: a randomized controlled trial. Obstet Gynecol. 2012;120(2, Part 1):302–10.
205. Price BB, Amini SB, Kappeler K. Exercise in pregnancy: effect on fitness and obstetric outcomes—a randomized trial. Med Sci Sports Exerc. 2012;44(12):2263–9.
206. Barakat R, Pelaez M, Montejo R, Refoyo I, Coteron J. Exercise throughout pregnancy does not cause preterm delivery: a randomized, controlled trial. J Phys Act Health. 2014;11(5):1012–7.
207. US. Department of health and Human Services. Physical activity guidelines for Americans. 2nd ed. Washington, DC: DHHS; 2018. p. 118.

208. WHO. WHO guidelines on physical activity and sedentary behaviour. Geneva: World Health Organization; 2020. https://www.who.int/publications/i/item/9789240015128.
209. Cordero Y, Mottola MF, Vargas J, Blanco M, Barakat R. Exercise is associated with a reduction in gestational diabetes mellitus. Med Sci Sports Exerc. 2015;47(7):1328–33.
210. Barakat R, Pelaez M, Cordero Y, Perales M, Lopez C, Coteron J, et al. Exercise during pregnancy protects against hypertension and macrosomia: randomized clinical trial. Am J Obstet Gynecol. 2016;214(5):649.e1–8.
211. Magro-Malosso ER, Saccone G, Di Tommaso M, Roman A, Berghella V. Exercise during pregnancy and risk of gestational hypertensive disorders: a systematic review and meta-analysis. Acta Obstet Gynecol Scand. 2017;96(8):921–31.
212. Muktabhant B, Lawrie TA, Lumbiganon P, Laopaiboon M. Diet or exercise, or both, for preventing excessive weight gain in pregnancy. Cochrane Database Syst Rev. 2015;(6):CD007145. https://doi.wiley.com/10.1002/14651858.CD007145.pub3. Accessed 20 Sep 2021.
213. Kołomańska-Bogucka D, Mazur-Bialy AI. Physical activity and the occurrence of postnatal depression—a systematic review. Medicina. 2019;55(9):560.
214. Nakamura A, van der Waerden J, Melchior M, Bolze C, El-Khoury F, Pryor L. Physical activity during pregnancy and postpartum depression: systematic review and meta-analysis. J Affect Disord. 2019;246:29–41.
215. Marín-Jiménez N, Acosta-Manzano P, Borges-Cosic M, Baena-García L, Coll-Risco I, Romero-Gallardo L, et al. Association of self-reported physical fitness with pain during pregnancy: the GESTAFIT project. Scand J Med Sci Sports. 2019;29:1022.
216. Seneviratne SN, McCowan LME, Cutfield WS, Derraik JGB, Hofman PL. Exercise in pregnancies complicated by obesity: achieving benefits and overcoming barriers. Am J Obstet Gynecol. 2015;212(4):442–9.
217. Wang S-M, Dezinno P, Maranets I, Berman MR, Caldwell-Andrews AA, Kain ZN. Low back pain during pregnancy: prevalence, risk factors, and outcomes. Obstet Gynecol. 2004;104(1):65–70.
218. Tennfjord MK, Engh ME, Bø K. The influence of early exercise postpartum on pelvic floor muscle function and prevalence of pelvic floor dysfunction 12 months postpartum. Phys Ther. 2020;100(9):1681–9.
219. Mota P, Pascoal AG, Carita AI, Bø K. The immediate effects on inter-rectus distance of abdominal crunch and drawing-in exercises during pregnancy and the postpartum period. J Orthop Sports Phys Ther. 2015;45(10):781–8.
220. Sancho MF, Pascoal AG, Mota P, Bø K. Abdominal exercises affect inter-rectus distance in postpartum women: a two-dimensional ultrasound study. Physiotherapy. 2015;101(3):286–91.

Biomechanical Adaptations of Gait in Pregnancy: Implications for Physical Activity and Exercise

5

Marco Branco, Rita Santos-Rocha, Liliana Aguiar, Filomena Vieira, and António Prieto Veloso

M. Branco (✉)
Sport Sciences School of Rio Maior - ESDRM, Polytechnic Institute of Santarém, Rio Maior, Portugal

Laboratory of Biomechanics and Functional Morphology, Interdisciplinary Centre for the Study of Human Performance - CIPER, Faculty of Human Kinetics – FMH, University of Lisbon, Cruz Quebrada-Dafundo, Portugal
e-mail: marcobranco@esdrm.ipsantarem.pt

R. Santos-Rocha
Sport Sciences School of Rio Maior - ESDRM, Polytechnic Institute of Santarém, Rio Maior, Portugal

Laboratory of Biomechanics and Functional Morphology, Interdisciplinary Centre for the Study of Human Performance - CIPER, Faculty of Human Kinetics - FMH, University of Lisbon, Lisbon, Portugal
e-mail: ritasantosrocha@esdrm.ipsantarem.pt

L. Aguiar
Laboratory of Biomechanics and Functional Morphology, Interdisciplinary Centre for the Study of Human Performance - CIPER, Faculty of Human Kinetics – FMH, University of Lisbon, Cruz Quebrada-Dafundo, Portugal

European University (Universidade Europeia), Lisbon, Portugal

School of Health Technology – ESTeSL, Polytechnic Institute of Lisbon, Lisbon, Portugal
e-mail: LAGUIAR@fmh.ulisboa.pt

F. Vieira · A. P. Veloso
Laboratory of Biomechanics and Functional Morphology, Interdisciplinary Centre for the Study of Human Performance - CIPER, Faculty of Human Kinetics – FMH, University of Lisbon, Cruz Quebrada-Dafundo, Portugal
e-mail: fvieira@fmh.ulisboa.pt; apveloso@fmh.ulisboa.pt

R. Santos-Rocha (ed.), *Exercise and Physical Activity During Pregnancy and Postpartum*, https://doi.org/10.1007/978-3-031-06137-0_5

Abstract

During pregnancy, women experience several changes in the body's physiology, morphology, and hormonal system. These changes may affect the balance and body stability and can cause discomfort and pain. The adaptations of the musculoskeletal system due to morphological changes during pregnancy are not fully understood. Few studies clarify the biomechanical changes of gait that occur during pregnancy and in postpartum. The purpose of this chapter is to analyze the available evidence on the biomechanical adaptations of gait that occur throughout pregnancy and in postpartum, specifically regarding the temporal, spatial, kinematic, and kinetic parameters of gait and balance.

The highlights of this chapter are the following: (1) pregnancy requires biomechanical adjustments as shown by several publications in the last 20 years; (2) adaptations due to pregnancy are recognized to provide safety and stability; (3) most studies performed a temporal, spatial and kinematic analysis, and few studies performed a kinetic analysis; (4) there is lack of consistency in the results of biomechanical studies due to different methodological approaches; (5) the adaptation strategies to the anatomical and physiological changes throughout pregnancy are still unclear, particularly in a longitudinal perspective and regarding kinetic parameters; (6) the main biomechanical adaptations during pregnancy are gait speed reduction, longer double-support time, and increased step width, and ground reaction forces decrease; (7) there is lack of information regarding the effects of physical activity and exercise, risk of falls, and low back pain on the biomechanical adjustments; and (8) exercise adaptations can be provided in order to increase adherence, safety, and effectiveness.

Keywords

Pregnancy · Postpartum · Biomechanics · Loading · Gait · Balance · Exercise

5.1 Introduction

In the last two decades, the literature has been supporting the recommendation to initiate or continue exercise in most pregnancies [1–3]. Several benefits of physical activity are evidence-based [4], and pregnant women with absence of medical or obstetric complications, are advised to accumulate 30 min or more of moderate-intensity activity per day on most, if not all, days of the week [2]. Moreover, an increase in sedentary behavior during pregnancy has been associated with adverse perinatal health outcomes [2, 5, 6].

Pregnancy is not only a window of opportunity, but also a remarkable period for the adoption of an active and healthy lifestyle since women are more focused on her own health [2, 7]. However, it is also a risk period for sedentariness, musculoskeletal disorders, and other discomforts [8–17].

Pregnancy leads to several changes in the pregnant physiology [18] (see Chap. 3), which in these days carry an increased risk and are potentially vulnerable to severe SARS-CoV-2 infections [19]. In addition, many other changes are felt during pregnancy, namely, body's anatomy [20], body composition and morphology (see Chap. 4), hormonal [21], and musculoskeletal systems of women [20, 22]. Over 38–42 weeks, women experience several changes which are especially visible in increased weight (10–15 kg) [23], an adaptation of the musculoskeletal system, and skeletal alignment. The maternal weight gain, the growth in size and weight of the fetus, and the increase in maternal abdominal and breasts weight and volume lead to an increase in lumbar lordosis, resulting in a shift in the woman's center of gravity, in the anterior direction until the end of the second trimester, and then in the posterior direction during the third trimester [24, 25].

One of the aspects that most influence the musculoskeletal system is the increase in maternal weight. The weight gain during pregnancy is related to several factors, such as the amount of blood, the increased volume of the breasts, and the increased fat mass and extracellular fluid [26]. The fetal tissues, the placenta, and the amniotic fluid are related to the weight gain of the fetus [23]. The variation in weight gain during pregnancy is related to the accretion of protein, fat, water, and minerals, not only in maternal components (blood, mammary and uterine tissues, body composition) but also in the fetal components (fetus, placenta, and amniotic fluid).

The ideal weight gain during pregnancy is related to the women's weight or body mass index (BMI) before pregnancy. The weight gain may range between 12.5 and 18 kg for women underweight (BMI < 18.5 kg/m^2); between 11.5 and 16 kg for women with normal weight ($18.5 \leq$ BMI < 25 kg/m^2); between 7 and 11.5 kg for women who are overweight ($25 \leq$ BMI < 30 kg/m^2); and between 5 and 9 kg for obese women [23]. Further explanation on this topic can be found in Chap. 4.

Anatomical adaptations during pregnancy are related to the 10–15 kg increase in body mass, the enormous size augmentation of the uterus and breasts, and the rib cage expanding laterally [20]. Additionally, the alterations in the hormonal context will influence the musculoskeletal system [21] leading to ligament laxity.

Maternal morphological adaptations to pregnancy are more evident in the trunk, due to enlarged uterus and breasts. Specifically it is referred an increment of abdominal girth and anterior–posterior [22] and transverse trunk breadths [27]. These dimensional increases are also accompanied by adaptations in abdominal muscle structure with increased abdominal muscle length and Diastasis Recti Abdominis [28].

The physical symptoms are common in pregnancy and are predominantly associated with normal physiological changes that occur during this time. However, most women experience some degree of musculoskeletal discomfort [7]. The enlarged uterus will anteriorly displace the center of mass which, in turn, lengthens the moment arm of the pelvic stabilizers, increasing stress in the stabilizers of the pelvic girdle and spine [20]. The changes in spinal curves and pelvic posture are related to increased lumbar lordosis and thoracic and cervical kyphosis. These adaptations will, in turn, stretch the abdominal muscles [20].

There are many anatomical changes during pregnancy that could potentially lead to gait alterations, and those alterations may contribute to musculoskeletal overuse conditions such as back and lower limb pain [29]. Low back pain is more prevalent in pregnant women (25%) than in the general population (6.3%); however, only the pelvic girdle pain (a subgroup of low back pain) is associated with pregnancy [30]. Low back pain is one of the most prevalent conditions during pregnancy [31]. In fact, Mogren and Pohjanen [32] and more recently Ng et al. [33] point that around 80% of women have complaints about low back pain during pregnancy, and of which 40% maintain complaints in the postpartum period. Aldabe et al. [34] stated that the onset of low back pain suggests that there is more influence of biomechanical factors than hormonal adaptations. Further explanation of these topics (low back pain and pelvic girdle pain) can be found in Chap. 6.

Several authors [35, 36] suggested that body composition is associated with alterations of the gait pattern. Thus, it is important to characterize the changes in morphology and gait pattern, which will affect the functionality of the pregnant women.

The changes in human foot morphology and foot function occur throughout the whole life and the foot has to bear loads during all kinds of bipedal locomotion. Furthermore, disease-dependent modifications can also have an influence on plantar loading and it is reasonable to assume that foot function will undergo changes in life [37]. Nevertheless, during pregnancy, alterations in the morphology of the foot were found in different measures, except for the length of the foot [38]. In other study, Varol et al. [39] found that foot pain is related to changes in the foot morphology observed by an increased foot area, force distributions in midfoot and forefoot, contact pressure in midfoot, and force-time integral in midfoot.

Other less visible changes are the increased joint laxity and change in the center of gravity. Altogether, these changes affect the balance and body stability and can cause discomfort and pain [40]. The hormonal and anatomic alterations lead to lower limb adaptations as a kinetic chain, in order to enhance postural stability [20].

Several authors focused on the possible alterations of gait during pregnancy. Such alterations may compromise the dynamic stability of walking and balance. On the other hand, a more variable gait pattern suggests poorer neuromuscular control, possibly leading to a fall [41].

Figure 5.1 shows the main anatomical, morphologic, and musculoskeletal adaptations that occur during pregnancy.

Thus, it is of utmost importance the knowledge about the biomechanical adaptations during the pregnancy period and its consequences on women' gait and physical activity ability.

The purpose of this chapter is to analyze the available evidence on the biomechanical adaptations of gait that occur throughout pregnancy and in postpartum, specifically with regard to the temporal, spatial, kinematic, and kinetic parameters of gait, as well as the potential implications for exercise prescription.

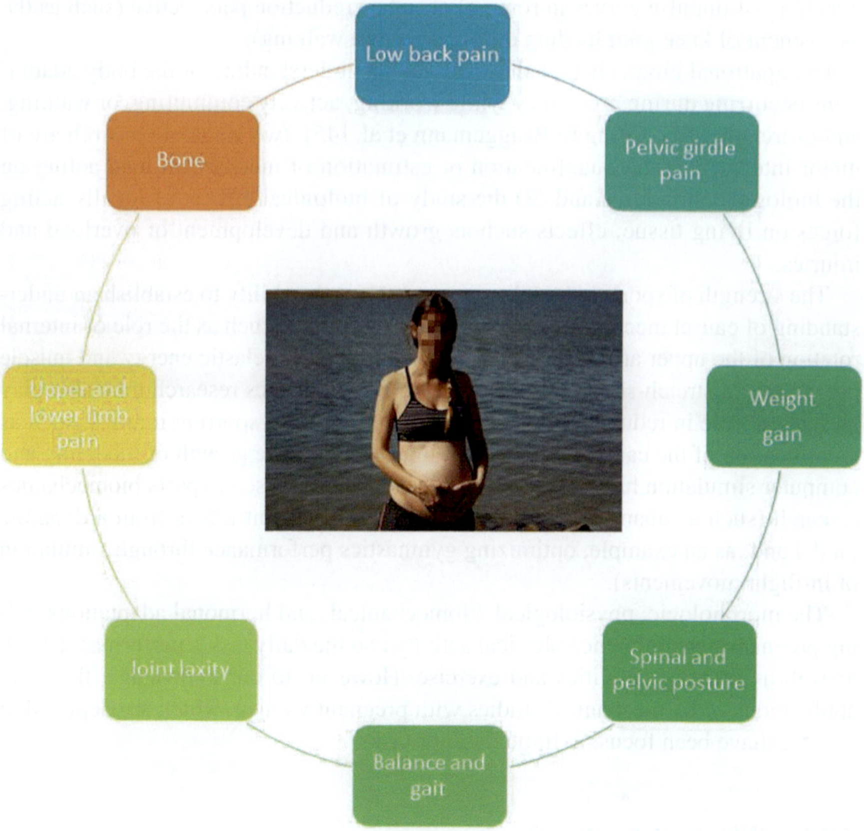

Fig. 5.1 Main anatomical, morphologic, and musculoskeletal adaptations that occur during pregnancy

5.2 Understanding the Biomechanical Variables

Biomechanics is one of the disciplines in the field of Human Movement and Exercise Science, and can be defined as the study of the motion and causes of motion of living things [3]; as the science that examines forces acting upon and within a biological structure and effects produced by such forces [42]; or as the study of the structure and function of biological systems by means of the methods of mechanics [43].

According to Elliott [44], biomechanics can be divided into three broad categories from a research perspective: (1) Clinical biomechanics involves research in the areas of gait, neuromuscular control, tissue mechanics, and movement evaluation during rehabilitation from either injury or disease; (2) Occupational biomechanics typically involves research in the areas of ergonomics and human growth or morphology as they influence movement; (3) Research in sports biomechanics may take the form of describing movement from a performance enhancement (such as matching of impulse curves in rowing) or injury reduction perspective (such as the assessment of knee joint loading during downhill walking).

Occupational biomechanics may provide an understanding of the body adaptations occurring during pregnancy while working, actively commuting, or walking, and exercising. According to Brüggemann et al. [45], two areas of research are of major interest: (1) the quantification or estimation of mechanical load acting on the biological structures and (2) the study of biological effects of locally acting forces on living tissue; effects such as growth and development or overload and injuries.

The strength of sports biomechanics research is the ability to establish an understanding of causal mechanisms for selected movements (such as the role of internal rotation of the upper arm in striking, and the influence of elastic energy and muscle pre-stretch in stretch-shorten-cycle actions). Biomechanics research may also play an integral role in reducing the incidence and severity of sporting injuries, such as identification of the causes of knee joint injuries [44]. The growth of modeling and computer simulation has further enhanced the potential use of sports biomechanics research (such as quantification of the knee joint ligament forces from a dynamic model and, as an example, optimizing gymnastics performance through simulation of in-flight movements).

The morphologic, physiological, biomechanical, and hormonal adaptations during pregnancy can influence physical activity and the daily task's performance [46], as well as sporting activities and exercise. However, to our knowledge, the main applications of biomechanical studies with pregnant women, which are depicted in Fig. 5.2, have been focusing limited motor tasks.

5.2.1 Why Gait Analysis?

Gait analysis or motion analysis of human gait, as one branch of biomechanics, has developed since early studies in the late 1900s of the twentieth century. Motion analysis has been extended during the past two decades to investigate many other activities in addition to gait analysis.

Nevertheless, one of the most studied human movements is gait, once it is the basic natural form of locomotion and it is used throughout the life. Thus, since childhood to elderly, walking is the functional way of moving from one place to another. With growing, the human body will change anatomically, going through different stages of growth and in adulthood, there is a possible stabilization of its development. From another perspective, as the mechanics of gait throughout life is very well known, this task can be considered as a reference for the study of mechanical changes that occur in different pathologies or situations, namely in the special phases of life.

The human body can percept and react in order to adapt to various kinds of environments, like stairs, different surfaces or obstacles. The lower limb segments optimize the energy conservation to exhibit a normal kinematical pattern. And this depends on muscle activation, which is responsible for producing a certain angular

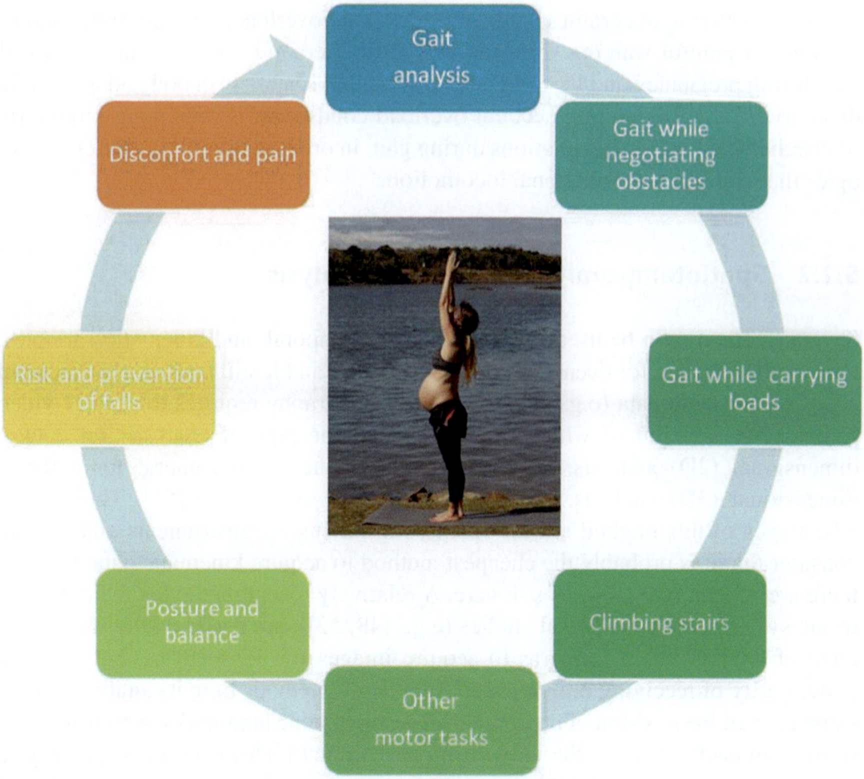

Fig. 5.2 Main applications of biomechanics studies with pregnant women

joint displacement in order to provide an accurate and necessary range of motion [47]. Biomechanical methods, as the three-dimensional motion capture synchronized with the ground reaction forces platforms, can be used in order to obtain joint kinematic and kinetic data, which represent a pattern to be interpreted quantitatively or qualitatively. When pathologies occur, the human body muscular efficiency is compromised, and compensatory reactions of the adjacent segments can happen, resulting in a mixture of normal and abnormal motions, compromising the functional versatility and increasing energy costs [47]. These pathologies can be detected by analyzing curve patterns of certain biomechanical parameters as the joints range of motion or ground reaction forces produced by the impact between the feet and a surface. In biomechanics, populations with a specific characteristic have particular attention regarding gait analysis. The human body can suffer physical changes as consequences of a physiological process, which in turn may affect locomotion [48]. Pregnancy, as a natural and physiological process, produces in women changes involving the motor system. Walking is a common way of physical exercise during pregnancy and daily physical activity during almost 40 weeks that can cause injuries by overuse of certain specific muscles, joint overload, asymmetries, uncomfortable, or painful walking. There is very little literature on the biomechanics of gait during pregnancy and lack of consensus among scientists in body adaptation in this period [48]. Taking into account overload conditions, is important to quantify biomechanical load and adaptations during gait, in order to prevent or detect pathologies that compromise functional locomotion.

5.2.2 Spatiotemporal and Kinematic Analysis

Several methods can be used to collect spatial, temporal, and kinematic variables. One method known for decades is the videography and it still is used to collect and analyze kinematic data (e.g., [29, 49, 50]). Videography requires the use of video cameras, the amount of which will depend on the type of analysis: for a two-dimensional (2D) analysis, it is only required one video camera; for a three-dimensional (3D) analysis, at least two cameras are needed [51]. The biggest advantages of this method are the easiness in having the instruments and we can consider that it is probably the cheapest method to acquire kinematic data, because there are several free analysis software. A relatively recent method is the optoelectronic systems, used in several studies (e.g., [48, 52]), are based on the same principle of having several cameras to acquire images for 3D analysis, but with the particularity of receiving only infrared light. Both methods base its analysis on the estimation of the position of predefined anatomical bone landmarks, which are digitized from each image of the video from each camera. However, the capability to digitize the landmark with high precision in a regular video image or in an infrared image can be quite different. The standard error in videography is around 3 cm, while in optoelectronic systems, the error might stand below 1 mm. One factor that also contributes to the error is the calibration method. In videography, calibration is based in the digitalization of a structure with well-known dimensions, of at least four coplanar points for 2D analysis, or at least six noncoplanar points for 3D analysis, in order to associate the real coordinates to the digital coordinates in the video image. Then the reconstruction of the trajectory is made through the Direct Linear Transformation (DLT) algorithm [53]. In optoelectronic systems, the 3D space is calibrated by wand type, with a wand of an exact length which is moved randomly across the recorded field. A static trial enables segment reconstruction and allows defining the dimensions, joint centers, and the segment coordinate system.

Kinematic variables are divided into linear and angular and are based on time and position of collected markers. Many variables can be computed, including displacement, velocity, and acceleration, either linear or angular, for segments, joints, and center of mass. Each of these has its own pattern, which can be analyzed qualitatively, by observing the data curve, or quantitatively through a detailed selection of values that characterize the time series of values, namely the mean, standard deviation, maximum and minimum peaks, amplitudes, and others. For more details about the kinematic methods and algorithms, further readings of Bartlett [54], Richards [55], Robertson et al. [56], and Winter [57] are suggested.

5.2.3 Kinetic Analysis and Biomechanical Loading

5.2.3.1 Ground Reaction Forces

Ground reaction forces (GRF) reflect the acceleration of the total body center of gravity (CG) and can be obtained using a force plate (Fig. 5.3). Force plates have been one of the most important measuring devices used in biomechanics for many years for quantifying external forces during human and animal locomotion [58]. GRF is most accurately measured with one of the proven force platforms available commercially, such as the Kistler force platform (Kistler AG, Winterthur, Switzerland) which utilizes piezoelectric transducers and the AMTI force platform (Advanced Mechanical Technology, Inc, Watertown, MA) which uses strain gauge technology [59].

Typically, the gait cycle is defined as the amount of time from the initial foot contact with the ground to the next instant when the same foot starts the following initial contact [60]. As a cyclical locomotor task, gait provides several impacts on the ground. Ground reaction forces produce joint reaction and moments of force, and some internal forces like bone-on-bone, ligament, and muscle forces [57]. To analyze human gait, ground reaction forces and motion data are measured, synchronized in time. Both parameters are used to calculate other variables, as joint moments which are calculated by the inverse dynamics method and add more information about the stress imposed in the joints and the necessary muscle control [47]. When GRF are unobtainable, simulation models can predict these data and can add more information for the understanding of interactions of the musculoskeletal system with the physical environment, such as the foot floor contact. In a clinical context, applied to the pregnant population, this methodology can be important to provide

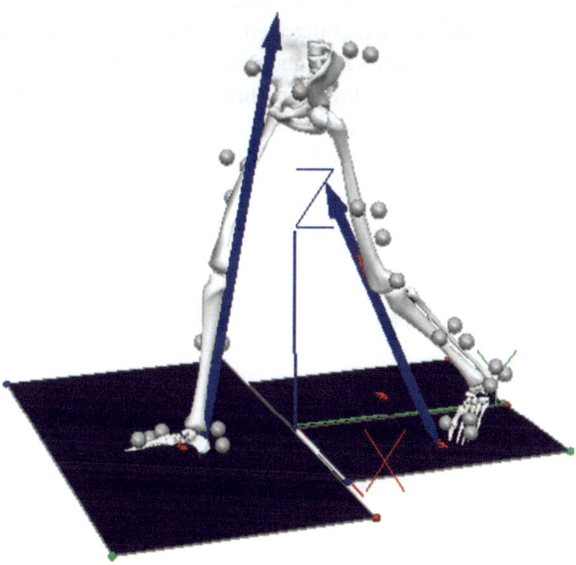

Fig. 5.3 Representation of the biomechanical model of the lower limb, in contact with the force platforms

more important biomechanical information that could not be collected in another way and to monitoring the foot contact during the pregnancy.

The GRF acts at a point usually called the center of pressure (CoP), under the area of the foot. Like the weight and most other contact forces, GRF is actually a distributed force that acts over the entire contact surface. As a force, the GRF is a vector quantity that can most conveniently be defined in terms of the magnitude, direction, and point of application of its resultant [59].

Most force platforms give a full three-dimensional description of the GRF vector. The sign convention is the one where the GRF is positive upwards, forwards, and to the right [59, 61]. It is important not to lose sight that the vertical, anterior–posterior, and mediolateral GRF are three components of a single force that changes in magnitude, direction, and point of application, during the course of support [59]. The description of these three components is useful in motion analysis.

The anterior–posterior (FX) GRF trace from the right foot shows "braking" during the first half of the stance phase and "propulsion" during the second half, concerning walking. The left foot shows the same pattern, but with the direction of the lateral force reversed [61]. Thus, the anterior–posterior component is first a braking force to mid-stance, followed by propulsion, and usually represents a sine curve with an amplitude of 25% of the body weight (BW), as shown in Whittle [61].

The lateral or mediolateral GRF (FY) is of lower magnitude in most situations and relates to balance during walking. This component of force initially acts in the medial direction with a magnitude of 10% BW or less and then acts laterally during the balance of stance phase [62]. The mediolateral component has been studied to better understand ankle instability. This lateral component of force is generally very small. It is the smallest of the three components and falls in the neighborhood of 10% to 20% BW. As an example, if a runner is to maintain a straight-line running path, the resultant side-to-side GRF impulse elicited during right and left foot contacts will have to equal zero when averaged over several footfalls [59].

Considering each component of the GRF separately (Fig. 5.4), the largest is the vertical component (FZ) and accounts for the acceleration of the body's center of mass in the vertical direction during walking. The vertical force shows a characteristic double hump, which results from an upward acceleration of the center of gravity during early stance, a reduction in downward force as the body "flies" over the leg in mid-stance, and a second peak due to deceleration, as the downward motion is checked in late stance [61]. The vertical curve of the GRF is sometimes called the "M

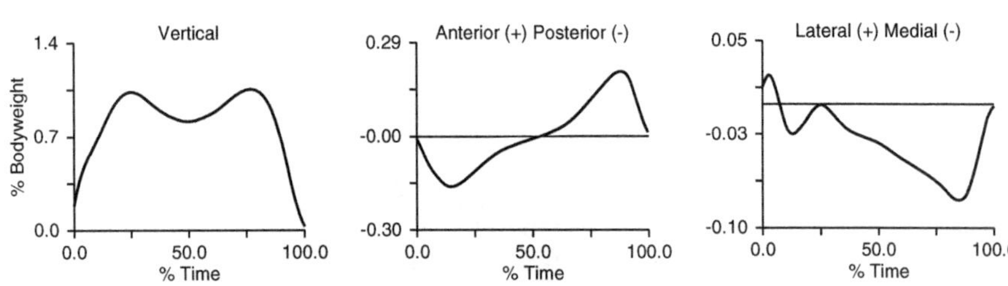

Fig. 5.4 Vertical, anterior–posterior, and medial-lateral ground reaction forces, during an entire gait cycle

curve" because it resembles that letter. During the first 100 ms, the GRF goes to a maximum of 120% BW during the double stance phase. During single stance phase, the vertical GRF drops to about 80% BW or for the more dynamic walker to 60–70% BW. When the acceleration is positive, the GRF must be greater than BW. The positive acceleration occurs during double stance when the center of mass is at its lowest point. The vertical component has received the greatest attention from a research standpoint. Because of its magnitude, it dominates the resultant GRF and can barely be distinguished from that of the resultant if one is superimposed on the other [59].

The true value of the force platform is only appreciated when the GRF data are combined with kinematics data. This combination provides a much more complete description of the gait than either by itself, and permits the calculation of joint moments of force and powers [61]. Image analysis can provide kinematics data. Although describing motion can be an end in itself, the most important reason for collecting kinematics data is to derive various kinetic quantities [56].

5.2.3.2 Biomechanical Loading

One particular source of loading on the body is the ground reaction force [56]; thus, GRFs are a common indicator of external biomechanical load. The major biological effects of forces include changes in the development of biological tissue and transportation of nutrients through the human body [63]. The major mechanical effects produced by forces include the ability to accelerate a mass and the ability to deform a material [63].

The effects of biomechanical loading applied to the Musculoskeletal System can be either biopositives or bionegatives. Bionegative effects can result from situations of insufficient loading or from excessive loading. Before maturity, insufficient loading might result in cases of abnormal growing and development of the musculoskeletal system. In the adult, insufficient loading might result in a decrease of functional capacity. Excessive loading before maturity can also lead to abnormal growing and development and injuries, independently of age. The biopositive effects before maturity include the harmonious growing of the musculoskeletal system and the increase of functional capacity in all ages [64].

Despite not yet defined, it has been suggested that there is an optimal window of loading that healthy individuals should maintain and that loading above this window presents the risk of injury [42]. The information derived from GRF measures is also important in gait research for diagnosing lower limb problems and injury prevention [63]. The intensity of skeletal exercise has been suggested to be defined by the loads applied to the bone [65]. Based upon the literature and preliminary laboratory studies, high skeletal loading intensity has been defined as ground reaction forces of greater than four times the body weight (BW), moderate intensity as 2–4 BW, and low intensity as GRF less than 2 BW [66]. Nevertheless, the result of the loading on the body depends on three factors: the magnitude of the force, the rate at which the force is applied, and the repetition of load application [56].

Biomechanical studies, although in small number, can contribute to improving knowledge about the effect of the anatomical and functional changes on the musculoskeletal system, which occurs during pregnancy and influence pregnant motor tasks and daily physical activity. The laboratory setting provides accurate data and more kinematical and kinetic data, necessary for biomechanical modeling. However, data collecting takes longer time and the pregnant women are required to visit the laboratory several times.

5.2.3.3 Plantar Pressure

Plantar pressure is reflected by the ability to measure the force exerted by area of the foot, which allows detecting excessive pressures in each region of the foot and, in turn, allows preventing tissue damage [55]. Pressure is therefore a scalar quantity, and as such is not dependent on direction but instead of magnitude [67]. Plantar pressure also shows the shape of the foot contact with the ground.

Pressure is commonly measured in gait analysis by either using force plates or in-shoe pressure monitor devices [68]. Pedography is an accurate and reliable pressure distribution measuring system for monitoring local loads between the foot (Fig. 5.5) and the shoe or the floor in the field context [69]. Pressure systems also allow calculating the vertical component of GRF.

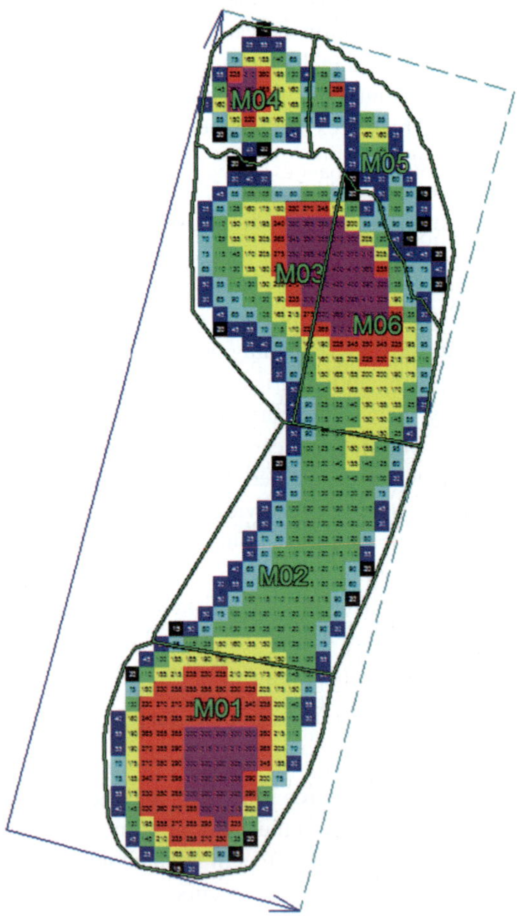

Fig. 5.5 Example of plantar pressure distribution by six foot regions: M01—hindfoot (heel); M02—midfoot; M03—medial forefoot; M04—hallux; M05—toes; M06—lateral forefoot

The use of a pressure platform (e.g., Novel EMED-X system, Münich, Germany) placed on the floor, is quite easy, allows obtaining several biomechanical parameters of barefoot gait, and enables its use in exercise and health centers. In-shoe plantar pressure measurement systems are capable of measuring pressures at the interface between the shoe and the foot. This equipment can be used in clinical, rehabilitation, and sports fields in order to assess patterns of forces between the agent and the ground [69, 70].

Compared to force platforms, pressure insoles have the advantage of measuring the plantar pressure directly applied to the foot during less constrained tasks and may be used to assess other parameters like force distribution along the plantar region or between right and left foot, including outside the laboratory, with relative ease.

The information derived from podobarometric measures is also important in gait and posture research for diagnosing lower limb problems and injury prevention [71–74]. Several factors have been associated with high levels of plantar pressure (i.e., peak pressure and pressure-time integral) generated during gait, such as increased body weight [75], foot structure (arch type) [76], foot pain and risk of falls [77], active diabetic foot ulcers [78], and walking strategy [79]. In recent years, some studies have been published that verify the effect of exercise intervention on plantar pressure variables, namely in the elderly [35, 80, 81], in recreational runners [82], patients with stroke [83], and in obese children [84]. However, to our knowledge, there are still no studies that assess the effect of exercise intervention on plantar pressure of pregnant or postpartum women.

Pregnant women' feet undergo morphological changes with the advancement of pregnancy and postpartum. Thus, it is important to understand the structural changes of the foot during pregnancy and postpartum because these changes may alter the foot biomechanics and the plantar pressure pattern. However, the current literature on plantar pressure in pregnancy is sparse.

5.3 Biomechanical Gait and Balance Adaptations During Pregnancy

So far, there are nine review studies in the literature, whose main objective was to research the biomechanical changes that occur in women during pregnancy and in postpartum. Although the objective is similar, the focus of the reviews differed to verify the complex adaptations in the temporal [85–91], spatial [85, 87–91], kinematic [85–87, 89, 91, 92], kinetic [87, 89, 93], and plantar pressure [85, 86, 88, 89, 92] parameters of gait, and also for the static and dynamic parameters of balance [85, 86, 91], posture [85, 86, 91–93], and morphology [85, 88, 91, 93] of pregnant women. Regarding the biomechanical measurement methods for this population, only two reviews focus on the methodological differences between the studies, considering the problems that arise from there for the correct comparison of results [90, 93]. In addition to these reviews, another study was found that identify the risk factors for accidental falls during pregnancy [94], in which the authors identify 13 intrinsic risk factors and 11 extrinsic risk factors, highlighting the physical activity maternity support bells and education as a negative risk factor or possible fall prevention strategy.

Since the last edition, several original research papers have been published considering biomechanical changes of gait and balance, considering women during pregnancy and in the postpartum period. In order to complete the review, with studies published after October 2017, the search was replicated via PubMed, web of Science and Scopus, in August 2021, that match the following criteria: (1) subjects were healthy pregnant and postpartum women; (2) studies were performed by means of optoelectronic systems, image analysis, force and plantar pressure systems; (3) outcome measures related to biomechanical variables of gait including, spatial (stride length, step length and stride width), temporal (single and double support time), kinematic (velocity and cadence), and kinetic (plantar pressure, ground reaction forces, joint moment and joint power) parameters; (4) any observational and controlled trials that evaluated biomechanical variables of gait; and (5) papers published after 1997 in the English, Portuguese, Spanish, and French languages.

The following combination of terms was used: "pregnancy" and "gait," "walking," and "biomechanics" (restriction: humans). Papers were excluded if they were reviews, congress abstracts, or letters. Papers were first selected by reading the titles and abstracts, followed by reading the full text. The final analysis included 38 studies published between 1997 and 2021. Table 5.1 shows the biomechanical studies published in the last 24 years, listed by chronological order of publication, regarding authors, sample size, data collection phases, sample mean age, outcome variables, and biomechanical instruments used.

5.3.1 General Characteristics of the Biomechanical Studies with Pregnant and Postpartum Women

Table 5.1 shows the information about the publications focused on the biomechanical analysis of gait in women during pregnancy and in the postpartum period. The first paper considered in this analysis was published in 1997. The sample sizes across the studies ranged from 2 to 73. All studies reported the mean age and standard deviation, with exception for the study of Catena, Wolcott [127]. Different periods of pregnancy were analyzed. Majority of the studies were designed to observe the walking pattern throughout two or three trimesters of pregnancy [50, 52, 96–99, 102–106, 109–118, 120, 121, 123, 124, 126, 127], and some of them also described the walking pattern after delivery [29, 48–50, 52, 99, 100, 102, 109, 114, 115, 118, 124]. Almost all authors considered the third trimester of pregnancy. Control group was usually observed only once, except for the study by Sunaga et al. [107], where the group was registered twice within 16 weeks, and the analysis of Gilleard [50] where two studies of non-pregnant were carried out within 32 weeks.

Researchers performed different approaches in the selection of experimental groups: some of them focused on the observation of the same group of women

Table 5.1 Biomechanical studies published in the last two decades, listed by chronological order of publication, including authors, sample size, data collection phases, sample mean age, outcome variables, and biomechanical instruments used

Authors	Sample size (*N*) and groups	Data collection phase(s) of pregnancy and postpartum	Sample mean age (years)	Biomechanical outcome variables	Biomechanical instruments
Nyska et al. [95]	28 pregnant	…	28 years	…	EMED System
	28 non-pregnant				
Foti et al. [29]	2—Before pregnancy	Third trimester	32 years	Time and distance	60 Hz video cameras
	15—Third trimester	1 year postpartum		Kinematic	1 AMTI force platform
	13—Postpartum			Kinetic	
Goldberg et al. [96]	13 pregnant	First trimester	…	Plantar Pressure	…
		Second trimester			
		Third trimester			
Huang et al. [97]	10 experimental group	First trimester	…	Joint Moments	EVA motion analysis system
	10 control group	Second trimester			
		Third trimester			
Lymbery and Gilleard [49]	13 pregnant	Third trimester	27.8 ± 1.2	Spatial	60 Hz EVA motion analysis system
		8 weeks postpartum		Temporal	1 Kistler force platform
				Ground Reaction Forces	

(continued)

Table 5.1 (continued)

Authors	Sample size (N) and groups	Data collection phase(s) of pregnancy and postpartum	Sample mean age (years)	Biomechanical outcome variables	Biomechanical instruments
Ribas and Guirro [98]	15—First trimester	First trimester	23.3 ± 25.5	Peak contact pressure, width support distance, contact area	Plantar pressure analysis Matscan5.1
	15—Second trimester	Second trimester			40 Hz
	15—Third trimester	Third trimester			
	15—Non-pregnant				
Carpes et al. [99]	7 pregnant	Second trimester	23–35	Spatial	60 Hz Video cameras
		Third trimester		Temporal	
		Until fourth month postpartum		3D Kinematics	
Gaymer et al. [100]	22 pregnant	38 weeks	…	Mean and maximum plantar pressures	Plantar pressure analysis (Fscan system)
	20 non-pregnant	4 months post-natal			500 Hz
Karadag-Saygi et al. [101]	35 pregnant	Third trimester	Pregnant: 29.5 ± 4 years	Static and dynamic	Plantar pressure analysis
	35 non-pregnant		Non-pregnant: 30 ± 5 years	pedobarographic parameters	(PMD-S System)
Hagan and Wong [102]	2 pregnant	Before pregnancy	21 and 39	Spatial	30 Hz Video Cameras
		First trimester		Temporal	
		Second trimester		2D Kinematics	
		Third trimester			
		12–16 weeks postpartum			

Ribeiro et al. [103]	6 pregnant	First trimester	32 ± 6.3 years	Plantar pressure (contact time, contact area, peak pressure, and maximum force)	Capacitive insoles from the pedar-X system
		Second trimester			
		Third trimester			
McCrory et al. [104]	41 pregnant,	29 weeks	Pregnant: 26.5 ± 6.4	GRF	Vicon 120 Hz
	40 non-pregnant controls	35 weeks	Non-pregnant: 29.5 ± 4.9	fallers and non-fallers	Bertec force plate 1080 Hz
Forczek and Staszkiewicz [48]	13 pregnant	Before	29.15 ± 3.5	Time and Distance	Vicon 250 3D system
		Third trimester		ROM	
		Half year postpartum		Base of Support	
Moccellin and Driusso [105]	13 pregnant	First trimester	29.15 ± 5.64	Statokinesigram	2 Bertec force platforms
	20 non-pregnant	Second trimester		GRF	
		Third trimester			
Branco et al. [106]	22 pregnant	Second and Third trimester	32.5 ± 2.6	Spatial	200 Hz Qualisys Oqus 300
	12 non-pregnant			Temporal	
				3D Kinematics	
Gilleard [50]	9 pregnant	18, 24, 32, 38 weeks	32.6 ± 4.3	Spatial	60 Hz EVA motion analysis system
		8 weeks postpartum		Temporal	1 Kistler force platform
				Trunk Kinematics	
Sunaga et al. [107]	12 pregnant	16, 24 and 32 gestational weeks	Pregnant—30.1 ± 4.0 years	Spatiotemporal	1 digital video camera (Sony), 30 Hz
	10 nulliparous		Nulliparous—31.2 ± 3.0 years	2D Kinematics	
Aguiar et al. [108]	18 pregnant	27 weeks	Pregnant 32.6 years	Spatial	200 Hz Qualisys Oqus 300, Kistler and AMTI force platforms
	18 non-pregnant		Non-pregnant: 20.4 years	Temporal	
				3D Kinematics	

(continued)

Table 5.1 (continued)

Authors	Sample size (*N*) and groups	Data collection phase(s) of pregnancy and postpartum	Sample mean age (years)	Biomechanical outcome variables	Biomechanical instruments
Branco et al. [109]	11	First trimester	33.20 ± 1.62 years	3D GRF	200 Hz Qualisys Oqus 300, Kistler and AMTI force platforms
		Second trimester		3D Joint Moments, 3D Joint Power	
		Third trimester			
		postpartum			
Yoo et al. [110]	19 pregnant women	Second trimester	29.54 ± 3.45 years	Posturography	GAITRite system
	15 non-pregnant	Third trimester			
Gimunova et al. [111]	9 pregnant women	First trimester	30.90 ± 2.56 years	GRF	Pedar Insole System
		Second trimester			
		Third trimester			
Bertuit et al. [112]	58 pregnant women	Sixth, seventh, eighth, ninth month pregnancy	29 ± 6 years	Plantar Pressure	GAITRite electronic walkway
	9 postpartum				
	23 control				
Branco et al. [52]	11	First trimester	33.20 ± 1.62 years	Spatial and temporal parameters	200 Hz Qualisys Oqus 300
		Second trimester		3D Joint kinematics	
		Third trimester			
		Postpartum			
Branco et al. [113]	24 pregnant	Second trimester	Pregnant: 32.4 ± 2.6 years	GRF, Joint Moments, Joint Power	200 Hz Qualisys Oqus 300, Kistler and AMTI force platforms
	12 non-pregnant	Third trimester	Non-Pregnant: 20.58 ± 1.73		
Blaszczyk et al. [114]	28	First trimester	28.2 ± 3.4 years	Spatiotemporal	Axotape v.2.0
		Third trimester			1 kHz
		2 and 6 months Postpartum			

Ramachandra et al. [115]	70	First trimester	27.98 ± 3.65 years	Static plantar pressure	Plantar pressure analysis
		Second trimester			
		Third trimester			
		3 days after partum			
		6 months postpartum			
Elsayed et al. [116]	11 pregnant	Second trimester	Pregnant: 26.9 ± 5.2 years	Plantar Pressure	Global Postural System (version4.7.16, Italy)
	11 non-pregnant	Third trimester	Non-Pregnant: 26 ± 5.3 years		
Krkeljas [117]	14—First trimester	First trimester	27.5 ± 6.1 years	Spatiotemporal, kinematics of COP and COG	Visual 3D
	20—Second trimester	Second trimester			
	10—Third trimester	Third trimester			
Mei et al. [118]	16 pregnant	Second trimester	32.5 ± 3.64 years	3D Joint Kinematics	8 Vicon cameras 200 Hz
		Third trimester		Plantar pressure	Novel platform 100 Hz
		Postpartum			
Christensen et al. [119]	25—Pregnant with PGP	Pregnant with PGP—23 weeks	Pregnant with PGP—30.9 ± 2.2 years	Spatiotemporal	12 Qualisys pro-reflex cameras 300 Hz
	24—Asymptomatic pregnant	Asymptomatic Pregnant—23 weeks	Pregnant—31.5 ± 3.7 years		2 AMTI LG6 Force plates 1500 Hz
	24—Asymptomatic non-pregnant		Asymptomatic non-pregnant—31.4 ± 4.0 years		

(continued)

Table 5.1 (continued)

Authors	Sample size (*N*) and groups	Data collection phase(s) of pregnancy and postpartum	Sample mean age (years)	Biomechanical outcome variables	Biomechanical instruments
Martínez-Martí et al. [120]	62 pregnant	First trimester	31.42 ± 4.44 years	Plantar Pressure	Custom-made insoles;
		Second trimester			F-Scan (TekScan)
		Third trimester			40 Hz
Mikeska et al. [121]	73 pregnant	27, 32 and 36 gestational weeks	30.34 ± 4.78 years	Plantar Pressure	Emed Walkway (Novel), 100 Hz
Forczek et al. [122]	15 pregnant	Before pregnancy	30.2 ± 3.05 years	Spatiotemporal	Vicon 250, 120 Hz
		First trimester		3D kinematics (Pelvis)	FreeMED force plate
				BOS	
Forczek et al. [123]	30 pregnant	First trimester	30.3 ± 3.4 years	3D kinematics	Vicon 250, 120 Hz
		Second trimester			
		Third trimester			
Bagwell et al. [124]	20 pregnant	Second trimester	Pregnant—31.6 ± 3.4 years	3D Kinematics	8 Qualisys cameras, 100 Hz
	20 Nulliparous	Third trimester	Nulliparous—32.1 ± 4.7 years	3D Kinetics	Bertec force plate, 2000 Hz
		Postpartum		EMG	EMG Delsys, 2000 Hz

Song et al. [125]	21 pregnant	28 ± 1.5 gestational weeks	Pregnant—31.5 ± 3.04 years	3D Kinematics	8 Vicon cameras, 100 Hz
	23 non-pregnant		Non-pregnant—30.5 ± 2.86 years	COP	2 Kistler force plates
Pauk et al. [126]	Pregnant:	11th, 25th, 38th gestational weeks	Normal-weight—27.1 ± 4.7 years	Spatiotemporal	Shoe insoles (T&T Medilogic), 60 Hz
	29 normal-weight		Overweight—27.0 ± 4.9 years	Plantar Pressure	
	26 overweight			GRF	2 Kistler force plates, 1000 Hz
Catena and Wolcott [127]	20 Pregnant	18th, 22nd, 26th, 30th, 34th gestational weeks	22–37 years	Spatiotemporal	1 Kistler force plate, 1000 Hz
				3D Kinematics	10 Motion analysis cameras, 100 Hz
				3D Kinetics	
				GRF	

2D two-dimensional analysis, *3D* three-dimensional analysis, *ROM* range of motion, *BOS* base of support, *GRF* ground reaction forces, *COP* center of pressure, *COG* center of gravity, EMG electromyography throughout pregnancy [50, 52, 99, 102–106, 109–111, 113–115, 117, 118, 120, 121, 123, 124, 126, 127]; some observed three non-dependent groups of women in each trimester [97, 98, 112]; some papers were designed to investigate the same group of women (self-controlled) before pregnancy [48, 102, 122] or/and postpartum [29, 48–50, 99, 100, 102, 109, 113–115, 118, 124], and some articles involved non-pregnant women in the control group [97, 100, 101, 104–106, 108, 110, 112, 113, 116, 119, 124, 125]. The range of age groups of the participants varied from 18 to 50 years old. Some studies have follow-up design and other studies were cross-sectional.

Regarding equipment, the most recent studies used optoelectronic systems for kinematic analysis, as opposed to studies prior to 2017 that most performed video-based kinematic analysis. Only six studies report a kinetic analysis [29, 97, 109, 113, 124, 127] and most studies provide an analysis of the kinematic, spatial, and temporal parameters, as follows.

Considering the specific methodological issues, in addition to the systematic reviews mentioned above, two studies of Aguiar et al. [128, 129] discuss considerations for collecting and processing kinematic and kinetic data from pregnant women.

5.3.2 Spatiotemporal and Kinematic Adaptations During Pregnancy and Postpartum

5.3.2.1 Centre of Gravity and Balance

The displacement of the center of gravity (in the static position) has been discussed over the years with different statements. Some studies indicate that the center of gravity (CG) shifts upper and anteriorly (e.g., [29, 130]). Other studies state that the CG shifts on the upper and posterior direction (e.g., [131, 132]). Whitcome et al. [25] evaluated the evolution of lumbar lordosis in bipedal hominids, and the results elucidate that the CG moves anteriorly until the fetus reaches 40% of the expected final weight. From that moment, the woman increases the lordotic adjustment which in turn enables the control of the CG, but with greater biomechanical costs [29].

Hormonal changes in women are quite variable throughout pregnancy. However, the hormone relaxin may have a more decisive role in the mechanics of movement, as it provides greater ligament laxity in the pelvis and in the peripheral joints [40, 133, 134]. The concentration peak of relaxin occurs around the 12th week of gestation, which means that there is enough time to act on osteoarticular structures until the end of pregnancy.

Jang et al. [135] referred that pregnant woman often remark that their balance degrades during pregnancy. They measured monthly the postural sway in 30 pregnant women and controls. They concluded that the perceived degradation in balance during pregnancy was strongly related to increasing postural sway instability in the anterior–posterior direction. Also, the lateral stability during pregnancy was maintained and likely accomplished by increasing stance width. In a recent study, Sancar et al. [136] assessed the static balance in three different tests (postural stability, limits of stability, and sensory integration and balance) during the three trimesters of pregnancy. Their results showed that although there were no changes in the women's postural stability values, it happens probably due to mechanical compensations, such as increased tonic activity of the ankle plantar flexors, increased ankle stiffness, and the duration of body swings, among others. However, changes were found in the limits of stability between the first and third trimesters, with progressive increases between these phases. These authors suggest that this increase in limits of stability may be due to the increase in the size of the abdomen, allowing pregnant women to achieve better control of the center of gravity and to be able to move lightly beyond the base of support. In the last test, significant increases in sway were found in the third trimester, when the test was performed with eyes closed, which seems to indicate that pregnant women with lack of vision tend to compensate with an increase in body sway [136].

5.3.2.2 Spatial and Temporal Parameters During Gait

The variables of gait velocity, stride length, step length, stride width and base of support, single and double support time are the spatial and temporal parameters analyzed by the papers reviewed. Table 5.2 summarizes the main spatial and temporal results and conclusions of the reviewed papers.

Most papers reviewed showed changes in spatial and temporal parameters in late pregnancy, specifically, a significant decrease in speed [48, 102], a significant reduction in the gait cadence [48], a significant decrease in the length of the gait cycle [50, 99, 102, 106, 114], and in step length [48, 99, 102, 106], and a significant increase in the double support time [29, 99, 106, 108, 114]. Pauk et al. [126] also found an increased double-step duration, both for normal-weight and overweight pregnant women, between first and third trimesters. Other studies showed a significant reduction in the single support time [29, 99], and a significant increase in step width [49, 50, 108, 122]. Forczek and Staszkiewicz [48] also found a significant increase in the base of support. Krkeljas [117], in a study that investigates the changes in postural dynamics during walking, found that although no changes were found in the spatiotemporal parameters of the women throughout pregnancy, they found associations that allow to state that increased step length reflected a decreased margin of stability, and an increased horizontal distance between center of pressure and center of gravity lead to a decreased step length and an increased step width, promoting in that way to a better stability. Nevertheless, the remaining studies suggest that pregnant women have the need to increase the body stability, and use the parameters listed above to meet those demands.

Table 5.2 Objectives, main results, and conclusions of studies with spatial and temporal analysis on gait, during pregnancy

Study	Main goals/objectives	Main results and conclusions
Foti et al. [29]	To objectively analyze gait during pregnancy	Decreased single-support time^{3T} Increased double-support time^{3T}
Lymbery and Gilleard [49]	To investigate selected temporospatial and GRF parameters in the stance phase of gait during late pregnancy	Increased step width^{3T}
Carpes et al. [99]	To describe the kinematic changes during pregnancy and in postpartum	Increased time in double-support and stance phase^{3T} Decreased time in single support^{3T} Decreased mean stride length and step length^{3T}
Hagan and Wong [102]	To study pregnancy-related changes in women's gait	Decreased gait speed^{3T} Decreased stride length^{3T}
Forczek and Staszkiewicz [48]	To measure the selected gait parameters	Decreased velocity, frequency of steps, step length^{3T} Increased base of support width^{3T}
Branco et al. [106]	To describe spatial and temporal parameters and quantify the kinematic variables on the structures of the lower limb during gait	Decreased stride length, left and right step length^{3T} Increased double support time$^{2T \text{ and } 3T}$
Gilleard [50]	To investigate the linear trends for change in the range of motion of the thoracic and pelvic segments and thoracolumbar spine, and the temporospatial characteristics for walking at a self-determined natural speed as the pregnancy progressed and in the early post-birth period using a longitudinal retest design	Decreased stride length^{3T} Increased step width^{3T}
Aguiar et al. [108]	To understand which gait adaptations may be related to an increased trunk mass or more associated with other factors such as the girth of the thigh during pregnancy	Increased stride width^{3T} Increased Left step time^{3T} Increased right and left stance time^{3T} Increased double support time^{3T}
Blaszczyk et al. [114]	To assess precisely spatiotemporal gait diagrams	Decreased gait velocity$^{1T \text{ and } 3T}$ Decreased stride length$^{1T \text{ and } 3T}$ Increased stance phase time$^{1T \text{ and } 3T}$ Increased double support time$^{1T \text{ and } 3T}$ Increased swing phase^{3T}

Table 5.2 (continued)

Study	Main goals/objectives	Main results and conclusions
Krkeljas [117]	To investigate the changes in postural dynamics during walking, and determine its effect on gait stability during pregnancy	Increased lateral movement of COG$^{2T \text{ and } 3T}$
		Increased COG/COP, decreased step length^{3T}
		Increased COG/COP, increased step width^{3T}
Forczek et al. [122]	To perform a kinematic analysis of the gait pattern in the first trimester of pregnancy	Increase of the mean inter-ankle distance^{1T}
Pauk et al. [126]	To analyze changes in spatiotemporal gait parameters, GRFs, and plantar pressure distribution in overweight pregnant women	Increased double-step duration^{3T}
Catena and Wolcott [127]	To understanding coevolution of lumbopelvic sexual dimorphism and bipedalism, and understanding clinical implications of intervening in gestational posture changes	No changes found

5.3.2.3 Gait and Joint Kinematics

Based on reviewed studies (Table 5.3), the joint kinematics of the lower limb, only were found decreases in pelvis obliquity and rotation during the first trimester, more changes were found in the second trimester, and the third trimester have most of the reported changes. Figures 5.6 and 5.7 show kinematic adaptations during walking reported in the studies found, respectively, for second and third trimesters.

Considering the sagittal plane, the angular displacement of the pelvis increases in the anterior tilt of approximately 5° [29, 52, 102, 106, 108, 118]. Forczek et al. [123] also found an increased pelvis tilt range of motion. The joints of the lower limb shows an increase in hip flexion during stance phase [29, 52, 102, 106, 108, 118], and a decrease in hip extension at the end of stance phase [29, 52, 106, 118, 124]; an increase of knee flexion during the terminal stance phase [52, 99, 106, 124], and a decrease of knee extension at the end of swing phase [52, 108]; and a decrease of ankle dorsiflexion and plantar flexion [102, 106].

In the frontal plane, Gilleard [50], Aguiar et al. [108], and Branco et al. [52] found a reduction in the amplitude of the unilateral elevation of the pelvis. The hip joint had different results considering the four studies performed: Foti et al. [29] and Mei et al. [118] found a peak with greater magnitude in the hip adduction, while Branco et al. [106] and Branco et al. [52] found a decrease of this peak; the ankle joint only show an increased peak inversion and peak eversion, respectively, in the pre-swing and initial swing phases [52, 108, 118]. The same results were found by Song et al. [125] focusing on the forefoot and hindfoot regions.

Table 5.3 Objectives, main results, and conclusions of studies with kinematic analysis on gait during pregnancy and postpartum

Study	Main goals/objectives	Main results and conclusions
Foti et al. [29]	To objectively analyze gait during pregnancy	Increased maximum anterior pelvic tilt^{3T}
		Increased maximum hip flexion^{3T}
		Increased maximum hip adduction during stance^{3T}
		Decreased maximum hip extension^{3T}
Carpes et al. [99]	To describe the kinematic changes during pregnancy and in postpartum	Increased knee flexion^{3T}
Hagan and Wong [102]	To study pregnancy-related changes in women's gait	Decreased dorsiflexion$^{2T \text{ and } 3T}$
		Increased pelvic tilt^{3T}
Branco et al. [106]	to describe spatial and temporal parameters and quantify the kinematic variables on the structures of the lower limb during gait and compare it between the later stages of second and third trimesters of pregnancy and with a control group of non-pregnant women	Pregnancy influences the biomechanical changes^{3T}
		Decreased hip extension$^{2T \text{ and } 3T}$
		Increased knee flexion^{3T}
		Decreased plantar flexion^{3T}
		Decreased hip abduction$^{2T \text{ and } 3T}$
Gilleard [50]	To investigate the linear trends for change in the range of motion of the thoracic and pelvic segments and thoracolumbar spine, and the temporospatial characteristics for walking at a self-determined natural speed as the pregnancy progressed and in the early post-birth period using a longitudinal retest design	Decreased range of motion in lateral rotations for pelvis and thoracolumbar spine through pregnancy with no reversal in PP
		Decreased range of motion in pelvic lateral motion^{a}
		Decreased range of motion in flexion/extension for pelvis and thoracolumbar spine^{3T}
Aguiar et al. [108]	To understand which gait adaptations may be related to an increased trunk mass or more associated with other factors such as the girth of the thigh during pregnancy	Increased peak eversion and peak inversion and therefore foot rotation ROM^{3T}
		Decreased maximum knee extension and Knee ROM during swig phase^{3T}
		Increased knee extension during stance phase^{3T}
		Increased maximum hip flexion^{3T}
		Decreased hip extension peak^{3T}
		Increased pelvis anterior tilt^{3T}
		Decreased maximum pelvic lateral motion and lateral ROM^{3T}
Branco et al. [52]	To describe the kinematic variables in the joints of the lower limb during gait at the end of the first, second and third trimesters of pregnancy and in the postpartum period	Increased Knee Flexion^{2T}
		Decreased Knee Extension^{2T}
		Decreased hip extension$^{2T \text{ and } 3T}$
		Increased hip flexion$^{2T \text{ and } 3T}$
		Increased pelvis anterior tilt$^{2T \text{ and } 3T}$
		Increased ankle inversion^{3T}
		Decreased hip adduction^{3T}
		Decreased pelvis right elevation^{2T}
		Increased pelvis right elevation^{3T}
		Increased hip internal rotation$^{2T \text{ and } 3T}$

Table 5.3 (continued)

Study	Main goals/objectives	Main results and conclusions
Mei et al. [118]	To analyze gait of pregnant individuals throughout pregnancy and postpartum	Decreased ankle eversion^{3T}
		Increased ankle eversion^{PP}
		Increased pelvis anterior tilt^{3T}
		Decreased pelvis anterior tilt^{PP}
		Increased Hip Flexion^{PP}
		Decreased Hip Extension^{PP}
		Increased Hip Adduction^{PP}
		Increased Hip External rotation^{3T}
Forczek et al. [122]	To perform a kinematic analysis of the gait pattern in the first trimester of pregnancy	Decreased Pelvis Obliquity^{1T}
		Decreased Pelvis Rotation^{1T}
Forczek et al. [123]	To get further insight into how morphology correlates with the kinematic pattern	Increased pelvis tilt RoM$^{2T\text{ and }3T}$
		Increased pelvis Tilt max$^{2T\text{ and }3T}$
Bagwell et al. [124]	To compare lower extremity joint loading and muscle activation during over-ground walking	Decreased Hip extension^{2T}
		Increased Knee flexion^{2T}
		Decreased Knee adduction^{2T}
Song et al. [125]	To investigate differences in forefoot, rearfoot and tibial motion during daily walk	Decreased Forefoot plantar flexion^{2T}
		Decreased Forefoot inversion^{2T}
		Increased Forefoot eversion^{2T}
		Increased Rearfoot plantar flexion^{2T}
		Decreased Rearfoot Dorsiflexion^{2T}
		Increased Rearfoot eversion^{2T}
		Decreased Rearfoot inversion^{2T}
		Increased Rearfoot internal rotation^{2T}
		Increased Rearfoot external rotation^{2T}
		Decreased Tibia forward tilt^{2T}
		Increased Tibia external rotation^{2T}
Catena and Wolcott [127]	To understanding coevolution of lumbopelvic sexual dimorphism	Increased Ankle RoM^{3T}
	and bipedalism, and understanding clinical implications of intervening in gestational posture changes	Increased Knee Flexion^{3T}

Few studies have done an analysis of the transverse plane. Gilleard [50] and Forczek et al. [122] found a decrease in the range of motion of the pelvis, Mei et al. [118] found an increased hip external rotation in loading response phase, and Branco et al. [52] found an increased in the peak of hip internal rotation during terminal stance phase. Finally, Song et al. [125] found an increased internal rotation and external rotation of rearfoot, respectively, during initial contact and mid-stance phase.

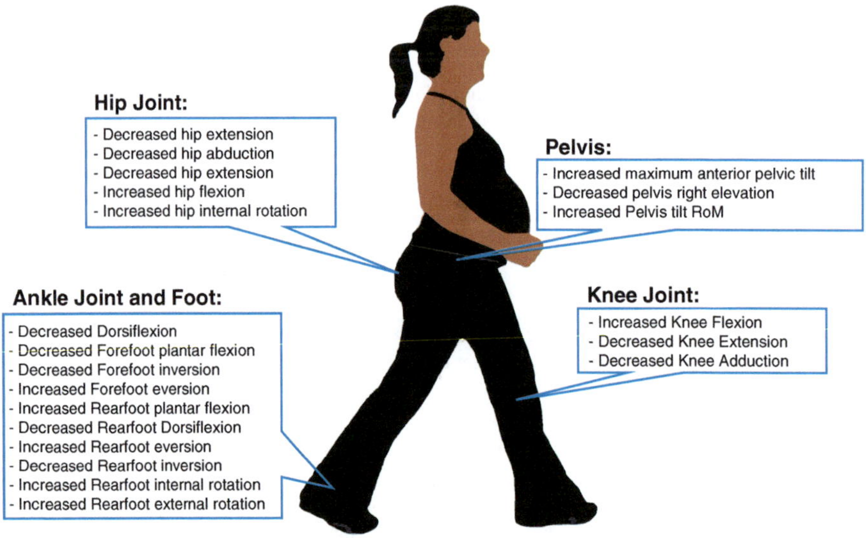

Fig. 5.6 Gait kinematic adaptations of pregnant women at the end of the second trimester

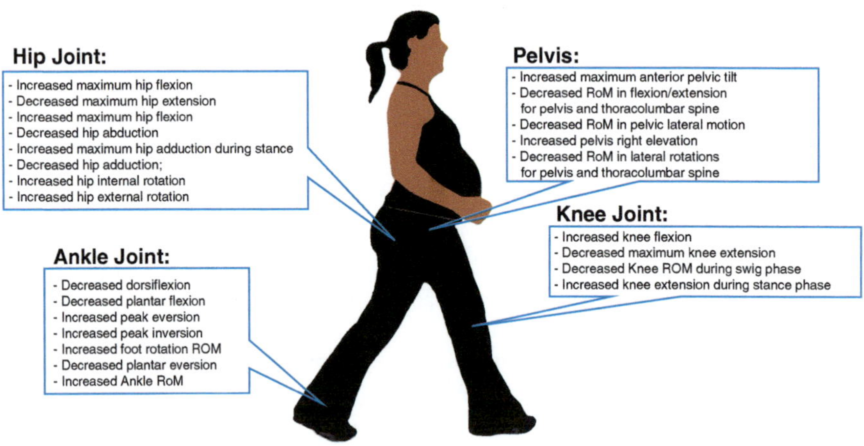

Fig. 5.7 Gait kinematic adaptations of pregnant women at the end of the third trimester

5.3.3 Biomechanical Loading During Pregnancy and Postpartum

5.3.3.1 Ground Reaction Forces

Changes in the different components of GRF were found during pregnancy. Table 5.4 summarizes the main results and conclusions of those studies. Significant decreases were found in the vertical component of the GRF [105, 109, 111, 113,

Table 5.4 Objectives, main results, and conclusions of studies with ground reaction forces analysis during pregnancy and postpartum

Study	Main goals/objectives	Main results and conclusions
Lymbery and Gilleard [49]	To investigate selected temporospatial and GRF parameters in the stance phase of gait during late pregnancy	Increased mediolateral GRF[3T]
		Increased lateral COP[3T]
		Less anteriorly COP[3T]
Moccellin and Driusso [105]	To evaluate static and dynamic postural control during the three trimesters of pregnancy and to check the quality of life in each trimester	Decreased magnitudes of vertical reaction force[3T]
		Decreased magnitudes of anterior–posterior reaction forces[3T]
		Increased lateral COP[3T]
Branco et al. [109]	To assess the gait kinetics, in order to check if there are any changes in the dynamics of the load of women from the beginning of pregnancy until the postpartum period	Decreased magnitudes of posterior reaction forces[1T]
		Decreased magnitudes of vertical reaction force[3T]
		Decreased magnitudes of anterior reaction forces[3T]
Branco et al. [113]	To quantify the lower limb kinetics of gait and draw a comparison between women in the second and third trimesters of pregnancy, and a non-pregnant group	Decreased magnitudes of vertical reaction force[3T]
		Decreased magnitudes of anterior reaction forces[3T]
		Increased medial reaction forces[3T]
Pauk et al. [126]	To analyze changes in spatiotemporal gait parameters, GRFs, and plantar pressure distribution in overweight pregnant women	No changes throughout pregnancy
Catena and Wolcott [127]	To understanding coevolution of lumbopelvic sexual dimorphism and bipedalism, and understanding clinical implications of intervening in gestational posture changes	Decreased magnitudes of vertical reaction force[3T]

137], also in the anterior and posterior components of GRF showed lower magnitudes [105, 109, 113].

Lymbery, Gilleard [49] investigated the GRF variables in the stance phase of walking during late pregnancy, and they concluded that in late pregnancy, mediolateral GRF tended to be increased in a medial and lateral directions. These results were corroborated in the studies of Branco et al. [109] and Branco et al. [113]. They suggested that women might adapt their gait to maximize stability in the stance phase of walking and to control mediolateral motion. Similar results were found in CoP, where an increase in lateral displacement [49, 105], and a decrease in anterior displacement [49] were found.

5.3.3.2 Plantar Pressure

The plantar pressure allows determining how the pressure is distributed through the regions of the foot. In Table 5.5 are summarized the main plantar pressure results and conclusions of the reviewed studies. Regarding the forefoot, there

Table 5.5 Objectives, main results, and conclusions of studies with plantar pressure analysis during pregnancy and postpartum

Study	Main goals/objectives	Main results and conclusions
Nyska et al. [95]	To measure plantar foot pressure distribution statically and dynamically in pregnant women	Decreased maximal pressures in forefoot^{3T}
		Increased maximal pressures in hindfoot^{3T}
		Increased total contact area^{3T}
		Increased total maximal force^{3T}
		Decreased contact time in medial side of the forefoot^{3T}
		Increased peak pressures in midfoot for booth feet and in lateral side of the right forefoot^{3T}
		Decreased peak pressures in medial side of the forefoot^{3T}
Goldberg et al. [96]	To determine changes in foot use and foot pressure patterns during pregnancy	Decreased floor contact times, Impulse and hindfoot peak pressure increases; forefoot peak pressure^{1T}
		Increased contact times, Impulse and peak pressure in hindfoot^{3T}
		Decreased forefoot peak pressure^{3T}
Ribas and Guirro [98]	To analyze plantar pressure and postural balance during the three trimesters of pregnancy and correlate these with anthropometric characteristics	Positive correlation between Centre of force and size of support base$^{1T\ and\ 3T}$
Gaymer et al. [100]	To quantify the plantar pressure of women in late pregnancy and assess the persistence of these changes after normalization of the patients' hormone profile postpartum	Increased peak plantar pressure for forefoot and midfoot^{3T}
		Decreased maximum peak plantar pressure in the hindfoot^{3T}
Karadag-Saygi et al. [101]	To evaluate plantar pressure changes and postural balance differences in pregnant women	Increased forefoot pressure on the right side for standing and Walking^{3T}
		Increased contact times in the Forefoot^{3T}
		Increased contact times^{3T}
Ribeiro et al. [103]	Describe longitudinally, and compare the plantar pressure distribution in orthostatic posture and gait throughout pregnancy	Decreased contact area of Lateral rearfoot^{2T}
		Decreased Peak pressure of Medial rearfoot
		Increased contact area of midfoot^{3T}
		Increased contact time for midfoot and medial forefoot^{3T}
		Decreased absolute maximum force for medial rearfoot$^{2T\ and\ 3T}$
		Increased absolute maximum force for medial forefoot^{2T}
Bertuit et al. [112]	To investigate plantar pressures during gait in the last 4 months of pregnancy and in the postpartum period. A comparison with nulliparous women was conducted to investigate plantar pressure modifications during pregnancy	Decreased Peak Pressure and contact area for the forefoot and rearfoot^{3T}
		Increased Peak Pressure and contact area for the midfoot^{3T}

Table 5.5 (continued)

Study	Main goals/objectives	Main results and conclusions
Ramachandra et al. [115]	Study the structural changes of foot and static plantar pressure patterns in women across various trimesters of pregnancy and postpartum	Increased forefoot and hindfoot pressure for both feet^{3T}
		Increased total contact area^{3T}
		Increased average pressure^{3T}
		Increased maximum pressure for right foot^{3T}
Elsayed et al. [116]	To investigate the plantar pressure distribution during pregnancy.	Asymmetry of weight bearing^{3T}
		Increased pressure in fifth metatarsal for both feet^{3T}
Mei et al. [118]	To analyze gait of pregnant individuals throughout pregnancy and postpartum	Lateral shift of COP$^{2T \text{ and } 3T}$
		Increased COP Deviation in initial contact^{3T}
		Decreased COP Deviation in forefoot$^{2T \text{ and } 3T}$
Martínez-Martí et al. [120]	To better understand the relationship between low back pain and gait	Increased heel peak pressure^{2T}
		Increased first metatarsal peak pressure^{2T}
		Increased fifth metatarsal peak pressure^{2T}
		Increased medially shifted CoP in right foot^{2T}
		Increased anteriorly shifted CoP in right foot^{3T}
		Decreased heel peak pressure in left foot^{3T}
		Increased first metatarsal peak pressure^{3T}
		Increased fifth metatarsal peak pressure in right foot^{3T}
Mikeska et al. [121]	To analyze the distribution of plantar pressure and foot characteristics during walking	**Left Foot:**
		Increased Hindfoot peak pressure^{3T}
		Increased Hindfoot contact area^{3T}
		Increased Midfoot peak pressure^{3T}
		Increased second Metatarsal Head contact area^{3T}
		Increased second Metatarsal Head contact area^{3T}
		Increased third Metatarsal Head contact area^{3T}
		Increased Big toe contact area^{3T}
		Right Foot:
		Increased Hindfoot peak pressure^{3T}
		Increased Hindfoot contact area^{3T}
		Increased third Metatarsal Head contact area^{3T}
		Increased Big toe contact area^{3T}
Pauk et al. [126]	To analyze changes in spatiotemporal gait parameters, GRFs, and plantar pressure distribution in overweight pregnant women	Increased lateral pressure^{3T}

are distinct results between studies, as some studies point to a decrease in peak pressures [95, 96, 112, 120] and others point to an increase in peak pressure for that region of the foot [100, 101, 115, 116, 120, 121]. For midfoot region, the results are more consensual, whose peak pressure is higher during pregnancy [95, 100, 112, 121]. In posterior region of the pregnant women foot (referred to in the various studies as hindfoot or rearfoot), dissimilar results were also found where Nyska et al. [95], Goldberg et al. [96], Ramachandra et al. [115], and recently Mikeska et al. [121] report an increased peak pressure. However, although Martínez-Martí et al. [120] has found an increase of the heel peak in second trimester, he also reported a decrease of this peak in the third trimester, which were also found by Gaymer et al. [100] and Bertuit et al. [112]. Relatively to contact time of the different regions of the foot with floor, only Nyska et al. [95] report a decrease of this variable in the medial side of forefoot; however, in the other studies, an increased contact time for hindfoot [96], midfoot [103], and forefoot [101, 103, 118] was found.

Other variables were studied based on plantar pressure data, namely, an increased contact force in the medial forefoot [103, 121] and in rearfoot [121]. However, Ribeiro et al. [103] for medial rearfoot reported a decreased magnitude. It was also found a positive correlation between the center of force and the size of the base of support [98]. In general, authors refer that those changes may be responsible for complaints of musculoskeletal pain in feet, lower limbs [95], and lower back [120] in pregnant women. In any case, pressure distribution can be alleviated by exercise and shoe modifications [101, 121]. Also, that those adjustments suggest that pregnant women keep the dynamic stability during walking gait [103, 112].

5.3.3.3 Joint Reaction Forces

In Table 5.6 are summarized the main findings and conclusions of joint reaction forces found in the studies, and Figs. 5.8, 5.9, and 5.10 show kinetic adaptations reported in the reviewed studies, respectively for first, second, and third trimesters.

Few studies have evaluated the kinetic parameters of gait during pregnancy. Foti et al. [29] analyzed the joint moments of force and joint powers with and without normalizing the weight of the women in late pregnancy. Although they found several changes in these parameters without normalization, the authors recommend the analysis with normalization [29]. Analyzes performed with normalized data for joint moments have had somewhat contradictory results. Huang et al. [97] found a significant increase in the hip extensors moment, while Catena, Wolcott [127] reported a decrease in hip extensors moment. In other studies, a significant decrease in the knee extensors moment [97] and in the ankle plantar flexors moment was found [29, 97], while Bagwell et al. [124] have found increased ankle plantar flexors and in dorsiflexors moments for the sagittal plane. In the frontal plane, there was an increase of the hip abductors moment [29, 124], in the knee adductors moment [97], and also in knee abductors moment [124].

Table 5.6 Objectives, main results, and conclusions of studies with kinetic analysis on gait during pregnancy and postpartum

Study	Main goals/objectives	Main results and conclusions
Foti et al. [29]	To objectively analyze gait during pregnancy	Increased hip abduction moment^{3T}
		Decreased ankle plantar flexion moment^{3T}
Huang et al. [97]	To find a reasonable model to compensate the lack of the anthropometric data and compare the pregnant data with the normal data	Increased hip extension moment^{3T}
		Decreased knee extension moment^{3T}
		Increased knee adduction moment^{3T}
		Decreased ankle plantar flexion moment^{3T}
Branco et al. [109]	To assess the gait kinetics, in order to check if there are any changes in the dynamics of the load of women from the beginning of pregnancy until the postpartum period	Decreased hip extensors moment^{3T}
		Decreased hip flexors moment$^{2T \text{ and } 3T}$
		Increased hip external rotators moment$^{2T \text{ and } 3T}$
		Increased eccentric contraction of the hip external rotators$^{2T \text{ and } 3T}$
		Decreased eccentric contraction of hip flexors^{3T}
		Decreased concentric contraction of the knee extensors^{1T}
		Decreased ankle plantar flexors moment^{3T}
		Decreased eccentric contraction of ankle abductors^{3T}
Branco et al. [113]	To quantify the lower limb kinetics of gait and draw a comparison between women in the second and third trimesters of pregnancy, and a non-pregnant group	Decreased participation of the hip flexors^{2T}
		Increased participation of hip external rotators^{2T}
		Decreased participation and asymmetry of hip flexors^{3T}
		Increased concentric contraction of hip extensors^{3T}
		Decreased eccentric contraction of hip flexors^{3T}
		Increased concentric contraction of hip abductors^{3T}
		Increased concentric contraction of hip external rotators^{3T}
		Decreased participation of the knee extensors^{2T}
		Increased participation of the knee flexors^{2T}
		Decreases participation of the ankle dorsiflexors^{2T}
		Decreased participation of the ankle eversors^{2T}
		Decreased participation of ankle dorsiflexors^{3T}
		Decreased concentric contraction and asymmetry in ankle dorsiflexors^{3T}

(continued)

Table 5.6 (continued)

Study	Main goals/objectives	Main results and conclusions
Bagwell et al. [124]	To compare lower extremity joint loading and muscle activation during over-ground walking	Increased Hip abductor moments^{2T}
		Increased Ankle sagittal negative work^{2T}
		Increased Hip abductor moments^{3T}
		Increased Knee abductors moments^{3T}
		Increased Ankle dorsiflexors moments^{3T}
		Increased Ankle plantar flexors moments^{3T}
		Increased Ankle sagittal negative work^{3T}
Catena and Wolcott [127]	To understanding coevolution of lumbopelvic sexual dimorphism and bipedalism, and understanding clinical implications of intervening in gestational posture changes	Decreased Hip extensors moment^{3T}

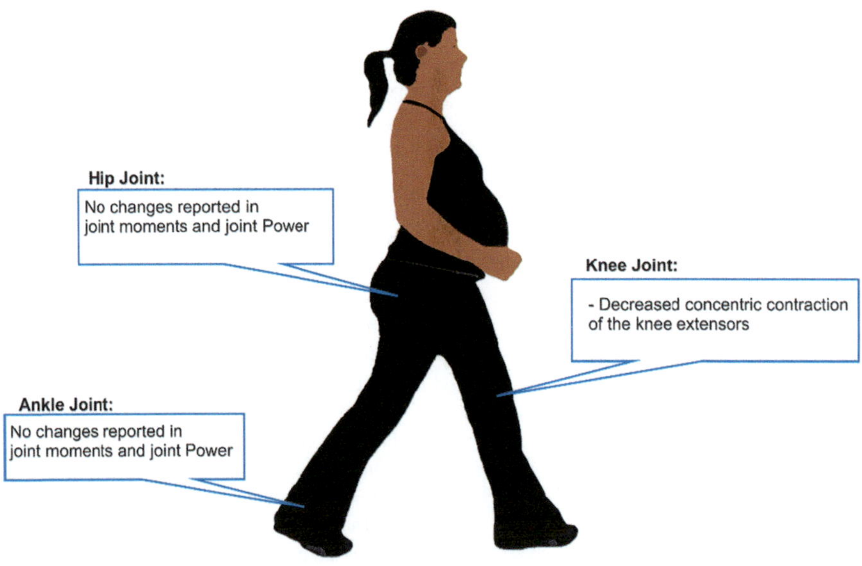

Fig. 5.8 Joint kinetic adaptations of pregnant women at the end of the first trimester, during gait

The body composition [35, 36, 126, 138], the increased loading in the trunk anterior area [139, 140], and the higher foot pressures in the pregnant women [95, 100, 120, 121] are associated with alterations of the gait pattern. The joint laxity increases, and consequently, there is an increase in the joints amplitude [133].

At the end of pregnancy, the adoption of strategies such as increasing the width of the base of support caused by the other body segments allows minimizing the increased weight and trunk girth effects. Indeed, such changes can substantially modify the gait pattern, contributing to an overload of the musculoskeletal system, causing lower limbs, hip, and lower back pain [29, 39, 101, 120, 141–143].

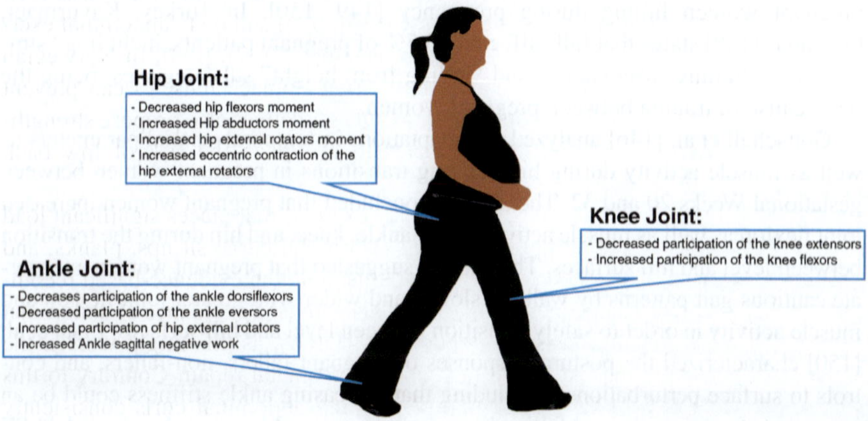

Fig. 5.9 Joint kinetic adaptations of pregnant women at the end of the second trimester, during gait

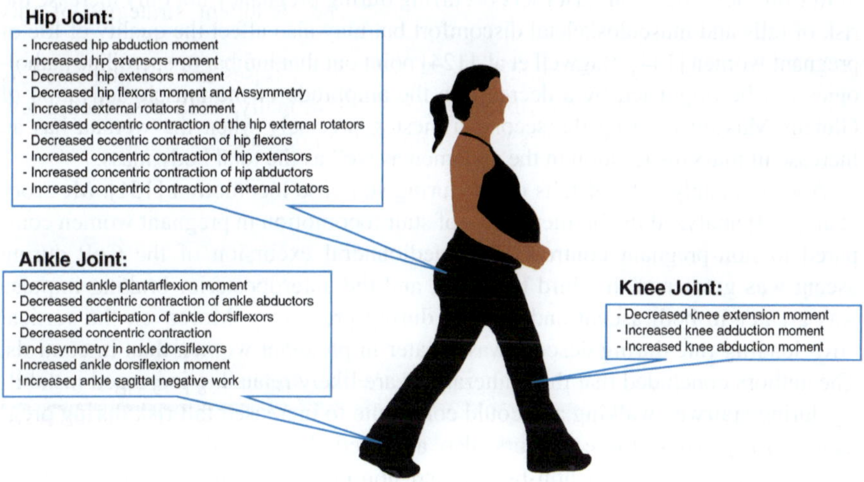

Fig. 5.10 Joint kinetic adaptations of pregnant women at the end of the third trimester, during gait

5.4 Other Biomechanical Adaptations During Pregnancy

5.4.1 Balance and Fall Risk

Throughout pregnancy, women experience hormonal, anatomical, and physiological alterations that are often accompanied by increased weight and ankle edema [144] and decreased postural control which increase the risk of falling during this period [40, 144, 145]. Falls are the leading cause of nonfatal injury across all age groups and a common incident for pregnant women [146–148], with nearly 27% of pregnant women falling during pregnancy [149, 150]. In Turkey, Kavurmaci, Gulbahar [148] states that falls affected 60.5% of pregnant patients, including "simple falls," "falling from stairs," and "falling from height" subcategories, being the main cause of trauma between pregnant women.

Gottschall et al. [146] analyzed the adaptations in temporal–spatial parameters as well as muscle activity during hill walking transitions in pregnant women between gestational Weeks 20 and 32. The authors concluded that pregnant women increased joint flexion as well as muscle activity at the ankle, knee, and hip during the transition between level and hill surfaces. The authors suggested that pregnant women exaggerate cautious gait patterns by walking slower and wider with greater joint flexion and muscle activity in order to safely transition between level and hill surfaces. Ersal et al. [150] characterized the postural responses of pregnant fallers, non-fallers, and controls to surface perturbations, concluding that increasing ankle stiffness could be an important strategy to prevent falling by pregnant women. Moreover, Inanir et al. [145] prospectively evaluated pregnant women regarding their dynamic postural stability, concluding that pregnancy has a negative effect on postural stability, especially in the third trimester. These gait disorders occurring during pregnancy not only increase the risk of falls and musculoskeletal discomfort but may also affect the quality of life of pregnant women [144]. Bagwell et al. [124] point out that lumbar or sacroiliac pathologies can be originated by a decrease in the amplitude of the muscle activation of Gluteus Maximus during the second trimester, precisely when the woman has an increase in mass distribution in the abdomen as well as the total body mass.

Approximately 40% of falls occur during staircase locomotion [151]. McCrory et al. [149] analyzed the biomechanics of stair locomotion in pregnant women compared to non-pregnant controls. The mediolateral excursion of the CoP during ascent was greater in the third trimester, and the anteroposterior braking impulse was greater in both ascent and descent during pregnancy. Moreover, the vertical GRF loading rate during descent was greater in pregnant women than in controls. The authors concluded that these alterations are likely related to increased instability during stairway walking and could contribute to increased fall risk during pregnancy [149]. Thus, these authors also analyzed the ground reaction forces in pregnant fallers, pregnant non-fallers, and non-pregnant controls to determine if pregnant fallers display alterations to ground reaction forces that increase their risk of falling on stairs [151]. The authors found that pregnant fallers increase stability during staircase locomotion. Pregnant fallers had an increased anterior–posterior braking impulse, medial impulse, and minimum between vertical peaks during ascent [151]. Also, during descent, pregnant fallers demonstrated a smaller anterior–posterior propulsive peak and propulsive impulse and a greater minimum between vertical peaks. In another study, Takeda et al. [152] compared pregnant women who fall with pregnant women who do not fall, verifying that in the second trimester the fallers had a significant higher increase of the abdominal girth over the non-fallers. In addition, in third trimester, the pregnant fallers had lower limits of stability over the non-fallers. These results seem to show that higher increases and probably faster increase of abdominal volume influence the woman's limits of stability that in turn decreases the pregnant capacity to recover from imbalances.

5.4.2 Trunk Motion and Load Transportation

Gilleard [50] investigated the systematic changes in the range of motion for the pelvic and thoracic segments of the spine, the motion between these segments (thoracolumbar spine) and temporospatial characteristics of step width, stride length, and velocity during walking as pregnancy progresses and post-birth. The author concluded that as pregnancy progresses, there were significant linear trends for an increase in step width and a decrease in stride length. Regarding trunk motion, there was a significant linear trend for a decrease in the range of motion of the pelvic segment and thoracolumbar spine about a vertical axis (side-to-side rotation), and the pelvic segment range of motion around an anterior–posterior axis (i.e., side tilt). Moreover, not all adaptations were resolved by 8 weeks post-birth [50]. Sawa et al. [153] also compared the gait characteristics and the functional ability of the trunk between women before and during the third trimester of pregnancy, suggesting that the functional ability of the trunk during gait declines in late pregnancy. Wu et al. [154] also suggest that pregnant women experience difficulties in realizing the more anti-phase pelvis-thorax coordination that is required at higher walking velocities.

McCrory et al. [151] were the first to investigate the thoracic and pelvic kinematics of gait regarding the "waddle" way of walking during pregnancy. The authors concluded that pregnant women demonstrate a lateral shifting of the body during gait, which accompanied a greater step width. The increased thoracic extension and anterior pelvic tilt, along with decreased sagittal plane ROM, are likely adaptations to increased abdominal size [27].

Sunaga et al. [107] analyzed the changes in the pattern of rising from a chair and walking forward as pregnancy progresses. The authors found that the peak trunk-flexion angle during rising was smaller in pregnant women than in controls. Moreover, the hip-extension angle during the stance phase was larger than in controls. Also, the peak horizontal and vertical velocities of the center of mass were lower, and appeared earlier, in pregnant women than in controls. The authors conclude that pregnant women should not initiate gait until reaching a stable standing position after rising, in order to ensure safety.

5.5 Implications for Exercise Prescription and Intervention

A strategy to promote health and control weight gain during pregnancy is by performing structured or recreational physical activity. The guidelines for exercise prescription of the American College of Obstetricians and Gynecologists recommend to engage aerobic and strength-conditioning exercises before, during, and after pregnancy [2], as well as flexibility and neuromotor exercises [3]. Further discussion on this topic is addressed in Chaps. 7 and 8. The adaptations of the exercise programs based on effectiveness and safety must take into consideration the morphological, biomechanical, physiological, and psychological alterations that occur during pregnancy. Moreover, in order to better develop safe and effective exercise programs, it is necessary to understand, among other variables, the physical activity patterns of pregnant women and the characteristics of proper exercise. These issues are addressed in Chaps. 1, 7, 8, and 9. As an example, walking is one of the movements most commonly performed by people in the day-to-day tasks, easy to control exercise intensity, and emerges as a highly recommended physical activity for pregnant women (see Chaps. 1, 7, and 8). Chapter 9 provides guidance on the specific adaptations of several recreational activities such as aerobics, step, strength training, stretching, and water exercise, among others, that might be adapted to healthy pregnant women.

The anatomic and biomechanical changes, together with hormonal changes, on the one hand, increase joint forces, and, on the other hand, increase the laxity of joints. These factors may contribute to joint pain, reduced coordination, and increased injury risk [20]. Moreover, these consequences may vary from mild to severe discomfort that resolves postpartum, to clinically significant musculoskeletal disorders contributing to future health problems. During pregnancy and postpartum, these factors may prevent women from either being physically active or practicing exercise. Regarding musculoskeletal health, the importance of exercise prescription for both preventive and rehabilitation programs should be emphasized. Thus, exercise prescription during the different phases of pregnancy and in the postpartum period must not only include the forms of adaptation of the type of exercise, of the intensity, duration, and frequency but also take in consideration the biomechanical adaptations and its consequences.

Physical exercise should provide adequate levels of mechanical loading, fundamental for bone health, minimizing the adverse effects such as pain and injury. One important characteristic of most of the recreational physical activities is the repetition of movements that induce GRF of low magnitude (1–2 BW) and high frequency (around 3000–4000 times on a 30-min session).

Considering the pregnant woman's increase in body weight, Alberton et al. [155] found that when statically immersed in water, pregnant women in third trimester had a weight reduction in the order of 82.9% in body weight. During the performance of aquatic exercises, the amplitude of the GRF varied between 67% and 72% of the body weight, which puts physical exercise in water, an alternative for women who suffer from joints or low back pain due to mechanical load.

Mechanical loading is related to the magnitude of the external and internal forces; with the frequency of the forces applied to the body; with the repetition of the load application; and with the way musculoskeletal structures deal with the internal forces [64], and could be truly related to musculoskeletal injuries, reported in the back, hip, knee, and ankle. Thus, the assessment of biomechanical loading in the musculoskeletal system of pregnant women is of particular interest. Also, the quantification or estimation of the mechanical load is essential to understand how much we need to maintain and improve the morphological and functional quality of biological structures [45]. This might give a major contribution to exercise prescription (see Chaps. 8 and 9) and injury prevention (see Chap. 12).

On the one hand, the level of discomfort or the diagnosed disorder may be a good indicator for a specific exercise program during pregnancy aiming to decrease back pain intensity and increase functional ability [156, 157] or a referral to a physiotherapeutic program (see Chaps. 6 and 12). On the other hand, promoting good posture and regular exercise can be recommended as a method to relieve back pain in pregnant women [157]. Thus, exercise prescription must be adapted to the morphological and biomechanical alterations that occur during pregnancy and contribute to pain relief and treatment. Nevertheless, it is not fully understood whether exercise programs can prevent pain, falls, or injury. The results of the present analysis may be useful to develop recommendations for pregnancy and postpartum-specific exercise programs, and eventually for foot, pelvic, and lumbar pain prevention.

The following questions are of major importance:

- How can exercise programs contribute to health, functional ability, pain relief or treatment?
- How can the pregnant body be best protected while exercising?

Based on the data available, some practical recommendations for exercise prescription and intervention can be provided to health and exercise professionals, in order to improve the well-being of women throughout pregnancy by means of an active and healthy lifestyle:

- Musculoskeletal health adaptations should be further addressed in the national and international guidelines for physical activity and exercise during pregnancy and postpartum.
- The benefits of exercise on the musculoskeletal health of pregnant women should also be further developed in those guidelines.
- Neuromotor (balance[1] and coordination[2]) exercise and posture training should be included in any exercise intervention throughout pregnancy and postpartum.
- Combined weight-bearing exercise with several types of weight-supported exercise (water or cycling) may be included in any exercise intervention throughout pregnancy.
- Exercise planning should avoid very fast movements and quick changes of position in group exercise with music, walking classes, or dynamic strength training, in order to avoid falls and stress to the joints.
- All pregnant women should be advised to be careful with wearing proper sports shoes regarding cushioning and impact attenuation, especially in what is concerned with the type of floor (indoor and outdoor).
- All pregnant women should be advised to be careful with the type and the conditions of the floor when exercising outdoor in order to avoid falls.
- All pregnant women should enhance visibility around the feet during exercise (e.g., mirror).

[1] Coordination is defined by the ability to use the senses, such as sight and hearing, together with body parts in performing tasks smoothly and accurately. In [3].

[2] Balance is defined by the maintenance of equilibrium while stationary or moving [3].

5.6 Further Research

Further research is required using common outcome measures and standard follow-up periods of data collection (weeks of gestation and postpartum period). Most of the results presented in this review are consistent between studies. However, there is a great scarcity of studies addressing the gait biomechanics of pregnant women in a longitudinal perspective.

Very few studies analyzed the kinetics of gait of pregnant women. Nevertheless, these data are seen as essential to understand the magnitude and implications of changes in the welfare of women. In future research, there must be a special focus on the analysis of moments of force and joint powers to understand the changes in muscle participation and type of contraction, regarding the direction of angular motion of the joints.

It is not possible to understand the influence of morphological changes, if body composition and anthropometric variables are not quantified throughout pregnancy. Further research is required to understand to which extent these variables influence the biomechanical parameters.

No studies were found addressing the effects of physical activity, low back and pelvic pain, or maternal weight control on the gait biomechanical adaptations of gait throughout pregnancy and postpartum. It would be of particular interest to understand either the impact of an active lifestyle or the effect of different types of exercise on the biomechanical adaptations occurring during pregnancy.

Gait analysis is a useful tool for understanding movement impairments or discomfort, which may impact on pregnant women well-being. The use of gait analysis in pregnant women, especially those with gestational diabetes and lower limb pain may lead to improvements in healthcare including the treatment and prevention, as well as to the development of targeted exercise interventions. On the one hand, there is a critical demand for research to evaluate if walking strategies in pregnant women change throughout pregnancy in order to effectively intervene and minimize the incidence rate [146]. On the other hand, it is also of particular importance to understand whether exercise intervention would have an effect on those walking strategies. Moreover, postural stability tests may detect pregnant women with a high fall risk [145].

Future research could address the influence of specific exercise interventions and footwear on the plantar pressure pattern in pregnant women, especially in the increased plantar pressures in hindfoot with the advancement of pregnancy.

There is sparse evidence on the effects of targeted exercise interventions on plantar pressure and ground reaction forces variables, especially in pregnant women. Thus, it would be interesting to understand how active women deal with increased mechanical loading from physical activity and in comparison with sedentary women. Moreover, there is a lack of evidence on the effect of exercise on quality of life and musculoskeletal health.

More specific questions could assess whether there are any significant imbalances between the right and left sides of the pregnant women' body; how long does it take to recover in the postpartum period; what are the adaptations in other locomotion-related tasks such as negotiating obstacles and stairs, and carrying loads; what is the real impact of weight gain.

Overall, future research should be focused on strengthening evidence by increasing the number of participants and better explain the characteristics of recruitment and of the women. Other focus should be the development of prospective studies to minimize bias in estimating the prevalence of falls and back and lower limb pain, regarding the biomechanical adaptations and the effects of an active lifestyle.

5.7 Conclusion

In this chapter, we have reviewed the musculoskeletal and biomechanical changes of gait during pregnancy and in the postpartum period. Although the dedicated literature is limited, the available evidence suggests biomechanical adaptations of gait throughout pregnancy and the postpartum period. However, no studies were found addressing the effects of physical activity, low back and pelvic pain or maternal weight control on the gait biomechanical adaptations of gait throughout pregnancy and postpartum.

In order to better develop safe and effective exercise programs, it is necessary to understand the physical activity patterns of pregnant women, the characteristics of proper exercise in terms of mechanical loading and its effects in the pregnant women in terms of gait, functionality, morphology, and treatment of low back pain. Thus, the assessment of biomechanical loading in the musculoskeletal system of pregnant women is of particular interest. This information becomes very important to implement exercise programs for pregnant women and to develop strategies to increase adherence.

References

1. Paisley TS, Joy EA, Price RJ Jr. Exercise during pregnancy: a practical approach. Curr Sports Med Rep. 2003;2(6):325–30.
2. A.C.O.G. Physical activity and exercise during pregnancy and the postpartum period: ACOG committee opinion, number 804. Obstet Gynecol. 2020;135(4):e178–e88. https://doi.org/10.1097/aog.0000000000003772.
3. American College of Sports Medicine, Riebe D, Ehrman JK, Liguori G, Magal M. ACSM's guidelines for exercise testing and prescription. 10th ed. Philadelphia, PA: Wolters Kluwer; 2018.
4. Bø K, Artal R, Barakat R, Brown W, Davies GAL, Dooley M, et al. Exercise and pregnancy in recreational and elite athletes: 2016 evidence summary from the IOC expert group meeting, Lausanne. Part 1—exercise in women planning pregnancy and those who are pregnant. Br J Sport Med. 2016;50(10):571.
5. Oken E, Ning Y, Rifas-Shiman SL, Radesky JS, Rich-Edwards JW, Gillman MW. Associations of physical activity and inactivity before and during pregnancy with glucose tolerance. Obstet Gynecol. 2006;108(5):1200–7. https://doi.org/10.1097/01.aog.0000241088.60745.70.
6. Foxcroft KF, Callaway LK, Byrne NM, Webster J. Development and validation of a pregnancy symptoms inventory. BMC Pregnan Childb. 2013;13(1):3. https://doi.org/10.1186/1471-2393-13-3.

7. Borg-Stein J, Dugan SA, Gruber J. Musculoskeletal aspects of pregnancy. Am J Phys Med Rehabil. 2005;84(3):180–92.
8. Domingues MR, Barros AJ. Leisure-time physical activity during pregnancy in the 2004 Pelotas Birth Cohort Study. Rev Saude Publica. 2007;41(2):173–80.
9. Pereira MA, Rifas-Shiman SL, Kleinman KP, Rich-Edwards JW, Peterson KE, Gillman MW. Predictors of change in physical activity during and after pregnancy: project Viva. Am J Prev Med. 2007;32(4):312–9. https://doi.org/10.1016/j.amepre.2006.12.017.
10. Borodulin K, Evenson KR, Monda K, Wen F, Herring AH, Dole N. Physical activity and sleep among pregnant women. Paediatr Perinat Epidemiol. 2010;24(1):45–52. https://doi.org/10.1111/j.1365-3016.2009.01081.x.
11. DiNallo JM, Williams NI, Downs DS, Le Masurier GC. Walking for health in pregnancy. Res Q Exerc Sport. 2008;79(1):28–35. https://doi.org/10.1080/02701367.2008.10599457.
12. Owe KM, Nystad W, Bø K. Correlates of regular exercise during pregnancy: the Norwegian Mother and Child Cohort Study. Scand J Med Sci Sports. 2009;19(5):637–45. https://doi.org/10.1111/j.1600-0838.2008.00840.x.
13. Evenson KR, Wen F. National trends in self-reported physical activity and sedentary behaviors among pregnant women: NHANES 1999–2006. Prev Med. 2010;50(3):123–8. https://doi.org/10.1016/j.ypmed.2009.12.015.
14. Walsh JM, McGowan CA, Mahony R, Foley ME, McAuliffe FM. Low glycaemic index diet in pregnancy to prevent macrosomia (ROLO study): randomised control trial. BMJ. 2012;345:e5605.
15. Hegaard HK, Damm P, Hedegaard M, Henriksen TB, Ottesen B, Dykes A-K, et al. Sports and leisure time physical activity during pregnancy in nulliparous women. Matern Child Health J. 2011;15(6):806–13. https://doi.org/10.1007/s10995-010-0647-y.
16. Tinloy J, Chuang CH, Zhu J, Pauli J, Kraschnewski JL, Kjerulff KH. Exercise during pregnancy and risk of late preterm birth, cesarean delivery, and hospitalizations. Womens Health Issues. 2014;24(1):e99–e104. https://doi.org/10.1016/j.whi.2013.11.003.
17. Liu L, Su H, Yu M. Full-term delivery in a pregnant breast cancer patient. Acta Obstet Gynecol Scand. 2011;90(12):1454. https://doi.org/10.1111/j.1600-0412.2011.01095.x.
18. Barakat R, Perales M, Garatachea N, Ruiz JR, Lucia A. Exercise during pregnancy. A narrative review asking: what do we know? Br J Sports Med. 2015;49(21):1377–81. https://doi.org/10.1136/bjsports-2015-094756.
19. Wastnedge EAN, Reynolds RM, van Boeckel SR, Stock SJ, Denison FC, Maybin JA, et al. Pregnancy and COVID-19. Physiol Rev. 2020;101(1):303–18. https://doi.org/10.1152/physrev.00024.2020.
20. Segal NA, Chu SR. Musculoskeletal anatomic, gait, and balance changes in pregnancy and risk for falls. In: Fitzgerald CM, Segal NA, editors. Musculoskeletal health in pregnancy and postpartum: an evidence-based guide for clinicians. Cham: Springer International Publishing; 2015. p. 1–18.
21. Reese ME, Casey E. Hormonal influence on the neuromusculoskeletal system in pregnancy. In: Fitzgerald CM, Segal NA, editors. Musculoskeletal health in pregnancy and postpartum: an evidence-based guide for clinicians. Cham: Springer International Publishing; 2015. p. 19–39.
22. Anselmo DS, Love E, Tango DN, Robinson L. Musculoskeletal effects of pregnancy on the lower extremity: a literature review. J Am Podiatr Med Assoc. 2017;107(1):60–4. https://doi.org/10.7547/15-061.
23. Institute of Medicine and National Research Council of the National Academies. Weight gain during pregnancy: reexamining the guidelines. Washington, DC: The National Academies Press; 2009.
24. Wang TW, Apgar BS. Exercise during pregnancy. Am Fam Physician. 1998;57(8):1846–52, 57.
25. Whitcome KK, Shapiro LJ, Lieberman DE. Fetal load and the evolution of lumbar lordosis in bipedal hominins. Nature. 2007;450(7172):1075–U11. https://doi.org/10.1038/nature06342.
26. Cunningham FG. Williams obstetrics. 25th ed. New York, NY: McGraw-Hill; 2018.
27. Ostgaard HC, Andersson GB, Schultz AB, Miller JA. Influence of some biomechanical factors on low-back pain in pregnancy. Spine (Phila Pa 1976). 1993;18(1):61–5.

28. Gilleard WL, Brown JM. Structure and function of the abdominal muscles in primigravid subjects during pregnancy and the immediate postbirth period. Phys Ther. 1996;76(7):750–62.
29. Foti T, Davids JR, Bagley A. A biomechanical analysis of gait during pregnancy. J Bone Joint Surg Am. 2000;82A(5):625–32.
30. Gutke A, Ostgaard HC, Oberg B. Predicting persistent pregnancy-related low back pain. Spine (Phila Pa 1976). 2008;33(12):E386–93. https://doi.org/10.1097/BRS.0b013e31817331a4.
31. Wang SM, Dezinno P, Maranets I, Berman MR, Caldwell-Andrews AA, Kain ZN. Low back pain during pregnancy: prevalence, risk factors, and outcomes. Obstet Gynecol. 2004;104(1):65–70. https://doi.org/10.1097/01.AOG.0000129403.54061.0e.
32. Mogren IM, Pohjanen AI. Low back pain and pelvic pain during pregnancy: prevalence and risk factors. Spine (Phila Pa 1976). 2005;30(8):983–91. https://doi.org/10.1097/01.brs.0000158957.42198.8e.
33. Ng BK, Kipli M, Abdul Karim AK, Shohaimi S, Abdul Ghani NA, Lim PS. Back pain in pregnancy among office workers: risk factors and its impact on quality of life. Horm Mol Biol Clin Invest. 2017;32(3) https://doi.org/10.1515/hmbci-2017-0037.
34. Aldabe D, Milosavljevic S, Bussey MD. Is pregnancy related pelvic girdle pain associated with altered kinematic, kinetic and motor control of the pelvis? A systematic review. Eur Spine J. 2012;21(9):1777–87. https://doi.org/10.1007/s00586-012-2401-1.
35. Monteiro M, Gabriel R, Aranha J, Neves e Castro M, Sousa M, Moreira M. Influence of obesity and sarcopenic obesity on plantar pressure of postmenopausal women. Clin Biomech. 2010;25(5):461–7. https://doi.org/10.1016/j.clinbiomech.2010.01.017.
36. Woo J, Leung J, Kwok T. BMI, body composition, and physical functioning in older adults. Obesity. 2007;15(7):1886–94. https://doi.org/10.1038/oby.2007.223.
37. Bosch K, Nagel A, Weigend L, Rosenbaum D. From "first" to "last" steps in life – pressure patterns of three generations. Clin Biomech. 2009;24(8):676–81. https://doi.org/10.1016/j.clinbiomech.2009.06.001.
38. Ramachandra P, Kumar P, Kamath A, Maiya AG. Do structural changes of the foot influence plantar pressure patterns during various stages of pregnancy and postpartum? Foot Ankle Spec. 2017;10(6):513–9. https://doi.org/10.1177/1938640016685150.
39. Varol T, Göker A, Cezayirli E, Özgür S, Tuç Yücel A. Relation between foot pain and plantar pressure in pregnancy. Turk J Med Sci. 2017;47(4):1104–8. https://doi.org/10.3906/sag-1601-185.
40. Butler EE, Druzin M, Sullivan EV. Gait adaptations in adulthood: pregnancy, aging, and alcoholism. In: Rose J, Gamble JG, editors. Human walking. 3rd ed. Philadelphia, PA: Lippincott Williams & Wilkins; 2006. p. 131–48.
41. Hong Y, Bartlett R. Routledge handbook of biomechanics and human movement science. Routledge international handbooks. London; New York, NY: Routledge; 2010.
42. Nigg BM, Herzog W. Biomechanics of the musculo-skeletal system. 3rd ed. Hoboken, NJ: John Wiley & Sons; 2007.
43. Flanagan SP. Biomechanics: a case-based approach. 2nd ed. Burlington, MA: Jones & Bartlett Learning; 2019.
44. Elliott B. Biomechanics: an integral part of sport science and sport medicine. J Sci Med Sport. 1999;2(4):299–310. https://doi.org/10.1016/S1440-2440(99)80003-6.
45. Brüggemann G-P, Potthast W, Braunstein B, Niehoff A. Effect of increased mechanical stimuli on foot muscles functional capacity. In: Cavanagh PR, Crago PE, editors. XXth Congress of the International Society of Biomechanics and 29th Annual Meeting of the American Society of Biomechanics. Cleveland, OH: International Society of Biomechanics; 2005.
46. Nicholls JA, Grieve DW. Performance of physical tasks in pregnancy. Ergonomics. 1992;35(3):301–11. https://doi.org/10.1080/00140139208967815.
47. Perry J. Gait analysis: normal and pathological function. Thorofare, NJ: SLACK; 1992.
48. Forczek W, Staszkiewicz R. Changes of kinematic gait parameters due to pregnancy. Acta Bioeng Biomech. 2012;14(4):113–9. https://doi.org/10.5277/abb120413.

49. Lymbery JK, Gilleard W. The stance phase of walking during late pregnancy - temporospatial and ground reaction force variables. J Am Podiat Med Assoc. 2005;95(3):247–53. https://doi.org/10.7547/0950247.
50. Gilleard WL. Trunk motion and gait characteristics of pregnant women when walking: report of a longitudinal study with a control group. BMC Pregnan Childb. 2013;13:71. https://doi.org/10.1186/1471-2393-13-71.
51. Bartlett R. Introduction to sports biomechanics: analysing human movement patterns. 3rd ed. Abingdon: Routledge; 2019.
52. Branco M, Santos-Rocha R, Vieira F, Aguiar L, Veloso AP. Three-dimensional kinematic adaptations of gait throughout pregnancy and postpartum. Acta Bioeng Biomech. 2016;18(2):153. https://doi.org/10.5277/ABB-00418-2015-05.
53. Abdel-Aziz YI, Karara HM, Hauck M. Direct linear transformation from comparator coordinates into object space coordinates in close-range photogrammetry*. Photogramm Eng Remote Sens. 2015;81(2):103–7. https://doi.org/10.14358/PERS.81.2.103.
54. Bartlett R. Introduction to sports biomechanics: analysing human movement patterns. 2nd ed. Abingdon, Oxon; New York, NY: Routledge; 2007.
55. Richards J. Biomechanics in clinic and research: an interactive teaching and learning course. Edinburgh; New York, NY: Churchill Livingstone/Elsevier; 2008.
56. Robertson DGE, Caldwell GE, Hamill J, Kamen G, Whittlesey SN. Research methods in biomechanics. 2nd ed. Champaign, IL: Human Kinetics; 2014.
57. Winter DA. Biomechanics and motor control of human movement. 4th ed. Hoboken, NJ: Wiley; 2009.
58. Nigg BM, Liu W. The effect of muscle stiffness and damping on simulated impact force peaks during running. J Biomech. 1999;32(8):849–56. https://doi.org/10.1016/S0021-9290(99)00048-2.
59. Miller D. Ground reaction forces in distance running. In: Cavanagh P, editor. Biomechanics of distance running. Champaign, IL: Human Kinetics; 1990.
60. Peterson DR, Bronzino JD. Biomechanics: principles and applications. Boca Raton, FL. London: CRC, Taylor & Francis; 2008.
61. Whittle M. Gait analysis: an introduction. 4th ed. Edinburgh; New York, NY: Butterworth-Heinemann; 2007.
62. Inman DJ, Soutas-Little R. Engineering mechanics: dynamics. Hoboken, NJ: Prentice Hall PTR; 1998.
63. Nigg BM, MacIntosh BR, Mester J. Biomechanics and biology of movement. Champaign, IL: Human Kinetics; 2000.
64. Watkins J. Structure and function of the musculoskeletal system. 2nd ed. Champaign, IL: Human Kinetics; 2010.
65. Turner CH, Robling AG. Designing exercise regimens to increase bone strength. Exerc Sport Sci Rev. 2003;31(1):45–50.
66. Witzke KA, Snow CM. Effects of plyometric jump training on bone mass in adolescent girls. Med Sci Sports Exerc. 2000;32(6):1051–7.
67. Hohmann E, Reaburn P, Tetsworth K, Imhoff A. Plantar pressures during long distance running: an investigation of 10 marathon runners. J Sports Sci Med. 2016;15(2):254–62.
68. Hennig EM, Milani TL. Shoe pressure distribution for running in various types of footwear. J Appl Biomech. 1995;11(3):299–310. https://doi.org/10.1123/jab.11.3.299.
69. Hughes J, Pratt L, Linge K, Clark P, Klenerman L. Reliability of pressure measurements: the EM ED F system. Clin Biomech. 1991;6(1):14–8. https://doi.org/10.1016/0268-0033(91)90036-P.
70. Santos-Rocha R, Veloso A. Comparative study of plantar pressure during step exercise in different floor conditions. J Appl Biomech. 2007;23(2):162–8. https://doi.org/10.1123/jab.23.2.162.
71. Abdul Razak AH, Zayegh A, Begg RK, Wahab Y. Foot plantar pressure measurement system: a review. Sensors. 2012;12(7):9884.
72. Robinson CC, Balbinot LF, Silva MF, Achaval M, Zaro MA. Plantar pressure distribution patterns of individuals with prediabetes in comparison with healthy individuals

and individuals with diabetes. J Diabetes Sci Technol. 2013;7(5):1113–21. https://doi.org/10.1177/193229681300700503.
73. Keijsers NLW, Stolwijk NM, Louwerens JWK, Duysens J. Classification of forefoot pain based on plantar pressure measurements. Clin Biomech. 2013;28(3):350–6. https://doi.org/10.1016/j.clinbiomech.2013.01.012.
74. Amemiya A, Noguchi H, Oe M, Ohashi Y, Ueki K, Kadowaki T, et al. Elevated plantar pressure in diabetic patients and its relationship with their gait features. Gait Posture. 2014;40(3):408–14. https://doi.org/10.1016/j.gaitpost.2014.05.063.
75. Butterworth PA, Landorf KB, Gilleard W, Urquhart DM, Menz HB. The association between body composition and foot structure and function: a systematic review. Obes Rev. 2014;15(4):348–57. https://doi.org/10.1111/obr.12130.
76. O'Brien DL, Tyndyk M. Effect of arch type and Body Mass Index on plantar pressure distribution during stance phase of gait. Acta Bioeng Biomech. 2014;16(2):131–5.
77. Mickle KJ, Munro BJ, Lord SR, Menz HB, Steele JR. Foot pain, plantar pressures, and falls in older people: a prospective study. J Am Geriatr Soc. 2010;58(10):1936–40. https://doi.org/10.1111/j.1532-5415.2010.03061.x.
78. Fernando M, Crowther R, Lazzarini P, Sangla K, Cunningham M, Buttner P, et al. Biomechanical characteristics of peripheral diabetic neuropathy: a systematic review and meta-analysis of findings from the gait cycle, muscle activity and dynamic barefoot plantar pressure. Clin Biomech. 2013;28(8):831–45. https://doi.org/10.1016/j.clinbiomech.2013.08.004.
79. Justin S, Joshua B, Roger A, Evangelos P, Jack C. Musculoskeletal and activity-related factors associated with plantar heel pain. Foot Ankle Int. 2014;36(1):37–45. https://doi.org/10.1177/1071100714551021.
80. Ramalho F, Santos-Rocha R, Branco M, Moniz-Pereira V, André H-I, Veloso A, et al. Effect of 6-month community-based exercise interventions on gait and functional fitness of an older population: a quasi-experimental study. Clin Interv Aging. 2018;13:595–606. https://doi.org/10.2147/cia.s157224.
81. Shin Jin H, Lee Joong S, Han Ki H, Bae Kang H. Effects of foot strengthening exercises and functional insole on range of motion and foot plantar pressure in elderly women. J Kor Soc Kinesiol. 2018;28(1):45–54. https://doi.org/10.5103/KJSB.2018.28.1.45.
82. Rowlands C, Plumb MS. The effects of a 4-week barefoot exercise intervention on plantar pressure, impact, balance and pain in injured recreational runners: a pilot study. Int J Osteopath Med. 2019;33:1–7. https://doi.org/10.1016/j.ijosm.2019.10.005.
83. Lee NK, Kwon JW, Son SM, Nam SH, Choi YW, Kim CS. Changes of plantar pressure distributions following open and closed kinetic chain exercise in patients with stroke. Neurorehabilitation. 2013;32:385–90. https://doi.org/10.3233/NRE-130859.
84. Molina-Garcia P, Miranda-Aparicio D, Molina-Molina A, Plaza-Florido A, Migueles JH, Mora-Gonzalez J, et al. Effects of exercise on plantar pressure during walking in children with overweight/obesity. Med Sci Sports Exerc. 2020;52(3):654.
85. Jimenez EMM, Velazquez JID, Gomez RS, Nuno FS, Hernandez IC, Castells XG. Experimental studies of gait biomechanics during pregnancy: systematic review of clinical trials. (2000-2018). Revista Internacional De Ciencias Podologicas. 2019;13(2):77–86. https://doi.org/10.5209/ricp.64723.
86. Ribeiro AP, João SMA, Sacco ICN. Static and dynamic biomechanical adaptations of the lower limbs and gait pattern changes during pregnancy. Women Health. 2013;9(1):99–108. https://doi.org/10.2217/whe.12.59.
87. Branco M, Santos-Rocha R, Vieira F. Biomechanics of gait during pregnancy. Sci World J. 2014;2014:5. https://doi.org/10.1155/2014/527940.
88. Anselmo DS, Love E, Tango DN, Robinson L. Musculoskeletal effects of pregnancy on the lower extremity: a literature review. J Am Podiat Med Assoc. 2017;107(1):60–4. https://doi.org/10.7547/15-061.
89. Forczek W, Ivanenko YP, Bielatowicz J, Wacławik K. Gait assessment of the expectant mothers - systematic review. Gait Posture. 2018;62:7–19. https://doi.org/10.1016/j.gaitpost.2018.02.024.

90. Wong JKL, McGregor AH. Spatiotemporal gait changes in healthy pregnant women and women with pelvic girdle pain: a systematic review. J Back Musculoskelet Rehabil. 2018;31(5):821–38. https://doi.org/10.3233/bmr-170828.
91. Conder R, Zamani R, Akrami M. The biomechanics of pregnancy: a systematic review. J Funct Morphol Kinesiol. 2019;4(4):72. https://doi.org/10.3390/jfmk4040072.
92. Ribeiro AP. Posture and gait biomechanical aspects during pregnancy and the importance of therapeutic exercise: literature review. Curr Women's Health Rev. 2015;11(1):51–8. https://doi.org/10.2174/157340481101150914201529.
93. Salazar NQ. Alteraciones musculoesqueléticas y adaptaciones biomecánicas durante los trimestres de embarazo: una revisión sistemática. Pensar en Movimiento: Revista de Ciencias del Ejercicio y la Salud. 2021;19(1):e44961. https://doi.org/10.15517/pensarmov.v19i1.44961.
94. Hrvatin I, Rugelj D. Risk factors for accidental falls during pregnancy - a systematic literature review. J Matern Fetal Neonatal Med. 2021:1–10. https://doi.org/10.1080/14767058.2021.1935849.
95. Nyska M, Sofer D, Porat A, Howard CB, Levi A, Meizner I. Planter foot pressures in pregnant women. Isr J Med Sci. 1997;33(2):139–46.
96. Goldberg J, Besser MP, Selby-Silverstein L. Changes in foot function throughout pregnancy. Obstet Gynecol. 2001;97(4):S39. https://doi.org/10.1016/S0029-7844(01)01235-2.
97. Huang T-H, Lin S-C, Ho C-S, Yu C-Y, Chou Y-L. The gait analysis of pregnant women. Biomed Eng Appl Basis Commun. 2002;14(2):4. https://doi.org/10.4015/s1016237202000103.
98. Ribas SI, Guirro ECO. Analysis of plantar pressure and postural balance during different phases of pregnancy. Rev Bras Fis. 2007;11(5):391–6.
99. Carpes F, Griebeler D, Kleinpaul J, Mann L, Mota C. Women able-bodied gait kinematics during and post pregnancy period. Brazilian. J Biomech. 2008;9(16):33.
100. Gaymer C, Whalley H, Achten J, Vatish M, Costa ML. Midfoot plantar pressure significantly increases during late gestation. Foot. 2009;19(2):114–6. https://doi.org/10.1016/j.foot.2009.02.001.
101. Karadag-Saygi E, Unlu-Ozkan F, Basgul A. Plantar pressure and foot pain in the last trimester of pregnancy. Foot Ankle Int. 2010;31(2):153–7. https://doi.org/10.3113/FAI.2010.0153.
102. Hagan L, Wong CK. Gait in pregnant women: spinal and lower extremity changes from pre- to postpartum. J Women's Health Phys Therapy. 2010;34(2):46–56. https://doi.org/10.1097/jwh.0b013e3181e8fd4d.
103. Ribeiro AP, Trombini-Souza F, Sacco IDN, Ruano R, Zugaib M, Joao SMA. Changes in the plantar pressure distribution during gait throughout gestation. J Am Podiat Med Assoc. 2011;101(5):415–23.
104. McCrory JL, Chambers AJ, Daftary A, Redfern MS. Ground reaction forces during gait in pregnant fallers and non-fallers. Gait Posture. 2011;34(4):524–8. https://doi.org/10.1016/j.gaitpost.2011.07.007.
105. Moccellin AS, Driusso P. Adjustments in static and dynamic postural control during pregnancy and their relationship with quality of life: a descriptive study. Fisioterapia. 2012;34(5):196–202. https://doi.org/10.1016/j.ft.2012.03.004.
106. Branco M, Santos-Rocha R, Aguiar L, Vieira F, Veloso AP. Kinematic analysis of gait in the second and third trimesters of pregnancy. J Pregnancy. 2013;2013:718095. https://doi.org/10.1155/2013/718095.
107. Sunaga Y, Anan M, Shinkoda K. Biomechanics of rising from a chair and walking in pregnant women. Appl Ergon. 2013;44(5):792–8. https://doi.org/10.1016/j.apergo.2013.01.010.
108. Aguiar L, Santos-Rocha R, Vieira F, Branco M, Andrade C, Veloso A. Comparison between overweight due to pregnancy and due to added weight to simulate body mass distribution in pregnancy. Gait Posture. 2015;42(4):511–7. https://doi.org/10.1016/j.gaitpost.2015.07.065.
109. Branco M, Santos-Rocha R, Vieira F, Aguiar L, Veloso AP. Three-dimensional kinetic adaptations of gait throughout pregnancy and postpartum. Scientifica. 2015;2015:580374. https://doi.org/10.1155/2015/580374.

110. Yoo H, Shin D, Song C. Changes in the spinal curvature, degree of pain, balance ability, and gait ability according to pregnancy period in pregnant and nonpregnant women. J Phys Ther Sci. 2015;27(1):279–84.
111. Gimunova M, Kasović M, Zvonar M, Turčínek P, Matković B, Ventruba P, et al. Analysis of ground reaction force in gait during different phases of pregnancy. Kinesiology. 2015;47(2):236–41.
112. Bertuit J, Leyh C, Rooze M, Feipel V. Plantar pressure during gait in pregnant women. J Am Podiat Med Assoc. 2016;106(6):398–405.
113. Branco M, Santos-Rocha R, Aguiar L, Vieira F, Veloso AP. Kinetic analysis of gait in the second and third trimesters of pregnancy. J Mech Med Biol. 2016;16(4):1. https://doi.org/10.1142/S021951941650055x.
114. Blaszczyk JW, Opala-Berdzik A, Plewa M. Adaptive changes in spatiotemporal gait characteristics in women during pregnancy. Gait Posture. 2016;43:160–4. https://doi.org/10.1016/j.gaitpost.2015.09.016.
115. Ramachandra P, Kumar P, Kamath A, Maiya AG. Do structural changes of the foot influence plantar pressure patterns during various stages of pregnancy and postpartum? Foot Ankle Spec. 2016;10:513. https://doi.org/10.1177/1938640016685150.
116. Elsayed E, Devreux I, Embaby H, Alsayed A, Alshehri M. Changes in foot plantar pressure in pregnant women. J Back Musculoskelet Rehabil. 2017;30(4):863–7. https://doi.org/10.3233/BMR-160555.
117. Krkeljas Z. Changes in gait and posture as factors of dynamic stability during walking in pregnancy. Hum Mov Sci. 2018;58:315–20. https://doi.org/10.1016/j.humov.2017.12.011.
118. Mei Q, Gu Y, Fernandez J. Alterations of pregnant gait during pregnancy and post-partum. Sci Rep. 2018;8(1):2217. https://doi.org/10.1038/s41598-018-20648-y.
119. Christensen L, Veierod MB, Vollestad NK, Jakobsen VE, Stuge B, Cabri J, et al. Kinematic and spatiotemporal gait characteristics in pregnant women with pelvic girdle pain, asymptomatic pregnant and non-pregnant women. Clin Biomech. 2019;68:45–52. https://doi.org/10.1016/j.clinbiomech.2019.05.030.
120. Martínez-Martí F, Ocón-Hernández O, Martínez-García MS, Torres-Ruiz F, Martínez-Olmos A, Carvajal MA, et al. Plantar pressure changes and their relationships with low back pain during pregnancy using instrumented insoles. J Sensors. 2019;2019:1567584. https://doi.org/10.1155/2019/1567584.
121. Mikeska O, Gimunova M, Zvonar M. Assessment of distribution of plantar pressures and foot characteristics during walking in pregnant women. Acta Bioeng Biomech. 2019;21(3):49–56. https://doi.org/10.5277/abb-01373-2019-04.
122. Forczek W, Masłoń A, Frączek B, Curyło M, Salamaga M, Suder A. Does the first trimester of pregnancy induce alterations in the walking pattern? PLoS One. 2019;14(1):e0209766. https://doi.org/10.1371/journal.pone.0209766.
123. Forczek W, Ivanenko Y, Salamaga M, Sylos-Labini F, Frączek B, Masłoń A, et al. Pelvic movements during walking throughout gestation - the relationship between morphology and kinematic parameters. Clin Biomech. 2020;71:146–51. https://doi.org/10.1016/j.clinbiomech.2019.11.001.
124. Bagwell JJ, Reynolds N, Walaszek M, Runez H, Lam K, Armour Smith J, et al. Lower extremity kinetics and muscle activation during gait are significantly different during and after pregnancy compared to nulliparous females. Gait Posture. 2020;81:33–40. https://doi.org/10.1016/j.gaitpost.2020.07.002.
125. Song Y, Liang M, Lian W. A comparison of foot kinematics between pregnant and non-pregnant women using the Oxford foot model during walking. Int J Biomed Eng Technol. 2020;34(1):20–30. https://doi.org/10.1504/IJBET.2020.110335.
126. Pauk J, Swinarska D, Daunoraviciene K. Mechanisms of gait adaptation in overweight pregnant women. J Am Podiat Med Assoc. 2020;110(4):2. https://doi.org/10.7547/17-177.
127. Catena RD, Wolcott WC. Self-selection of gestational lumbopelvic posture and bipedal evolution. Gait Posture. 2021;89:7–13. https://doi.org/10.1016/j.gaitpost.2021.06.022.

128. Aguiar L, Andrade C, Branco M, Santos-Rocha R, Vieira F, Veloso A. Global optimization method applied to the kinematics of gait in pregnant women. J Mech Med Biol. 2016;16(6):1. https://doi.org/10.1142/S0219519416500846.
129. Aguiar L, Santos-Rocha R, Branco M, Vieira F, Veloso A. Biomechanical model for kinetic and kinematic description of gait during second trimester of pregnancy to study the effects of biomechanical load on the musculoskeletal system. J Mech Med Biol. 2014;14(1):1450004. https://doi.org/10.1142/S0219519414500043.
130. Rodacki CL, Fowler NE, Rodacki AL, Birch K. Stature loss and recovery in pregnant women with and without low back pain. Arch Phys Med Rehabil. 2003;84(4):507–12. https://doi.org/10.1053/apmr.2003.50119.
131. Fries EC, Hellebrandt FA. The influence of pregnancy on the location of the center of gravity, postural stability, and body alignment. Am J Obstet Gynecol. 1943;46:374–80.
132. Opala-Berdzik A, Bacik B, Cieślińska-Świder J, Plewa M, Gajewska M. The influence of pregnancy on the location of the center of gravity in standing position. J Hum Kinet. 2010;2010(26):5–11. https://doi.org/10.2478/v10078-010-0042-1.
133. Calguneri M, Bird HA, Wright V. Changes in joint laxity occurring during pregnancy. Ann Rheum Dis. 1982;41(2):126–8. https://doi.org/10.1136/ard.41.2.126.
134. Schauberger CW, Rooney BL, Goldsmith L, Shenton D, Silva PD, Schaper A. Peripheral joint laxity increases in pregnancy but does not correlate with serum relaxin levels. Am J Obstet Gynecol. 1996;174(2):667–71. https://doi.org/10.1016/S0002-9378(96)70447-7.
135. Jang J, Hsiao KT, Hsiao-Wecksler ET. Balance (perceived and actual) and preferred stance width during pregnancy. Clin Biomech. 2008;23(4):468–76. https://doi.org/10.1016/j.clinbiomech.2007.11.011.
136. Sancar Ş, Atalay Güzel N, Çobanoğlu G, Özdemir Y, Bayram M. The changes in static balance during pregnancy: a prospective longitudinal study. Clin Exp Health Sci. 2021;11:127. https://doi.org/10.33808/clinexphealthsci.744603.
137. Catena RD, Connolly CP, McGeorge KM, Campbell N. A comparison of methods to determine center of mass during pregnancy. J Biomech. 2018;71:217–24. https://doi.org/10.1016/j.jbiomech.2018.02.004.
138. Branco M, Santos-Rocha R, Vieira F, Silva MR, Aguiar L, Veloso AP. Influence of body composition on gait kinetics throughout pregnancy and postpartum period. Scientifica. 2016;2016:3921536. https://doi.org/10.1155/2016/3921536.
139. Paisley JE, Mellion MB. Exercise during Pregnancy. Am Fam Physician. 1988;38(5):143–50.
140. Gilleard W, Crosbie J, Smith R. Effect of pregnancy on trunk range of motion when sitting and standing. Acta Obstet Gynecol Scand. 2002;81(11):1011–20.
141. Vullo VJ, Richardson JK, Hurvitz EA. Hip, knee, and foot pain during pregnancy and the postpartum period. J Fam Pract. 1996;43:63.
142. Bertuit J, Leyh C, Feipel V. Center of plantar pressure during gait in pregnancy-related pelvic girdle pain and the effect of pelvic belts. Acta Bioeng Biomech. 2018;20(3):69–76. https://doi.org/10.5277/abb-01141-2018-02.
143. Vico Pardo FJ, López Del Amo A, Pardo Rios M, Gijon-Nogueron G, Yuste CC. Changes in foot posture during pregnancy and their relation with musculoskeletal pain: a longitudinal cohort study. Women Birth. 2018;31(2):e84–e8. https://doi.org/10.1016/j.wombi.2017.08.114.
144. Albino MA, Moccellin AS, Firmento Bda S, Driusso P. [Gait force propulsion modifications during pregnancy: effects of changes in feet's dimensions]. Revista Brasileira de Ginecologia e Obstetricia 2011;33(7):164–9.
145. Inanir A, Cakmak B, Hisim Y, Demirturk F. Evaluation of postural equilibrium and fall risk during pregnancy. Gait Posture. 2014;39(4):1122–5. https://doi.org/10.1016/j.gaitpost.2014.01.013.
146. Gottschall JS, Sheehan RC, Downs DS. Pregnant women exaggerate cautious gait patterns during the transition between level and hill surfaces. J Electromyogr Kinesiol. 2013;23(5):1237–42. https://doi.org/10.1016/j.jelekin.2013.04.011.

147. Wallberg CD, Smart DM, Mackelprang JL, Graves JM. Stair-related injuries among pregnant women treated in united states emergency departments. Matern Child Health J. 2021;25(6):892–9. https://doi.org/10.1007/s10995-021-03141-3.
148. Kavurmaci SA, Gulbahar A. Physical trauma etiologies in pregnancy in Turkey. Clin Exp Obstet Gynecol. 2021;48(2):292–8. https://doi.org/10.31083/j.ceog.2021.02.2268.
149. McCrory JL, Chambers AJ, Daftary A, Redfern MS. Ground reaction forces during stair locomotion in pregnancy. Gait Posture. 2013;38(4):684–90. https://doi.org/10.1016/j.gaitpost.2013.03.002.
150. Ersal T, McCrory JL, Sienko KH. Theoretical and experimental indicators of falls during pregnancy as assessed by postural perturbations. Gait Posture. 2014;39(1):218–23. https://doi.org/10.1016/j.gaitpost.2013.07.011.
151. McCrory JL, Chambers AJ, Daftary A, Redfern MS. Ground reaction forces during stair locomotion in pregnant fallers and non-fallers. Clin Biomech. 2014;29(2):143–8. https://doi.org/10.1016/j.clinbiomech.2013.11.020.
152. Takeda K, Yoshikata H, Imura M. Changes in posture control of women that fall during pregnancy. Int J Womens Health Reprod Sci. 2018;6(3):255–62. https://doi.org/10.15296/ijwhr.2018.43.
153. Sawa R, Doi T, Asai T, Watanabe K, Taniguchi T, Ono R. Differences in trunk control between early and late pregnancy during gait. Gait Posture. 2015;42(4):455–9. https://doi.org/10.1016/j.gaitpost.2015.07.058.
154. Wu WH, Meijer OG, Lamoth CJC, Uegaki K, van Dieen JH, Wuisman PIJM, et al. Gait coordination in pregnancy: transverse pelvic and thoracic rotations and their relative phase. Clin Biomech. 2004;19(5):480–8. https://doi.org/10.1016/j.clinbiomech.2004.02.003.
155. Alberton CL, Bgeginski R, Pinto SS, Nunes GN, Andrade LS, Brasil B, et al. Water-based exercises in pregnancy: apparent weight in immersion and ground reaction force at third trimester. Clin Biomech. 2019;67:148–52. https://doi.org/10.1016/j.clinbiomech.2019.05.021.
156. Kluge J, Hall D, Louw Q, Theron G, Grove D. Specific exercises to treat pregnancy-related low back pain in a South African population. Int J Gynaecol Obstet. 2011;113(3):187–91. https://doi.org/10.1016/j.ijgo.2010.10.030.
157. Shim MJ, Lee YS, Oh HE, Kim JS. Effects of a back-pain-reducing program during pregnancy for Korean women: a non-equivalent control-group pretest-posttest study. Int J Nurs Stud. 2007;44(1):19–28. https://doi.org/10.1016/j.ijnurstu.2005.11.016.

Specific Musculoskeletal Adaptations in Pregnancy: Pelvic Floor, Abdominal Muscles, Pelvic Girdle, and Lower Back—Implications for Physical Activity and Exercise

6

Kari Bø, Britt Stuge, and Gunvor Hilde

Abstract

Pregnancy and childbirth bring along several changes to a woman's body, especially to the musculoskeletal system. On one hand, pregnancy and childbirth not only represents a window of opportunity for the adoption of an active and healthy lifestyle, but it is also a risk period for the development of musculoskeletal disorders that may negatively affect ability to participate in physical activity both during pregnancy, in the postpartum period and for some, if the conditions are not treated, the rest of their lives. This chapter addresses the most prevalent musculoskeletal complaints related to pregnancy and the postpartum period: pelvic floor dysfunction; urinary incontinence, diastasis recti abdominis, and low back pain and/or pelvic girdle pain.

Keywords

Diastasis recti abdominis · Exercise · Low back pain · Pelvic floor pelvic girdle pain · Physical activity · Postpartum · Pregnancy

---

K. Bø (✉)
Department of Sports Medicine, Norwegian School of Sport Sciences, Oslo, Norway

Department of Obstetrics and Gynecology, Akershus University Hospital, Lørenskog, Norway
e-mail: kari.bo@nih.no

B. Stuge
Division of Orthopaedic Surgery, Oslo University Hospital, Oslo, Norway
e-mail: britt.stuge@medisin.uio.no

G. Hilde
Department of Physiotherapy, OsloMet-Oslo Metropolitan University (former: Oslo and Akershus University College of Applied Sciences), Oslo, Norway
e-mail: ghilde@oslomet.no

R. Santos-Rocha (ed.), *Exercise and Physical Activity During Pregnancy and Postpartum*, https://doi.org/10.1007/978-3-031-06137-0_6

6.1 Introduction

Pregnancy and childbirth bring along several changes to a woman's body, especially to the musculoskeletal system. Pregnancy represents a window of opportunity for the adoption of an active and healthy lifestyle, but it is also a risk period for development of musculoskeletal disorders. This chapter addresses the most prevalent musculoskeletal complaints during pregnancy and after childbirth; pelvic floor muscle dysfunction; urinary incontinence, diastasis recti abdominis, and low back pain and/or pelvic girdle pain. These conditions are reported to have a negative effect on activity of daily living and quality of life, and especially participation in physical activities.

6.2 The Pelvic Floor

The urethra, bladder, vagina, uterus, and bowel situated within the pelvis are given structural support by pelvic floor structures arranged into a superficial and a deep layer of muscles and connective tissue (ligaments and fascia) [1]. In addition to pelvic organ support, the pelvic floor maintains continence, permit urination, defecation, intercourse, and vaginal birth [1].

The superficial layer of the pelvic floor includes the perinal muscles (ischiocavernosus, bulbospongiosus, and transversus perinea superficialis), and the deep layer includes the levator ani (LA) muscle [1]. The pelvic floor muscles (PFM) in addition to the urethral and anal sphincter system (external and internal sphincter muscles and vascular elements within the submucosa) play a significant role in maintaining pelvic organ support and continence [1–3].

The PFM interact with the supportive ligaments and fasciae in order to maintain support of the pelvic organs, and protect the pelvic floor connective tissue from excessive loads [3–5]. The function of this supportive system is illustrated by the "boat in dry dock theory" by Norton [5], where the PFM act as water in the dock floating the boat (pelvic organs) unloading the mooring (ligaments and fasciae) holding the boat in place. If the water is removed (loss of pelvic floor muscle tone), the moorings (pelvic ligaments and fasciae) are placed under excessive strain.

A voluntary PFM contraction can best be described as an inward lift and squeeze around the urethra, vagina, and rectum [6, 7]. During a voluntary PFM contraction, the urethra is compressed against adjacent tissues, which creates increased urethral pressure and stabilization of the urethra and bladder neck [2, 3].

The area surrounding the pelvic openings (urethra, vagina, and rectum) is named the levator hiatus (LH). The normal baseline activity of the PFM keeps the pelvic openings and the LH closed and keeps the pelvic floor elevated inside the pelvis [4, 8]. In situations where abdominal pressure increases, during physical exertions such as coughing, laughing, high impact activities etc., a simultaneous well-timed PFM contraction may counteract the increased abdominal pressure by increased structural support and compression of the urethra [2–4, 9].

The PFM is supposed to react automatically when the abdominal pressure increases. The pelvic floor works like a "firm trampoline" giving a quick response when loads are put onto it [10]. This is one theory. Another, and maybe more likely, theory is that a well-functioning pelvic floor implies an adequately located and firm pelvic floor musculature that keeps the LH closed and with no or little downward movement during increases in intra-abdominal pressure, thus preventing hypermobility and opening of the urethra.

Together with the urethral sphincter muscles, the PFM play an important role for maintaining urinary continence [2–4, 9]. The mechanical supportive potential of the PFM is demonstrated by Miller et al. [11]. By perineal ultrasound assessment, they found that a voluntary contraction of the PFM prior to and during a cough (a manoeuvre called the "Knack") resulted in a significant reduced displacement of the bladder neck [11]. Use of the "Knack" manoeuvre has also shown to significantly reduce urine loss among women with SUI [12, 13].

6.2.1 Pelvic Floor Dysfunction and Risk Factors

The understanding of the development of pelvic floor muscle dysfunction is far from complete. Rather than a single factor, the most common types of pelvic floor dysfunction (UI, faecal incontinence, and pelvic organ prolapse) probably have a complex list of risk factors [14–16]. Factors that may lead to the development of pelvic floor impairment and dysfunction in women can, according to Bump and Norton [14], be classified into the following four categories:

- **Predisposing factors:** e.g., gender, racial, neurologic, anatomic, collagen, muscular, cultural, and environmental.
- **Inciting factors:** e.g., childbirth, nerve damage, muscle damage, radiation, tissue disruption, and radical surgery.
- **Promoting factors:** e.g., constipation, occupation, recreation, obesity, surgery, lung disease, smoking, menstrual cycle, infection, medication, and menopause.
- **Decompensating factors:** e.g., aging, dementia, debility, disease, environment, and medication.

DeLancey et al. [16] integrate factors affecting pelvic floor dysfunction into a "Integrated Lifespan Model," in which pelvic floor function is plotted into three major life phases: (1) development of functional reserve during growth, influenced by predisposing factors, e.g., genetic constitution; (2) amount of injury and potential recovery occurring during and after childbirth; and (3) deterioration occurring with advancing age. Throughout the lifespan, a decline of the functional reserve of the pelvic floors may be accelerated by other factors, e.g., obesity and chronic coughing, medications, and dementia.

Knowledge about the various risk factors and their relative importance in relation to type of pelvic floor dysfunction is essential for primary and secondary prevention strategies [14, 16].

6.2.2 Urinary Incontinence

UI has been defined by the International Continence Society as "the complaint of any involuntary leakage of urine," and can further be classified into subtypes with the following definitions [17]:

- Stress urinary incontinence (SUI): "the complaint of involuntary leakage on effort or exertion, or on sneezing or coughing."
- Urgency urinary incontinence (UUI): "the complaint of involuntary leakage accompanied by or immediately proceeded by urgency."
- Mixed urinary incontinence (MUI): "the complaint of involuntary leakage associated with urgency and also with exertion, effort, sneezing or coughing."

6.2.2.1 Prevalence

A systematic literature review by Milsom et al. [18] including epidemiological studies from many different countries, showed a prevalence of any UI within the range 5–69% among the general female population. However, most of these studies showed a UI prevalence within the range 25–45% [18]. A wide range in UI prevalence might be explained by differences in the population studied, definition of UI, type of UI, and assessment of UI [19–21]. The most common type of UI reported by young and middle-aged women is SUI, while older women are more likely to report MUI and UUI [18, 22].

6.2.2.2 Prevalence During Pregnancy

Studies of prevalence of UI during pregnancy have shown period prevalence within the range 32–64% for any type of UI, and 40–59% for the combination SUI/MUI [18, 22]. Parity is associated with increased risk of UI. Higher period prevalence has been reported in parous than in nulliparous women [23–27]. A single delivery is associated with adjusted OR of around 1.3–1.6 for UI, and further deliveries linearly increasing the risk up to an adjusted OR of 1.5–2.0 [18]. Wesnes et al. [27] reported the results of a study being part of the Norwegian Mother and Child Cohort Study. Results showed that prevalence of UI increased from 15% before pregnancy to 48% at gestational Week 30 for nulliparous women, and from 35% before pregnancy to 67% at gestational Week 30 for parous women. SUI was the most common type of UI with figures showing an increase from 9% before pregnancy to 31% at gestational Week 30 for nulliparous women, and from 24% to 42% for parous women [28].

6.2.2.3 Prevalence After Childbirth

The estimation of postpartum UI is, according to Milsom et al. [22], challenged by study heterogeneity (study design and method, definition of UI, and sample studied). Milsom et al. [18] concluded that the prevalence of UI in the first 3 months post-delivery was 30%, with infrequent stress UI being the most common. The difference in UI rates between women delivering vaginally and those delivering by caesarean is evident immediately after delivery. There is a gradual decrease in prevalence during the first postpartum year. Instrumental delivery (vacuum and forceps) and perineal tears increases the risk of UI.

6.2.3 Etiology and Pathophysiology of Urinary Incontinence

UI also occurs in women who never have gone through pregnancy and childbirth and is common in nulliparous elite athletes of almost all sports [29]. However, pregnancy and childbirth are considered main etiological factors for the development of UI [30]. Connective tissue, peripheral nerves, and muscular structures are already during pregnancy subjected to hormonal, anatomical, and morphological changes. During vaginal delivery, the above mentioned structures are forcibly stretched and compressed. This may initiate changed tissue properties, which may contribute to altered pelvic floor function and increased risk of UI [30]. The picture of possible causative factors and the pathophysiology of UI is complex, some factors are studied more than others, and the importance of factors associated by the pregnancy itself versus factors associated childbirth is still under discussion [30].

6.2.3.1 Pregnancy

Prospective observational studies have shown increased prevalence of UI from the first trimester to the second, and further into the third trimester [26, 31, 32]. One hypothesis of increased prevalence during pregnancy is linked to increased bladder pressure due to the growing uterus and weight of the fetus, and another is linked to hormonal changes altering the viscoelastic properties [26]. In the observational study by Hvidman et al. [26], the authors suggest that UI may not be provoked by the onset of pregnancy, but by its progressive concentration of pregnancy hormones which may lead to local tissue changes. They found no association between UI and the birth weight of the child, and state less support for the theory linking UI to increased pressure on the bladder caused by weight of the fetus. Studies have shown an association between UI and maternal obesity both during pregnancy [27] and after childbirth [33–35], which could be caused by increased intra-abdominal pressure and increased bladder pressure [36].

The PFM is considered to play a significant role in the continence control system [2–4, 9], and urine loss may be linked to impaired PFM function, e.g., weak PFM. Several observational studies have demonstrated significantly higher PFM strength in continent women than in women having UI [37–44], while some studies did not find such difference [45, 46]. Three of the above-mentioned studies were on pregnant women [37, 41, 44]. In addition to significantly higher PFM strength, Mørkved et al. [41] also report a significantly thicker PFM among the continent pregnant women.

UI during pregnancy is transient in some women but may become long lasting in others. Prospective observational studies have shown that antenatal UI may increase the risk of postpartum UI [35, 47–49].

6.2.3.2 Childbirth

Parity seems to be an increased risk factor for UI [15, 24, 32, 50–52]. In a cross-sectional study of 27,900 women, Rørtveit et al. [51] report a relative risk (RR) of UI of 2.2 (95% CI: 1.8–2.6) for primiparus women and 3.3 (95% CI: 2.4–4.4) for grand multiparous women. Altman et al. [49] included 304 primiparous women and followed them 10 years prospectively. They found vaginal delivery to be independently associated with a significant long-term increase in SUI and UUI, regardless of maternal age and number of deliveries. This is supported by Viktrup et al. [35] following 241 primiparous women 12 years after their first delivery.

The protective effects of caesarean section have been and still are much debated. In a systematic review by Press et al. [53], the prevalence of postpartum SUI after caesarean section was compared with vaginal delivery. Based on data from six cross-sectional studies, caesarean section reduced the risk of postpartum SUI from 16% to 10% (OR 0.56; 95% CI: 0.45–0.68), while data from 12 cohort studies gave a reduction from 22% to 10% (OR 0.48; 95% CI: 0.39–0.58). However, risk of severe SUI and UUI did not differ by mode of birth.

6.2.3.3 Bladder Neck and Urethral Hypermobility

Impaired structural support of the urethra may cause increased bladder neck mobility and reduced compression of the urethra which again may lead to UI [3]. Peschers et al. [54] investigated change in bladder neck mobility, during the Valsalva manoeuvre, from late pregnancy to 6–10 weeks postpartum. They found increased mobility in women who delivered vaginally ($p < 0.001$), but found no such change in women with elective caesarean section ($p = 0.28$). Their findings are supported by Meyer et al. [55] and Dietz et al. [56].

Meyer et al. [57] found significantly higher bladder mobility, during the Valsalva maneuver, in women with SUI (mean parity 2.4, SD 0.8) when compared to nulliparous continent women. However, the association between increased bladder neck mobility and SUI may not solely be explained by vaginal childbirth. King and Freeman [58] followed nulliparous pregnant women with no pre-existing UI from gestational Week 15–17 to 10–14 weeks postpartum. They found that primiparous women with SUI postpartum had significantly greater antenatal bladder neck mobility than continent counterparts, which could be explained by a predisposed weak connective tissue, aggravated by pregnancy hormones and collagen remodelling [58, 59].

A study on bladder neck mobility and tissue stiffness was performed by Howard et al. [60]. Results from their study showed that primiparous women with SUI displayed similar bladder neck mobility during a cough and during a Valsalva manoeuvre ($p = 0.49$), while significantly less mobility was displayed during a cough than during the Valsalva both for continent nulliparous women ($p = 0.001$) and for continent primiparous women (0.002). When controlling for abdominal pressures, their calculations showed that nulliparous women displayed a significantly greater pelvic floor stiffness during a cough than the continent and incontinent primiparous women ($p = 0.001$).

6.2.3.4 Neural Denervation

Neuromuscular impairment is associated with the development of incontinence. Smith et al. [61] found that terminal branches of the pudendal nerve had a delayed conduction both to the striated urethral muscle and to the PFM in women with SUI when compared to continent women. Such denervation seems to be related to parity and vaginal childbirth [62–65]. In a biomechanical study by Lien et al. [66], lengthening of pudendal nerve branches was simulated by using a 3D computer model. The results from this study showed that the inferior rectal branch of the pudendal nerve may exhibit a strain of 35%. Pudendal nerve neuropathy appears to be associated with both a long second stage and high birth weight [64, 67, 68]. Such neural impairment may alter the muscle morphology. In a study by Gilpin et al. [69], biopsy samples from women with SUI showed a significant higher number of muscle fibers with pathological damage when compared to biopsy samples from continent women.

6.2.3.5 Weakening of the Pelvic Floor Muscles

Vaginal delivery is considered as a main risk factor for weakening of the PFM [64, 67, 70–75]. Due to the extensive stretching of muscle fibers and the likelihood of muscle denervation, it is not surprising that vaginal delivery may lead to reduced vaginal resting pressure and impaired PFM strength and endurance, and that caesarean section may protect the PFM. A PubMed search gave seven studies [37, 55, 76–80] investigating change in PFM strength from pregnancy to shortly after childbirth in relation to mode of delivery. Except from one study [78], the other six studies showed a significant reduction in PFM strength after vaginal delivery, but no significant decline after caesarean section.

6.2.4 Levator Ani Muscle Defects

Vaginal delivery may stretch and load beyond the physiological properties of the PFM, which may lead to muscle fibre tearing and reduced contractile force. The biomechanical study by Lien et al. [81] showed that muscle fibers of the most medial part of the LA muscle might be stretched up to three times their resting length as the fetal head is crowning. Their findings showing a pronounced stretch and deformation of the medial part of the LA muscle is confirmed by Hoyte et al. [82] and Parente et al. [83].

During recent years, technical advancement within magnetic resonance and ultrasound imaging has enabled diagnosis of defects of the LA muscle [84]. Major defects of the LA muscle are often defined as an abnormal insertion of this muscle toward the pubic bone, visually seen as a complete loss of visible muscle attachment at this specific site either unilaterally or bilaterally [70, 73, 84]. Imaging studies have shown that major LA muscle defects among primiparous women delivering vaginally could appear in 20–36% of the women [70, 85]. The use of forceps [71] and length of the second stage [71, 86] are associated with major LA muscle defects, whereas the importance of fetal head circumference and high fetal birth weight seems to be less clear [85–87].

Decreased strength is one of the most common symptoms following muscle tears within sport injuries [88]. Hence, decreased PFM strength in women with major LA muscle defects is expected, but has been sparsely investigated. A PubMed search revealed five observational studies [89–93] in which PFM strength in women with and without LA muscle defects was assessed. Results from all five studies showed significantly reduced PFM strength in women with LA muscle defects when compared to women without such defects. Dynamometer was used for the assessment of PFM strength in two of these five studies [89, 92], digital palpation in one study [90], transperineal ultrasound in one [91], and manometer in one [93]. These studies did also differ in age and parity of the women included.

Major LA muscle defects have shown a marked effect on hiatal dimensions [94–96] and pelvic organ support [96] which in turn could be explanatory factors for pelvic floor dysfunction. Major defect of the LA muscle has been linked to pelvic organ prolapse in particular [84, 89, 97, 98], while the link between LA muscle defects and UI is debated. Two studies [70, 85] report a significant association between LA muscle defects and SUI in the postpartum period. However, contradictory findings are reported for the link between LA muscle defects and SUI in studies on women with mixed parity and mean age >50 years [87, 99, 100].

6.2.5 Muscle Injury Regeneration

The healing process of a torn muscle has three phases: (1) the destruction phase, (2) the repair phase, and (3) the remodeling phase [88, 101, 102]. In the destruction phase, the rupture is followed by necrosis and formation of a hematoma. In the repair phase, a phagocytosis of necrotised tissue takes place, followed by proliferation of skeletal muscle satellite cells which induce regeneration of myofibrils. Along with this is formation of scar tissue and revascularization of the injured area initiated. During the remodeling phase, a further maturation of the regenerated myofibrils is implemented together with remodeling of the scar tissue, followed by recovery to functional capacity [88, 101, 102].

6.2.5.1 Treatment Principles for Skeletal Muscle Injuries

Recommendations for the treatment of muscle injuries and how to recover functional capacity are most often based on theoretical framework from epidemiological studies, clinical practice, and findings from experimental research [103]. Early mobilization is a standard treatment after muscle injury within sports medicine, and training is believed to be important in speeding up tissue healing (repair and remodelling). This approach is supported by experimental studies showing that early mobilisation after a muscle injury may facilitate the following: more rapid capillary ingrowths, improved parallel orientation of the regenerating myofibrils, and improved tensile properties [88, 101, 102, 104].

6.3 Diastasis Recti Abdominis

The most obvious change to the musculoskeletal system during pregnancy is related to the growth of the fetus and the stretching of the abdominal muscles, which may influence the mother's posture and balance [105]. Today there is a strong focus on the pregnant woman's appearance, especially through social media. Webpages and apps recommend how women should stay thin and get back into shape and "a flat tummy" at an early stage of the postpartum period. In addition, there are easily available advices on how to get rid of what is named "the mum's belly" (e.g., www.mammamage.se, www.breakingmuscle.com, www.befitmom.com, www.babybellybelt.com, http://tummyzip.com/). A systematic review of the scientific literature has found none or very weak evidence behind any of these advices [106].

A strong focus on an area of the body that is naturally changed during pregnancy and after childbirth, and that may recover by itself over time, maybe a risk factor for development of an unhealthy attitude towards exercise, appearance, body shape and image, and new mothers may become dissatisfied with their bodies and especially their abdomen. On the other hand, pregnancy and childbirth is a risk period for the development of obesity and musculoskeletal complaints such as low back and pelvic girdle pain [107] and pelvic floor dysfunctions including urinary and anal incontinence and pelvic organ prolapse [108]. A possible link between these conditions and injuries and weakness of the abdominal muscles has been postulated [109].

Diastasis recti abdominis (DRA) is defined as an impairment with midline separation of the two rectus abdominis muscles along the *linea alba*. The condition affects a significant number of women during the antenatal and postnatal period [110]. Prevalence rates (with and without protrusion/hernia) during pregnancy varies between 27% and 100% in the second and third trimesters [111, 112]. Postpartum, the prevalence rates of DRA vary between 30% and 68% [113, 114]. In a longitudinal study of 300 first-time pregnant women at Akershus University Hospital in Norway, Sperstad et al. [115] found that prevalence rates changed from 33% at gestational Week 21 to 60%, 45.4%, 32.6%, 6 weeks, 6 months, and 12 months postpartum, respectively. However, DRA has been found to be common in middle-aged women [116] and may also be present in men [117]. Whether strong abdominal muscles can prevent or is a risk factor for development of the condition is not known. To date, there are no prevalence studies or assessments of this condition among recreational exercisers and elite athletes [105].

DRA is diagnosed by measuring the distance between the median borders of the two rectus abdominis; inter-rectus distance (IRD), and measurement methods in use are palpation with fingerbreadths, caliper, or ultrasound [118]. Palpation is the most used method in clinical practice [119] and has an intra and inter-tester ICC of 0.5 and 0.7, respectively [120]. However, ultrasound has been found to have the best intra- and inter-tester reliability with ICC > 0.9 [121]. To date, there is no consensus on where to measure IRD along the *linea alba* (frequently used locations are 4.5 cm above the umbilicus, at the umbilicus and 4.5 cm below the umbilicus), or the cutoff point for diagnosing the condition [118]. A commonly used cutoff point is two fingerbreadths on palpation [118]. Candido et al. [122] have classified severity of the diastasis as follows: mild (2.5–3.5 cm or visible protrusion with diastasis less than 2.5 cm), moderate (3.5–5 cm), and substantial (>5 cm). Mota et al. [123] did a longitudinal study of 84 first-time pregnant women following them from gestational Week 35–41 and then 6–8, 12–14, and 24–26 weeks postpartum. They found higher values in these women compared to studies on nulliparous women at all measuring points and suggested a cutoff point for DRA of >28 mm in parous women.

The etiology and risk factors for DRA are not clear [124]. Fernandes da Mota et al. [125] found that neither age, BMI, weight gain during pregnancy, hypermobility, birthweight, abdominal circumference at gestational Week 35 nor exercise level before and during pregnancy were risk factors for diastasis 6 months postpartum. This was in agreement with the results of Sperstad et al. [115] comparing women with and without diastasis 12 months postpartum. Spitznagle et al. [116] found higher prevalence of DRA in older multiparous women, while Candido et al. [122] did not find any relationship with parity. None of the above mentioned studies found any relationship with mode of delivery (vaginal versus caesarean section) and diastasis.

6.3.1 Consequences of Diastasis Recti Abdominis

It has been postulated that DRA, in addition to being a cosmetic concern for many women, may reduce low back and pelvic stability and cause low back and pelvic girdle pain and be related to pelvic floor dysfunctions such as urinary incontinence, anal incontinence, and pelvic organ prolapse [116, 126]. However, to date, there is scant scientific knowledge on this topic. An association between DRA and abdominal muscle strength has not yet been substantiated with strong evidence. In a longitudinal small study following six women from gestational Week 14 to 8 weeks postpartum, Gilleard and Brown [127] found that women with IRD > 3.5 cm measured with palpation had reduced curl-up "capacity." This was supported by a study following 40 women postpartum, which found that postpartum women had weaker abdominal muscles than a control group [128]. However, at 6 months postpartum, there was no correlation between IRD and reduced abdominal muscle strength. Benjamin et al. [129], in a systematic review, found only weak evidence that DRA severity may be associated with impaired abdominal muscle strength. This was supported by a recent study of Gluppe et al. [130].

No strong link between DRA and low back pain has been found [129]. Parker et al. [131] found that women at least 3 months postpartum with DRA had more abdominal and pelvic pain than women without. Gluppe et al. [130] conferred more reported abdominal pain in women with DRA compared to matched controls. However, three studies did not find any difference in prevalence of low back or pelvic girdle pain in primiparous women 6–12 months postpartum between women with and without DRA [112, 115, 130]. Most of these studies included women with light and moderate diastasis. Hence, it is important to investigate the association between severe diastasis and low back and pelvic girdle pain.

Benjamin et al. [129] found no relationship between DRA and urinary incontinence and this confers with newer studies [130, 132, 133].

6.4 Pregnancy-Related Low Back Pain and Pelvic Girdle Pain

Pregnancy-related low back pain (LBP) and/or pelvic girdle pain (PGP) are common across many countries, irrespective of socioeconomic factors [134–138], and are reported to have a negative effect on daily activities such as walking, lifting, climbing stairs, lying flat on the back, turning in bed, housework, exercise, employment, leisure, sexual life, hobbies, and personal relationships [139]. Women with LBP and PGP report a significantly lower health-related quality of life than that reported by healthy women and a major factor affecting their quality of life is found to be lack of physical ability [140, 141]. PGP during pregnancy greatly affects a woman's experience of her pregnancy, her roles in relationships and her social context [142, 143]. These women are struggling with enduring pain that disturbs most aspects of their lives [142, 144], and the pain is perceived as an unpredictable and potentially disabling condition [145]. While most women recover after delivery, a number of women continue living with disabling PGP. Postpartum PGP may influence women's lives for months and years after delivery. Discouragement, isolation, and loneliness may be part of a daily life with pain and limited physical activity [146].

The prevalence rates of pregnancy-related LBP and PGP vary depending on the criteria used and mode of reporting but are estimated to be about 50% during pregnancy [147]. While LBP is usually defined as pain between the 12th rib and the gluteal fold, PGP is defined as pain experienced between the posterior iliac crest and the gluteal fold, particularly in the vicinity of the sacroiliac joints [107]. PGP generally arises in relation to pregnancy and is defined as pain in the pelvic musculoskeletal system that does not derive from gynecological and urological disorders. A diagnosis of PGP can be reached after the exclusion of lumbar causes and the pain or functional impairments in relation to PGP must be reproducible by specific clinical tests [107]. Although similar and overlapping features may be ascribed to LBP and to PGP, it is argued that a distinction should be made [107, 147]. PGP has more impact on pain intensity and disability than LBP [148, 149]. While the normal progression of LBP during pregnancy peaks between 12 and 30 weeks [150, 151], PGP increases progressively with advancing pregnancy [152]. Most probably about 20–25% of all pregnant women suffer from PGP sufficiently seriously to require medical help [107, 153]. Although the majority of women with PGP recover spontaneously soon after delivery, 3–7% report having serious problems from persistent PGP years after delivery [147, 154]. In the only study among elite athletes, 12.6% reported retrospectively that they experienced PGP 6 weeks postpartum and 9.7% experienced LBP. The prevalence increased to 19.4% for PGP and 29% for LBP at the time of completing the questionnaire 0–17 years after delivery [155].

The etiology and pathogenesis of PGP are unclear and probably multifactorial. Possible underlying causes include hormonal and biomechanical aspects, inadequate motor control and stress on ligament structures [156]. PGP often occurs during the early stages of pregnancy [158] and the symptoms typically regress shortly after delivery [154]. A possible association between serum relaxin levels and PGP is debated [154, 157, 158]. The exact movements that occur in the pelvic joints have been traced [159, 160]. Recently, it was shown that the movement in the sacroiliac joints is small and almost undetectable by precise radiostereometric analysis [161]. Even though small, any increased motion in the pelvic joints may diminish the efficiency of load transfer and increase the shear forces across the joints. Increased shear forces have been suggested to be one factor for pain in women with PGP

[108]. The self-locking mechanism of the sacroiliac joints with the principles of form and force closure, based on a theoretical model from anatomical and biomechanical studies was introduced in 1997 by Snijders and co-workers [162]. Failure of the self-locking mechanism and load transfer through the pelvis have been suspected in patients with sacroiliac pain [163, 164], and asymmetric laxity of the sacroiliac joints has been shown to correlate with moderate to severe levels of symptoms in subjects with postpartum PGP [165].

The sacrospinous ligament and superficial sacroiliac joint structures, such as the long dorsal sacroiliac ligament, are a potential source of pain in PGP [166–169]. An impaired load transfer during activities may result in overload of the ligaments of the pelvis and hence have an influence on PGP [170, 171]. Frequent or sustained pain-provoking postures might influence the pelvic ligaments and in turn link to other symptoms. Changes in spinal curvature and posture may be caused by pregnancy. Both increased lumbar lordosis [172] and a tendency for lumbar kyphosis or a flattening of the lumbar spine are reported to be prevalent during pregnancy [173, 174].

There is some evidence that PGP is related to an altered pelvic mechanism and/or motor control [175]. PGP disorders have been associated with an alteration in the strategy for lumbopelvic stabilization with excessive as well as insufficient motor activation of the lumbopelvic and surrounding musculature [176]. Impaired motor control patterns may be a possible mechanism for ongoing pain and disability in patients with persistent PGP [177]. Attention has been paid to motor control of local muscles, especially the transverse abdominals [178, 179]. In addition, the pelvic floor muscles are considered to be an important part of the local muscle system, and Stuge and co-workers found significantly smaller levator hiatus area in women with PGP than in controls both at rest, during voluntary contraction, and during automatic contraction [180].

While the role of muscle function in LBP in the general population is debated, an association between reduced muscle function and the development of LBP and/or PGP in pregnant women is reported [181]. Indications exist that pregnant women with gluteus medius weakness are more likely to have LBP than those without this weakness [182]. In pregnant women with LBP and/or PGP, both lower levels of trunk muscle endurance and hip extension muscle strength [183], and increased muscle activity during the active straight leg raise test are reported [184]. Consequently, an association between muscle dysfunction and LBP and/or PGP during and after pregnancy may exist.

Recently, a consensus-based core outcome set for evaluating the effectiveness of interventions in PGP during pregnancy and postpartum for use in research and clinical practice was developed. Consensus was achieved on five outcomes for inclusion in the final PGP-COS. All outcomes are grouped under the "life impact" domain and include: pain frequency, pain intensity/severity, function/disability/activity limitation, health-related quality of life, and fear avoidance. It is advocated that all trials, other non-randomized studies and clinicians in this area, use this COS by reporting these outcomes as a minimum [185].

References

1. Healey CH, Borley NR, Mundy A. True pelvis, pelvic floor and perineum. In: Standring S, Ellis H, Healy JC, Johnson D, Williams A, editors. Gray's anatomy: the anatomical basis of clinical practice. Edinburgh: Elsevier Churchill livingstone; 2005. p. 1357–71.
2. Delancey JO. Structural aspects of the extrinsic continence mechanism. Obstet Gynecol. 1988;72(3 Pt 1):296–301.
3. Delancey JO. Structural support of the urethra as it relates to stress urinary incontinence: the hammock hypothesis. Am J Obstet Gynecol. 1994;170(6):1713–20.
4. Ashton-Miller JA, Delancey JO. Functional anatomy of the female pelvic floor. Ann N Y Acad Sci. 2007;1101:266–96.
5. Norton PA. Pelvic floor disorders: the role of fascia and ligaments. Clin Obstet Gynecol. 1993;36(4):926–38.
6. Kegel AH. Stress incontinence and genital relaxation; a nonsurgical method of increasing the tone of sphincters and their supporting structures. Ciba Clin Symp. 1952;4(2):35–51.
7. Bø K, Lilleas F, Talseth T, Hedland H. Dynamic MRI of the pelvic floor muscles in an upright sitting position. Neurourol Urodyn. 2001;20(2):167–74.
8. Taverner D, Smiddy FG. An electromyographic study of the normal function of the external anal sphincter and pelvic diaphragm. Dis Colon Rectum. 1959;2(2):153–60.
9. Ashton-Miller JA, Howard D, Delancey JO. The functional anatomy of the female pelvic floor and stress continence control system. Scand J Urol Nephrol Suppl. 2001;207:1–7.
10. Bø K, Aschehoug A. Pelvic floor and exercise science: strength training. In: Bø K, Berghmans B, Mørkved S, Van Kampen M, editors. Evidence-based physical therapy for the pelvic floor. Edinburgh: Churchill Livingstone Elsevier; 2007. p. 119–32.
11. Miller JM, Perucchini D, Carchidi LT, DeLancey JO, Ashton-Miller J. Pelvic floor muscle contraction during a cough and decreased vesical neck mobility. Obstet Gynecol. 2001;97(2):255–60.
12. Miller JM, Ashton-Miller JA, DeLancey JO. A pelvic muscle precontraction can reduce cough-related urine loss in selected women with mild SUI. J Am Geriatr Soc. 1998;46(7):870–4.
13. Miller JM, Sampselle C, Ashton-Miller J, Hong GR, Delancey JO. Clarification and confirmation of the Knack maneuver: the effect of volitional pelvic floor muscle contraction to preempt expected stress incontinence. Int Urogynecol J Pelvic Floor Dysfunct. 2008;19(6):773–82.
14. Bump RC, Norton PA. Epidemiology and natural history of pelvic floor dysfunction. Obstet Gynecol Clin N Am. 1998;25(4):723–46.
15. MacLennan AH, Taylor AW, Wilson DH, Wilson D. The prevalence of pelvic floor disorders and their relationship to gender, age, parity and mode of delivery. BJOG. 2000;107(12):1460–70.
16. DeLancey JO, Kane LL, Miller JM, Patel DA, Tumbarello JA. Graphic integration of causal factors of pelvic floor disorders: an integrated life span model. Am J Obstet Gynecol. 2008;199(6):610–5.
17. Abrams P, Cardozo L, Fall M, Griffiths D, Rosier P, Ulmsten U, et al. The standardisation of terminology in lower urinary tract function: report from the standardisation sub-committee of the International Continence Society. Urology. 2003;61(1):37–49.
18. Milsom I, Altman D, Cartwright R, Lapitan M, Nelson R, Sjöström S, et al. Epidemiology of urinary incontinence [UI] and other lower urinary tract symptoms [LUTS], pelvic organ prolapse [POP] and anal [AI] incontinence. In: Abrams P, Wagg A, Wein A, editors. Incontinence. 6th international consultation on incontinence, Tokyo; 2017.
19. Thom D. Variation in estimates of urinary incontinence prevalence in the community: effects of differences in definition, population characteristics, and study type. J Am Geriatr Soc. 1998;46(4):473–80.
20. Botlero R, Urquhart DM, Davis SR, Bell RJ. Prevalence and incidence of urinary incontinence in women: review of the literature and investigation of methodological issues. Int J Urol. 2008;15(3):230–4.

21. Minassian VA, Stewart WF, Wood GC. Urinary incontinence in women: variation in prevalence estimates and risk factors. Obstet Gynecol. 2008;111(2 Pt 1):324–31.
22. Milsom I, Altman D, Lapitan MC, Nelson R, Sillén U, Thom D. Epidemiology of urinary (UI) and faecal (FI) incontinence and pelvic organ prolapse (POP). In: Abrams P, Cardozo L, Khoury S, Wein A, editors. Incontinence: 4th International Consultation on Incontinence. 4th ed. Paris: Health Publication Ltd; 2009. p. 35–111.
23. Dimpfl T, Hesse U, Schussler B. Incidence and cause of postpartum urinary stress incontinence. Eur J Obstet Gynecol Reprod Biol. 1992;43(1):29–33.
24. Marshall K, Thompson KA, Walsh DM, Baxter GD. Incidence of urinary incontinence and constipation during pregnancy and postpartum: survey of current findings at the Rotunda Lying-In Hospital. Br J Obstet Gynaecol. 1998;105(4):400–2.
25. Mørkved S, Bo K. Prevalence of urinary incontinence during pregnancy and postpartum. Int Urogynecol J Pelvic Floor Dysfunct. 1999;10(6):394–8.
26. Hvidman L, Hvidman L, Foldspang A, Mommsen S, Bugge NJ. Correlates of urinary incontinence in pregnancy. Int Urogynecol J Pelvic Floor Dysfunct. 2002;13(5):278–83.
27. Wesnes SL, Rortveit G, Bo K, Hunskaar S. Urinary incontinence during pregnancy. Obstet Gynecol. 2007;109(4):922–8.
28. Borello-France D, Burgio KL, Richter HE, Zyczynski H, Fitzgerald MP, Whitehead W, et al. Fecal and urinary incontinence in primiparous women. Obstet Gynecol. 2006;108(4):863–72.
29. Bø K, Nygaard IE. Is Physical activity good or bad for the female pelvic floor? A narrative review. Sports Med. 2020;50:471. https://doi.org/10.1007/s40279-019-01243-1.
30. Koelbl H, Nitti V, Baessler K, Salvatore S, Sultan A, Yamaguchi O. Pathophysiology of urinary incontinence, faecal incontinence and pelvic organ prolapse. In: Abrams P, Cardozo L, Khoury S, Wein A, editors. Incontinence: 4th International Consultation on Incontinence. 4th ed. Paris: Helarh Publication Ltd; 2009. p. 255–330.
31. Thorp JM Jr, Norton PA, Wall LL, Kuller JA, Eucker B, Wells E. Urinary incontinence in pregnancy and the puerperium: a prospective study. Am J Obstet Gynecol. 1999;181(2):266–73.
32. Burgio KL, Locher JL, Zyczynski H, Hardin JM, Singh K. Urinary incontinence during pregnancy in a racially mixed sample: characteristics and predisposing factors. Int Urogynecol J Pelvic Floor Dysfunct. 1996;7(2):69–73.
33. Wilson PD, Herbison RM, Herbison GP. Obstetric practice and the prevalence of urinary incontinence three months after delivery. Br J Obstet Gynaecol. 1996;103(2):154–61.
34. Rasmussen KL, Krue S, Johansson LE, Knudsen HJ, Agger AO. Obesity as a predictor of postpartum urinary symptoms. Acta Obstet Gynecol Scand. 1997;76(4):359–62.
35. Viktrup L, Rortveit G, Lose G. Risk of stress urinary incontinence twelve years after the first pregnancy and delivery. Obstet Gynecol. 2006;108(2):248–54.
36. Sugerman H, Windsor A, Bessos M, Wolfe L. Intra-abdominal pressure, sagittal abdominal diameter and obesity comorbidity. J Intern Med. 1997;241(1):71–9.
37. Sampselle CM. Changes in pelvic muscle strength and stress urinary incontinence associated with childbirth. J Obstet Gynecol Neonatal Nurs. 1990;19(5):371–7.
38. Hahn I, Milsom I, Ohlsson BL, Ekelund P, Uhlemann C, Fall M. Comparative assessment of pelvic floor function using vaginal cones, vaginal digital palpation and vaginal pressure measurements. Gynecol Obstet Investig. 1996;41(4):269–74.
39. Samuelsson E, Victor A, Svardsudd K. Determinants of urinary incontinence in a population of young and middle-aged women. Acta Obstet Gynecol Scand. 2000;79(3):208–15.
40. Morin M, Bourbonnais D, Gravel D, Dumoulin C, Lemieux MC. Pelvic floor muscle function in continent and stress urinary incontinent women using dynamometric measurements. Neurourol Urodyn. 2004;23(7):668–74.
41. Mørkved S, Salvesen KA, Bo K, Eik-Nes S. Pelvic floor muscle strength and thickness in continent and incontinent nulliparous pregnant women. Int Urogynecol J Pelvic Floor Dysfunct. 2004;15(6):384–9.
42. Thompson JA, O'Sullivan PB, Briffa NK, Neumann P. Assessment of voluntary pelvic floor muscle contraction in continent and incontinent women using transperineal ultrasound, man-

ual muscle testing and vaginal squeeze pressure measurements. Int Urogynecol J Pelvic Floor Dysfunct. 2006;17(6):624–30.

43. Shishido K, Peng Q, Jones R, Omata S, Constantinou CE. Influence of pelvic floor muscle contraction on the profile of vaginal closure pressure in continent and stress urinary incontinent women. J Urol. 2008;179(5):1917–22.
44. Hilde G, Staer-Jensen J, Ellstrom EM, Braekken IH, Bo K. Continence and pelvic floor status in nulliparous women at midterm pregnancy. Int Urogynecol J. 2012;23(9):1257–63.
45. Bø K, Stien R, Kulseng-Hanssen S, Kristofferson M. Clinical and urodynamic assessment of nulliparous young women with and without stress incontinence symptoms: a case-control study. Obstet Gynecol. 1994;84(6):1028–32.
46. Sartore A, Pregazzi R, Bortoli P, Grimaldi E, Ricci G, Guaschino S. Assessment of pelvic floor muscle function after vaginal delivery. Clinical value of different tests. J Reprod Med. 2003;48(3):171–4.
47. Hvidman L, Foldspang A, Mommsen S, Nielsen JB. Postpartum urinary incontinence. Acta Obstet Gynecol Scand. 2003;82(6):556–63.
48. Foldspang A, Hvidman L, Mommsen S, Nielsen JB. Risk of postpartum urinary incontinence associated with pregnancy and mode of delivery. Acta Obstet Gynecol Scand. 2004;83(10):923–7.
49. Altman D, Ekstrom A, Gustafsson C, Lopez A, Falconer C, Zetterstrom J. Risk of urinary incontinence after childbirth: a 10-year prospective cohort study. Obstet Gynecol. 2006;108(4):873–8.
50. Groutz A, Gordon D, Keidar R, Lessing JB, Wolman I, David MP, et al. Stress urinary incontinence: prevalence among nulliparous compared with primiparous and grand multiparous premenopausal women. Neurourol Urodyn. 1999;18(5):419–25.
51. Rortveit G, Hannestad YS, Daltveit AK, Hunskaar S. Age- and type-dependent effects of parity on urinary incontinence: the Norwegian EPINCONT study. Obstet Gynecol. 2001;98(6):1004–10.
52. Lukacz ES, Lawrence JM, Contreras R, Nager CW, Luber KM. Parity, mode of delivery, and pelvic floor disorders. Obstet Gynecol. 2006;107(6):1253–60.
53. Press JZ, Klein MC, Kaczorowski J, Liston RM, von DP. Does cesarean section reduce postpartum urinary incontinence? A systematic review. Birth. 2007;34(3):228–37.
54. Peschers U, Schaer G, Anthuber C, Delancey JO, Schuessler B. Changes in vesical neck mobility following vaginal delivery. Obstet Gynecol. 1996;88(6):1001–6.
55. Meyer S, Schreyer A, De GP, Hohlfeld P. The effects of birth on urinary continence mechanisms and other pelvic-floor characteristics. Obstet Gynecol. 1998;92(4 Pt 1):613–8.
56. Dietz HP, Clarke B, Vancaillie TG. Vaginal childbirth and bladder neck mobility. Aust N Z J Obstet Gynaecol. 2002;42(5):522–5.
57. Meyer S, De GP, Schreyer A, Caccia G. The assessment of bladder neck position and mobility in continent nullipara, mulitpara, forceps-delivered and incontinent women using perineal ultrasound: a future office procedure? Int Urogynecol J Pelvic Floor Dysfunct. 1996;7(3):138–46.
58. King JK, Freeman RM. Is antenatal bladder neck mobility a risk factor for postpartum stress incontinence? Br J Obstet Gynaecol. 1998;105(12):1300–7.
59. Lavin JM, Smith ARB, Anderson J, Grant M, Buckley H, Critchley H, et al. The effect of the first pregnancy on the connective tissue of the rectus sheath. Neurourol Urodyn. 1997;16:381–2.
60. Howard D, Miller JM, DeLancey JO, Ashton-Miller JA. Differential effects of cough, valsalva, and continence status on vesical neck movement. Obstet Gynecol. 2000;95(4):535–40.
61. Smith AR, Hosker GL, Warrell DW. The role of pudendal nerve damage in the aetiology of genuine stress incontinence in women. Br J Obstet Gynaecol. 1989;96(1):29–32.
62. Snooks SJ, Setchell M, Swash M, Henry MM. Injury to innervation of pelvic floor sphincter musculature in childbirth. Lancet. 1984;2(8402):546–50.
63. Smith AR, Hosker GL, Warrell DW. The role of partial denervation of the pelvic floor in the aetiology of genitourinary prolapse and stress incontinence of urine. A neurophysiological study. Br J Obstet Gynaecol. 1989;96(1):24–8.

64. Allen RE, Hosker GL, Smith AR, Warrell DW. Pelvic floor damage and childbirth: a neurophysiological study. Br J Obstet Gynaecol. 1990;97(9):770–9.
65. Snooks SJ, Swash M, Mathers SE, Henry MM. Effect of vaginal delivery on the pelvic floor: a 5-year follow-up. Br J Surg. 1990;77(12):1358–60.
66. Lien KC, Morgan DM, Delancey JO, Ashton-Miller JA. Pudendal nerve stretch during vaginal birth: a 3D computer simulation. Am J Obstet Gynecol. 2005;192(5):1669–76.
67. Snooks SJ, Swash M, Henry MM, Setchell M. Risk factors in childbirth causing damage to the pelvic floor innervation. Int J Color Dis. 1986;1(1):20–4.
68. Sultan AH, Kamm MA, Hudson CN. Pudendal nerve damage during labour: prospective study before and after childbirth. Br J Obstet Gynaecol. 1994;101(1):22–8.
69. Gilpin SA, Gosling JA, Smith AR, Warrell DW. The pathogenesis of genitourinary prolapse and stress incontinence of urine. A histological and histochemical study. Br J Obstet Gynaecol. 1989;96(1):15–23.
70. Delancey JO, Kearney R, Chou Q, Speights S, Binno S. The appearance of levator ani muscle abnormalities in magnetic resonance images after vaginal delivery. Obstet Gynecol. 2003;101(1):46–53.
71. Kearney R, Miller JM, Ashton-Miller JA, Delancey JO. Obstetric factors associated with levator ani muscle injury after vaginal birth. Obstet Gynecol. 2006;107(1):144–9.
72. Dietz HP. Pelvic floor trauma following vaginal delivery. Curr Opin Obstet Gynecol. 2006;18(5):528–37.
73. DeLancey JO, Ashton-Miller JA. Measurement of pelvic floor muscle function and strength and pelvic organ prolapse: MRI of intact and injured female pelvic floor muscles. In: Bø K, Berghmans B, Mørkved S, Van Kampen M, editors. Evidence-based physical therapy for the pelvic floor. Edinburgh: Churchill Livingstone Elsevier; 2007. p. 93–105.
74. Ashton-Miller JA, Delancey JO. On the biomechanics of vaginal birth and common sequelae. Annu Rev Biomed Eng. 2009;11:163–76.
75. Turner CE, Young JM, Solomon MJ, Ludlow J, Benness C. Incidence and etiology of pelvic floor dysfunction and mode of delivery: an overview. Dis Colon Rectum. 2009;52(6):1186–95.
76. Peschers UM, Schaer GN, Delancey JO, Schuessler B. Levator ani function before and after childbirth. Br J Obstet Gynaecol. 1997;104(9):1004–8.
77. Botelho S, Riccetto C, Herrmann V, Pereira LC, Amorim C, Palma P. Impact of delivery mode on electromyographic activity of pelvic floor: comparative prospective study. Neurourol Urodyn. 2010;29(7):1258–61.
78. Caroci AS, Riesco ML, Sousa WS, Cotrim AC, Sena EM, Rocha NL, et al. Analysis of pelvic floor musculature function during pregnancy and postpartum: a cohort study: (a prospective cohort study to assess the PFMS by perineometry and digital vaginal palpation during pregnancy and following vaginal or caesarean childbirth). J Clin Nurs. 2010;19(17–18):2424–33.
79. Sigurdardottir T, Steingrimsdottir T, Arnason A, Bo K. Pelvic floor muscle function before and after first childbirth. Int Urogynecol J. 2011;22:1497.
80. Hilde G, Staer-Jensen J, Siafarikas F, Engh ME, Braekken IH, Bo K. Impact of childbirth and mode of delivery on vaginal resting pressure and on pelvic floor muscle strength and endurance. Am J Obstet Gynecol. 2013;208(1):50–7.
81. Lien KC, Mooney B, Delancey JO, Ashton-Miller JA. Levator ani muscle stretch induced by simulated vaginal birth. Obstet Gynecol. 2004;103(1):31–40.
82. Hoyte L, Damaser MS, Warfield SK, Chukkapalli G, Majumdar A, Choi DJ, et al. Quantity and distribution of levator ani stretch during simulated vaginal childbirth. Am J Obstet Gynecol. 2008;199(2):198–5.
83. Parente MP, Jorge RM, Mascarenhas T, Fernandes AA, Martins JA. Deformation of the pelvic floor muscles during a vaginal delivery. Int Urogynecol J Pelvic Floor Dysfunct. 2008;19(1):65–71.
84. Dietz HP. Quantification of major morphological abnormalities of the levator ani. Ultrasound Obstet Gynecol. 2007;29(3):329–34.
85. Dietz HP, Lanzarone V. Levator trauma after vaginal delivery. Obstet Gynecol. 2005;106(4):707–12.

86. Valsky DV, Lipschuetz M, Bord A, Eldar I, Messing B, Hochner-Celnikier D, et al. Fetal head circumference and length of second stage of labor are risk factors for levator ani muscle injury, diagnosed by 3-dimensional transperineal ultrasound in primiparous women. Am J Obstet Gynecol. 2009;201(1):91–7.
87. Krofta L, Otcenasek M, Kasikova E, Feyereisl J. Pubococcygeus-puborectalis trauma after forceps delivery: evaluation of the levator ani muscle with 3D/4D ultrasound. Int Urogynecol J Pelvic Floor Dysfunct. 2009;20(10):1175–81.
88. Jarvinen TA, Jarvinen TL, Kaariainen M, Aarimaa V, Vaittinen S, Kalimo H, et al. Muscle injuries: optimising recovery. Best Pract Res Clin Rheumatol. 2007;21(2):317–31.
89. Delancey JO, Morgan DM, Fenner DE, Kearney R, Guire K, Miller JM, et al. Comparison of levator ani muscle defects and function in women with and without pelvic organ prolapse. Obstet Gynecol. 2007;109(2 Pt 1):295–302.
90. Dietz HP, Shek C. Levator avulsion and grading of pelvic floor muscle strength. Int Urogynecol J Pelvic Floor Dysfunct. 2008;19(5):633–6.
91. Steensma AB, Konstantinovic ML, Burger CW, de Timmerman RD, Deprest J. Prevalence of major levator abnormalities in symptomatic patients with an underactive pelvic floor contraction. Int Urogynecol J. 2010;21(7):861–7.
92. Brincat CA, Delancey JO, Miller JM. Urethral closure pressures among primiparous women with and without levator ani muscle defects. Int Urogynecol J. 2011;22(12):1491–5.
93. Hilde G, Staer-Jensen J, Siafarikas F, Gjestland K, Ellstrom EM, Bo K. How well can pelvic floor muscles with major defects contract? A cross-sectional comparative study 6 weeks after delivery using transperineal 3D/4D ultrasound and manometer. BJOG. 2013;120(11):1423–9.
94. Shek KL, Dietz HP. The effect of childbirth on hiatal dimensions. Obstet Gynecol. 2009;113(6):1272–8.
95. Majida M, Braekken IH, Bo K, Engh ME. Levator hiatus dimensions and pelvic floor function in women with and without major defects of the pubovisceral muscle. Int Urogynecol J. 2012;23:707.
96. Morgan DM, Larson K, Lewicky-Gaupp C, Fenner DE, Delancey JO. Vaginal support as determined by levator ani defect status 6 weeks after primary surgery for pelvic organ prolapse. Int J Gynaecol Obstet. 2011;114(2):141–4.
97. Dietz HP, Steensma AB. The prevalence of major abnormalities of the levator ani in urogynaecological patients. BJOG. 2006;113(2):225–30.
98. Dietz HP, Simpson JM. Levator trauma is associated with pelvic organ prolapse. BJOG. 2008;115(8):979–84.
99. Tunn R, Goldammer K, Neymeyer J, Gauruder-Burmester A, Hamm B, Beyersdorff D. MRI morphology of the levator ani muscle, endopelvic fascia, and urethra in women with stress urinary incontinence. Eur J Obstet Gynecol Reprod Biol. 2006;126(2):239–45.
100. Dietz HP, Kirby A, Shek KL, Bedwell PJ. Does avulsion of the puborectalis muscle affect bladder function? Int Urogynecol J Pelvic Floor Dysfunct. 2009;20(8):967–72.
101. Bodine-Fowler S. Skeletal muscle regeneration after injury: an overview. J Voice. 1994;8(1):53–62.
102. Jarvinen TA, Jarvinen TL, Kaariainen M, Kalimo H, Jarvinen M. Muscle injuries: biology and treatment. Am J Sports Med. 2005;33(5):745–64.
103. Orchard JW, Best TM, Mueller-Wohlfahrt HW, Hunter G, Hamilton BH, Webborn N, et al. The early management of muscle strains in the elite athlete: best practice in a world with a limited evidence basis. Br J Sports Med. 2008;42(3):158–9.
104. Lovering R. Physical therapy and related interventions. In: Tiidus PM, editor. Skeletal muscle damage and repair. Champaign, IL: Human Kinetics; 2007. p. 219–30.
105. Bø K, Artal R, Barakat R, Brown W, Davies GA, Dooley M, et al. Exercise and pregnancy in recreational and elite athletes: 2016 evidence summary from the IOC expert group meeting, Lausanne. Part 1-exercise in women planning pregnancy and those who are pregnant. Br J Sports Med. 2016;50(10):571–89. https://doi.org/10.1136/bjsports-2016-096218.

106. Benjamin DR, van der Water ATM, Peiris CL. Effects of exercise on diastasis of the rectus abdominis muscle in the antenatal and postnatal periods: a systematic review. Physiotherapy. 2014;100:1–8.
107. Vleeming A, Albert HB, Ostgaard HC, et al. European guidelines for the diagnosis and treatment of pelvic girdle pain. Eur Spine J. 2008;17:794–819.
108. Koelbl H, Igawa TY, Salvatore S, et al. Pathophysiology of urinary incontinence, faecal incontinence and pelvic organ prolapse. In: Abrams P, Cardozo L, Khouy S, Wein A, editors. Incontinence. 5th ed. Cardiff: Health publication Ltd; 2013. p. 261–359. Committee 4.
109. Lee D, Hodges PW. Behavior of the linea alba during a curl-up task in diastasis rectus abdominis; An Observational Study. J Orthop Sports Phys Ther. 2016;46:580–9.
110. Venes D, Taber CW. Taber's cyclopedic medical dictionary 20, 2005, Philadelphia, PA: Davis
111. Boissonnault JS, Blaschak MJ. Incidence of diastasis recti abdominis during the childbearing year. Phys Ther. 1988;68(7):1082–6.
112. Mota PGF, Pascoal AG, Carita AI, Bo K. The immediate effects on inter-rectus distance of abdominal crunch and drawing in exercises during pregnancy and the postpartum period. J Orthop Sports Phys Ther. 2015;45:781–8.
113. Rett MT, Braga MD, Bernardes NO, Andrade SC. Prevalence of diastasis of the rectus abdominis muscles immediately postpartum: comparison between primiparae and multiparae. Revista Brasileira De Fisioterapia. 2009;13(4):275–80.
114. Turan V, Colluoglu C, Turkyilmaz E, Korucuoglu U. Prevalence of diastasis recti abdominis in the population of young multiparous adults in Turkey. Ginekol Pol. 2011;82(11):817–82.
115. Sperstad JB, Tennfjord MT, Hilde G, Engh ME, Bø K. Diastasis recti abdominis and risk of low back and pelvic girdle pain. Br J Sports Med. 2016;50:1092–6.
116. Spitznagle TM, Leong FC, Van Dillen LR. Prevalence of diastasis recti abdominis in a urogynecological patient population. Int Urogynecol J. 2007;18:321–8.
117. Lockwood T. Rectus muscle diastasis in males: primary indication for endoscopically assisted abdominoplasty. Plast Reconstr Surg. 1998;101:1685–91; discussion 1692–1684.
118. van de Water AT, Benjamin DR. Measurement methods to assess diastasis of the rectus abdominis muscle (DRAM): a systematic review of their measurement properties and meta-analytic reliability generalisation. Man Ther. 2016;21:41–53.
119. Keeler J, Albrecht M, Eberhardt L, Horn L, Donelly C, Lowe D. Diastasis recti abdominis; a survey of women's health specialists for current physical therapy clinical practice for postpartum women. J Womens Health Phys Ther. 2012;36:131–42.
120. Mota P, Pascoal AG, Sancho F, Carita AI, Bo K. Reliability of the inter-rectus distance measured by palpation. Comparison of palpation and ultrasound measurements. Man Ther. 2013;18(4):294–8.
121. Mota P, Pascoal AG, Sancho F, Bø K. Test-retest and intrarater reliability of 2-dimensional ultrasound measurements of distance between rectus abdominis in women. J Orthop Sports Phys Ther. 2012;42(11):940–6.
122. Candido G, Lo T, Janssen PA. Risk factors for diastasis of the recti abdominis. J Assoc Chart Physiother Women's Health. 2005;97:49–54.
123. Mota P, Pascoal AG, Carita AI, Bø K. Normal width of the inter-recti distance in pregnant and postpartum primiparous women. Musculoskelet Sci Pract. 2018;35:34–7. https://doi.org/10.1016/j.msksp.2018.02.004.
124. Lo T, Candido G, Janssen P. Diastasis of the Recti abdominis in pregnancy: risk factors and treatment. Physiother Can. 1999;51:32.
125. Fernandes da Mota PG, Pascoal AG, Carita AI, Bo K. Prevalence and risk factors of diastasis recti abdominis from late pregnancy to 6 months postpartum, and relationship with lumbo-pelvic pain. Man Ther. 2015;20(1):200–5.
126. Lee DG, Lee LJ, McLaughlin L. Stability, continence and breathing: the role of fascia following pregnancy and delivery. J Bodyw Mov Ther. 2008;12:333–48.
127. Gilleard WL, Brown JM. Structure and function of the abdominal muscles in primigravid subjects during pregnancy and the immediate postbirth period. Phys Ther. 1996;76:750–62.

128. Liaw LJ, Hsu MJ, Liao CF, Liu MF, Hsu AT. The Relationships between inter-recti distance measured by ultrasound imaging and abdominal muscle function in postpartum women: a 6-month follow-up study. J Orthop Sports Phys Ther. 2011;41(6):435–43.
129. Benjamin DR, Frawley HC, Shields N, van de Water ATM, Taylor NF. Relationship between diastasis of the rectus abdominis muscle (DRAM) and musculoskeletal dysfunctions, pain and quality of life: a systematic review. Physiotherapy. 2019;105(1):24–34.
130. Gluppe S, Engh ME, Bø K. Women with diastasis recti abdominis might have weaker abdominal muscles and more abdominal pain, but no higher prevalence of pelvic floor disorders, low back and pelvic girdle pain than women without diastasis recti abdominis. Physiotherapy. 2021;111:57. https://doi.org/10.1016/j.physio.2021.01.008.
131. Parker MA, Millar LA, Dugan SA. Diastasis rectus abdominis and lumbo-pelvic pain and dysfunction-are they related? J Women's Health Phys Therapy. 2009;33:15–22.
132. Braga A, Caccia G, Nasi I, Ruggeri G, Di Dedda MC, Lamberti G, et al. Diastasis recti abdominis after childbirth: is it a predictor of stress urinary incontinence? J Gynecol Obstet Hum Reprod. 2019:101657.
133. Wang Q, Yu X, Chen G, Sun X, Wang J. Does diastasis recti abdominis weaken pelvic floor function? A cross-sectional study. Int Urogynecol J. 2020;31(2):277–83.
134. Bjorklund K, Bergstrom S. Is pelvic pain in pregnancy a welfare complaint? Acta Obstet Gynecol Scand. 2000;79:24–30.
135. Charpentier K, Leboucher J, Lawani M, et al. Back pain during pregnancy and living conditions: a comparison between Beninese and Canadian women. Ann Phys Rehabil Med. 2012;55:148–59.
136. Mousavi SJ, Parnianpour M, Vleeming A. Pregnancy related pelvic girdle pain and low back pain in an Iranian population. Spine. 2007;32:E100–4.
137. Gutke A, Boissonnault J, Brook G, et al. The severity and impact of pelvic girdle pain and low-back pain in pregnancy: a multinational study. J Women's Health (Larchmt). 2017;27:510.
138. Gashaw M, Gedlu S, Janakiraman B, Gashaw M, et al. Burden of pelvic girdle pain during pregnancy among women attending ante-natal clinic, Ethiopia: a cross-sectional study. BMC Pregnan Childb. 2020;20(1):494.
139. Wormslev M, Juul AM, Marques B, et al. Clinical examination of pelvic insufficiency during pregnancy. An evaluation of the interobserver variation, the relation between clinical signs and pain and the relation between clinical signs and physical disability. Scand J Rheumatol. 1994;23:96–102.
140. Olsson C, Nilsson-Wikmar L. Health-related quality of life and physical ability among pregnant women with and without back pain in late pregnancy. Acta Obstet Gynecol Scand. 2004;83:351–7.
141. Stuge B, Veierød MB, Lærum E, et al. The efficacy of a treatment program focusing on specific stabilizing exercises for pelvic girdle pain after pregnancy. A two-year follow-up of a randomized clinical trial. Spine. 2004;29:E197–203.
142. Persson M, Winkvist A, Dahlgren L, et al. "Struggling with daily life and enduring pain": a qualitative study of the experiences of pregnant women living with pelvic girdle pain. BMC Pregnan Childb. 2013;13:111.
143. Pierce H, Homer CS, Dahlen HG, et al. Pregnancy-related lumbopelvic pain: listening to Australian women. Nurs Res Pract. 2012;2012:387428.
144. Gutke A, Bullington J, Lund M, et al. Adaptation to a changed body. Experiences of living with long-term pelvic girdle pain after childbirth. Disabil Rehabil. 2017;40:1–7.
145. Fredriksen EH, Moland KM, Sundby J. "Listen to your body". A qualitative text analysis of internet discussions related to pregnancy health and pelvic girdle pain in pregnancy. Patient Educ Couns. 2008;73:294–9.
146. Engeset J, Stuge B, Fegran L. Pelvic girdle pain affects the whole life--a qualitative interview study in Norway on women's experiences with pelvic girdle pain after delivery. BMC Res Notes. 2014;7:686.
147. Wu WH, Meijer OG, Uegaki K, et al. Pregnancy-related pelvic girdle pain (PPP), I: Terminology, clinical presentation, and prevalence. Eur Spine J. 2004;13:575–89.

148. Ostgaard HC, Zetherstrom G, Roos-Hansson E, et al. Reduction of back and posterior pelvic pain in pregnancy. Spine. 1994;19:894–900.
149. Gutke A, Ostgaard HC, Oberg B. Pelvic girdle pain and lumbar pain in pregnancy: a cohort study of the consequences in terms of health and functioning. Spine. 2006;31:E149–55.
150. Robinson HS, Mengshoel AM, Bjelland EK, et al. Pelvic girdle pain, clinical tests and disability in late pregnancy. Man Ther. 2010;15:280–5.
151. Kristiansson P, Svardsudd K, von Schoultz B. Back pain during pregnancy: a prospective study. Spine. 1996;21:702–9.
152. Ostgaard HC, Andersson GB. Previous back pain and risk of developing back pain in a future pregnancy. Spine. 1991;16:432–6.
153. Ostgaard HC, Andersson GB, Karlsson K. Prevalence of back pain in pregnancy. Spine. 1991;16:549–52.
154. Bjelland EK, Stuge B, Engdahl B, et al. The effect of emotional distress on persistent pelvic girdle pain after delivery: a longitudinal population study. BJOG. 2013;120:32–40.
155. Bø K, Backe-Hansen KL. Do elite athletes experience low back, pelvic girdle and pelvic floor complaints during and after pregnancy? Scand J Med Sci Sports. 2007;17:480–7.
156. O'Sullivan PB, Beales DJ. Diagnosis and classification of pelvic girdle pain disorders, Part 2: illustration of the utility of a classification system via case studies. Man Ther. 2007;12:e1–12.
157. Aldabe D, Ribeiro DC, Milosavljevic S, et al. Pregnancy-related pelvic girdle pain and its relationship with relaxin levels during pregnancy: a systematic review. Eur Spine J. 2012;21:1769–76.
158. Nielsen LL. Clinical findings, pain descriptions and physical complaints reported by women with post-natal pregnancy-related pelvic girdle pain. Acta Obstet Gynecol Scand. 2010;89:1187–91.
159. Goode A, Hegedus EJ, Sizer P, et al. Three-dimensional movements of the sacroiliac joint: a systematic review of the literature and assessment of clinical utility. J Man Manip Ther. 2008;16:25–38.
160. Mens JM, Vleeming A, Snijders CJ, et al. The active straight leg raising test and mobility of the pelvic joints. Eur Spine J. 1999;8:468–74.
161. Kibsgard TJ, Roise O, Sturesson B, et al. Radiosteriometric analysis of movement in the sacroiliac joint during a single-leg stance in patients with long-lasting pelvic girdle pain. Clin Biomech. 2014;29:406–11.
162. Snijders CJ, Vleeming A, Stoeckart R, et al. Biomechanics of the interface between spine and pelvis in different postures. In: Vleeming A, Mooney V, Dorman T, et al., editors. Movement, stability & low back pain. The essential role of the pelvis. Edinburgh: Churchill Livingstone; 1997. p. 103–14.
163. Hungerford B, Gilleard W, Hodges P. Evidence of altered lumbopelvic muscle recruitment in the presence of sacroiliac joint pain. Spine. 2003;28:1593–600.
164. Hungerford B, Gilleard W, Lee D. Altered patterns of pelvic bone motion determined in subjects with posterior pelvic pain using skin markers. Clin Biomech. 2004;19:456–64.
165. Damen L, Buyruk HM, Guler-Uysal F, et al. Pelvic pain during pregnancy is associated with asymmetric laxity of the sacroiliac joints. Acta Obstet Gynecol Scand. 2001;80:1019–24.
166. Palsson TS, Graven-Nielsen T. Experimental pelvic pain facilitates pain provocation tests and causes regional hyperalgesia. Pain. 2012;153:2233–40.
167. Palsson TS, Hirata RP, Graven-Nielsen T. Experimental pelvic pain impairs the performance during the active straight leg raise test and causes excessive muscle stabilization. Clin J Pain. 2015;31:642.
168. Torstensson T, Lindgren A, Kristiansson P. Corticosteroid injection treatment to the ischiadic spine reduced pain in women with long-lasting sacral low back pain with onset during pregnancy: a randomized, double blind, controlled trial. Spine. 2009;34:2254–8.
169. Torstensson T, Lindgren A, Kristiansson P. Improved function in women with persistent pregnancy-related pelvic pain after a single corticosteroid injection to the ischiadic spine: a randomized double-blind controlled trial. Physiother Theory Pract. 2013;29:371–8.

170. Eichenseer PH, Sybert DR, Cotton JR. A finite element analysis of sacroiliac joint ligaments in response to different loading conditions, vol. 36. Spine; 2011. p. E1446–52.
171. Snijders CJ, Vleeming A, Stoeckart R. Transfer of lumbosacral load to iliac bones and legs. 1. Biomechanics of Self-bracing of the sacroiliac joints and its significance for treatment and exercise. Clin Biomech. 1993;8:285–94.
172. Franklin ME, Conner-Kerr T. An analysis of posture and back pain in the first and third trimesters of pregnancy. J Orthop Sports Phys Ther. 1998;28:133–8.
173. Moore K, Dumas GA, Reid JG. Postural changes associated with pregnancy and their relationship with low-back pain. Clin Biomech. 1990;5:169–74.
174. Okanishi N, Kito N, Akiyama M, et al. Spinal curvature and characteristics of postural change in pregnant women. Acta Obstet Gynecol Scand. 2012;91:856–61.
175. Aldabe D, Milosavljevic S, Bussey MD. Is pregnancy related pelvic girdle pain associated with altered kinematic, kinetic and motor control of the pelvis? A systematic review. Eur Spine J. 2012;21:1777–87.
176. Beales DJ, O'Sullivan PB, Briffa NK. Motor control patterns during an active straight leg raise in chronic pelvic girdle pain subjects. Spine. 2009;34:861–70.
177. Richardson CA, Snijders CJ, Hides JA, et al. The relation between the transversus abdominis muscles, sacroiliac joint mechanics, and low back pain. Spine. 2002;27:399–405.
178. Stuge B, Morkved S, Dahl HH, et al. Abdominal and pelvic floor muscle function in women with and without long lasting pelvic girdle pain. Man Ther. 2006;11:287–96.
179. Stuge B, Saetre K, Braekken IH. The association between pelvic floor muscle function and pelvic girdle pain--a matched case control 3D ultrasound study. Man Ther. 2012;17:150–6.
180. Stuge B, Saetre K, Ingeborg HB. The automatic pelvic floor muscle response to the active straight leg raise in cases with pelvic girdle pain and matched controls. Man Ther. 2013;18:327.
181. Dumas GA, Leger A, Plamondon A, et al. Fatigability of back extensor muscles and low back pain during pregnancy. Clin Biomech. 2010;25:1–5.
182. Bewyer KJ, Bewyer DC, Messenger D, et al. Pilot data: association between gluteus medius weakness and low back pain during pregnancy. Iowa Orthop J. 2009;29:97–9.
183. Gutke A, Ostgaard HC, Oberg B. Association between muscle function and low back pain in relation to pregnancy. J Rehabil Med. 2008;40:304–11.
184. Pool-Goudzwaard ALGM, Spoor CW, et al. The active straight leg raising test (ASLR) in pregnant women: differences in muscle activity and force between patients and healthy subjects. Man Ther. 2008;13:68–74.
185. Remus A, et al. A core outcome set for research and clinical practice in women with pelvic girdle pain: PGP-COS. PLoS One. 2021;16(2):e0247466.

Further Reading

Bø K, Berghmans B, Mørkved S, Van Kampen M, editors. Evidence-based physical therapy for the pelvic floor. Churchill Livingstone Elsevier: Edinburgh; 2007.
Fitzgerald CM, Segal NA, editors. Musculoskeletal health in pregnancy and postpartum. Cham: Springer International Publishing Switzerland; 2015.

7 Evidence-Based and Practice-Oriented Guidelines for Exercising During Pregnancy

Anna Szumilewicz, Aneta Worska, Rita Santos-Rocha, and Miguel Ángel Oviedo-Caro

Abstract

Physical activity is associated with health benefits during pregnancy, delivery, and the postpartum period. The last three decades produced an increasing amount of scientific evidence on the positive effects of the prenatal physical activity on the maternal and fetal health, as well as in pregnancy outcomes. However, authors from different countries observe insufficient level of physical activity in pregnant women. The lack of information among women on the exercises during pregnancy, and lack of social support are two of the reasons hindering engagement in a prenatal exercise program. According to other studies, the knowledge of health benefits can lead to more favorable attitudes toward exercise during pregnancy, among women, exercise professionals, and healthcare providers. The purpose of this chapter is to review the information provided in the current guidelines for exercise during pregnancy in different countries, regarding the contents related to prenatal exercise programs. We analyzed the changes in recommendations over the past 4 years. Nowadays, experts emphasize the need to limit sedentary behaviors in

A. Szumilewicz (✉) · A. Worska
Gdansk University of Physical Education and Sport, Gdańsk, Poland
e-mail: anna.szumilewicz@awf.gda.pl; aneta.worska@awf.gda.pl

R. Santos-Rocha
Sport Sciences School of Rio Maior - ESDRM, Polytechnic Institute of Santarém, Rio Maior, Portugal

Laboratory of Biomechanics and Functional Morphology, Interdisciplinary Centre for the Study of Human Performance - CIPER, Faculty of Human Kinetics - FMH, University of Lisbon, Lisbon, Portugal
e-mail: ritasantosrocha@esdrm.ipsantarem.pt

M. Á. Oviedo-Caro
Department of Physical Education and Sport, University of Seville, Seville, Spain
e-mail: moviedo@us.es

R. Santos-Rocha (ed.), *Exercise and Physical Activity During Pregnancy and Postpartum*, https://doi.org/10.1007/978-3-031-06137-0_7

pregnant women and to individualize exercise, departing from the total limitation of physical activity and bed rest even in complicated pregnancies. There is a more open approach to the continuation of vigorous sports activities during pregnancy by previously physically active women or female athletes.

Keywords

Guidelines · Exercise · Physical activity · Pregnancy · Postpartum

7.1 Introduction

Physical activity is associated with many health benefits during pregnancy, delivery, and in the postpartum period. Research over the past 30 years has shown that regular physical activity during pregnancy has a positive effect on the physical and psychological conditions of the pregnant woman, pregnancy and fetal development, parturition, and the postpartum period [1–5]. Physical activity started in pregnancy may be the first step to a lifelong change to a health-promoting lifestyle [6]. Research has also proved that prenatal physical activity of mothers has a long-term effect on the health of the children, including a reduction in the risk of obesity in later life [3, 7, 8].

With the increasing amount of scientific evidence on the positive effects of the prenatal physical activity, the authors from different countries observe its insufficient level in pregnant women [9–19]. As the reasons for this phenomenon, the authors list among other things: lack of information among women on the exercises during pregnancy [13, 18] and lack of social support [20, 21]. For some women, pregnancy itself is a sufficient reason for not exercising [19, 20].

There have been few studies regarding the level of pregnant women's knowledge and their attitudes toward prenatal physical activity [22–25]. Gouveia et al. [25] noted that although most mothers in Portugal understand the benefits of physical activity in pregnancy, which does not seem to increase their participation. However, according to other studies, the knowledge of health benefits can lead to more favorable attitudes toward exercise during pregnancy among women from different countries [23, 24, 26]. Cannella et al. [23] showed that women who were informed about the benefits and risks of physical activity, risks of inactivity and also about the exercise techniques, displayed more favorable attitudes toward prenatal physical activity. Many of the women surveyed in their study reported that they had received information about the benefits of prenatal physical activity, but fewer answered that they had received information about how to exercise safely.

The importance of healthcare professionals in promoting the benefits of physical activity and exercise, and advising women on a healthy and active lifestyle during pregnancy, referring them to a prenatal exercise specialist is highlighted in Chap. 1 [27]. Official guidelines for exercise in pregnancy could be an effective tool in fulfilling this task. Tanha et al. [26] have proved that dissemination of such documents among pregnant women contributes significantly to the increase in their participation in prenatal exercise. Official guidelines published by national and international obstetrics, gynecology, or sports medicine institutions should be a trustworthy and comprehensive source of information on the safe and beneficial exercise program during pregnancy. They should be accessible to all interested in prenatal physical activity: pregnant women and their families, obstetric care providers, and exercise professionals to enable an effective cooperation in the exercise program design.

Pregnancy causes many changes in the woman's body: morphological, physiological, biomechanical, and psychological [28]. This should be taken into account in the planning of the intensity, frequency, and duration of the exercise sessions and also of their content—through a proper selection of the type of exercises and their technique [29–31]. Evenson et al. [32] have shown that nine out of ten guidelines on exercise in pregnancy from different countries contained information on the intensity and duration of exercise. Eight of these documents contained recommendations on the exercise frequency. In this chapter, we aimed to answer the question on what information on the contents of prenatal exercises is provided in the current guidelines for exercise during pregnancy in different countries. The second question was what significant changes have occurred in the approach to exercise in pregnancy in the last 4 years.

We have updated a review study published in 2015 [33] that was focused on detailed information on the contents of prenatal exercises presented in reliable guidelines. The methodological issues are fully described in the original paper. In the first edition of this book, we have analyzed 13 papers. In this edition, we included 11 recent documents, published after 2017. In the following part of this work, depending on the year of publication, we call these documents "old guidelines" (published until the end of 2017) or "new guidelines" (published after 2017). All documents included in the analysis are the official position of national obstetrics, gynecology, or sports medicine institutions on exercise in pregnancy. We have narrowed the documents to those published in English, which ensures their wide usage. The first stage of the update began with a search of documents in the scientific database MEDLINE, with full text. Bearing in mind that the guidelines need not have the character of scientific work, and only represent the official position of credible national institutions; in the second stage, we completed the search of documents in public search engines. We used the keywords: "exercise" or "physical activity" and "pregnancy" and "guidelines" or "statement." The 15th of July 2021 was the last date searched.

In the first stage of the analysis, we looked for the general recommendation on the type of exercise, information on the recommended and not recommended forms of exercise and sports activities for pregnant women. In the second stage of the analysis, we looked for detailed information that might be useful for designing the contents of targeted exercise classes for pregnant women, including special pregnant populations like elite athletes or women with specific health conditions.

7.2 General Features of the Guidelines on Physical Activity in Pregnancy

In the previous edition of this book, we have analyzed 13 documents from seven countries: Australia [34, 35], Canada [36, 37], Denmark [38], Norway [39], South Africa [40], United Kingdom [41], USA [42–45], and an international document supported by the International Olympic Committee [1, 2, 46] (Table 7.1). In this edition, we have added 11 documents from five countries: Australia [47–49], Canada [50], United Kingdom [51], USA [52–55], and New Zealand [49], and two international documents: one supported by the International Olympic Committee (IOC) [56] and one developed by the World Health Organization (WHO) [57] (Table 7.2). In five documents, authors presented the full methodology of scientific reports selection and evidence quality assessment. Those five documents were affiliated by The Royal Australian and New Zealand College of Obstetricians and Gynaecologists (RANZCOG), The Society of Obstetricians and Gynaecologists of Canada together with The Canadian Society for Exercise Physiology (SOGC/CSEP), The American College of Obstetricians and Gynecologists (ACOG), the IOC and WHO. Four documents, published by Sport Medicine Australia (SMA), Australian Government. Department of Health (AGDH), American College of Sports Medicine (ACSM), Exercise is Medicine/American College of Sports Medicine (EIM/ACSM) are layman-oriented brochures. National Health Service (NHS) guidelines are published entirely online and contain two short videos with exercise examples. All of these materials met our criteria for inclusion in the analysis (were published in English and were the most recent country-specific, official position of national obstetrics, gynecology, or sports medicine institutions).

In our previous guidelines, revision completed at the end of 2017, the year of their publication was a striking feature (Table 7.1). Only five of the 13 documents were published 5 years earlier than that date. For obvious reasons, they were based on scientific works that had been frequently 15 or more years old. Since 2018, 11 new documents on exercise in pregnancy have been released. The advances in the scientific evidence about the effect of physical activity on pregnant women's health have made necessary the update of the main guidelines on this issue.

Both in the scientific research on prenatal physical activity [26, 58, 59], and in educational standards [60], as well as in exercise programs [30], the authors refer to

Table 7.1 Characteristics of analyzed guidelines on exercise in pregnancy, published by the end of 2017

Country	Organization	Title	Year of publication
Australia	Sport Medicine Australia (SMA) [34]	SMA statement:	2002
		The benefits and risks of exercise during pregnancy	Updated 2016 [34]
Australia	Fitness Australia. The Health & Fitness Industry Association [35]	Pre and post-natal exercise guidelines	2013
Canada	Society of Obstetricians and Gynaecologists of Canada;	Exercise in pregnancy and the postpartum period	2003
	Canadian Society for Exercise Physiology SOGC/CSEP [36]		

Table 7.1 (continued)

Country	Organization	Title	Year of publication
Canada	Canadian Academy of Sport and Exercise Medicine (CASEM) [37]	Position statement:	2007
		Exercise and pregnancy	updated 2008
Denmark	National Board of Health [38]	Healthy habits before, during and after pregnancy. First English edition	2010
Norway	Directorate for Health and Social Affairs [39]	A National Clinical Guideline for Antenatal Care. Short Version—Recommendations	2005
South Africa	South African Sports Medicine Association (SASMA) [40]	South African Sports Medicine Association Position Statement on Exercise in Pregnancy	2012
United Kingdom	Royal College of Obstetricians and Gynaecologists (RCOG) [41]	Exercise in pregnancy	2006
United States	American College of Obstetricians and Gynecologists (ACOG) [42]	Committee Opinion: Exercise during	2002
		pregnancy and the postpartum period	Reaffirmed in 2009
			Updated in 2015 [42]
United States	U.S. Department of Health and Human Services (U.S. DHHS) [43]	Physical Activity for Women During Pregnancy and the Postpartum Period	2008
		Chapter in: 2008 Physical Activity Guidelines for Americans	
United States	American College of Nurse-Midwives (ACNM) [44]	Exercise in Pregnancy	2014
United States	American College of Sports Medicine (ACSM) [45]	Current Comment: Exercise during Pregnancy	Not reported
International	International Olympic Committee (IOC); three parts [1, 2, 46]	Exercise and pregnancy in recreational and elite athletes: 2016 evidence summary from the IOC expert group meeting, Lausanne.	2016

the official guidelines for exercise in pregnancy. Although it is difficult to estimate the extent of their impact, the contribution of these documents to change the perception on prenatal physical activity in the past decades is indisputable.

The guidelines issued 30 years ago suggested that exercising women reduce their habitual levels of exertion in pregnancy and that non-exercising women refrain from initiating strenuous exercise program [61]. Such conservative recommendations were based, among others, on the results of scientific studies demonstrating the

Table 7.2 Characteristics of analyzed guidelines on exercise in pregnancy, published after 2017

Country	Organization	Title	Year of publication
Australia	Sport Medicine Australia (SMA) [47]	Exercise in pregnancy (layman oriented brochure)	Not reported Access 2021
Australia	Australian Gavernment. Department of Health (AGDH) [48]	Guidelines for physical activity during pregnancy (layman oriented brochure)	2021
Australia and New Zealand	Royal Australian and New Zealand College of Obstetricians and Gynaecologists (RANZCOG) [49]	Exercise in Pregnancy	2020
Canada	Society of Obstetricians and Gynaecologists of Canada; Canadian Society for Exercise Physiology SOGC/CSEP [50]	2019 Canadian guideline for physical activity throughout pregnancy	2018
United Kingdom	National Health Service NHS [51]	Exercise in pregnancy (online materials on the official webpage)	2020
United States	American College of Obstetricians and Gynecologists (ACOG) [52]	Committee Opinion: Exercise during pregnancy and the postpartum period	2020
United States	American College of Sports Medicine (ACSM) [53]	ACSM information on Pregnancy Physical Activity (layman oriented brochure)	2020
United States	Exercise is Medicine/ American College of Sports Medicine (EIM/ ACSM) [54]	Being Active during Pregnancy (layman oriented brochure)	2019
United States	U.S. Department of Health and Human Services (U.S. DHHS) [55]	Key Guidelines for Women During Pregnancy and the Postpartum Period; Section in: Physical Activity Guidelines for Americans, second edition	2018
International	International Olympic Committee (IOC) [56]	Exercise and pregnancy in recreational and elite athletes: 2016/2017 evidence summary from the IOC expert group meeting, Lausanne. Part 5. Recommendations for health professionals and active women	2018
International	World Health Organization WHO [57]	World Health Organization 2020 guidelines on physical activity and sedentary behavior	2020

negative effects of hard physical work, combined with undernutrition, on the development of pregnancy in laboratory animals [62, 63]. However, the results of research conducted on pregnant women have proved that those assumptions do not apply to people [1, 13, 64–66]. With the current evidence about the positive impact of prenatal exercise on maternal and child health, increasingly, the question is not "if" but "how" pregnant woman should exercise [61].

The breakthrough was the recommendation published in Canadian guidelines in 2003 that "All women without contraindications should be encouraged to participate in aerobic and strength-conditioning exercises as part of a healthy lifestyle during their pregnancy" [36]. ACOG [67] and SMA [68] issued similar recommendations in 2002 and in their latest updates [34, 42]. Finally, in 2015, the ACOG recommendations were updated emphasizing that physical activity in pregnancy has minimal risk and highlighting that women who exercised regularly prior to pregnancy, in the absence of contraindications, can continue and engage in moderate to strenuous activities [42]. Also in this update, several activities were introduced as recommended activities if pregnant women practiced them prior to pregnancy (i.e., aerobics, jogging, running, or stationary cycling). It should be emphasized that it was the first document where physical inactivity has been treated as a risky behavior leading among others to maternal obesity and related pregnancy complications, including gestational diabetes mellitus.

The Sports Medicine Australia recommendations were first updated in 2016 [34], increasing the specification of the recommended physical activities during pregnancy (i.e., resistance training, swimming, or jogging) and introducing pelvic floor exercises as a recommended activity to include in exercise programs during pregnancy. In 2016 and 2017, Bø et al. and the Medical and Scientific Commission of the International Olympic Committee (IOC) drove a discussion about the management of pregnancy for elite athletes, and produced comprehensive evidence summary on exercise during pregnancy [1, 2] and postpartum [46], as well as recommendations for future research [69]. The last part of this report series, published in 2018, has been directed at health professionals and very active women [56].

All new guidelines are in agreement that physical activity in pregnancy is safe and desirable in the absence of obstetrics and medical complications or contraindications and that pregnant women should be encouraged to continue or initiate safe physical activities. Interestingly, the SMA experts emphasized that "there are currently NO known adverse risks associated with meeting the recommended guidelines of at least 150 min of moderate-vigorous physical activity per week" ([47], p. 1). Experts are clearly changing the approach to exercise in complicated pregnancy. In the event of complications, it is more and more often recommended to consult a specialist and individualize physical activity, rather than limiting it completely [48–50, 52, 53].

The fact that for the first time in 2020 the World Health Organization provides specific recommendations on physical activity for pregnant and postpartum women [57] highlights the increasing importance of this topic. For the first time, specific international guidelines emphasizing the need to reduce sedentary behaviors by pregnant women have been presented.

7.3 Exercise Prescription Considering Pre-pregnancy Habits Related to Physical Activity and the Course of Pregnancy

Two of the old guidelines [34, 42] highlighted the importance of considering the habits of pregnant women related to physical activity and exercise prior to pregnancy in order to individualize the prescription of exercise during pregnancy. Since 2018, the experts differentiate recommendations on prenatal exercise for women with different pre-pregnancy physical activity habits in all documents.

7.3.1 Previously Inactive Pregnant Women

According to the old guidelines, the prescription of an exercise program in previously inactive pregnant women should commence with low-intensity activities such as walking or swimming, initially accumulated in short bouts, and follow a gradual progression up to the minimum level of the physical activity and exercise recommendations [42]. A walking program may be a good option for previously inactive pregnant women to become physically active [70], because it has been demonstrated that even mild walking (30% of peak aerobic capacity) improves fitness levels in sedentary women during pregnancy [71]. In the new guidelines, it is emphasized that previously inactive pregnant women should start with a small amount of physical activity and gradually increase the amount and intensity over time based on their own possibilities. Walking and swimming are still the recommended forms of exercise for previously inactive pregnant women.

7.3.2 Previously Active Pregnant Women

Two of the old guidelines [34, 42] addressed the issue of continuing physical activity by previously active women. According the ACOG and SMA experts, pregnant women with habits of physical activity or exercise prior to pregnancy and without obstetrics complications could continue their physical activity or exercise habits throughout pregnancy or until it caused any discomfort [34, 42]. Already in 2015, ACOG stated that pregnant women who were regular exercisers before pregnancy and do not present obstetrics complications were able to engage in high-intensity exercise programs. When high-intensity or prolonged exercise exceed 45 min, they should take into account a proper caloric intake and hydration before, during, and after exercise to minimize the risk of hypoglycemia [42].

Recommendations on the potential continuation of a physical activity exceeding the recommended minimum level or of high intensity are much more popular in the new documents. They were mentioned in 10 of 11 guidelines analyzed [47–50, 52–57].

7.3.3 Elite or Competitive Athletes

The statements endorsed by IOC [1, 2, 46] include scientific evidence about endurance and strength training in elite athlete during pregnancy. In addition, the IOC pointed out that future research should focus on the effects and obstetric risks of specific types of exercise, training place, or strenuous exercise. There is also a need to improve the knowledge on the influence of physiological and anatomical changes related to pregnancy on the training development, or influence of training during pregnancy on the return to the competitive level in the postpartum period. The last part of IOC work [56] is focused on the recommendations for female athletes who want to combine their training regimes with motherhood and to compete during the years of optimal fertility.

Pregnant women who are elite or competitive athletes need to maintain a more strenuous training schedule throughout pregnancy and resume high-intensity postpartum training sooner as compared to non-athlete pregnant women [42]. Their training program should be managed by experts that ensure the safety and well-being of the mother and the child [34]. Although an upper level of safe exercise intensity has not been established, women who were regular exercisers before pregnancy and who have uncomplicated, healthy pregnancies should be able to engage in high-intensity exercise programs. Particular attention should be paid to avoid weight loss and hyperthermia through a proper caloric intake and hydration before, during, and after exercise [42].

Studies show transient fetal bradycardia when the pregnant elite athlete exercises at above 90% of maximal maternal heart rate (HR), but whether these transient fetal HR changes influence neonatal outcomes is unknown. However, to be appropriately cautious, IOC does not recommend maximum rate of oxygen consumption (VO_{2max}) testing and exercise above 90% of VO_{2max}, except in highly supervised (research) settings. Until more data are available in respect of strength training, athletes who prior to pregnancy developed heavy strength training should avoid Valsalva maneuver and large increases in intra-abdominal pressure which may temporarily decrease uteroplacental blood flow [1]. The repercussions to the fetus of these temporary changes remain unknown. Avoiding Valsalva maneuver by exhaling with an open airway also seems prudent [72].

In the absence of studies in elite athletes, IOC agreed that female athletes might consider refraining from repetitive heavy lifting efforts in the first trimester of pregnancy to avoid the potential risk of miscarriage. However, as IOC emphasized, these recommendations are based on low-quality evidence. Available studies were retrospective and based on participant's self-reports, conducted to assess the influence of lifting loads in occupational tasks, not in sport training. Indeed, Juhl et al. [73] observed that women with occupational lifting were more likely to have a first-trimester miscarriage than women with no lifting. Nevertheless, they also noted that women with occupational lifting were more likely to smoke and less likely to engage in physical exercise. Undoubtedly, there is a need for well-designed research on the course of pregnancy, labor and delivery, and fetus development in heavy-lifting athletes to support them with reliable information in terms of the safety of their training process.

The latest update of the ACOG document [52] still emphasizes maintaining proper hydration, avoiding hyperthermia and sustaining adequate caloric intake to prevent weight loss that may affect fetal growth. The ACOG experts stated that pregnant elite athletes should consider a reduction of the pre-pregnancy resistance load and avoid high-impact activities with increased risk of blunt trauma.

Currently, the participation of pregnant women in strenuous sports training and competitions is becoming more and more acceptable. Under some of the new guidelines, when considering athletic competition, or exercising significantly above the recommended levels, pregnant women should seek supervision from a specialist health-care provider [47, 48, 50, 52, 53, 56, 57]. On the other hand, the RANZCOG experts mentioned that regardless of baseline level of fitness and previous exercise routine, pregnancy is not a time for serious competition or aiming to reach peak lifetime fitness [49].

7.3.4 Pregnant Women with Obesity

In three new documents from: Australia and New Zealand [49], Canada [50], and USA [52], the experts individualized recommendations on exercise for pregnant women with obesity. In line with the ACOG guidelines [42, 52], women with obesity should be encouraged to engage in exercise and nutritional interventions aimed at a healthier lifestyle. To start such interventions, low-intensity and short periods of exercise should be considered and gradually increased adequately to the women's exercise capacities. For overweight or obese women, RANZCOG also recommends a shorter duration of exercise (15–20 min) at the commencement of a program, before slowly building up to 30 min.

7.3.5 Exercising in Complicated Pregnancy

What is a completely new approach, in 2020 the ACOG experts removed the list of absolute or relative contraindications to exercise in pregnancy. Instead, they recommend consultation with specialist (i.e., obstetrics and gynecology, maternal-fetal medicine, cardiology, pulmonology) when questions regarding exercise safety exist [52]. In case of obstetric or medical comorbidities, exercise regimens should be individualized. Finally, this ACOG guidelines update advises against activity restrictions in the primary prevention of preeclampsia or preterm birth, which was a common practice in the obstetric care.

According to the RANZCOG guidelines [49] for those women with pregnancy complications, the promotion of exercise may still be appropriate under some circumstances with appropriate medical evaluation and suitable modification of the exercise prescription. In line with the Canadian recommendations, "women with absolute contraindications may continue their usual activities of daily living but should not participate in more strenuous activities. Women with relative contraindications should discuss the advantages and disadvantages of moderate-to-vigorous intensity physical activity with their obstetric care provider prior to participation"

([50], p. 1340). The Canadian experts listed the absolute and relative contraindications to exercise during pregnancy. However, they are far from completely limiting physical activity in the event of these contraindications. A similar approach is presented in the AGDH guidelines [48].

Importantly, the list of contraindications to prenatal physical activity have been substantially modified [50], based on scientific evidence. Meah et al. [74] found that a majority of medical conditions listed as contraindications were based on expert opinion. They identified 11 complications (e.g., gestational hypertension, twin pregnancy) previously classified as contraindications where women may in fact benefit from regular prenatal physical activity with or without modifications.

The routinely prescribed "bed rest" has been strongly criticized by the ACOG experts since 2015 [42, 52]. They highlight the negative health consequences of this practice, such as the risk of thromboembolism, bone demineralization, and deconditioning of the pregnant patient and also the negative psychosocial effects impacting not only the mother but the whole family as well. So far, there are no studies documenting an improvement in outcomes in women at risk for preterm birth who are placed on activity restriction, including bed rest. Taking the above into account, Jain [75] appeals that bed rest should not be treated "as a panacea for all that ails the gravida." Based on available evidence from multiple Cochrane reviews, prescribing bed rest to pregnant patients was even called unethical [76].

7.3.6 Recommendations to Reduce Time Spent in Sedentary Behavior

The WHO guidelines [57] emphasize that in pregnant women, as in all adults, higher levels of sedentary behavior are associated with the following poor health outcomes: all-cause mortality, cardiovascular disease mortality and cancer mortality and incidence of cardiovascular disease, cancer, and incidence of type 2 diabetes. Therefore, pregnant women should be encouraged to reduce the sedentary time.

The WHO experts advise pregnant women to replace sedentary time with any intensity of physical activity, including light intensity. This general recommendation "moving more and sitting less" [77] is exactly the same as for others populations. Furthermore, the previous recommendation for exercise bouts of at least 10-min duration has been removed. Scientific evidence shows that physical activity of any bout duration is associated with improved health outcome [78]. The WHO experts underline that "doing some physical activity is better than doing none" ([57], p. 8), which is in line with the public message "every step counts."

Similar approach has been presented in NHS, EIM, and U.S. DHHS guidelines [51, 54, 55]. The EIM experts suggest pregnant women add more steps by taking the stairs or parking farther away, go for a 10-min walk after two of daily meals and try "walking meetings" when women need no computer or pen and paper. They also add that activities like raking the lawn or heavy vacuuming count toward the weekly activity. Likewise, the AGDH [48] and RANZCOG [49] guidelines state that it is important to reduce sedentary behavior by minimizing the amount of time spent in prolonged sitting or standing still and breaking up long motionless periods as often as possible. Nowadays, there is growing evidence that breaking up prolonged sedentary time leads to health benefits [79].

When individuals do not meet the minimum physical activity levels, they should start with small amounts of physical activity and gradually increase frequency, intensity, and duration over time. However, more physical activity is better for optimal health. The Canadian guidelines [50] advise pregnant women to undertake more than the recommended levels of moderate-to-vigorous physical activity for greater health benefits. This is in line with the public message that not just the fulfillment of the minimum recommendations is important. Undertaking more than the recommended levels of physical activity may reduce the detrimental potential effects of high levels of sedentary behaviors on health [80].

7.4 Recommended Types of Exercise and Forms of Sports Activities for Pregnant women

For an exercise program to be effective, it must take into account four training components: intensity, frequency, duration, and proper type of exercise [29]. The work by Evenson et al. [32] shows that the guidelines for exercise in pregnancy contain much more information on the intensity, frequency, and duration than on the contents of exercise programs. In fact, the contents of prenatal exercise seem to be particularly important for pregnant women, because during this period, through physical activity, they should pursue both their overall objectives of promoting their own health and maternity.

In Tables 7.3, 7.4, 7.5, and 7.6, we presented the results regarding the general recommendation on the type of exercise and information on the recommended and not recommended forms of exercise and sports activities for pregnant women.

All guidelines published by the end of 2017 contained general recommendations to perform aerobic exercises, 12 of them—to perform resistance exercises and two of them—flexibility exercises (Table 7.3). All new guidelines also advised pregnant women to participate in aerobic activities, as well as in resistance exercise; eight of them—to perform flexibility exercises. The forms of physical activity recommended for pregnancy were listed in 11 old and in eight new documents. In the old guidelines, the most frequently mentioned were walking and swimming (in 9 out of 13). Other recommendations included inter alia: aerobics, water exercise, jogging, cycling (especially stationary), running, and cross-country skiing. The new guidelines also listed walking most frequently (in 8 out of 11 documents). New mentioned forms were stretching [50, 52, 54] and everyday activities [50, 54], like climbing the stairs, raking the lawn or heavy vacuuming. Certainly, in terms of biomechanical analysis, these forms of exercise are very beneficial for pregnancy, but it can be expected that they would not meet the interests and needs of all pregnant women of different countries. And here comes the controversial question

Table 7.3 Guidelines on the type of exercise and forms of sports activities recommended in pregnancy, published by the end of 2017

	Australia (SMA) 2016	Australia (FA) 2013	Canada (SOGC/ CSEP)	Canada (CASEM)	Denmark	Norway	South Africa (SASMA)	United Kingdom (RCOG)	United States (ACOG) 2015	United States (ACNM)	United States (ACSM)	United States (U.S. DHHS)	Interna-tional (IOC) 2016
General recommendation on the type[a] of exercise:													
Aerobic exercise[b]	+	+	+	+	+	+	+	+	+	+[c]	+[c]	+	+
Strengthening exercise[d]	+	+	+	+	+	+	+	+	+	+[c]		+	+
Flexibility exercise		+											+
Recommended forms[e] of exercise and sports activities:													
Aerobics[f]	+	+				+	+	+	+	+	+		
Cross-country skiing			+	+			+						
Cycling	+				+	+	+			+			
Dancing						+	+						
Exercise in water	+	+	+		+			+	+		+		
Gymnastics						+							
Hiking							+						
Jogging	+					+	+	+	+[g]		+		
Pilates									Modified +				
Racquet sports									+[h]				
Rowing							+						
Running	+						+		+[g]				
Stationary cycling	+		+	+			+		+		+		

(continued)

Table 7.3 (continued)

	Australia (SMA) 2016	Australia (FA) 2013	Canada (SOGC/ CSEP)	Canada (CASEM)	Denmark	Norway	South Africa (SASMA)	United Kingdom (RCOG)	United States (ACOG) 2015	United States (ACNM)	United States (ACSM)	United States (U.S. DHHS)	International (IOC) 2016
Strengthening training	+	+			+				+[g]	+			
Swimming	+		+	+	+	+	+		+	+	+		
Targeted prenatal classes	+	+						Aqua natal					
Walking	+		+	+	+	+	+		+	+	+		
Yoga									Modified +	+			
An advice to consult health care provider on the type of exercise:	+	+	+		+				+	+	+	+	

[a]Based on the provided health benefits

[b]Also called an endurance exercise or cardio exercise; in this kind of exercise, the body's large muscles move in a rhythmic manner for a sustained period of time. Brisk walking, running, bicycling, jumping rope, and swimming are all examples

[c]Based on the recommended forms of sports activities

[d]We searched for the information on muscle-strengthening exercise, also called resistance exercise (this kind of exercise causes the body's muscles to work or hold against an applied force or weight)

[e]Based on the specific nature of the movements, skills, equipment, the environment and the rules that determine participation in it

[f]Is a form of exercise that combines rhythmic aerobic exercise with stretching and strength training routines with the goal of improving all elements of fitness (flexibility, muscular strength, and cardiovascular fitness). It is usually performed to music and may be practiced in a group setting

[g]Recommended if a pregnant woman developed this activity prior to pregnancy

[h]Racquet sports wherein a pregnant woman's changing balance may affect rapid movements and increase the risk of falling should be avoided as much as possible

Table 7.4 Guidelines on the type of exercise and forms of sports activities recommended in pregnancy, published after 2017

	Australia (SMA) 2021	Australia AGDH 2021	Australia and New Zealand 2020	Canada (SOGC/ CSEP) 2018	United Kingdom (NHS) 2021	United States (ACOG) 2020	United States (ACSM) 2020	United States (EIM/A CSM) 2019	United States (U.S. DHHS) 2018	International (IOC) 2018	International (WHO) 2020
General recommendation on the type[a] of exercise:											
Aerobic exercise[b]	+	+	+	+	+	+	+	+	+	+	+
Strengthening exercise[c]	+	+	+	+	+	+	+	+	+	+	+
Flexibility exercise	+		+	+	+	+	+	+			+
Recommended forms[a] of exercise and sports activities:											
Aerobics[d]	+[e]				+	+	+[e]				
Cycling		+									
Dancing		+			+	+		+			
Everyday activity				+				+			
Exercise classes		+									
Exercise in water/Aquafit/ in a pool			+	+		+		+			
Jogging	+						+[f]				
Pilates						+[g]	+[g]				
Running				+[f]	+		+[f]				
Stationary cycling	+		+	+		+		+			

(continued)

Table 7.4 (continued)

	Australia (SMA) 2021	Australia AGDH 2021	Australia and New Zealand 2020	Canada (SOGC/ CSEP) 2018	United Kingdom (NHS) 2021	United States (ACOG) 2020	United States (ACSM) 2020	United States (EIM/A CSM) 2019	United States (U.S. DHHS) 2018	International (IOC) 2018	International (WHO) 2020
Racket sports							+[f]				
Resistance training						+[f]	+				
Stretching				+		+		+			
Swimming	+	+	+	+	+		+				
Walking	+	+	+	+	+	+	+	+			
Yoga				+	+	+[g]	+[g]				

[a]Based on the provided health benefits
[b]Also called an endurance exercise or cardio exercise; in this kind of exercise, the body's large muscles move in a rhythmic manner for a sustained period of time. Brisk walking, running, bicycling, jumping rope, and swimming are all examples
[c]We searched for the information on muscle-strengthening exercise, also called resistance exercise (this kind of exercise causes the body's muscles to work or hold against an applied force or weight)
[d]Is a form of exercise that combines rhythmic aerobic exercise with stretching and strength training routines with the goal of improving all elements of fitness (flexibility, muscular strength, and cardio-vascular fitness). It is usually performed to music and may be practiced in a group setting
[e]Low⁻ impact aerobics was recommended
[f]Recommended if a pregnant woman participated in this activity prior to pregnancy
[g]Modified

Table 7.5 Guidelines on the type of exercise and forms of sports activities not recommended in pregnancy, published by the end of 2017

	Australia (SMA) 2016	Australia (FA) 2013	Canada (SOGC/CSEP)	Canada (CASEM)	Denmark	Norway	South Africa (SASMA)	United Kingdom (RCOG)	United States (ACOG) 2015	United States (ACNM)	United States (ACSM)	United States (U.S. DHHS)	International (IOC) 2016
Sports mentioned as risky in pregnancy:													
"Hot yoga" or "hot Pilates"									+				
Basketball						+			+	+		+	
Bobsledding													+
Cricket	+												
Cycling											+		
Diving/Scuba diving	+		+		+	+	+	+	+	+	+		+
Downhill skiing	+			+		+	+		+	+		+	+[a]
Generally contact sports	+	+						+	+				
Gymnastics	+			+			+		+	+	+		
Handball						+							
Hang gliding							+						
Heavy weightlifting	+				+				+[b]	+			+[b]
Horseback riding	+			+		+	+		+	+		+	

(continued)

Table 7.5 (continued)

	Australia (SMA) 2016	Australia (FA) 2013	Canada (SOGC/ CSEP)	Canada (CASEM)	Denmark	Norway	South Africa (SASMA)	United Kingdom (RCOG)	United States (ACOG) 2015	United States (ACNM)	United States (ACSM)	United States (U.S. DHHS)	International (IOC) 2016
Ice hockey	+					+			+	+			+
Luge													+
Martial arts	+												
Off-road cycling									+				
Pole vaulting													+
Skating	+						+						
Sky-diving	+								+				
Soccer	+						+		+	+		+	
Softball	+												
Surfing									+				
Vigorous racket games							+		+	+			
Water skiing	+						+		+				

[a]Downhill ski racing

[b]Referring to low to moderate level of evidence for a negative effect of occupational lifting, female athletes may consider refraining from repetitive heavy lifting efforts in the first trimester to avoid the potential risk of miscarriage

Table 7.6 Guidelines on the type of exercise and forms of sports activities not recommended in pregnancy, published after 2017

	Australia (SMA) 2021	Australia (AGDH) 2021	Australia and New Zealand 2020	Canada (SOGC/CSEP) 2018	United Kingdom (NHS) 2021	United States (ACOG) 2020	United States (ACSM) 2020	United States (EIM/ACSM) 2019	United States (U.S. DHHS) 2018	International (IOC) 2018	International (WHO) 2020
Sports listed as "to be avoided" in pregnancy:											
"Hot yoga" or "hot Pilates"						+	+	+			
Artistic gymnastics										+[a]	
Basketball							+	+	+	+[a]	
Bobsledding										+[a]	
Cycling				+							
Diving/Scuba diving	+	+		+	+	+	+	+		+	
Downhill skiing				+			+	+	+	+[a]	
Equestrian										+[a]	
Field hockey										+[a]	
Freestyle skiing and ski jumping										+[a]	
Figure skating (some events)										+[a]	
Generally contact sports	+				+	+	+	+	+		

(continued)

Table 7.6 (continued)

	Australia (SMA) 2021	Australia (AGDH) 2021	Australia and New Zealand 2020	Canada (SOGC/ CSEP) 2018	United Kingdom (NHS) 2021	United States (ACOG) 2020	United States (ACSM) 2020	United States (EIM/A CSM) 2019	United States (U.S. DHHS) 2018	International (IOC) 2018	International (WHO) 2020
Gymnastics				+			+	+		+[a]	
Handball										+[a]	
Heavy weightlifting/ Olympic lifts		+	+	+				+			
Horseback riding				+			+	+	+		
Ice hockey				+		+	+	+		+[a]	
Luge										+[a]	
Martial arts (e.g., boxing, judo, kickboxing, taekwondo, wrestling)					+		+			+[a]	
Off-road cycling/ mountain cycling/BMX							+			+[a]	
Rugby										+[a]	

Short track speed skating										+[a]	
Sky-diving		+					+			+[a]	
Snowboard										+[a]	
Soccer (football)						+	+	+	+	+[a]	
Some track and field events										+[a]	
Squash						+					
Surfing							+				
Trampoline										+[a]	
Volleyball										+[a]	
Water skiing							+	+			

[a]Where there is the possibility for contact with other athletes or the environment and subsequent damage to the fetus/placenta. Non-contact training may be continued

related to sports activities, which generally are classified as hazardous for pregnant women.

All old guidelines contained information on the forms of exercise to avoid in pregnancy. It was suggested that women should avoid sports activities with high risks of falling or loss of balance or with high risk of abdominal trauma. Those 14 documents provided specific examples of forms of sports to avoid. For example, in 2015 ACOG guidelines [42] we found: gymnastics, horseback riding and downhill skiing or with a high potential for contact, such as ice hockey, soccer, and basketball (Table 7.5).

All new documents, apart from the WHO guidelines, also mentioned activities to avoid (Table 7.6). However, the experts' approach to the participation of pregnant women in the so-called risky sports is becoming more and more open. For example, in the RANZCOG document, we found that "although there is no strong scientific evidence regarding the risk of participation in activities with an inherent risk of falling (e.g., horse-riding, learning to ski) or impact trauma to the abdomen (i.e., team sport games), common-sense suggests that these activities may be best avoided, or at least undertaken with awareness and serious consideration of the potential risks" ([49], p. 10). According to latest guidelines by SMA [47], women active before pregnancy can continue with their regular sport as long as associated risks and recommended modifications are considered (e.g., contact sports and downhill skiing, rapid changes in direction, etc.). Although IOC [56] published a long list of sports to be avoided, at the same time, they mentioned that non-contact training might be continued in such sports as: artistic gymnastics, equestrian, field hockey, freestyle skiing, ski jumping, figure skating, rugby, short track speed skating, snowboard, some track and field events, trampoline, and volleyball.

It should be noted that there is no reliable research showing that some sports activities are indeed dangerous for pregnancy and fetal development. The classification of the forms of activities as "not recommended for pregnant women" is rather due to the cautious attitude of the authors of the guidelines. For example, in RCOG document, we found that: "Prudence dictates that activities such as contact sports should be avoided" ([41], p. 2). There are more and more studies that change the view of the so-called risky sports in pregnancy. For instance, research has cast doubts on the earlier assumptions that women should not scuba dive in pregnancy, as the fetus is not protected from decompression sickness and gas embolism [36, 41]. Results by Conger and Magann [81] prove that if the woman dived when she did not know she was pregnant, there was usually a normal outcome. Based on recently published review by Reid and Lorenzo, human data on the scuba diving effects on pregnancy outcomes are of poor quality. Nevertheless, scuba diving is the most frequently mentioned form of activity to be avoided during pregnancy, both in the old and new documents (Tables 7.5 and 7.6). To reassure women who have already dived while pregnant, it would be good to add in these guidelines that "inadvertent exposure to recreational diving in early pregnancy is not a reason for pregnancy termination" ([82], p. 1).

It seems reasonable to classify forms of exercise or physical activity, as safe for pregnancy or not, on the basis of multidimensional research analysis. Information to be included in official guidelines for exercise in pregnancy should be treated with extreme caution. Based on the studies of Tanha et al. [26] it can be assumed that these documents significantly influence the choice of the form of exercise by pregnant women. Listing certain forms of activity as potentially dangerous may result in women giving them up. In the case where they decide to continue participation in such sports, they may have to overcome the pressure of society. In the study by Fieril et al. [20], "social reproach was cited as a barrier to exercise. Some women recounted that relatives, friends or colleagues demonstrated their lack of understanding about exercising during pregnancy or questioned a particular type of exercise, such as resistance training" (p. 1140). The research by Krans and Chang also corresponds to this observation [83]. They concluded that health care providers should be aware of cultural myths that prevent many African American women from performing certain activities during pregnancy. Changing social perceptions of various forms of prenatal physical activity can be of key importance for its development.

In the analyzed guidelines, we have noted certain inconsistency in classifying sport activities as recommended to perform or to avoid. Cross-country skiing, cycling, or racket sports that have been proposed to pregnant women (Tables 7.2 and 7.3) may be associated with a high risk of fall for a complete novice. Nevertheless, it will depend on the cultural and social aspects of the country, as well as on the woman's skills in a particular sport. In this vein, a more reasonable position in relation to all forms of activity is presented in the guidelines from South Africa that "the type of exercise needs to be individualized in accordance with the woman's skills, abilities and preference" ([40], p. 70). The latest update of US guidelines includes some activities (i.e., racquet sports or running) as safe if pregnant women usually practiced this activities prior to pregnancy [42]. The need to adapt or modify the exercises for pregnancy was also mentioned in other documents [41, 45, 47, 49, 50, 52, 53, 56]. In the old guidelines, there were no specific guidance on how to implement this task. We found only very brief advice like "Exercise should be safe—there should be minimum injury risk to both mother and fetus" and that "Exercise should be comfortable—especially as the pregnancy progresses" ([40], p. 70). Some more detailed tips appear in the new guidelines [49, 56].

From a practical point of view, it would be valuable to develop guidelines on adaptation of exercises to different needs of pregnant women and action to minimize the risk of participating in various sports activities during pregnancy. This would allow women to self-assess the benefits and risks of a particular physical activity, so that they can make informed decisions about participation. Fieril et al. [20] report that modifying the type of exercise, altering exercise goals and being extra attentive during performance are recommended strategies to overcome exercise barriers in pregnancy.

7.5 Targeted Exercise Classes for Pregnant Women

In Tables 7.7 and 7.8, we presented the detailed information that might be useful for designing the contents of targeted exercise classes for pregnant women. Selecting variables for this analysis, we took into account that they should pursue goals specific to health-related physical activity, as well as specific targets for pregnant women, i.e., positive impact on pregnancy and child development, psychophysical preparation for childbirth and postpartum and to the tasks of motherhood [29–31, 84–88]. For this reason, our analysis of the documents focused on the specific content related to: aerobic exercises (cardio part of the exercise classes), resistance (strengthening) exercises, stretching (flexibility) exercises, specific exercises for pregnancy: abdominal, pelvic floor and body posture exercises[1] and exercises preparing for childbirth: breathing exercises, birth positions, relaxation, pregnancy and birth visualization. Additionally, we searched for any tips on how to exercise when the common pregnancy complaints appear (e.g., diastasis recti abdominis, stress urinary incontinence, lumbopelvic, or back pain). We also analyzed the organizational instructions useful in the implementation of the targeted exercise classes for pregnant women.

The main assumption of the targeted exercise classes for pregnant women should be such a selection of exercises that they are not only safe for the mother and fetus but also bring women the most health benefits, among others by alleviating common complaints of pregnancy [58, 89–91]. To be able to respond to the needs of all participants of the course, it is necessary to propose various versions of the exercises, considering trimester of pregnancy and its progress, the level of skills and abilities of women. Pregnant women should be informed, both what is the correct technique of each exercise, but also how to modify it in case of discomfort during its execution. Fieril et al. [20] recorded that in the opinion of pregnant women participating in resistance training "(…), besides length and intensity, a focus on the quality of the exercise performance was of paramount importance" (p. 1140).

The guidelines analyzed contained surprisingly little information on the exercise technique and other tips that might be useful for designing the contents of the targeted exercise classes for pregnant women (Tables 7.5 and 7.6). Both old Australian documents [34, 35] mentioned pregnancy-specific exercise classes and RCOG [41] recommended aqua natal classes. Only the guidelines of Fitness Australia suggested what such classes should include [35], e.g., gradual warm ups and cool downs for pre-natal circulation and avoidance of blood pooling, general strengthening plus particular focus on pregnancy specific muscles such as pelvic floor core and postural muscle strengthening, modified strength training according to the Fitness Australia Safety Guidelines for Strength Training, modifications for standing and supine positions such as four point kneeling, sitting on a fitball and side lying, flexibility training limited to a comfortable range of movement, relaxation, and labor

[1] Abdominal, pelvic floor exercises, and body posture are especially important in pregnancy, so for the purposes of this work we have included them in exercises specific to pregnancy. However, differently oriented, they should be performed in all programs of physical activity.

Table 7.7 Guidelines useful for designing the contents of targeted prenatal exercise classes published by the end of 2017

	Australia (SMA) 2016	Australia (FA) 2013	Canada (SOGC/ CSEP)	Canada (CASEM)	Denmark	Norway	South Africa (SASMA)	United Kingdom (RCOG)	United States (ACOG) 2015	United States (ACNM)	United States (ACSM)	United States (U.S. DHHS)	International (IOC) 2016
Aerobic exercises (cardio part):													
General recommendations[a]	+	+				+	+	+	+	+	+		+
Detailed instructions[b]		+				+							+
Muscle-strengthening exercises:													
General recommendations	+	+	+	+	+	+	+	+		+		+	+
Detailed instructions	+	+		+	+	+	+						+
Flexibility exercises:													
General recommendations		+											+
Detailed instructions	+	+											
Abdominal, pelvic floor and body posture exercises:													
General recommendations	+	+			+	+	+		+				+
Detailed instructions	+	+											

(continued)

Table 7.7 (continued)

	Australia (SMA) 2016	Australia (FA) 2013	Canada (SOGC/ CSEP)	Canada (CASEM)	Denmark	Norway	South Africa (SASMA)	United Kingdom (RCOG)	United States (ACOG) 2015	United States (ACNM)	United States (ACSM)	United States (U.S. DHHS)	International (IOC) 2016
Exercises preparing to childbirth:													
General recommendations		+											
Detailed instructions													
Exercises addressing common pregnancy complaints:													
General recommendations	+		+	+	+	+			+				+
Detailed instructions	+				+	+							
Organizational recommendations:													
Structure of the exercise class	+	+	+					+		+			
Exercise positions	+	+	+		+		+	+	+	+	+	+	
Other	+	+						+			+		+

[a] Related to the particular element of the targeted exercise classes for pregnant women
[b] Any tips related to the quality of exercise execution

Table 7.8 Guidelines useful for designing the contents of targeted prenatal exercise classes published after 2017

	Australia (SMA) 2021	Australia (AGDH) 2021	Australia and New Zealand 2020	Canada (SOGC/CSEP)	United Kingdom (NHS) 2021	United States (ACOG) 2020	United States (ACSM) 2020	United States (EIM/ACSM) 2019	United States (U.S. DHHS) 2018	International (IOC) 2018	International WHO 2020
Aerobic exercises (cardio part):											
General recommendations[a]	+	+	+	+	+	+	+	+	+	+[b]	+
Detailed instructions[c]	+	+	+			+	+	+	+	+[b]	
Muscle-strengthening exercises:											
General recommendations	+	+	+	+	+	+	+	+	+	+[b]	+
Detailed instructions	+[d]		+		+		+	+	+	+[b]	
Flexibility exercises:											
General recommendations	+		+	+			+	+			+
Detailed instructions	+		+				+				
Abdominal, body posture exercises:											
General recommendations				+	+	+				+[b]	
Detailed instructions				+	+						
Pelvic floor exercises:											
General recommendations	+	+	+	+	+		+	+		+[b]	+

(continued)

Table 7.8 (continued)

	Australia (SMA) 2021	Australia (AGDH) 2021	Australia and New Zealand 2020	Canada (SOGC/ CSEP)	United Kingdom (NHS) 2021	United States (ACOG) 2020	United States (ACSM) 2020	United States (EIM/A CSM) 2019	United States (U.S. DHHS) 2018	International (IOC) 2018	International WHO 2020
Detailed instructions	+			+	+ Video			+		+[b]	
Exercises preparing to childbirth:											
General recommendations					+						
Detailed instructions					+ Video						
Exercises addressing common pregnancy complaints:											
General recommendations	+	+	+	+	+	+	+	+		+[b]	+
Detailed instructions										+[b]	
Organizational recommendations:											
Structure of the exercise class	+		+	+	+	+	+				
Exercise positions	+	+	+	+	+	+		+	+	+[b]	+
Other		+	+	+	+			+		+[b]	

[a]Related to the particular element of the targeted exercise classes for pregnant women
[b]Related to very active and elite athletes
[c]Any tips related to the quality of exercise execution
[d]Link to examples of strengthening exercises was provided

preparation. The new guidelines did not mention targeted prenatal exercise classes at all. However, they contained some useful information to design it.

7.5.1 Aerobic, Resistance, and Stretching Exercises

In eight old documents, we found only general recommendation to perform aerobics [34, 35, 39–42, 44, 45]; in six documents specified to low impact [35, 39, 40, 42, 44, 45], which is one of the basic modes of aerobic exercise in prenatal exercise classes. There were no tips on the selection and the technique of the aerobics moves and their usage. In the new guidelines, the low-impact aerobics was mentioned only once [53]. There is a growing evidence that pregnant women can safely participate in high-impact aerobics [92].

In relation to the muscle-strengthening (or resistance) exercises, 12 old documents contained only general advice to perform them [1, 34–44]. More detailed tips were inter alia: to pay attention to correct technique [40], to consider that exercises requiring balance and agility may become more difficult while the pregnancy progresses [34, 42, 45] and to work with an instructor or use equipment to reduce the risk of overexertion [38]. It was also recommended to avoid breath holding [35, 37] and the Valsalva maneuver during resistance exercises [35, 40]. For safe and effective training, the guidelines from South Africa [40] and Australia [34] advised pregnant women to use relatively low weights. Other documents also discouraged the use of heavy weights in pregnancy [29, 38, 44].

All new documents mentioned muscle-strengthening exercises as recommended for pregnant women (Table 7.4). To provide examples of strengthening exercises, the SMA guidelines [47] included link to an electronic version of the Canadian PARmed-X for Pregnancy. The RANZCOG advised that movements should be slow and steady and performed with proper breathing technique. Other sensible precautions include avoiding activities that involve straining, holding the breath, or that are isometric in nature [49]. According to the IOC, in general, athletes are advised to pay attention to technique and safety. If there is a feeling of muscle strain or excessive fatigue, exercises should be modified to avoid injury. Strenuous strength training should be adjusted to avoid the Valsalva maneuver and excessive pressure toward the pelvic floor [56]. Two Australian institutions did not recommend heavy weight lifting [48, 49]. Two other guidelines [50, 54] did not advise the Olympic lifts to be performed during pregnancy. However, the upper load limit for resistance exercises has not yet been established. "Heavy" is rather a very relative term, depending on the individual's fitness level prior to pregnancy.

According to the old SMA document, pregnant women should avoid wide squats, lunges, or any unilateral leg exercises that place excessive shearing forces on the pubic symphysis [34]. Fitness Australia excluded some exercises that significantly involved abdominal muscles [35]. In the new guidelines, RANZCOG stated that walking lunges were best avoided to prevent injury to pelvic connective tissue [49]. However, so far, there was no study published which could indicate negative influences of the above exercises on pregnant woman's body.

Only the old Australian guidelines [34, 35] provided short practical instructions on stretching exercises. We found recommendations that flexibility training should be limited to a comfortable range of movement [35] and also that it should be controlled and not "over-extended" as joints and ligaments are already loose due to the release of the hormone relaxin in preparation for birth [34]. The Canadian guidelines from 2003 stated that "stretching and strength training exercises such as yoga and Pilates have not been studied in a pregnant population" ([36], p. 4). Nevertheless, in recent years, there have been several scientific publications on yoga [93–95] and Pilates classes [96, 97] for pregnant women. The outcomes of those studies should be disseminated in public sources of information by credible institutions. A change in this aspect is visible in the new guidelines. They recommended pregnant women practice yoga, stretching, or Pilates, sometimes in modified versions [50, 52–54]. According to SMA [47], stretching exercises should be done gently due to the increased joint laxity during pregnancy. The RANZCOG mentioned that "stretching should always be performed in a slow and controlled manner" ([49], p. 9), which is a general advice for all exercisers.

7.5.2 Specific Exercises for Pregnancy and in Selected Pregnancy Complaints

In the old guidelines, we found very limited guidance on how to perform abdominal exercises. The only information available was that "the ability to perform abdominal strengthening exercises may be impeded by the development of diastasis recti and associated abdominal muscle weakness" ([36], p. 4) and that "abdominal exercises are not recommended if diastasis recti develops" ([37], p. 3). In Norwegian guidelines, it was only generally stated that strong stomach muscles can prevent pain in the lower back and bad posture [39]. ACOG guidelines also propose strengthening of both abdominal and back muscles to minimize the risk of low back pain [42].

In 2013 Fitness Australia suggested that any exercise that places significant load on the abdominals or pelvic floor including abdominal curls, sit ups, planks, and hovers should be avoided [35]. Nevertheless, this is not an evidence-based recommendation. The new Canadian guidelines [50] also advised avoidance of abdominal curls for women with diastasis recti abdominis (DRA), as this might worsen the condition, increasing the likelihood of requiring postnatal repair. Contrary to this statement, Mota et al. [98] proved that performing abdominal curls consistently produced a significant narrowing of the inter-rectus distance both in pregnant and postpartum women (IRD). IOC expert group, both in the older and newer documents, presented available scientific data on the diastasis recti abdominis, concluding that the etiology and possible preventive and treatment strategies of this condition were not clear [1, 56].

In the new guidelines, strengthening abdominal exercises are still indicated as prevention or treatment of back pain [51, 52]. Additionally, NHS described a few examples of abdominal exercises to perform during pregnancy.

As regards the pelvic floor exercises, in the old guidelines they were mentioned by Danish [38], Norwegian [39] and Australian experts [34, 35]. They were generally recommended for the prevention of stress urinary incontinence [38] and presented as particularly important during pregnancy and after the birth [39]. Australia Fitness [35] underlined its significance for pregnant women. The Sport Medicine Australia guidelines included instruction to design pelvic floor exercise program for pregnant women. The exercise technique recommended in this document was to contract pelvic floor muscles maximally with an inward and upward squeezing movement, mixing slow and fast controlled contraction in a sitting, kneeling, standing, lying down, or standing with leg astride position. The prevalence of pelvic floor dysfunctions and suggestions for their prevention and treatment, e.g., through supervised training in combination with home exercise were discussed in the IOC summary [1].

All new guidelines, apart from ACOG and U.S. DHHS, recommended that women perform pelvic floor muscle exercises (Table 7.8), highlighting their role in the prophylaxis of urinary incontinence. The ACOG experts [52] addressed this recommendation only to the postpartum women. Three documents [47, 51, 56] provided detailed instructions on how to perform pelvic floor muscle exercises. NHS [51] included a short video with explanations how these muscles work and tips for the exercise performance. EIM [54] recommended visiting a pelvic health specialist during pregnancy to learn the best way to train the muscles of the pelvic floor. IOC [56] emphasized the importance of the pelvic floor muscle training for female elite athletes. They were advised to contract the pelvic floor muscles before and during heavy lifting to counteract the impact on the pelvic floor from increased intra-abdominal pressure.

In the old analyzed documents very little attention was devoted to the body posture, except the note that strengthening exercises would help to maintain it [39, 40]. Pregnant women with pelvic or back problems were advised to cycle [38] or to exercise in the water [38, 39]. Fitness Australia generally recommended postural muscle strengthening [35]. According to the IOC "changes in spinal curvature during pregnancy as well as frequent or sustained pain-provoking postures might influence the pelvic ligaments, causing pain" ([1], p. 582). The experts suggested that women should be aware of their body positions while pregnant to avoid unnecessary load and stress on joint, ligaments and muscles, during exercise and daily activities. They also showed the relationship between pregnancy, exercise and the low back pain or pelvic girdle pain. Other common conditions, illnesses, and complaints typical for pregnancy and the chances of their treatment through prenatal exercise were summarized in the IOC document, as well. The Part 5 of the IOC work [56] contains detailed recommendations for health professionals and active women in this subject.

All new documents, apart from U.S. DHHS (Table 7.8), provided some information on physical activity for women with pregnancy complaints. Experts generally recommended modifying or individualizing the exercise program and consult physical activity pattern with highly qualified specialists. However, more detailed recommendations on how to implement exercise for pregnant patients with specific complaints should be developed, based on available scientific evidence.

In our previous review, the Fitness Australia was the only one organization which presented labor preparation as an important part of activities for pregnant women [35]. Until 2018, the breathing exercises, birth positions, relaxation, pregnancy and birth visualization were not even mentioned in any analyzed document. In guidelines published after 2017, only the NHS [51] emphasizes the importance of exercise in preparing for childbirth. A short instructional video presenting the birthing positions and breathing exercises has for pregnant women been included.

7.5.3 Exercise Positions, Structure of the Exercise Class, and Other Organizational Recommendations

Eleven old guidelines [1, 34–37, 40–42, 44, 45] recommended avoiding or limiting the supine position after the first trimester, or after 16 weeks of gestation, or after the fourth month of gestation. As an alternative solution it was proposed to change the exercises [40] or to put a pillow or towel underneath one hip [44]. ACSM also suggested avoiding prone position until more information becomes available [45].

The information on the potential need to limit the supine position while exercising during pregnancy was mentioned in ten new documents [47–52, 54–57]. The Canadian guidelines explained that some pregnant women may experience lightheadedness, nausea or feel unwell when they exercise flat on their back. The experts from other countries complemented this information with tips like to tilt the upper body to a 45-degree angle or to perform the exercises in different positions, like a side-lying, sitting or standing positions [48–50, 54]. However, IOC experts [56] pointed that some studies report no adverse effect with exercise in the supine position for 2–3 min at a time.

With regard to the structure of the exercise classes in five old documents we found the advice to include a warm up and cool down in any exercise regimen [34–36, 41, 44] and in two documents—to avoid motionless standing [40–42]. Other organizational tips were, e.g., to use properly adjusted exercise equipment and a smooth floor surface [45] and to use pelvic support belts for the weight-bearing exercise in women affected by joint laxity changes [41].

Six new documents [47, 49–51, 53] mentioned the warm up or cool down, as important parts of exercise session for pregnant women. Other recommendations were to use body weight, hand weights, elastic bands, or weight machines in resistance exercises [49, 52–54]. The Canadian experts stated that: "Although the majority of the evidence base for these recommendations used supervised exercise, physical activity during pregnancy does not need to be done in a supervised setting or with any specific equipment" ([50], p. 1344).

7.6 Exercise Professionals and Obstetrics Care Providers

Exercise professionals are supposed to play the most important role in providing information on exercise selection and techniques. However, in our previuos work, we have proved [99] that although the future exercise professionals are generally aware of the positive impact of prenatal physical activity, they lack detailed knowledge, allowing the implementation of exercise sessions with pregnant clients. Those results demonstrate that there is a need to educate them on the exercise in pregnancy. An attempt at international discussion on how to prepare professionals to conduct exercises for pregnant women was undertaken during the fifth International Standards Meeting in Amsterdam in 2014, organized by the EuropeActive (former European Health and Fitness Association). Representatives from 12 European countries interested in the development of an international educational standard for the Pregnancy and Postnatal Exercise Specialists participated in this work. It is the first document of this type specifying the learning outcomes necessary for design and delivery of a prenatal exercise program, and set within the concept of the European Qualifications Framework [60]. The educational standard should correspond to the official and up to date guidelines for exercise in pregnancy. Thanks to this, professional tasks performed by Pregnancy and Postnatal Exercise Specialists would have a better chance to meet with the approval of pregnant women and medical staff.

In the old guidelines, only the experts from Denmark stated that the exercise during pregnancy should be supervised by an "instructor" [38], especially for the beginners [68]. The analyzed documents did not pay much attention to the exercise professionals' skills and competencies necessary to promote and implement exercise programs, foster women's adherence to exercise, evaluate their training progress and, if needed, to cooperate with a health professional. Only guidelines from The Health & Fitness Industry Association indicated that exercise professionals who offer specific services to pregnant or postpartum women were required to complete a Fitness Australia Continuing Education program [35]. In nine of the 11 new guidelines, experts recommend pregnant women consult with a physical activity or exercise specialist, or exercise physiologist [47, 49, 51, 53–57]. It is clearly visible that the role of this professional group has been strengthening in the last few years.

In eight of 13 old guidelines, pregnant women were advised to consult the health care providers regarding their exercise program [34–36, 38, 42–45]. This recommendation appears in all new documents analyzed. The ACOG guidelines [52] still emphasizes the need for a thorough clinical evaluation before recommending an exercise program, to ensure that there is no medical reason preventing participants from engaging in exercise. Women with medical or obstetric complications should be carefully assessed by obstetricians beforehand to determine an individual physical activity plan. Additionally, women should be advised to stay well hydrated and to stop exercising if any warning symptoms develop (e.g., vaginal bleeding, abdominal pain, regular painful contractions, leakage of amniotic fluid, etc.). The ACOG listed several warning signs to discontinue exercise during pregnancy. Healthcare professionals should inform their patients that as soon as these warning signs appear, pregnant women should stop or significantly reduce physical activity and immediately contact their obstetric care providers. According to some guidelines, pregnant athletes or women exercising significantly above the recommended level should be supervised by a specialist healthcare provider [47, 48, 50, 52, 53, 56, 57].

Such a recommendation seems justified only under the condition that the obstetricians and midwives would be well educated in this area, including the knowledge of the impact of vigorous-intensity physical activity on maternal, fetal, and neonatal outcomes. However, research shows that medical staff often remain at the former conservative position and do not support exercises during pregnancy. Only 1% of doctors in Poland recommend physical activity to pregnant women. What is more, 11% of them recommend that pregnant women limit their physical activity without any medical reason [15]. In the research by Hagen Haakstad et al. [6] only 36% of Norwegian pregnant women surveyed reported that they had received advice about physical activity at least once during their pregnancy from a physician or a midwife. Similarly, Schmidt et al. [100] showed that only 48% of pregnant women surveyed had received information on the subject of physical exercise in pregnancy from their general practitioner or gynecologist.

As noted by Evenson and Bradley [22] more work is needed to understand what advice is being given to pregnant women by their health care providers. In another study Jukic et al. [101] observed that health professionals' advice was associated with the level of prenatal physical activity of their patients. Because health care providers have great influence on patients' health behavior, it is critical that they give pregnant women accurate and sufficient information [23]. In the study by Padmanabhan et al. [102] women felt that their midwives provided detailed information on what they should not do during pregnancy but were rarely given information about what they should do in relation to diet and physical activity for weight management. Consequently, women often used information from a variety of sources which they filtered using "common sense." According to Watson [103] the majority of South African medical practitioners (98%) believe that exercise during pregnancy is beneficial, and were knowledgeable on most of the expected benefits, but at the same time most of them (83%) were unaware of the recommended exercise guidelines. These results highlight the need to educate health care professionals in this topic. Malta et al. [104] proved that after an educational intervention health care professionals were more likely to give their pregnant patients proper guidance regarding leisure-time walking and healthy eating comparing to the control group. In order to prepare obstetricians and midwives to answer pregnant women's questions regarding exercise in pregnancy, they must be given reliable and comprehensive sources of information. The new guidelines seem to be good sources of general information on exercise in pregnancy. Still, close cooperation between obstetric care providers and exercise professionals is essential.

The Canadian guidelines by SOGC/CSEP [36, 50], Australian by Fitness Australia [35] and Sport Medicine Australia [34, 47], American by ACSM [53] and by IOC [56] proposed PARmed-X for pregnancy as a tool for collaboration between a pregnant woman, her obstetric care provider and an exercise professional in terms of the exercise program design [105]. Watson et al. [103] observed that only 24% of health practitioners referred pregnant women to exercise specialists. In the area of prenatal physical activity there is dynamically growing reliable information, both from research and practical experience, in the implementation of various programs of exercise for pregnant women. This should be the basis of educational standards and materials for pregnancy exercise specialists. Unfortunately, the training providers still rely too often on information that is 20 or more years old.

Another important issue is to prepare professionals, both from the fitness and health sector to supervise pregnant elite athletes. Given the infrequency of pregnancy in athletes competing at the national or international level in any given time period, enrolling these women from around the globe in prospective research trials seems a very challenging task. Therefore, Bø et al. [56] recommend that the IOC develop a prospective international registry of elite competitive athletes who plan to become or are pregnant to allow for the collection and analysis of maternal and neonatal consequences of extreme levels of exercise before, during, and after gestation. This solution would enable the collection of relevant data to develop a specific educational standard for the entire training staff and help female athletes combine both sports and maternal goals.

7.7 Limitations

One of the limitations of the work is the selection of documents for the analysis. Owing to the fact that the guidelines for exercise in pregnancy do not always have the character of scientific work, and only represent the official position of credible national institutions, sometimes it was impossible to find them in the scientific databases. Nevertheless, we have tried to adopt a procedure in seeking material for analysis that would ensure its effectiveness and repeatability. We realize that we might have missed some of the documents that meet the inclusion criteria.

The procedure adopted for qualifying documents for the analysis excludes material published in other languages and not available on the Internet. Because of that, the presented picture of the current guidelines on exercise during pregnancy is incomplete and is not global. It seems justified to continue and expand the international cooperation started by Evenson et al. [32] in order to collect the material published in other languages, understanding their contents, as well as their historical and cultural context. It is necessary to follow the analysis of official guidelines with international implementation activities, promoting exercise in pregnancy. One of them seems to be the development and dissemination of international educational standards for professionals involved in the implementation of programs of prenatal exercise. This task has already been started by EuropeActive in 2014, and published in 2015 [60]. Currently, work is underway in the international team to update this document, as well as to develop an educational program and educational materials for future pregnancy exercise specialists.

Notwithstanding these limitations, the presented review can be a starting point for discussion in the work on updating the existing and creation of new documents in this area. We realize that the specific content that we propose for inclusion in a new version of the guidelines for exercise in pregnancy would significantly increase their volume. However, they would become a much more useful tool, supporting prenatal physical activity.

7.8 Conclusions

Since the last review of the guidelines in 2017, 11 new documents have appeared as official statements of national or international obstetrics, gynecology, or sports medicine bodies on physical activity in pregnancy. Almost half of these documents are evidence-based. There is a visible change in the approach to physical activity in pregnancy. There are more and more recommendations for women with a high level of physical activity and participating in high-intensity sports, including female elite athletes. It is becoming acceptable to continue sports training and participation in competitions. Nevertheless, experts emphasize that there is a lack of scientific data on this topic and that research of good quality is necessary in this area.

The approach to physical activity in complicated pregnancy has completely changed. The list of health conditions that were previously considered contraindications to physical activity during pregnancy has been verified. More and more often there is a recommendation to individualize exercise and maintain normal life activity in the case of a complicated pregnancy. The prescription to bed rest is strongly criticized as harmful to the physical and mental health of the future mother and the whole family.

The new guidelines are still very general in nature, although, compared to the documents published before 2018, there are more detailed provisions on the content of the exercise. It is worth noting that most of the documents contain recommendations on pelvic floor muscle training, mainly as a prevention of urinary incontinence. An innovative element in the British guidelines is the inclusion of short videos on exercise of pelvic floor muscles and preparation for childbirth.

Certainly, the current guidelines can be a good source of information for obstetric care providers who should advise their patients about physical activity during pregnancy. However, specific guidelines for exercise professionals on how to plan and conduct targeted prenatal exercise classes should be developed in separate, broader documents. According to the current trend, a lot of space should be devoted to exercise in complicated pregnancy. It is also important to develop rules for cooperation between obstetric care providers and exercise professionals to enable the safe implementation of exercise programs for pregnant women with different needs.

Analyzed guidelines should be disseminated among all parties interested in prenatal physical activity: pregnant women and their families, obstetric care providers and exercise professionals to enable their effective cooperation and to globally promote exercise in pregnancy. It is important that similar documents are developed and implemented by national maternity care organizations in all countries.

References

1. Bø K, Artal R, Barakat R, Brown W, Davies GAL, Dooley M, et al. Exercise and pregnancy in recreational and elite athletes: 2016 evidence summary from the IOC expert group meeting, Lausanne. Part 1-exercise in women planning pregnancy and those who are pregnant. Br J Sports Med. 2016;50(10):571–89.

2. Bø K, Artal R, Barakat R, Brown W, Dooley M, Evenson KR, et al. Exercise and pregnancy in recreational and elite athletes: 2016 evidence summary from the IOC expert group meeting, Lausanne. Part 2-the effect of exercise on the fetus, labour and birth. Br J Sports Med. 2016;50(21):1297–305.
3. Davenport MH, Meah VL, Ruchat S-M, Davies GA, Skow RJ, Barrowman N, et al. Impact of prenatal exercise on neonatal and childhood outcomes: a systematic review and meta-analysis. Br J Sports Med. 2018;52(21):1386–96.
4. Davenport MH, Ruchat S-M, Sobierajski F, Poitras VJ, Gray CE, Yoo C, et al. Impact of prenatal exercise on maternal harms, labour and delivery outcomes: a systematic review and meta-analysis. Br J Sports Med. 2019;53:99.
5. Cai C, Ruchat S-M, Sivak A, Davenport MH. Prenatal exercise and cardiorespiratory health and fitness: a meta-analysis. Med Sci Sports Exerc. 2020;52(7):1538–48.
6. Hagen Haakstad LA, Voldner N, Bø K. Stages of change model for participation in physical activity during pregnancy. J Pregnancy. 2013;2013:1–7.
7. Ruchat S-M, Mottola MF. Preventing long-term risk of obesity for two generations: prenatal physical activity is part of the puzzle. J Pregnancy. 2012;2012:470247.
8. Perales M, Valenzuela PL, Barakat R, Cordero Y, Pelaez M, Lopez C, et al. Gestational exercise and maternal and child health: effects until delivery and at post-natal follow-up. J Clin Med. 2020;9(2):14.
9. Evenson KR, Savitz DA, Huston SL. Leisure-time physical activity among pregnant women in the US. Paediatr Perinat Epidemiol. 2004;18(6):400–7.
10. Petersen AM, Leet TL, Brwonson RC. Correlates of physical activity among pregnant women in the United States. Med Sci Sports Exerc. 2005;37(10):1748–53.
11. Liu J, Blair SN, Teng Y, Ness AR, Lawlor DA, Riddoch C. Physical activity during pregnancy in a prospective cohort of British women: results from the Avon longitudinal study of parents and children. Eur J Epidemiol. 2011;26(3):237–47.
12. Amezcua-Prieto C, Lardelli-Claret P, Olmedo-Requena R, Mozas-Moreno J, Bueno-Cavanillas A, JiméNez-Moleón JJ. Compliance with leisure-time physical activity recommendations in pregnant women. Acta Obstet Gynecol Scand. 2011;90(3):245–52.
13. Nascimento SL, Surita FG, Cecatti JG. Physical exercise during pregnancy: a systematic review. Curr Opin Obstet Gynecol. 2012;24(6):387–94.
14. Juhl M, Madsen M, Andersen AMN, Andersen PK, Olsen J. Distribution and predictors of exercise habits among pregnant women in the Danish National Birth Cohort. Scand J Med Sci Sports. 2012;22(1):128–38.
15. Wojtyła A, Kapka-Skrzypczak L, Paprzycki P, Skrzypczak M, Biliński P. Epidemiological studies in Poland on effect of physical activity of pregnant women on the health of offspring and future generations - adaptation of the hypothesis development origin of health and diseases. Ann Agric Environ Med. 2012;19(2):315–26.
16. Gaston A, Vamos C. Leisure-time physical activity patterns and correlates among pregnant women in Ontario, Canada. Maternal Child Health J. 2013;17(3):477–84.
17. Santos PC, Abreu S, Moreira C, Lopes D, Santos R, Alves O, et al. Impact of compliance with different guidelines on physical activity during pregnancy and perceived barriers to leisure physical activity. J Sports Sci. 2014;32(14):1398–408.
18. Christopher PC, Deborah LF, James MP. Overcoming barriers to physical activity during pregnancy and the postpartum period: the potential impact of social support. Kinesiol Rev. 2014;3(2):135–48.
19. Atkinson L, Parsons J, Jackson BR. Exercise in pregnancy - UK women's views and experiences: results of an online survey. Pregnan Hypertens. 2014;4(3):231.
20. Petrov Fieril K, Fagevik Olsén M, Glantz A, Larsson M. Experiences of exercise during pregnancy among women who perform regular resistance training: a qualitative study. Phys Ther. 2014;94(8):1135–43.

21. Thornton PL, Kieffer EC, Salabarria-Pena Y, Odoms-Young A, Willis SK, Kim H, et al. Weight, diet, and physical activity-related beliefs and practices among pregnant and postpartum Latino women: the role of social support. Matern Child Health J. 2006;10(1):95–104.
22. Evenson KR, Bradley CB. Beliefs about exercise and physical activity among pregnant women. Patient Educ Couns. 2010;79(1):124–9.
23. Cannella D, Lobel M, Monheit A. Knowing is believing: information and attitudes towards physical activity during pregnancy. J Psychosom Obstet Gynecol. 2010;31(4):236–42.
24. Mbada CE, Adebayo OE, Adeyemi AB, Arije OO, Dada OO, Akinwande OA, et al. Knowledge and attitude of Nigerian pregnant women towards antenatal exercise: a cross-sectional survey. ISRN Obstet Gynecol. 2014;2014:1–8.
25. Gouveia R, Martins S, Sandes AR, Nascimento C, Figueira J, Valente S, et al. [Pregnancy and physical exercise: myths, evidence and recommendations]. Acta Medica Port. 2007;20(3):209–14.
26. Tanha FD, Ghajarzadeh M, Mohseni M, Shariat M, Ranjbar M. Is ACOG guideline helpful for encouraging pregnant women to do exercise during pregnancy? Acta Medica Iranica. 2014;52(6):458–61.
27. van Poppel M, Owe K, Santos-Rocha R, Dias H, Oviedo-Caro MA. Physical activity, exercise, and health promotion for the pregnant exerciser and the pregnant athlete. In: Santos-Rocha R, editor. Exercise and physical activity during pregnancy and postpartum. Evidence-based guidelines. 2nd ed. Cham: Springer International Publishing; 2022. Chapter 1.
28. Tan EK, Tan EL. Alterations in physiology and anatomy during pregnancy. Best Pract Res Clin Obstet Gynaecol. 2013;27(6):791–802.
29. ACSM. ACSM's Resources for the personal trainer. 5th ed. Philadelphia, PA: Wolters Kluwer Health; 2017. 632 p.
30. Berk B. Motherwell maternity fitness plan. Champaign, IL: Human Kinetics, Inc; 2005. 232 p.
31. Clapp JF, Cram C. Exercise through your pregnancy. 2nd ed. Omaha, NB: Addicus Books; 2012. 268 p.
32. Evenson KR, Barakat R, Brown WJ, Dargent-Molina P, Haruna M, Mikkelsen EM, et al. Guidelines for physical activity during pregnancy: comparisons from around the world. Am J Lifestyle Med. 2014;8(2):102–21.
33. Szumilewicz A, Worska A, Rajkowska N, Santos-Rocha R. Summary of guidelines for exercise in pregnancy – are they comprehensive enough for designing the contents of a prenatal exercise program? Curr Women's Health Rev. 2015;11(1):3–12.
34. Hayman M, Brown W, Ferrar K, Marchese R, Tan J. SMA position statement for exercise in pregnancy and the postpartum period. Sydney Olympic Park, NSW: SMA; 2016. http://sma.org.au/wp-content/uploads/2016/09/SMA-Position-Statement-Exercise-Pregnancy.pdf.
35. Pre & post-natal exercise guidelines. 2013. https://fitnessaustralia.s3.amazonaws.com/uploads/uploaded_file/file/219/Pre-and-Post-Natal-Exercise-Guidelines.pdf.
36. Davies GAL, Wolfe LA, Mottola MF, MacKinnon C, Arsenault M-Y, Bartellas E, et al. Exercise in pregnancy and the postpartum period. J Obstet Gynaecol Can. 2003;25(6):516–29.
37. Alleyne J. Position statement: exercise and pregnancy. 2008. http://casem-acmse.org/wp-content/uploads/2013/07/Exercise-Pregnancy-Position-Paper-_2008_pdf.
38. Healthy habits – before, during and after pregnancy. 2010. https://www.sst.dk/en/health-and-lifestyle/~/media/BCB704A368E3404C8CEEAE057CDEDE26.ashx.
39. Holan S, Mathiesen M, Petersen K. A national clinical guideline for antenatal care. Short version. 2005. https://helsedirektoratet.no/Lists/Publikasjoner/Attachments/404/National-clinical-guideline-for-antenatal-care-short-version%20-IS-1339.pdf.
40. Barsky E, Smith T, Patricios J, Collins R, Branfield A, Ramagole M. South African Sports Medicine Association Position Statement on Exercise in Pregnancy. S A J Sports Med. 2012;24(2):69–71.
41. RCOG. Statement No. 4. Exercise in pregnancy. London: Royal College of Obstetricians and Gynaecologists (RCOG); 2006. https://www.rcog.org.uk/globalassets/documents/guidelines/statements/statement-no-4.pdf.

42. ACOG. Physical Activity and exercise during pregnancy and the postpartum period. Washington, DC: The American College of Obstetricians and Gynecologists (ACOG); 2015. Committee Opinion No. 650.
43. DHHS US. Physical activity guidelines for Americans. Washington, DC: U.S. Department of Human and Health Services; 2008. https://health.gov/paguidelines/pdf/paguide.pdf.
44. ACNM. Exercise in pregnancy. J Midwif Women's Health. 2014;59(4):473–4.
45. ACSM. Current comment. Exercise during pregnancy. Indianapolis, IN: ACSM.
46. Bø K, Artal R, Barakat R, Brown WJ, Davies GAL, Dooley M, et al. Exercise and pregnancy in recreational and elite athletes: 2016/17 evidence summary from the IOC Expert Group Meeting, Lausanne. Part 3-exercise in the postpartum period. Br J Sports Med. 2017;51(21):1516–25.
47. SMA. Pregnancy and exercise. Women in sport. Sydney Olympic Park, NSW: SMA. SMA_AWiS_Pregnancy_Exercise.pdf. Accessed 13 Jul 2021.
48. AGDH. Guidelines for physical activity during pregnancy. Guidelines for physical activity during pregnancy (health.gov.au). Indianapolis, IN: Australian Government. Department of Health; 2021.
49. RANZCOG. Exercise in pregnancy. Melbourne, VIC: The Royal Australian and New Zealand College of Obstetricians and Gynaecologists; 2020.
50. Mottola MF, Davenport MH, Ruchat S-M, Davies GA, Poitras VJ, Gray CE, et al. 2019 Canadian guideline for physical activity throughout pregnancy. Br J Sports Med. 2018;52(21):1339–46.
51. NHS. Exercise in pregnancy exercise in pregnancy. London: NHS; 2020. www.nhs.uk.
52. ACOG. ACOG Committee opinion no. 804: Physical activity and exercise during pregnancy and the postpartum period. Obstet Gynecol. 2020;135(4):e178–e88.
53. ACSM. ACSM information on pregnancy physical activity. Indianapolis, IN: American College of Sports Medicine; 2020.
54. EIM/ACSM. Being active during pregnancy. Exercise is medicine. Indianapolis, IN: American College of Sports Medicine; 2019.
55. DHHS. Physical activity guidelines for Americans. 2nd ed. Washington, DC: U.S. Department of Health and Human Services; 2018.
56. Bø K, Artal R, Barakat R, Brown WJ, Davies GAL, Dooley M, et al. Exercise and pregnancy in recreational and elite athletes: 2016/2017 evidence summary from the IOC expert group meeting, Lausanne. Part 5. Recommendations for health professionals and active women. Br J Sports Med. 2018;52(17):1080–5.
57. WHO. WHO guidelines on physical activity and sedentary behaviour. Geneva: World Health Organization; 2020.
58. Beyaz EA, Özcan E, Ketenci A, Beyaz MM. The Effectiveness of pregnancy rehabilitation: effects on low back pain and calf cramps during pregnancy and pregnancy outcomes. Gebelik Rehabilitasyonunun Etkinliği: Gebelik Sirasindaki Bel Ağrisi ve Baldir Kramplarina ve Gebelik Sonuçlarina Etkileri. 2011;7(2):67–74.
59. Piper TJ, Jacobs E, Haiduke M, Waller M, McMillan C. Core training exercise selection during pregnancy. Streng Condition J. 2012;34(1):55–62.
60. Santos-Rocha R, Szumilewicz A, Perales M, Pajaujiene S. EuropeActive standards EQF level 5 - pregnancy and postnatal exercise specialist. EuropeActive. 2016;
61. Kehler AK, Heinrich KM. A selective review of prenatal exercise guidelines since the 1950s until present: written for women, health care professionals, and female athletes. Women Birth. 2015;28(4):E93–E8.
62. Tafari N, Naeye RL, Gobezie A. Effects of maternal undernutrition and heavy physical work during pregnancy on birth-weight. Br J Obstet Gynaecol. 1980;87(3):222–6.
63. Terada M. Effect of physical activity before pregnancy on fetuses of mice exercised forcibly during pregnancy. Teratology. 1974;10(2):141–4.
64. Kader M, Naim-Shuchana S. Physical activity and exercise during pregnancy. Eur J Physiother. 2014;16(1):2–9.
65. Bo K, Artal R, Barakat R, Brown W, Dooley M, Evenson KR, et al. Exercise and pregnancy in recreational and elite athletes: 2016 evidence summary from the IOC expert group meet-

ing, Lausanne. Part 2-the effect of exercise on the fetus, labour and birth. Br J Sports Med. 2016;50(21):1297–305.
66. Downs DS, Chasan-Taber L, Evenson KF, Leiferman J, Yeo S. Physical activity and pregnancy: past and present evidence and future recommendations. Res Q Exerc Sport. 2012;83(4):485–502.
67. ACOG. Committee opinion. Number 267, January 2002: exercise during pregnancy and the postpartum period. Obstet Gynecol. 2002;99(1):171–3.
68. SMA. SMA statement the benefits and risks of exercise during pregnancy. Sport Medicine Australia. J Sci Med Sport. 2002;5(1):11–9.
69. Bo K, Artal R, Barakat R, Brown WJ, Davies GAL, Dooley M, et al. Exercise and pregnancy in recreational and elite athletes: 2016/17 evidence summary from the IOC expert group meeting, Lausanne. Part 4-Recommendations for future research. Br J Sports Med. 2017;51(24):1724–6.
70. Mottola MF. Components of exercise prescription and pregnancy. Clin Obstet Gynecol. 2016;59(3):552–8.
71. Ruchat SM, Davenport MH, Giroux I, Hillier M, Batada A, Sopper MM, et al. Walking program of low or vigorous intensity during pregnancy confers an aerobic benefit. Int J Sports Med. 2012;33(8):661–6.
72. Artal R. Exercise during pregnancy and the postpartum period. Philadelphia, PA: Wolters Kluwer; 2017. https://www.uptodate.com/contents/exercise-during-pregnancy-and-the-postpartum-period.
73. Juhl M, Strandberg-Larsen K, Larsen PS, Andersen PK, Svendsen SW, Bonde JP, et al. Occupational lifting during pregnancy and risk of fetal death in a large national cohort study. Scand J Work Environ Health. 2013;39(4):335–42.
74. Meah VL, Davies GA, Davenport MH. Why can't I exercise during pregnancy? Time to revisit medical 'absolute' and 'relative' contraindications: systematic review of evidence of harm and a call to action. Br J Sports Med. 2020;54(23):1395–404.
75. Jain V. Choosing wisely: bedrest-a panacea for all that ails the gravida? J Obstet Gynaecol Can. 2019;41(7):971–3.
76. McCall CA, Grimes DA, Lyerly AD. "Therapeutic" bed rest in pregnancy: unethical and unsupported by data. Obstet Gynecol. 2013;121(6):1305–8.
77. Ozemek C, Arena R. Evidence supporting moving more and sitting less. Prog Cardiovasc Dis. 2021;64:3–8.
78. Jakicic JM, Kraus WE, Powell KE, Campbell WW, Janz KF, Troiano RP, et al. Association between bout duration of physical activity and health: systematic review. Med Sci Sports Exerc. 2019;51(6):1213–9.
79. Vandelanotte C, Van Itallie A, Brown W, Mummery WK, Duncan MJ. Every step counts: understanding the success of implementing the 10,000 steps project. Stud Health Technol Inf. 2020;268:15–30.
80. Ekelund U, Brown WJ, Steene-Johannessen J, Fagerland MW, Owen N, Powell KE, et al. Do the associations of sedentary behaviour with cardiovascular disease mortality and cancer mortality differ by physical activity level? A systematic review and harmonised meta-analysis of data from 850 060 participants. Br J Sports Med. 2019;53(14):886–94.
81. Conger J, Magann EF. Diving and pregnancy: what do we really know? Obstet Gynecol Surv. 2014;69(9):551–6.
82. Reid RL, Lorenzo M. SCUBA diving in pregnancy. J Obstet Gynaecol Can. 2018;40(11):1490–6.
83. Krans EE, Chang JC. Low-income African American women's beliefs regarding exercise during pregnancy. Matern Child Health J. 2012;16(6):1180–7.
84. Karowicz-Bilińska A, Sikora A, Estemberg D, Brzozowska M, Berner-Trabska M, Kuś E, et al. [Physiotherapy in obstetrics]. Ginekol Pol. 2010;81(6):441-5
85. Zwelling E. Overcoming the challenges: maternal movement and positioning to facilitate labor progress. MCN Am J Matern Child Nurs. 2010;35(2):72–8.

86. Artieta-Pinedo I, Paz-Pascual C, Grandes G, Espinosa M. Framework for the establishment of a feasible, tailored and effective perinatal education programme. BMC Pregnan Childb. 2017;17:1–10.
87. Miquelutti MA, Cecatti JG, Makuch MY. Antenatal education and the birthing experience of Brazilian women: a qualitative study. BMC Pregnan Childb. 2013;13(1):1–8.
88. Levett KM, Smith CA, Bensoussan A, Dahlen HG. The Complementary Therapies for Labour and Birth Study making sense of labour and birth - experiences of women, partners and midwives of a complementary medicine antenatal education course. Midwifery. 2016;40:124–31.
89. Shiri R, Coggon D, Falah-Hassani K. Exercise for the prevention of low back and pelvic girdle pain in pregnancy: a meta-analysis of randomized controlled trials. Eur J Pain. 2018;22(1):19–27.
90. Magro-Malosso ER, Saccone G, Di Tommaso M, Roman A, Berghella V. Exercise during pregnancy and risk of gestational hypertensive disorders: a systematic review and meta-analysis. Acta Obstet Gynecol Scand. 2017;96(8):921–31.
91. Lemos A, de Souza AI, Ferreira ALCG, Figueiroa JN, Cabral-Filho JE. Do perineal exercises during pregnancy prevent the development of urinary incontinence? A systematic review. Int J Urol. 2008;15(10):875–80.
92. Szumilewicz A, Dornowski M, Piernicka M, Worska A, Kuchta A, Kortas J, et al. High-low impact exercise program including pelvic floor muscle exercises improves pelvic floor muscle function in healthy pregnant women – a randomized control trial. Front Physiol. 2019;9:1867.
93. Jain S, Bhartiya N. Positive effects of antenatal yoga on pregnancy outcomes. Indian Obstet Gynaecol. 2017;7(4):27–31.
94. Riley K, Drake E. The effects of prenatal yoga on birth outcomes: a systematic review of the literature. J Prenat Perinat Psychol Health. 2013;28(1):3–19.
95. Jiang Q, Wu Z, Zhou L, Dunlop J, Chen P. Effects of yoga intervention during pregnancy: a review for current status. Am J Perinatol. 2015;32(6):503–14.
96. Muller A, Hammill H. The Effect of pilates and progressive muscle relaxation therapy (Mrt) on stress and anxiety during pregnancy: a literature review. S A J Sports Med. 2015;27:53.
97. Mazzarino M, Kerr D, Wajswelner H, Morris ME. Pilates method for women's health: systematic review of randomized controlled trials. Arch Phys Med Rehabil. 2015;96(12):2231–42.
98. Mota P, Pascoal AG, Carita AI, Bø K. The immediate effects on inter-rectus distance of abdominal crunch and drawing-in exercises during pregnancy and the postpartum period. J Orthop Sports Phys Ther. 2015;45(10):781–8.
99. Worska A, Szumilewicz A. Aktywność fizyczna kobiet w ciąży w świadomości przyszłych instruktorów rekreacji ruchowej [Physical activity of expecting mothers in the awareness of future exercise professionals]. J Educ Health Sport. 2015;5(8):91–102.
100. Schmidt T, Heilmann T, Savelsberg L, Maass N, Weisser B, Eckmann-Scholz C. Physical exercise during pregnancy - how active are pregnant women in germany and how well informed? Geburtshilfe Frauenheilkd. 2017;77(5):508–15.
101. Jukic AMZ, Evenson KR, Herring AH, Wilcox AJ, Hartmann KE, Daniels JL. Correlates of physical activity at two time points during pregnancy. J Phys Act Health. 2012;9(3):325–35.
102. Padmanabhan U, Summerbell CD, Heslehurst N. A qualitative study exploring pregnant women's weight-related attitudes and beliefs in UK: the BLOOM study. BMC Pregnan Childb. 2015;15:99.
103. Watson ED, Oddie B, Constantinou D. Exercise during pregnancy: knowledge and beliefs of medical practitioners in South Africa: a survey study. BMC Pregnan Childb. 2015;15:245.
104. Malta MB, Carvalhaes M, Takito MY, Tonete VLP, Barros AJD, Parada C, et al. Educational intervention regarding diet and physical activity for pregnant women: changes in knowledge and practices among health professionals. BMC Pregnan Childb. 2016;16:175.
105. PARmed-X for PREGNANCY (Physical Activity Readiness Medical Examination for Pregnancy). CSEP. 2013.

Exercise Testing and Prescription in Pregnancy

8

Rita Santos-Rocha, Isabel Corrales Gutiérrez, Anna Szumilewicz, and Simona Pajaujiene

Abstract

Physical exercise should be part of an active lifestyle during pregnancy and the puerperium, as shown by growing evidence on its benefits for the health of pregnant women and newborns. Appropriate exercise testing and exercise prescription are needed to tailor effective and safe exercise programs. Exercise testing and prescription in pregnancy is the plan of exercise and fitness-related activities designed to meet the health and fitness goals and motivations of the pregnant woman. It should address the health-related fitness components and the pregnancy-specific conditions, based on previous health and exercise assessments, and take into account the body adaptations and the pregnancy-related symptoms of each stage of pregnancy, in order to provide safe and effective exercise. This

R. Santos-Rocha (✉)
Sport Sciences School of Rio Maior - ESDRM, Polytechnic Institute of Santarém, Rio Maior, Portugal

Laboratory of Biomechanics and Functional Morphology, Interdisciplinary Centre for the Study of Human Performance - CIPER, Faculty of Human Kinetics - FMH, University of Lisbon, Lisbon, Portugal
e-mail: ritasantosrocha@esdrm.ipsantarem.pt

I. Corrales Gutiérrez
Fetal Medicine Unit, Department of Surgery, University Hospital Virgen Macarena, University of Seville, Seville, Spain
e-mail: icorrales@us.es

A. Szumilewicz
Gdansk University of Physical Education and Sport, Gdańsk, Poland
e-mail: anna.szumilewicz@awf.gda.pl

S. Pajaujiene
Lithuanian Sports University, Kaunas, Lithuania
e-mail: simona.pajaujiene@lsu.lt

R. Santos-Rocha (ed.), *Exercise and Physical Activity During Pregnancy and Postpartum*, https://doi.org/10.1007/978-3-031-06137-0_8

chapter reviews the guidelines for exercise testing and prescription of pregnant women to be developed by exercise professionals, following the health screening and medical clearance for exercise by healthcare providers.

Keywords

Pregnancy · Physical activity · Exercise · Health screening · Pre-exercise evaluation · Exercise testing · Exercise prescription · Safety

8.1 Introduction

The purpose of this chapter is to provide exercise and healthcare professionals an understanding about the planning of the several steps of health screening, pre-exercise evaluation, exercise testing, and exercise prescription during pregnancy.

Exercise prescription commonly refers to the specific plan of fitness-related activities that are designed for a specified purpose, which is often developed by a fitness or physiotherapy specialist for the client or patient [1]. An exercise training program ideally is designed to meet individual health and physical fitness goals [2] independently of the fact that the client in the group of the apparently healthy adult population, in a special stage of life (such as pregnancy) or has a determined clinical condition. An optimal exercise prescription should address the health-related physical fitness components, and also the neuromotor fitness[1] [2] in order to provide effective and safe training.

Physical fitness is defined as a set of attributes or characteristics individuals have or achieve that relates to their ability to perform physical activity, and these characteristics are usually separated into the health-related and skill-related components of physical fitness [3]. According to the ACSM [2], the *health-related* physical fitness components include the cardiorespiratory endurance, the body composition, the muscular strength and endurance, and the flexibility, while the *skill-related* components of physical fitness include agility, coordination, balance, power, reaction time, and speed. According to the USDHHS [4], the components of physical fitness include: cardiorespiratory fitness,[2] musculoskeletal fitness,[3] flexibility,[4] balance,[5] and speed.[6]

Appropriate exercise testing and prescription are needed to tailor effective and safe exercise programs. This Chapter reviews the guidelines and scientific papers for exercise testing and prescription of pregnant women to be developed by exercise

[1] *Neuromotor exercise* training involves motor skills such as balance, coordination, gait, and agility, and proprioceptive training and is sometimes called *functional fitness* training [2].

[2] *Cardiorespiratory fitness* is the ability to perform large-muscle, whole-body exercise at moderate-to-vigorous intensities for extended periods of time [4].

[3] *Musculoskeletal fitness* is the integrated function of muscle strength, muscle endurance, and muscle power to enable performance of work [4].

[4] *Flexibility* is the range of motion available at a joint or group of joints [4].

[5] *Balance* is the ability to maintain equilibrium while moving or while stationary [4].

[6] *Speed* is the ability to move the body quickly [4].

professionals, following the health screening and medical clearance for exercise by healthcare providers.

8.1.1 Previous Considerations Before Start Exercising

Being a special stage of life, pregnancy includes several phases that have specific needs and, although there are recommendations and guidelines for the exercise prescription during pregnancy, these should always be adapted to each case, and common sense should prevail. It should also be noted that pregnancy is a natural process, although complex, and occurs differently from woman to woman, and even among the potential pregnancies of the same woman. That is, every pregnancy is a unique and special case! Thus, when a pregnant woman intends to become involved in an exercise program or to give continuity to it, it becomes essential to distinguish between two situations in the first place:

- Pregnancy occurs normally, without problems or clinical complications
- Pregnancy is at risk or there is a certain clinical condition.

One frequent question is: When should a pregnant woman start exercising? The answer is that in the absence of clinical contraindications, every pregnant woman should start or continuing exercising. This statement is issued in all official documents supporting physical activity during pregnancy, as reviewed in the previous Chapter by Szumilewicz et al. [5]. Healthcare providers (i.e., gynecologists, general practitioners or midwives) are in charge of assessing women' health and their pregnancies, and answer the question, bearing in mind the benefits of an active lifestyle for all populations [4, 6]. According to Artal [7], pregnant women tend to be highly motivated to improve unhealthy behaviors and have frequent visits with their healthcare providers, which facilitates counseling, support, and supervision. Unfortunately, despite the increasing evidence on the important benefits of exercising during pregnancy [8], many women remain inactive, or significantly reduce their exercise participation during pregnancy [9, 10]. The probability of a woman exercising during pregnancy is increased if her gynecologist/obstetrician encourages her to exercise [11]. Thus, after making sure that there are no contraindications for exercising, healthcare providers should provide counseling on an active lifestyle and refer pregnant women to an exercise professional (e.g., exercise physiologist, exercise specialist, coach) with background and experience on pregnancy and postnatal exercise. In line with The Royal Australian and New Zealand College of Obstetricians and Gynaecologists (RANZCOG) [12] "Exercise prescription for the pregnant woman requires appropriate consideration of the frequency, intensity, duration and mode of exercise," thus, the National Health Service of the U.K. (NHS) [13] advises to pregnant women to "… make sure your teacher is properly qualified and knows that you're pregnant, as well as how many weeks pregnant you are."

The pregnancy exercise specialist role is to build exercise participation for beginners and already active women at all stages of pregnancy. In addition, this exercise professional will be expected to assess overall physical fitness, to develop proper exercise programs, to review participants' progress and to be able to report on adherence and outcomes to relevant stakeholders [14]. Thus, following medical clearance for exercising during pregnancy, it is very important to understand the motivations, facilitators, and barriers for exercising, as discussed by Atkinson et al. [15], and the type of exercise on which she is interested in, as well as the level of experience she has.

In summary, there are three types of pregnant women in terms of practicing exercise:

- Those who didn't practice any kind of exercise or physical activity prior to pregnancy: In them, we would advise to start with a light physical activity or exercise program.
- Those who did perform exercise regularly: In them, we would advise to maintain this regularity and control intensity and safety.
- Those who are athletes: In them, we would advise to continue with their training routine, possibly with some adaptations regarding exercise selection and safety.

On the other hand, a woman with any risk pregnancy or obstetric or clinical complications, with contraindications to exercise, is out of the scope of practice of the exercise professional, unless with medical supervision, prescription, and guidance. Nevertheless, a specific exercise program may be beneficial as an adjunct therapy or primary prevention of determined conditions [2]. The ACSM recommends that a pregnant woman that is severely obese or have gestational diabetes mellitus or hypertension should consult her physician before beginning an exercise program, and the exercise program must be adjusted to her medical condition, symptoms, and fitness level [2]. Moreover, as explained in Chap. 7 [5], the list of contraindications to prenatal physical activity have been substantially modified in the Canadian [16], RANZCOG [12], and the Australian Government—Department of Health (AGDH) [17] guidelines based on scientific evidence, and they are far from completely limiting physical activity in the event of these contraindications. For those women with pregnancy complications, the promotion of exercise may still be appropriate under some circumstances with appropriate medical evaluation and suitable modification of the exercise prescription [12]. According to the Canadian guidelines "women with absolute contraindications may continue their usual activities of daily living but should not participate in more strenuous activities. Women with relative contraindications should discuss the advantages and disadvantages of moderate-to-vigorous intensity physical activity with their obstetric care provider prior to participation" [16].

8.1.2 Contraindications for Exercising While Pregnant

Summarizing, pregnant women who performed exercise or physical activity regularly before pregnancy may continue with it, and previously sedentary women may start exercising during pregnancy [4–6, 12, 13, 16–22]. However, although this practice is safe and recommendable for them, in certain situations, it should be inadvisable, or, in accordance with recent guidelines by the American College of Obstetricians and Gynecologists (ACOG) [18], in case of obstetric or medical comorbidities, exercise regimens should be individualized. In fact, in 2020, the list of absolute or relative contraindications to exercise in pregnancy were removed from the ACOG guidelines. Instead, they recommend consultation with a specialist (i.e., obstetrics and gynecology, maternal-fetal medicine, cardiology, pulmonology) when questions regarding exercise safety exist [18].

Anyway, there are medical circumstances in which the sudden appearance of complications due to their pregnancy or a bad maternal health status contraindicates the practice in an absolute or in a relative way. The absolute or relative contraindications for exercising during pregnancy, as well as the signs and symptoms to stop exercise, issued in the recent guidelines [5] are summarized in Box 8.1. The appearance of any of these relative contraindications, may lead to stop performing the physical activity in order to avoid future complications and risks.

Once established these limitations under the supervision of the healthcare provider, it is of utmost importance to interact with the exercise physiologist or coach that will adapt the exercise program.

Box 8.1 Relative and Absolute Contraindications for Exercising During Pregnancy, According to Recently Published Guidelines (2017–2021)

Organization	Guidelines
Sport Medicine Australia [19]	**Signs and symptoms to cease exercise**: abdominal pain, any "gush" of fluid from the vagina, calf pain or swelling, chest pain, decreased fetal movement, dizziness or presyncope, dyspnea before exertion, excessive fatigue, headache, pelvic pain, excessive shortness of breath, painful uterine contractions, and vaginal bleeding.
Australian Government—Department of health [17]	**Pregnancy complications:** If you have any of the following you are advised not to exercise until you get individual advice from your health professional: incompetent cervix, ruptured membranes, preterm labor, persistent bleeding in the second or third trimester, placenta previa, pre-eclampsia, evidence of intrauterine growth restriction, multiple gestation (triplets or higher), poorly controlled type 1 diabetes, hypertension or thyroid disease, other serious cardiovascular, respiratory or systemic disorders.
The Royal Australian and New Zealand College of Obstetricians and Gynaecologists [12]	**Warning signs to stop exercise and seek medical attention**: chest pain, unexplained shortness of breath, dizziness, feeling faint or headache, muscle weakness, calf pain, swelling or redness, sudden swelling of the ankles, hands or face, vaginal bleeding or amniotic fluid loss, decreased fetal movement, uterine contractions or pain in the lower back, pelvic area or abdomen (potentially indicating pre-term labor).

(continued)

Organization	Guidelines
2019 Canadian guideline for physical activity throughout pregnancy [16]	**Absolute contraindications to exercise**: ruptured membranes, premature labor, unexplained persistent vaginal bleeding, placenta previa after 28 weeks' gestation, pre-eclampsia, incompetent cervix, intrauterine growth restriction, high-order multiple pregnancy (e.g., triplets), uncontrolled type I diabetes, uncontrolled hypertension, uncontrolled thyroid disease, other serious cardiovascular, respiratory or systemic disorder.
	Relative contraindications to exercise: recurrent pregnancy loss, gestational hypertension, a history of spontaneous preterm birth, mild/moderate cardiovascular or respiratory disease, symptomatic anemia, malnutrition, eating disorder, twin pregnancy after the 28th week, other significant medical conditions.
	Reasons to stop physical activity and consult a healthcare provider: persistent excessive shortness of breath that does not resolve on rest, severe chest pain, regular and painful uterine contractions, vaginal bleeding, persistent loss of fluid from the vagina indicating rupture of the membranes, persistent dizziness or faintness that does not resolve on rest.
American College of Obstetricians and Gynecologists [18]	**Reasons to stop physical activity and consult a healthcare provider**: persistent excessive shortness of breath that does not resolve on rest, severe chest pain, regular and painful uterine contractions, vaginal bleeding, persistent loss of fluid from the vagina indicating rupture of the membranes, persistent dizziness or faintness that does not resolve on rest.
American College of Sport Medicine [2]	**Stop physical activity and consult a medical professional if any of the following occur**: persistent excessive shortness of breath that doesn't resolve with rest, severe chest pain, regular and painful uterine contractions, vaginal bleeding, persistent loss of fluid from the vagina, persistent dizziness or faintness that doesn't resolve with rest.
Exercise is Medicine by ACSM [22]	**Reasons to stop physical activity and seek medical advice**: bleeding or fluid coming from your vagina, chest pain, dizziness or faintness that does not go away with rest, shortness of breath that does not go away with rest, regular painful uterine contractions, calf pain or swelling.

Organization	Guidelines
International Olympic Committee [20]	**Conditions that post a high risk to the fetus and in which aerobic exercise is absolutely contraindicated**: hemodynamically significant heart disease, intrauterine growth restriction in current pregnancy, poorly controlled hypertension, restrictive lung disease, cervical insufficiency/cerclage, multiple gestation at risk of premature labor, persistent second or third trimester bleeding, placenta previa after 26 weeks gestation, premature labor during the current pregnancy, ruptured membranes, pre-eclampsia/pregnancy-induced hypertension, severe anemia.
	Conditions that post a moderate risk to the fetus and in which aerobic exercise is relatively contraindicated: history of fetal growth restriction, miscarriage, premature birth or labor; cervical enlargement, unevaluated maternal cardiac arrhythmia, chronic bronchitis or other respiratory disorders, poorly controlled type I diabetes, extreme underweight, orthopedic limitations, poorly controlled seizure disorder.
World Health Organization [6]	Pregnant women should be informed by their health-care provider of the danger signs alerting them as to when to stop; or to limit physical activity and consult a qualified health-care provider immediately should they occur.

After medical clearance, pregnant women can begin or continue an exercise program, preferably, supervised by a qualified exercise professional. However, both participants and exercise professionals should be familiarized themselves with the absolute and relative contraindications to exercise during pregnancy, as well as with the signs and symptoms to terminate exercise.

8.2 Guidelines on Exercise During Pregnancy and Useful Sources of Information

When promoting physical activity and exercise during pregnancy, and developing exercise prescription plans, either health professionals or exercise professionals are supposed to follow specific guidelines for physical activity and exercise during pregnancy. These guidelines may be published by national or international organizations. The main international organizations supporting and publishing guidelines for physical activity and exercise during pregnancy are listed in Box 8.2.

Box 8.2 International Organizations Supporting and Publishing Guidelines for Physical Activity and Exercise During Pregnancy

ACOG—American Congress of Obstetricians and Gynecologists—https://www.acog.org/

ACSM—American College of Sports Medicine—http://www.acsm.org/ (http://www.acsm.org/public-information/roundtables)

AGDH—Australian Government. Department of Health—https://www.health.gov.au/

APA—American Pregnancy Association—http://americanpregnancy.org/ (http://americanpregnancy.org/pregnancy-health/exercise-guidelines/)

CSEP—Canadian Society Exercise Physiology—http://www.csep.ca/home (http://www.csep.ca/view.asp?ccid=519)

Department of Health—UK Government—https://www.gov.uk/ (https://www.gov.uk/government/publications)

ESSA—Exercise and Sports Science Australia—https://www.essa.org.au

EuropeActive—http://www.europeactive.eu (http://www.ehfa-standards.eu/es-standards)

IOC—International Olympic Committee—https://www.olympic.org/ (https://www.olympic.org/news/ioc-drives-discussions-on-pregnancy-and-elite-athletes)

Promotion Santé Suisse—https://promotionsante.ch/ (German, French, Italian)

RCOG—Royal College of Obstetricians and Gynaecologists—https://www.rcog.org.uk/

SASMA—South African Sports Medicine Association—https://www.sasma.org.za/

SMA—Sports Medicine Australia—http://sma.org.au/ (http://sma.org.au/publications-media/sma-position-statements/)

SOGC—Society of Obstetricians and Gynaecologists of Canada—https://sogc.org/

US-DHHS—U.S. Department of Health and Human Services—https://www.hrsa.gov/

WHO—World Health Organization—http://www.who.int/about/en/ (http://www.who.int/nutrition/publications/guidelines/antenatalcare-pregnancy-positive-experience/en/)

The American College of Obstetricians and Gynecologists was the organization that published in 1985, the first guidelines for pregnant and postpartum women [23], subsequently improved in 1994 [24]. In 2002, the ACOG published recommendations for physical exercise during pregnancy, promoting its benefits to the health and safety of exercise, both for active and inactive women prior to pregnancy, assuming the existence of medical authorization and the absence of contraindications [25]. These ACOG recommendations from 2002, stated that pregnant women should accumulate 30 min or more of moderate-intensity exercise on most, if not all, days of the week if no medical or obstetric complications are present, i.e., a minimum of three exercise sessions of at least 15 min each, gradually increasing to 30 min per day, preferably on all days of the week [25]. The recommendations were highlighted again in 2009, including the practice of 30 min or more of moderate exercise, mostly, if not every day of the week, in the absence of medical or obstetrical complications. According to the review paper on the available guidelines for exercising during pregnancy provided by Evenson et al. in 2013 [26], nine out of ten guidelines on exercise in pregnancy from different countries contained information on the intensity and duration of exercise, and eight of these documents contained recommendations on the exercise frequency. Evenson et al. [26], state that the program should consist of moderate-intensity exercise (including moderate-intensity aerobic exercise, light-intensity resistance training, Pilates and balance exercises, pelvic-floor training and stretching), performed three times per week, under the supervision of an exercise specialist. In a previous review by Szumilewicz et al. [27] we analyzed existing guidelines at that time. In 2015, we verify that the documents analyzed contain very general recommendations on exercise during pregnancy and little information that exercise professionals could use when programming the contents of targeted exercise classes for pregnant women.

In December 2015, the ACOG republished its recommendations on "Physical Activity and Exercise during Pregnancy and in the Postpartum Period" [28]. To be noted that this was the first document stating officially that moderate exercise during pregnancy does not cause miscarriage, fetal growth restriction, premature delivery, or musculoskeletal injury. Between 2016 and 2018, Bø et al. and the Medical and Scientific Commission of the International Olympic Committee (IOC) drove a discussion about the management of pregnancy for an elite athlete and produced comprehensive guidelines and recommendations on exercise during pregnancy and postpartum [20, 29–31], as well as for future research [32].

More recently, namely since 2018, these above-mentioned organizations published for the first time (i.e., WHO [6], ADGH [17], ACSM/EIM [21, 22], NHS [13]), endorsed (i.e., ACSM [2] endorsed ACOG, SOGC/CSEP, and USDHHS) or updated (i.e., ACOG [18], USDHHS [4], RANZCOG [12], SMA [19], SOGC/CSEP [16]) specific recommendations on physical activity during pregnancy. To be noted that the World Health Organization published for first time in 2020, specific international recommendations on physical activity for pregnant and postpartum women, as well as on the need to reduce sedentary behaviors. A general overview, further discussion, and update of the recent guidelines are provided in another Chapter of the present publication, by Szumilewicz et al. [5].

8.3 Health Screening of Pregnant Women Before Starting Exercise

The first step before planning to start or continuing an exercise program during pregnancy is the health screening of the woman by a healthcare provider, i.e., overall health and medical and obstetric risks should be reviewed [2, 4, 7, 12, 16, 18, 20].

The American College of Obstetricians and Gynecologists' Antepartum Records and Postpartum form [33] can assist healthcare providers in health screening.

To establish a prenatal fitness class for pregnant women, we have to know if she is going to be capable of following it in terms of prenatal fitness and health, intensity, type of pregnancy and exercise. In a normal healthy pregnancy, no study has found any negative effect of moderate-intensity aerobic training on the development of the fetus or the outcome of pregnancy. In fact, it appears that the benefits of exercise during pregnancy clearly outweigh the potential risks. Current research suggests that healthy pregnant women can begin or maintain moderate intensity aerobic exercise programs with little fear of adverse effects on their unborn fetus [34]. Moreover, recent systematic reviews show strong evidence on the effectiveness of (moderate intensity) physical activity on maternal cardiorespiratory fitness [35–37], reduced risk of excessive gestational weight gain [8, 37], reduced risk of gestational hypertensive disorders overall and gestational hypertension [8, 37, 38], prevention and treatment of gestational diabetes mellitus [8, 37–40], prevention of urinary incontinence [36], reduced cesarean delivery [38], and prevention of antenatal [41] and post-birth [8, 42] depression, as well as positive impact on offspring health in adulthood [37, 43]. The maternal-fetal physiological reserve is going to be the limiting factor for prescribing a safe prenatal exercise program, thus, before performing the fitness activities, there is the need to evaluate pregnant women with a convenient checklist. In this regard, after medical clearance regarding a regular healthcare protocol, healthcare providers should encourage pregnant women to start or continue with a fitness program suitable for their needs and gestational status.

Other important role of the healthcare providers is to promote the benefits of physical activity and exercise during pregnancy. Pregnant women should be educated on these benefits, and be aware of the normal symptoms, physiological and biomechanical adaptations related to pregnancy [6, 12, 19, 44]. They should be educated on the existence and contents of the documents referred as "guidelines," some of them, designed and produced in plain language in order to be more attractive for them (e.g., SMA [19], AGDH [17], EIM [22]), and also including videos (e.g., NHS [13]).

A convenient and worldwide used checklist is the Physical Activity Readiness Medical Examination (PARmed-X) for Pregnancy, which aims to facilitate the communication between the healthcare provider, the fitness professional, and the pregnant woman [45]. The PARmed-X for Pregnancy questionnaire was recently replaced by the Get Active Questionnaire for Pregnancy. This questionnaire is available from CSEP website (https://csep.ca/2021/01/20/pre-screening-for-physical-activity/) in the English and French languages, and it can also be found in the literature, its translations to other languages are required to fill in the four-page form:

1. Pregnant women should provide all the information about their general health status, their status of current pregnancy, and provide the information about the daily activity habits during the past month.
2. The healthcare provider must remark the absolute and relative contraindications based on the current medical information provided by the pregnant women.

3. Once the health evaluation form has been signed by the healthcare provider, and in the absence of contraindications, pregnant women should give it to their prenatal fitness professional.

If necessary, the Get Active Questionnaire for Pregnancy may be used together with other preliminary screening tools, such as the latest version of the Physical Activity Readiness Questionnaire for Everyone (PAR-Q+) available at the official website [46] (http://eparmedx.com/) and in the main ACSM's publications [2, 47]. This questionnaire helps on the decision of whether it is necessary to seek further advice before becoming more physically active or engaging in a fitness appraisal, and can be fulfilled by a doctor, another healthcare practitioner, or a qualified exercise professional. Another widely used tool is the ACSM Health Status & Health History Questionnaire [48] to assess safety or possible contraindications to exercise. According to ACSM, these tools can be used in the two basic approaches to preparticipation physical activity screening: the self-guided screening and the professionally supervised screening [2, 47]. In addition, ACSM provides the Exercise Preparticipation Health Screening Questionnaire for Exercise Professionals, which is a simple tool asking for symptoms, current activity, and medical conditions of the participants [49].

To be noted that health screening is of particular importance when these pregnant women are obese, have gestational diabetes mellitus, or hypertension. These women should consult the healthcare provider before beginning an exercise program, which, in turn, must be adjusted to her medical condition, symptoms, and physical fitness level [2].

8.4 Pre-exercise Evaluation with Pregnant Exercisers and Athletes

Following the medical clearance provided by the healthcare provider, the exercise professional develops the pre-exercise evaluation of the pregnant women. It is important to understand some personal factors regarding her health and fitness level that will affect the exercise program plan, namely the intensity, the complexity, and the adaptation of exercises. The fact that pregnant women are either sedentary or experienced in some exercise modes, will affect the exercise prescription significantly. Thus, the second step is to know her pattern, level, and experience with physical activity and exercise:

- For those who were sedentary prior to pregnancy, we need to plan a simpler exercise program, regarding the intensity (light) and complexity (low) of the exercises.
- For those who were active and perform exercise regularly, we need to plan an exercise program in order to maintain the intensity and complexity of the exercises she is motivated to do, or evaluate other options, regarding the safety of the program.
- For those who are athletes, we also need to plan an exercise program in order to maintain the intensity and complexity of the exercises she is motivated to do, to maintain her sports level as much as possible or evaluate other options, regarding the safety of the program for her to continue with the training routine, possibly with some adaptations regarding exercise selection.

An objective form of better understanding the physical activity pattern and/or volume is using basic equipment, such as pedometers or accelerometers. The advantages of using accelerometers compared to other techniques of gait analysis include: low-cost methods; testing is not restricted to a laboratory environment; accelerometers are small, and not restricting walking [50]. The use of wearable body sensors for measuring physical activity is quite useful and a growing field in health monitoring and sport assessment. From free mobile applications to expensive and extensive sports monitoring, plenty of wearables can be found nowadays. The conclusions from recent systematic reviews pointed that several healthcare interventions using feedback on objectively monitored physical activity had a moderately positive effect on levels of physical activity [51], and that the use of wearable trackers in healthy adults may be associated with modest short-term increases in physical activity [52].

Questionnaires such as the 7-day Physical Activity Recall interview (7-day PAR) [53, 54] (available from Professor James F. Sallis website: http://sallis.ucsd.edu/measures.html), and the Pregnancy Physical Activity Questionnaire (PPAQ) developed by Chasan-Taber et al. in 2004 [55], can also be used to recall physical activity pattern and volume. The PPAQ is a self-administered questionnaire regarding the current trimester of pregnancy. It assesses sedentary, light, moderate, and vigorous activity regarding household/caregiving, occupational, and sports/exercise activities. Pregnant women are asked to select the category that best approximates the amount of time spent in 32 activities and in inactivity during the current trimester. At the end of the questionnaire, an open-ended section allows the respondent to add activities not already listed.

Other questions regarding maternal health and pregnancy itself that will affect exercise prescription includes the following:

- What is woman's age?
- Is it the first pregnancy?
- On which stage of pregnancy is she?
- How were previous pregnancies?
- How is her self-perception of health?
- Is she aware of relative and absolute contraindications for exercising?
- Which are the main sign and symptoms related to pregnancy she is experiencing?
- What are her occupation and other leisure activities?
- When to start exercise during pregnancy?

In brief, age may be related to fatigue, as well as her perception of health, and the existence of any disability or discomfort when performing the exercises. The type of occupation, regarding stress and physical activity, and other leisure activities will influence the global level of physical activity. A first pregnancy will promote physiological and psychological changes that she is experiencing for the first time. If it is the second or third pregnancy, the tendency will be to compare it with the previous ones (which may not have any comparison!). It means that, in practice, we must not assume that different pregnancies in the same client will progress in the same way. The stage of pregnancy is of particular importance regarding exercise selection and adaptation, as well the main body adaptations and the signs and symptoms that can be more common and prevalent at each stage.

Regarding signs and symptoms related to pregnancy, exercise professionals and healthcare providers may objectively monitor them using a validated inventory available from Foxcroft et al. [56]. The authors developed a comprehensive inventory of pregnancy-related symptoms, with a mechanism for assessing their effect on function, providing a validated tool for assessing the impact of interventions in pregnancy [56]. Exercise professionals must be aware of the possible relative and absolute contraindications for exercising, as well as the signs for stopping exercise, as above-mentioned, in order to refer the client for a healthcare provider, as necessary.

Previous sedentary women can begin light activity anytime and progressively increase it. Previous active women can continue the exercise routine. Sometimes, the normal pregnancy-related symptoms, such as low back pain, tiredness or nauseousness, may interfere with the adoption of an active lifestyle, but pregnant women should start exercising anytime they feel comfortable.

Other important questions, regarding the exercise prescription plan, as well as establishing realistic objectives and promoting adherence to exercise are the following:

- What are the main motivations for exercising during pregnancy?
- Which are the women's preferences regarding exercise?
- What can be the main barriers and facilitators?

- Which strategies should but put in practice regarding adherence to exercise?

Assessing motivations and preferences of pregnant women, as well as identifying barriers and facilitators towards exercise is a very important stage in the prescription process to avoid failure and behavioral relapse. More development on these topics can be found in Chap. 2 by Atkinson et al. [15]. Finally, it is important to explain to a pregnant woman that physical activity and exercise, if tailored to her health and fitness level, will not bring any harmful effects neither for her nor for the baby. On the contrary, the participation in an exercise program may increase her perception of health [57], and there are several trustable sources of information from where she can learn about the general and specific benefits of exercise during pregnancy. For example, an interesting source of information is the infographic with new advice on "physical activity for pregnant women" published by the UK's chief medical officers (CMOs), aiming at providing health and exercise professionals, with the latest evidence on physical activity during pregnancy [58, 59].

In summary, addressing a pregnant woman at the beginning of an exercise program and developing a pre-exercise evaluation process is a key element to plan a tailored exercise prescription for an effective and safe exercise program. Exercise professionals must bear in mind that some of the above-described questions may be openly placed (or can be included in validated questionnaires) not only at the beginning of the exercise program, but whenever there is an alteration or adaptation regarding her health or fitness status. Furthermore, it is important to understand the normal process of pregnancy [60], as well as the psychological [15], physiological [61, 62], musculoskeletal [63, 64], and biomechanical [65] adaptations occurring during this period of life.

8.5 Exercise Testing with Pregnant Women

Although not harmful, and unless the pregnant woman desires and requires it, extensive exercise testing during pregnancy should only be performed for medical reasons or for research purposes [2]. An extensive assessment protocol will take a long time and maybe bore or without significance for a (monthly) changing body and mind. Unless the testing is useful for motivation and education purposes, as well as requested by the pregnant participant or athlete in order to evaluate aerobic fitness, or other fitness components. On the other hand, the assessment of cardiovascular fitness is important in pregnant women because it is linked to increased risk of cardiac disease but is rarely undertaken or studied [66]. However, cardiopulmonary exercise testing during pregnancy is valuable in identifying underlying cardiopulmonary conditions, stratifying the risk of adverse pregnancy outcomes, as well as establishing exercise tolerance/limitations [67]. Special care should be taken to ensure that the pregnant woman feels comfortable and there are no risk of falls or injuries.

In practice, there are several maximal and submaximal tests to evaluate the health-related physical fitness components (cardiorespiratory endurance, body composition, muscular strength and endurance, and flexibility), as well as the skill-related components of physical fitness (agility, coordination, balance, power, reaction time, and speed) [2]. Most tests were built for the apparently healthy adult population, and there are specific tests or adapted tests for the special populations. These tests can be used to objectively understand the effectiveness of an exercise intervention and to know the fitness status of the client. Nevertheless, simple tests could be used for motivation purposes, and to quantify the effects of physical activity and exercise programs for pregnant women.

Regarding ethical and legal considerations, before any exercise testing, adequate informed consent should be obtained from participants. An example of form can be found in ACSM [2] or from the website: https://certification.acsm.org/files/file/B_ExPrescripReferral_pdf.pdf.

However, this form may vary according to the objectives and methods of the exercise testing. The consent form, along with a verbal explanation, should include the following information: (1) purpose (either exercise prescription or research), and explanation on the test (equipment, procedures, etc.); (2) potential participant's risks and discomforts; (3) responsibilities of the participant (e.g., information about health status); (4) benefits to be expected (e.g., diagnosis of illness, fitness evaluation, or exercise progression); (5) inquiries (e.g., any concerns or questions about the test); (6) state the privacy of personal and health information (to be kept confidential); and (7) freedom of consent [2].

A comprehensive fitness testing includes in the first place, the measurements of heart rate[7] (HR) and blood pressure[8] (BP). Usually, in a fitness setting, HR can be determined using pulse palpation (for 30 or 60 s), or a heart rate monitor. Both methods can be used during the exercise session or to assess resting HR. Assessing resting heart rate requires allowing to the participant some time to relax at least 5 min in order to stabilize HR. The same principle applies to resting BP measure-

[7] Measurements in beats per minute (beats/min) or (bpm).

[8] Measurements in mmHg.

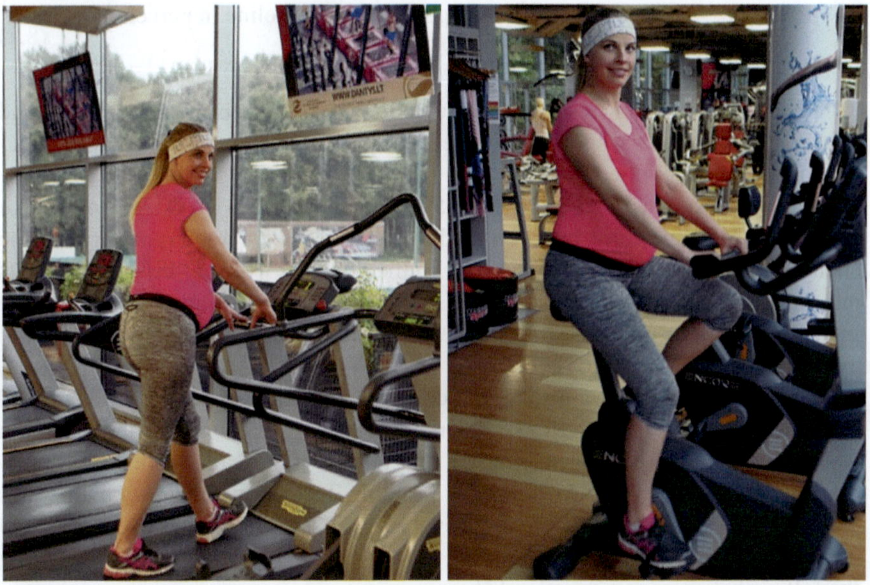

Fig. 8.1 Treadmill walking and upright leg cycling are the most useful testing modalities during pregnancy

ment. Further description of heart rate and blood pressure measurements and procedures can be found in ACSM [2].

Due to the limited amount of data on the use of maximal tests in pregnant women, ACSM [2, 47] does not recommend performing maximal exercise testing on pregnant women for the exercise program design, unless medically necessary, and with medical supervision. Submaximal exercise testing is appropriate and effective for this special population [2] in order to assess the maximum rate of oxygen utilization of muscles during exercise (VO_{2max}). We can find guidance on clinical exercise testing during pregnancy in other publications provided by O'Toole and Artal [68], and Wolfe [69], regarding cycle ergometer or graded treadmill exercise. Jędrzejko et al. [70] assessed a group of pregnant women with a submaximal cardiopulmonary exercise test up to 80% HRmax with a supine cycle ergometer, concluding that it is a safe and precise method for assessing work efficiency in term pregnancy women.

According to Wolfe [69], treadmill walking and upright leg cycling are the most useful testing modalities during pregnancy (Fig. 8.1), since the injury risk is low, the physiologic monitoring is easy (not much vertical movement), and the exercises require basic movements. On the contrary, both treadmill running and bench stepping tests are less convenient in these respects, as well as arm cranking ergometry because a relatively small muscle mass is employed [69].

A peak maximal oxygen consumption[9] predicted equation determined for pregnant women can be found in Mottola et al. [71]. This equation was developed using a treadmill modified Balke protocol:

[9] Measure of highest rate of oxygen consumption during an exercise test regardless of whether or not a VO_2 plateau is reached.

$$\begin{aligned} VO_{2peak} &= (0.055 \times \text{peak HR in bpm}) + (0.381 \times \text{incline in percent}) \\ &+ (5.541 \times \text{speed in mph}) + (-0.090 \times \text{BMI in kg/m}^2) - 6.846 \end{aligned} \tag{8.1}$$

Other recommended treadmill protocols include, e.g., the modified Bruce and the Naughton protocols, because most sedentary pregnant women have low capacity for non-weight-supported exercise [69].

Typically, a submaximal test (i.e., <75% of heart rate reserve) is used in place of a maximal test, and most research studies have selected cycle ergometry, due to changes in posture and center of gravity of the pregnant women [48]. Cycling tests may involve one or more steady-state submaximal power outputs or progressive increases in power output, while the pedaling frequency should be 60–80 rpm to avoid lower limb fatigue [69].

Another option may be a field test consisting of walking for a predetermined time or distance, such as the Rockport One-Mile Fitness Walking Test and the 6-min walk test. They are easy to administer and require little equipment. In the well-recognized Rockport One-Mile Fitness Walking Test the pregnant woman walks 1.6 km (1 mi) as fast as possible on a level surface, and HR is obtained in the final minute of completion of the walk. Then, the VO_{2max} of the woman is estimated using the following regression equation [2]:

$$\begin{aligned} VO_{2max}(\text{mL/kg/min}) &= 132.853 - (0.1692 \times \text{body mass in kg}) \\ &- (0.3877 \times \text{age in years}) \\ &- (3.2649 \times \text{time in min}) \\ &- (0.1565 \times \text{HR in bpm}) \end{aligned} \tag{8.2}$$

The 6-min walk test (6 MWT) has been used with older and clinical populations, and its results have been related to morbidity and mortality. Recently, Tinius et al. [72] have validated the 6-Minute Walk Test during midpregnancy. In this test the pregnant woman is assessed as the most distance she can walk in a 6 min time interval. Then, one of the equations used to estimate the VO_{2max} is the following [2]:

$$\begin{aligned} VO_{2max}(\text{mL/kg/min}) &= (0.02 \times \text{distance in m}) - (0.191 \times \text{age in years}) \\ &- (0.07 \times \text{body mass in kg}) \\ &+ (0.09 \times \text{height in cm}) + (0.26 \times \text{RPP} \times 10^{-3}) + 2.45; \\ &\text{where RPP} = \text{rate} - \text{pressure product:} \\ &\text{HR} \times \text{SBP in mmHg; SEE} = 2.68\ \text{mL/kg/min}. \end{aligned} \tag{8.3}$$

Dennis et al. [66] concluded that the 6 MWT is safe, feasible, and applicable in term pregnant women. Moreover, the authors generated reference intervals for resting HR and distance walked.

Unfortunately, the main publications on the guidelines for exercise during pregnancy (i.e., CSEP [16], ACOG [18], and IOC [20]) do not address submaximal and maximal exercise testing, but further description of these procedures can be found elsewhere [2, 47, 48, 68, 69].

After understanding the most appropriate tests for pregnant women, procedures should be selected according to the facilities and equipment available, the existence of appropriate environment, and the qualifications of the exercise professional performing the tests [48]. The exercise professional must ensure the proper conditions of the facility and thermal environment where the testing takes place, and must be aware of the proper conditions of the testing equipment, the full testing protocol (e.g., regarding the duration and the work rate of each stage, the monitoring of HR at least two times during each stage, the use of additional effort rating scales, etc.), as well as the subject appearance and symptoms, and the test termination criteria. All exercise test protocols should incorporate a 3–5 min low-intensity warm-up to acquaint the pregnant woman with the equipment, as well as a gradual cool-down to avoid venous pooling of maternal blood, arterial hypotension, and reduced uterine blood flow [2, 69]. Moreover, Wolfe [69] recommended that the total length of a progressive treadmill or cycling exercise test should not exceed 10–12 min in order to minimize the potential reduction of uterine blood flow. However, there is no scientific evidence to date to support this risk.

According to Szumilewicz et al. [73] there is some evidence that in the laboratory settings pregnant women may undergo progressive maximal exercise test and that they tolerate it well. However, due to the acute physiologic responses normally observed during pregnancy (which are increased during pregnancy compared to non-pregnancy) [74], submaximal protocols might be more useful in exercise professionals' practice in determining the effects of training rather than accurately estimating maximal aerobic power [2]. Other interesting and useful utilization of this data is to establish intensity and metabolic calculations to determine calorie expenditure.

There are no specific tests for proper assessment of musculoskeletal function—muscular strength and resistance, and flexibility—although these components of health-related physical fitness are addressed in the recommended guidelines for exercise during pregnancy. The same situation occurs regarding the skill-related fitness components, namely, agility, coordination, and balance. Nevertheless, the main purpose of a prenatal exercise program is to promote maternal-fetal health, rather than to maximize physical performance [69]. Nevertheless, fitness testing protocols might be useful in determining the effects of training, and to increase motivation.

To our knowledge, it is no established literature, for the safety and validity of maximal muscle strength assessment for pregnant women. In addition, commonly used tests for the strength evaluation of the upper and lower body, or abdominal muscles, such as the bench press, leg press, curl-ups and the push-ups tests, are not practically justified in this stage of life due to anatomical and musculoskeletal changes. Isometric and isotonic strength involves a pressure response, which is undesirable during pregnancy [69]. Further explanation of the musculoskeletal health adaptations during pregnancy can be found in Fitzgerald and Segal [64].

A good option may be static handgrip strength test. The static handgrip strength test is measured with a dynamometer and has been predicted mortality and functional status in older populations [2, 47]. After adjusting the grip, the participant holds the dynamometer in line with the forearm at the level of the thigh, away from the body, without touching the body or any other object. Then, the participant squeezes the handgrip as hard as possible, twice with each hand. The score is the highest of two readings with each hand (e.g., 58–62 would be a good score for women of 20–39 years). Other option is the modified push-up test which measures upper body strength and endurance (Fig. 8.2). A modified push-up begins with the hands touching the floor or an object (e.g., a step bench), the knees resting on the

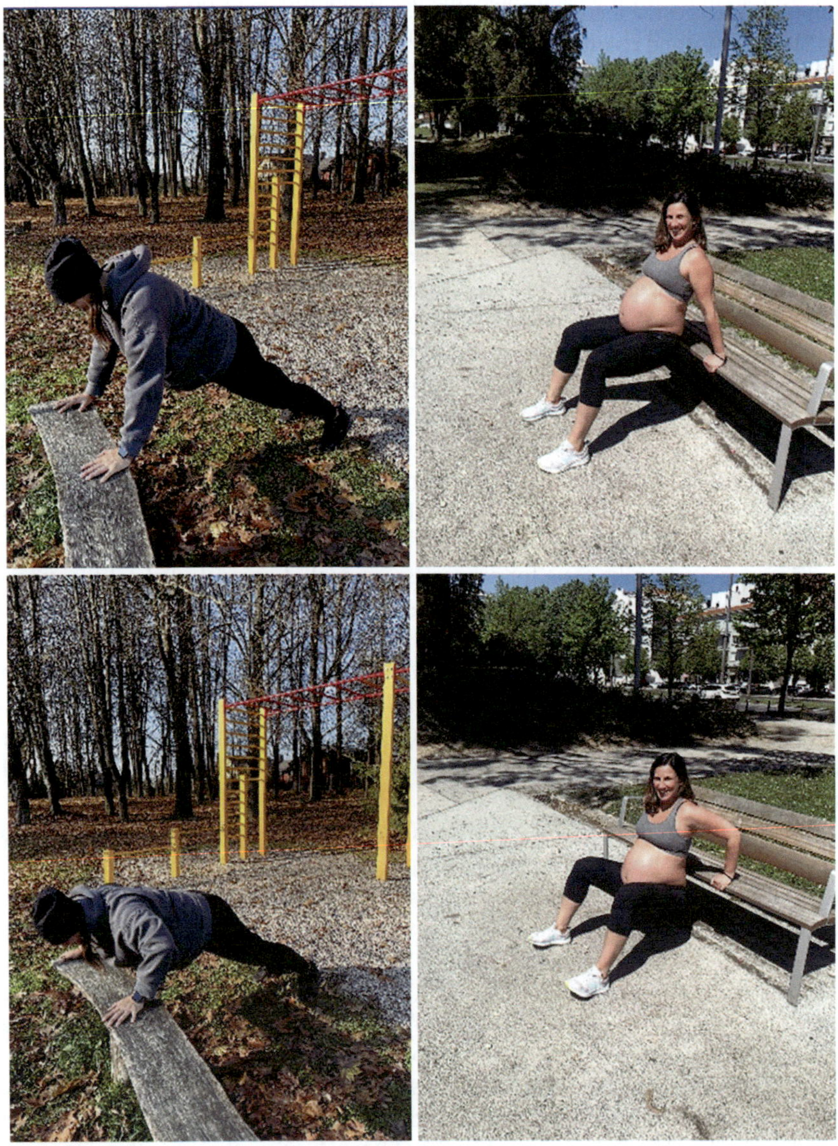

Fig. 8.2 The modified push-up test (left) and the reverse push up test (right)

ground, and the back straight. The flexion and extension of the arms is performed to the point of 90-degree flexion, during 1 or 2 min. The score corresponds to the maximal push-ups performed in this time interval. Further explanation of the procedures and fitness categories can be found in ACSM [2, 47].

Regarding flexibility, test procedures and fitness categories are also provided in ACSM [2]. Test procedures for goniometry assessment of joints commonly of concern to health and fitness professionals, and static stretches for the major muscle groups are provided in ACSM [47]. The range of motion of selected single-joint movements is provided in ACSM [2]. However, the value of specific flexibility tests during pregnancy is questionable because flexibility is temporarily altered, and because the anatomic changes will interfere mechanically with some common tests (e.g., sit-and-reach) [68]. Thus, no single test can characterize flexibility and there are no specific tests to be used during pregnancy. Due to anatomical changes, a good option may be the (modified) sit-and-reach test which is a reflection of hamstring, hip and lower back flexibility, which in turn, is important to prevent low back pain [48] (Fig. 8.3). However, specific procedures and norms regarding pregnant women are lacking [47]. The Back Scratch Test measures how close the hands can be brought together behind the back. It was designed to test the functional fitness of seniors [75], but could be a good option for pregnant woman.

Physical performance testing protocols that have been used for the assessment of functional status and fitness components of senior populations [75, 76], might be useful and safe for pregnant women, although there are no reference data to

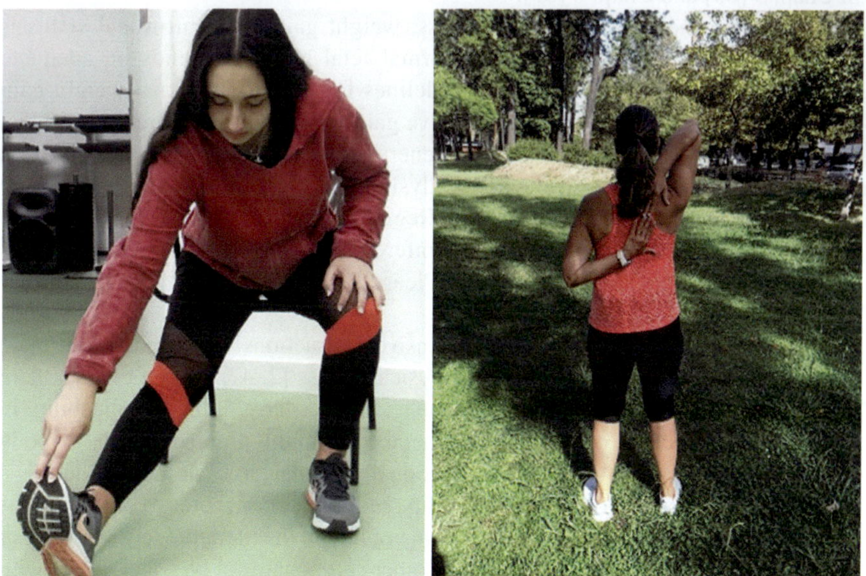

Fig. 8.3 The modified sit-and-reach test (left) and the back scratch test (right)

accurately interpret the results. Postural analysis and body alignment are also very important to be assessed in pregnant women. Physical performance testing is appealing since most performance tests require little space, equipment, and cost; can be administered by lay or health/fitness personnel with minimal training; and are considered extremely safe in healthy and clinical populations [2]. However, to our knowledge, there are no testing batteries validated for the pregnant population, regarding the static and dynamic assessment of posture, functionality, and overall autonomy in pregnant women. Chapter 6 in ACSM [47] provides a comprehensive functional movement assessment for apparently healthy participants.

One option is the Timed Up and Go (TUG) test which is a simple test used to assess a person's mobility and requires both static and dynamic balance [75]. The TUG is a commonly used screening tool to identify patients at risk of falling, sometimes used along with other outcome measures to assess functional mobility or balance. In this test, the time that a person takes to rise from a chair, walk 3 m, turn around, walk back to the chair, and sit down is recorded. Usually applied to older populations, it has been used with pregnant women.

Static changes to the body in pregnancy include anterior displacement of the center of mass, anterior tilt of the pelvis, increased lumbar lordosis, knee hyperextension, and increased length and width of the feet. Angular kinematics and spatiotemporal parameters of gait will suffer changes as well, due to increase body mass and musculoskeletal adaptations [62]. Gait alterations during pregnancy may contribute to pain, falls, and muscle fatigue. Thus, gait assessment may be useful to diagnose and prevent such situations. Further development on this topic is provided in Chap. 5 [65] and Chap. 6 [63].

Monitoring the maternal body fatness, weight gain, and nutritional status is very important. On the one hand, a normal fetal growth depends on adequate maternal energy stores and specific guidelines for optimal maternal weight gain are available. On the other hand, excessive gains in body fatness are undesirable. The exercise professional can provide general advice regarding healthy nutrition during pregnancy. However, dietary analysis and tailored nutrition plans should be conducted by a qualified nutritionist. Regarding the assessment of the pregnant women's body composition, body circumferences, body fat distribution markers and other body indexes can be used. Please refer to Chap. 4 [62] for further explanation.

Other publications provide comprehensive instructions for fitness assessment regarding the different components of physical fitness [2, 47, 48]. Of course, there are other assessment techniques, but those techniques have limited applicability in fitness settings because of the cost and the need of highly trained staff (e.g., body composition with DEXA or three-dimensional gait analysis). Moreover, there is a lack of knowledge regarding safety, validity, reliability, or accuracy considerations with pregnant populations. However, we do not find in the literature any evidence or guidelines regarding the evaluation of the other components of physical fitness with pregnant women.

The key point is that exercise testing does not need to be too much invasive with the pregnant client. Instead, it should aim to increase motivation, to objectively understand the effects of training, and to support the exercise prescription for the pregnant woman, since it should consider her baseline level of fitness as well as her previous exercise experience, as pointed as good practice by the RANZCOG [12].

8.6 Exercise Prescription for Pregnant Women

Exercise prescription and monitoring during pregnancy require knowledge and expertise from the fields of obstetrics and exercise physiology, and on the interactive effects of pregnancy and exercise on maternal-fetal biologic and psychologic functions [69]. For most adults, an exercise program including aerobics, body composition, resistance, flexibility, and neuromotor training is indispensable to improve and maintain physical fitness and health [77]. For pregnant women, we need to add pelvic floor training [78], and preparation for birth exercises [79, 80]. Pregnant women fall into the category of apparently healthy adults, although they are considered a special population. Thus, the general guidelines of ACSM regarding the "FITT-VP principle" apply to pregnant women, with some modifications [2, 47]. This principle states that there are recommended levels of the following elements that address mainly one or more physical fitness components:

- F—Frequency (how many exercise sessions per week?)
- I—Intensity (how hard or difficult is the exercise?)
- T—Time (how long is each exercise session?)
- T—Type of exercise (which mode of exercise?)
- V—Volume (which amount?)[10]
- P—Progression/Periodization (how to advance?).[11]

Thus, the recommended exercise prescription for pregnant women should be modified according to the woman's symptoms, discomforts, and abilities during pregnancy [2]. Table 8.1 resumes the exercise prescription components applied to pregnant women.

[10] Usually, the volume is considered to be the product of intensity, frequency and duration of the exercise sessions.

[11] With pregnant clients, the "progression" is assumed as the adaptation of exercise to each trimester of pregnancy, rather than focused on intensity and complexity, taking into account the physiological adaptations to pregnancy.

Table 8.1 Summary of exercise prescription components for pregnant women

Type	Intensity	Duration	Frequency	Progression/Adaptation
Aerobic				
Exercises that activate large muscle groups in a rhythmic and continuous fashion	Moderate intensity exercise (3–5.9 METs; RPE = 12–13; 40–60% $VO_{2reserve}$)	30 min/day of accumulated moderate intensity exercise to total at least 150 min/week	Previous sedentary: up to 3 days/week	The optimal time to progress is after the first trimester (13 week) because the discomforts and risks of pregnancy are lowest at that time
A variety of weight- and non-weight-bearing activities are well-tolerated during pregnancy	Vigorous intensity exercise (>6 METs; RPE = 14–17) for women who were highly active prior to pregnancy or for those who progress to higher fitness levels during pregnancy	or	Previous active: 3–5 days/week to most days of the week	Avoid activities with risk of fall and trauma
Aerobic exercises can be categorized by the intensity and skill demands	So far, there is not much evidence on the influence of exercise of high intensity (RPE > 17) on the course of pregnancy.	75 min/week of vigorous intensity		Activities that require jumping movements and quick changes in direction which can stress joints should be done with caution to—minimize the risk of joint injury
		Previous inactive women should progress from 15 to 30 min/day		

Resistance				
A variety of machines, free weights, and body weight exercises are well-tolerated during pregnancy	Intensity that permits multiple submaximal repetitions (i.e., 8–10 or 12–15 repetitions) to be performed to the point of moderate fatigue	1 set for beginners	2–3 nonconsecutive days/week	Consider exercising in the supine position after 16 weeks of pregnancy to ensure that venous obstruction does not occur, or if the pregnant woman feels uncomfortable
	(40–60% of estimated one repetition maximum)	2–3 sets for intermediate and advanced		Modifying the position of the exercise to instead be performed on one's side, sitting or standing is a safe alternative
		Target major muscles groups		Avoid performing the Valsalva maneuver during exercise
		A basic program includes 8–10 different exercises		Heavy-resistance weight lifting and intense repetitive isometric exercises should be performed with caution until more data is available
Flexibility				
A series of active or passive static and dynamic flexibility exercises for each muscle-tendon unit	Stretch to the point of feeling tightness or slight discomfort	Hold static stretch for 10–30 s (up to 60 s) 2–4 repetitions of each exercise	At least 2–3 up to 7 days/week	Avoid excessive joint stress

(continued)

Table 8.1 (continued)

Type	Intensity	Duration	Frequency	Progression/Adaptation
Neuromotor				
Exercises involving motor skill (e.g., balance, agility, coordination, gait), proprioceptive training, and multifaceted activities (e.g., Pilates, Yoga, tai chi)	Intensity in balance training refers to the degree of difficulty of the postures, movements, or routines practiced	20–30 to 60 min/day	At least 2–3 up to 7 days/week	Can be included in daily activities
	An effective intensity (and volume) of neuromotor exercise has not been determined			The only supervision requirement is the safety considerations and the level of fall risk
				Avoid positions that are uncomfortable or likely to result in loss of balance and falling
Pelvic floor training				
Complex training for pelvic-floor muscles should be focused both on their contraction and relaxation	An effective intensity (and volume) of pelvic floor exercise has not been determined	10–30 min/day	1–7 days/week	Can be done anywhere, anytime, everyday
Various devices can be used to increase the effectiveness and attractiveness of exercise (e.g. vaginal cones)				Should be incorporated in any prenatal exercise program
				Ensure proper technique
				Different exercises should be performed to improve pelvic floor muscle speed, strength, endurance and muscular coordination, and engaging both fast and slow twitch muscle fibers

RPE rating of perceived exertion (6–20 scale), *METs* metabolic equivalents, $VO_{2reserve}$ oxygen uptake reserve ($VO_{2max} - VO_{2rest}$)

8.6.1 Type and Mode of Exercise

There are plenty of physical activities to be performed alone or in group, indoor or outdoor, with or without equipment. In the first place it is important to understand the physical activity pattern of the pregnant women, as addressed in Chap. 1 [81], and choose an activity or activities for which the women are motivated for. Thus, the pregnant woman should select the physical activity or exercise program she is more motivated and able to do, having in mind that those activities or sessions may be adapted according to her health and fitness, and trimester of pregnancy (Fig. 8.4). According to the USDHHS [4] it is important to break up long periods of sitting and standing still, and understand that even a very low volume of physical activity is better than none, in line with WHO [6].

The development of safe and effective exercise programs is a main role and competence of exercise professionals. Each of the several activities available should respect the technical and progression issues of the activity, as well as the associated safety issues. As examples, indoor or outdoor cycling, aerobic and step exercise, or swimming, can be performed using a span of intensity and complexity, and require different pedagogical approaches. Each of the activities given as example can be performed by pregnant women who already practiced them and who already acquired the basic aspects inherent in their safety. For a pregnant woman who has never practiced these activities, the entire learning process must be kept in mind so as not to jeopardize her safety in the event of falls or collisions.

In the second place, the several recommended types of exercise for pregnant should address all health-related physical fitness components (i.e., aerobic, resistance training, and flexibility), as well as neuromotor exercises, pelvic floor training, and preparation for birth exercises. In other words, the type or mode of exercise should be selected first using the specificity principle of training [47]. A variety of exercise modes places different impact stresses on the body, i.e., walking, running, swimming, cycling, or stepping uses different muscles groups, and weight-bearing activities produce greater mechanical loading than non-weight-bearing activities. This loading from physical activity will impact bone metabolism and bone health across the lifespan [82]. Sañudo et al. [83] highlight the importance of quantifying loading intensity and frequency, as these parameters are determinants for bone adaptation. ACSM [77] also recommends loading exercises (i.e., weight-bearing and resistance exercise) to maintain bone health.

This means that on one hand, the exercise program may be focused on one or more types of exercise, and on the other hand, each session of the exercise program can be planned having in mind to include at least 30 min if aerobic exercise, and also strength and flexibility training (including posture and functional exercise), neuromotor exercise (especially, balance and coordination), and pelvic floor muscle training. For example, a step exercise session may combine aerobic, lower limb resistance, and neuromotor training, while a Pilates exercise session may combine upper, core and lower limb resistance, posture, flexibility, and neuromotor training.

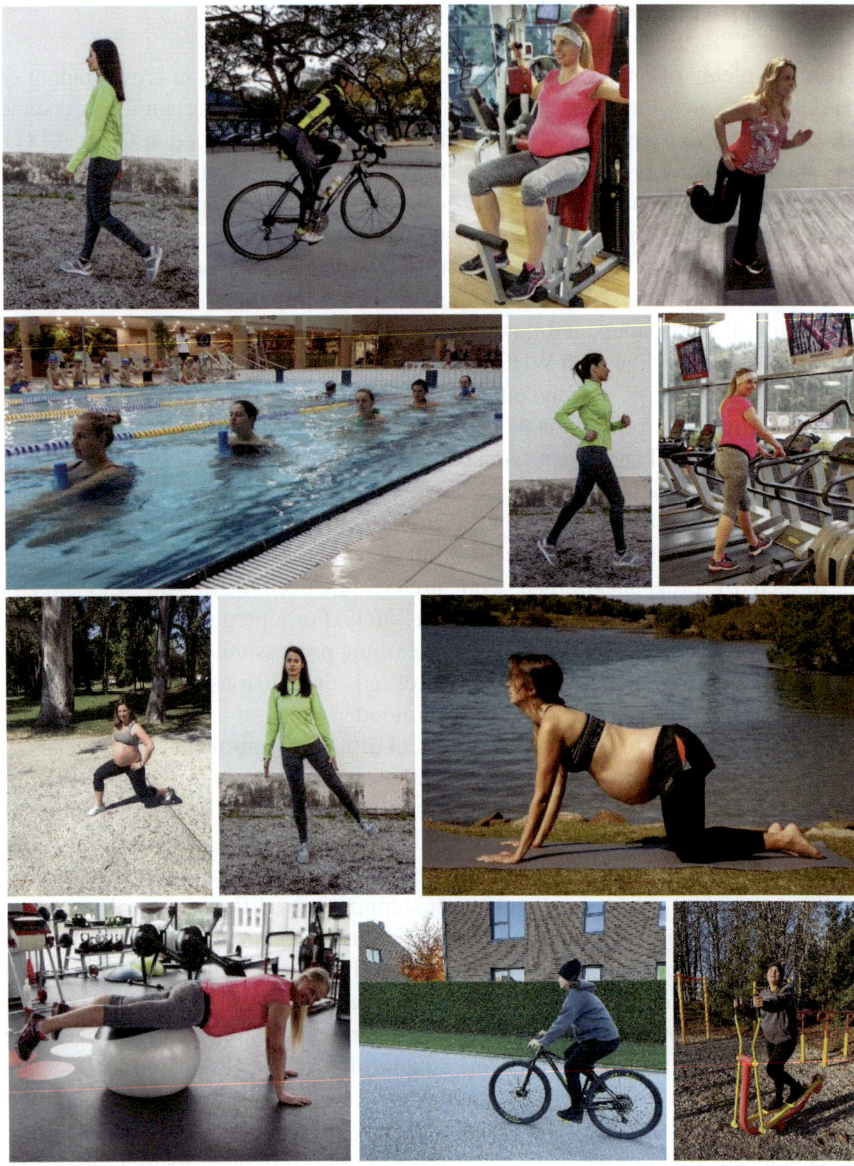

Fig. 8.4 Walking, jogging, running, cycling, swimming, water exercise, aerobics, Pilates, flexibility, and resistance training are among the recommended types of exercise during pregnancy

As discussed in the previous Chap. 7 [5], most of the existing guidelines [4, 6, 12, 13, 16–19, 21, 22] refer that the more appropriate and safe physical activities during pregnancy include walking, swimming, stationary cycling, cycling[12] [19], low-impact aerobics, dancing, modified yoga, and modified Pilates. Other physical activities, such as running, jogging, strength training and racquet sports, are considered safe for pregnant women who participated in these activities regularly before pregnancy, upon consultation with an obstetric care provider [12, 21]. Several study of review and trials available in the literature, on the potential benefits of different forms of exercise during pregnancy on health outcomes, can also help to acknowledge the effectiveness of different activities, such as pelvic-floor muscle training [78, 84], indoor cycling [85–87], resistance exercise [35, 88, 89], home exercise [90], Pilates [91–94], yoga [95–97], aquatic exercise [98–100], swimming [101–103], aerobic exercise [35, 38, 74, 104, 105], dancing [106, 107], and group exercise [108].

Regarding the pregnant athlete, vigorous intensity exercise appears to be safe in healthy pregnancies [18], and elite athletes who wish to become pregnant, should discuss specific issues with their medical team [16, 20]. According to the Australian Sports Commission [109], recreational and competitive athletes may train safely at higher intensities and volumes throughout pregnancy with the understanding that they are undergoing close obstetric supervision. They can continue their exercise programs or sports, unless prior to pregnancy, the women athletes were engaged in extreme sports [110]. However, although potential impact on neonatal outcomes is unknown, athletes may push beyond a threshold intensity at which fetal well-being may be compromised [110], and there may be a limit to how intense an elite performer should exercise during pregnancy [111]. Nevertheless, the key message from IOC [20] is that elite athletes with an uncomplicated pregnancy should be reassured that they can continue exercising, although some adjustments in intensity and activity may be required.

The USDHHS [4], Canadian [16], AGDH [17], ACOG [18], SMA [19], and EiM [22] guidelines also point non-recommended physical activities, including contact sports, activities with high risk of falling, activities at high altitude, scuba diving, skydiving, downhill skiing, water skiing, activities in excessive heat (e.g., hot Pilates, and hot yoga). It should be emphasized, however, that these forms are listed as deprecated based on expert opinion and not based on scientific evidence supporting the harmfulness of these forms of physical activity. Regarding exercise selection and adaptation, exercise specialists must be aware of the morphological, physiological, and musculoskeletal and biomechanical changes that occur during pregnancy (addressed in previous Chap. 3 [61], Chap. 4 [62], and Chap. 5 [65], respectively), such as increased ligament laxity, weight gain, change in the center of gravity, and carpal tunnel syndrome, that will affect the response to exercise. Moreover, the

[12] Outdoor cycling may be safe but requires regular participation prior to pregnancy. As any other activity, it requires balance and ability, depending on the purpose of use (e.g., sports, fitness, well-being, commuting), as well as appropriate equipment (i.e., there are several types of bikes). On the contrary, the Canadian guidelines are quite conservative regarding cycling [16].

typical signs and symptoms associated to each trimester of pregnancy, the motivations and objectives, the safety considerations, the fitness level, and the level of experience of the pregnant women, will also impact on exercise selection and adaptation. Chapter 9 [112] further develops the methods for planning an exercise program, including exercise selection and adaptation.

8.6.2 Exercise Duration, Frequency, and Intensity

Exercise time or duration is prescribed as a measure of the amount of time physical activity is performed, i.e., time per session, per day, and per week [2]. Frequency is prescribed in sessions per day and in days per week. Exercise duration typically ranges from 20 to 60 min. Most adults, including pregnant women are recommended to accumulate at least 150 min/week. Most guidelines for exercise during pregnancy [4, 6, 12, 13, 16–19, 21, 22] suggest 30 min of exercise daily, 5–7 days per week. Pregnant women who have not been regular exercisers should follow a gradual progression of increasing the duration of exercise and can begin with as little as 10 min. Previously sedentary women should begin with 10–20 min of continuous low-intensity exercise three times per week, increasing the intensity, frequency, and duration gradually.

According to the overload principle of training, exercising below a minimum intensity or threshold, will not challenge the body sufficiently to result in changes in physiologic parameters, including the increased maximal volume of oxygen consumed per unit of time [74]. The individual threshold depends on several factors, and it is important to bear in mind that, in general, the physiologic responses to acute exercise may be different in pregnancy compared to non-pregnancy, due to inter alia increased rest cardiac output, rest HR, and plasma volume, and decreased blood pressure [2, 18].

Several methods can be used to estimate intensity during exercise; however, the intensity is usually prescribed using heart rate reserve (%HRR) (Eq. 8.4) or oxygen uptake reserve (VO_2) (Eqs. 8.5 and 8.6) [2].

$$\text{HRR method}(\text{training}) = \left[(\text{HRmax} - \text{HRrest}) \times \text{intensity in percent}\right] + \text{HRrest}(\text{bpm}) \tag{8.4}$$

$$\text{Gross } VO_2 \text{ reserve method}(\text{training}) = \left[(VO_{2\text{max}} - VO_{2\text{rest}}) \times \text{intensity in percent}\right] + VO_{2\text{rest}}(\text{mL/kg/min}) \tag{8.5}$$

$$\text{Net } VO_2(\text{training}) = (VO_{2\text{max}} - VO_{2\text{rest}}) \times \text{intensity in percent}(\text{mL/kg/min}) \tag{8.6}$$

Because maximal exercise testing is rarely performed with pregnant women, Mottola et al. [71] developed and validated heart rate (HR) ranges that correspond to moderate intensity exercise for low-risk pregnant women based on age and body mass index (BMI) while taking fitness levels into account. The Canadian [16] and RANZCOG [12] guidelines, ACSM [2], and SMA [19], provide the HR ranges.

Regarding maximal heart rate the estimation equations by Gellish et al. [113] are more accurate than other formulas, and were estimated for men and women participants in an adult fitness program with a broad range of age and fitness levels, as follows:

$$HRmax = 207 - (0.7 \times age)(bpm) \tag{8.7}$$

$$HRmax = 192 - (0.007 \times age^2)(bpm) \tag{8.8}$$

Although the nonlinear predictor model (Eq. 8.8) was slightly more accurate than the linear equation (Eq. 8.7), the authors suggest that the linear model is easier to use.

However, due to HR variability during pregnancy, two other simpler and more practical methods may be used to monitor intensity [2, 12, 16, 19]:

- Monitoring perceived exertion: for moderate exercise, ratings of perceived exertion should be 13–14 (somewhat hard) on a Borg Rating of Perceived Exertion scale (Fig. 8.5), where 6 represents no exertion and 20 represents maximal exertion [114]. The participant is instructed to report the overall sensation of effort
- OMNI scales of perceived exertion for walking/running and cycling are also available [48]
- The "talk test": the individual should be able to carry on a normal conversation with moderate exercise intensity. By comparison, vigorous exercise is associated with substantial increases in breathing, inability to carry on a normal conversation easily, and perspiration [115]. The participant is asked to work at a level that causes a sensation of increased breathing but that still allows comfortable speaking in complete sentences [48].

Independently of the intensity monitoring methods, an exercise program should start slowly and gradually improve intensity. Throughout the exercise program, a pregnant woman should feel comfortable and avoid overexertion. The limits of intensity are

Fig. 8.5 Borg's Rating of Perceived Exertion (RPE) 6–20 scale [114]

20	**Maximal exertion**
19	Extremely hard
17-18	Very hard
15-16	Hard (heavy)
13-14	Somewhat hard
10-12	Light
8-9	Very light
7	Extremely light
1-6	**No exertion at all**

individual, depending on the previous physical activity patterns. Each body will naturally provide signals that it is time to reduce the level of exercise she is performing. Pregnant women should not exercise to the point of exhaustion or breathlessness.

8.6.3 Exercise Volume

Exercise volume is the product of frequency, intensity, and duration of exercise. Usually, the exercise volume is used to estimate the gross energy expenditure in metabolic equivalents (in MET-min/week or in kcal/week) with respect to body composition and weight management outcomes [2]. A target volume of 500–1000 MET-min/week is recommended for most adults because is associated with lower rates of cardiovascular disease and premature mortality. The calculation of exercise volume may use different methods, as follows [2]:

- Metabolic equivalents (METs): an index of energy expenditure. A MET is the ratio of the rate of energy expended during an activity to the rate of energy expended at rest. By convention, 1 MET = an oxygen uptake of 3.5 mL/kg/min
- MET-min: an index of energy expenditure that quantifies the total amount of physical activity performed in a standardized manner across individuals and types of activities, usually per week or per day (i.e., METs × min)
- Kilocalorie (kcal): by convention, the energy needed to increase the temperature of 1 kg of water by 1 °C. Usually standardize as kcal per week or per day. Conversion of METs to kcal:

$$\text{kcal}/\text{min} = \left[\left(\text{METs} \times 3.5\text{mL}/\text{kg}/\text{min} \times \text{body weight in kg}\right)/1000\right)] \times 5 \tag{8.9}$$

- Treadmill walking, running, and cycling metabolic equations: conventional equations to predict energy cost are probably valid during pregnancy [69]:

$$\begin{aligned} VO_2 \text{ walking}\left(\text{cadence of } 50-100\text{m}/\text{min}\right) = {} & \left(0.1 \times \text{speed in m}/\text{min}\right) \\ & +\left(1.8 \times \text{speed} \times \%\text{grade}\right) \\ & +3.5\left(\text{mL}/\text{kg}/\text{min}\right) \end{aligned} \tag{8.10}$$

$$\begin{aligned} VO_2 \text{ running}\left(\text{cadence over } 130\text{m}/\text{min}\right) = {} & \left(0.2 \times \text{speed in m}/\text{min}\right) \\ & +\left(0.9 \times \text{speed} \times \%\text{grade}\right) \\ & +3.5\left(\text{mL}/\text{kg}/\text{min}\right) \end{aligned} \tag{8.11}$$

$$VO_2 \text{ cycling}\begin{pmatrix} \text{work rate of } 50-200\text{W or } 300 \\ -1200\text{kgm}/\text{min} \end{pmatrix} = \begin{bmatrix} \left(1.8 \times \text{work rate}\right)/ \\ \text{body mass in kg} \end{bmatrix} + 7 \tag{8.12}$$

- Another form of estimating the exercise volume is the steps per day given by pedometers which are effective tools for promoting physical activity [116]. The goal of 10,000 steps/day is often cited regarding health benefits, but it appears that achieving a pedometer step count of at least 5400–7900 steps/day can meet recommended exercise targets [77, 117]. This step count volume is approximately equal to 1000 kcal/week or 150 min/week of moderate-intensity physical activity [2].

8.6.4 Other Forms of Physical Activity

Doing any physical activity is better than doing none [6, 19]. If the pregnant woman does not do any physical activity, she should be advised to start by doing some, and gradually build up to the recommended amount. Other forms of increasing the volume of physical activity or exercise are by integrating it into occupational activities, active commuting, and daily activities, such as (Fig. 8.6):

- Engaging in walking groups
- Using a pedometer
- Increasing the walking time to a minimum of 10,000 steps per day
- Playing with other children
- Walking or biking for active commuting
- Taking stairs instead of the elevator
- Parking far away from office or garage
- Doing housework
- Not standing in the same position for long periods of time
- Limiting the seating time

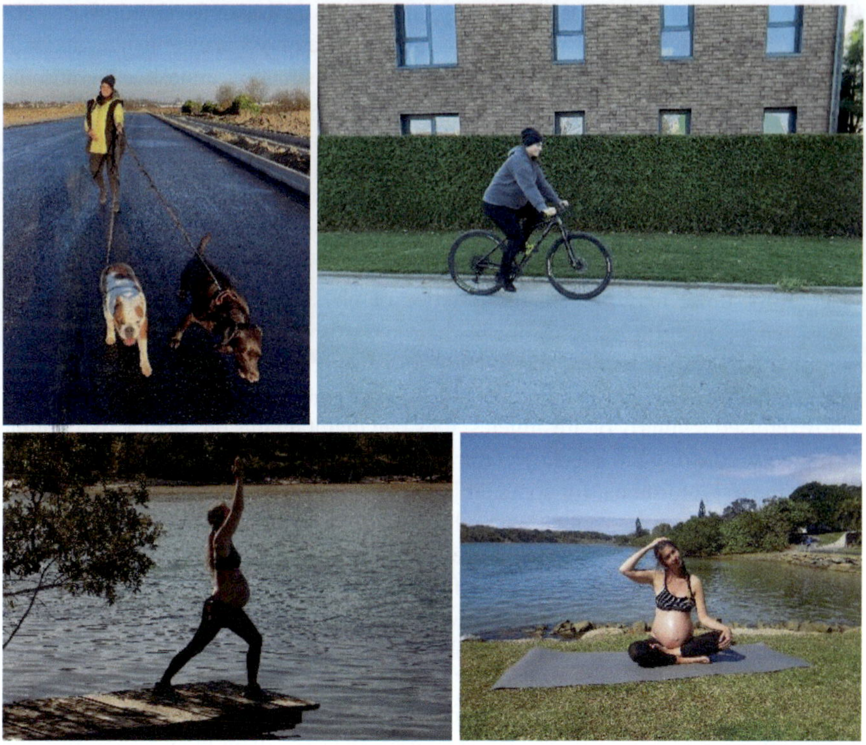

Fig. 8.6 Other forms of increasing the volume of physical activity or exercise are by integrating it into occupational activities, active commuting, and daily activities

- Doing stretching pauses while working in the seated position
- Using a standing desk
- Decreasing the time spent in sedentary activities (e.g., television watching, computer use, sitting in a car or at a desk).
- Taking short bouts of exercise at home (e.g., by following YouTube videos [118, 119])
- Using available apps that encourage physical activity
- Dancing with the music at home
- Walking the dog

8.6.5 Exercise Progression and Adaptation

Exercise goals and progression may vary at different time points during pregnancy, and exercise routines should remain flexible [2]. The progression of exercise during pregnancy may consist of increasing exercise volume or adapting the exercise routine in accordance with the physiological and biomechanical adaptations occurring over the time course of pregnancy [60].

The body undergoes major changes during the first trimester of pregnancy. During the first trimester, the initiation or continuity of physical activity should be established gradually by pregnant women, once the absence of risk is established, and will be adjusted in accordance with participants' clinical situation, fitness level, and the level of adaptation to their new state. In the first trimester, the pregnant woman experiences the typical symptoms of pregnancy, such as mood changes, nausea, vomiting, breast tenderness, dyspepsia, frequent urination, and constipation, which can limit her daily activity and therefore limit her capacity to carry out activities that could aggravate this symptomatology. Although these are common pregnancy symptoms, every woman has a different experience. Depending on the level of symptoms and discomfort, those may prevent the practice of physical activity or exercise (e.g., breast tender may limit exercising in the ventral position; frequent urination and vomiting may require a quick access bathroom during an exercise session). In sedentary pregnant women, it is recommendable to start gradually. Those pregnant women who exercised regularly or are athletes, they can maintain this physical activity uninterruptedly, adapting the intensity and frequency to their personal needs and abilities. Due to the risk of trauma, for some athletes of contact sports it may be necessary to plan a different exercise routine with other types of exercise that provide the maintenance of fitness level during this stage. Along with the other fitness components, pelvic floor training should be advised from the first trimester.

During the second trimester, the previously described discomforts of the first trimester are gone in most cases, and the physical limitations of the third trimester have not yet appeared. For many pregnant women the second trimester is the easiest 3 months of pregnancy. During this period, women feel emotionally better, since they are better adapted to pregnancy. The anatomic changes allow them to comfortably perform most of the types of exercise included in a program. However, it is important to bear in mind that throughout this trimester, the uterine volume increases, and in the supine position, the inferior vena cava syndrome can develop, which consists in the reduction of the venous return through said vessel, due to the pressure exerted by the pregnant uterus when the pregnant woman is lying on her back. That is why some women may feel discomfort or dizziness in the supine position and sometimes it is necessary to avoid it while exercising. In practice, it is rarely to observe this situation, and many women report sleeping lying on back. Nevertheless, some guidelines recommend avoiding this position after the first trimester of pregnancy [6, 13] or, states that pregnant women should be advised to avoid long periods lying flat on back weeks [13, 18]. The Canadian guidelines [16] are clearer when stating that "pregnant women who experience light-headedness, nausea or feel unwell when they exercise flat on their back should modify their exercise position to avoid the supine position." During the third trimester, the increase in the volume of the gravid uterus as well as the weight gain of the pregnant woman produces a compromise of space at the abdominal level as well as at the pulmonary level. That is why the pregnant woman tends to decrease the intensity and duration of their physical activity. To avoid this negative effect it is recommended the start of activities in the aquatic environment, which give the pregnant woman a situation of weightlessness. The aquatic environment also allows mobilizing joints with passive resistance. It is very important to also take into account the possibility of the appearance of inferior vena cava syndrome, which in water is attenuated by weightlessness. AGDH guidelines [17] recommend that after 28 weeks, the exercises should not be performed lying flat on back, and to, instead, tilt the upper body to a 45-degree angle or doing the exercises lying on side. Another aspect to take in consideration is the change in balance and coordination, which can lead to falls. Moreover, hormonal, and biomechanical adaptations may be related to the prevalence of joint and low back pain. Many pregnant women experience low back pain and strengthening of abdominal and back muscles could minimize this risk [18]. This is the period when pregnant women tend to reduce the intensity of exercise, although maintaining pelvic floor exercises [63, 73, 78, 84] and starting a preparation for birth program [79, 80, 120, 121]. However, reducing exercise intensity at this stage of pregnancy should be based on the individual well-being of the woman and is not a standard recommendation. If a woman in the third trimester wants to continue the current intensity of exercise, there are no contraindications for this provided that the pregnancy is progressing well.

8.6.6 Session Organization

- All exercise sessions should always start with a 5–10 min warm-up period, including slow walk, light stretching, or movements that will be performed during the main part of the session.
- All sessions should end with a cool-down period, which can include breathing exercises, light stretching, pelvic floor training, movements that were performed during the main part of the session (reinforcing the motor task learning), or movements that will be performed in the next sessions. Further development of this topic can be found in Chap. 9 [112].

8.7 Exercise Prescription in Special Conditions

Exercise can be planned in a recreational or competitive perspective, but also as an adjunct treatment for several disorders, such as gestational diabetes, excessive weight gain and obesity, hypertension and preeclampsia, low back pain, and antenatal depression. In these cases, it is of particular importance the communication between healthcare providers and exercise professionals. Pregnant women in special clinical conditions face substantial barriers to participating in exercise and require support to enable them to benefit from the increased physical activity. Under medical supervision, exercise professionals will need to select appropriate exercise interventions and behavioral strategies which will benefit the pregnant women regarding the disorder or disease. Independently of the level of evidence, the following issues should be addressed in antenatal care programs and supported by exercise programs. IOC guidelines [20] advise that special attention should be paid to screening for these conditions and referral to a gynecologist or sport/women's health physiotherapist for proper individual management.

8.7.1 Gestational Diabetes

A healthy pregnancy can be associated with resistance to the action of insulin on glucose uptake and utilization. This leads to more use of fats than carbohydrates for energy by mother and saves carbohydrates for the growing fetus [122]. In 1–14% of pregnant women this condition develops into gestational diabetes mellitus (GDM) [123]. GDM is associated with a wide range of adverse health consequences for women and their infants in the short and long term, including an increased risk of macrosomia, birth complications, and maternal diabetes after pregnancy. It may also increase the risk of obesity and type 2 diabetes in offspring later in life [124]. Thus, any strategy to prevent GDM should be considered.

Gestational diabetes is the most common metabolic disorder in pregnancy and its prevalence is nowadays increasing because there is a higher number of pregnant women with a body mass index (BMI) or weight gain level in the range of overweight or obesity, and also because childbearing age is increasing [125].

There is growing evidence in favor of the fact that exercise and physical activity are basic tools to be able to control this prevalent disorder, as they are easy to be carried out, effective and with minimum costs [126]. It is therefore been introduced a new tendency in this disorder's therapy that helps to preserve the glycemia levels in a normal range, by modifying pregnancy women's lifestyles in a salutary way thanks to maternal education, acquisition of healthy living habits such as balanced dietary patterns and performing exercise and physical activity, and finally, a fetal's close monitoring [127, 128]. If despite these circumstances, the glycemic control is not in the proper values, glucose-lowering drugs should be prescribed.

Observational studies strongly support the performance of exercise and physical activity not only as a tool that may control glycemia levels in pregnancy, but also as a preventive factor by reducing the risk of gestational diabetes. In the meta-analysis published by Russo et al. [129], in which there are described 10 interventional trials suitable for the risk group, has shown a significant reduction of developing a gestational diabetes of 28% (95% IC) in comparison to the control group ($R^2 = 0.72$, $p = 0.0005$), consenting to exercise and physical activity a protective factor.

The exercise that pregnant women with gestational diabetes can perform does not differ from that prescribed to a pregnant woman without this disorder. However, it is necessary to take into account that those pregnant women who need glucose-lowering drugs for the metabolic control of glycemia should be closely monitored, since exercise may misadjust the prescribed pharmacological regimen.

In the management of pregnant women with gestational diabetes, there is evidence that exercise, in particular aerobic and resistance is the most beneficial [130–132]. Another meta-analysis, which evaluated seven randomized trials, found that exercise and physical activity are helpful as a complement to good gestational follow-up, increasing postprandial blood glucose control, and decreasing the rapid passage of blood into the bloodstream in pregnant women with gestational diabetes compared with the control group [133]. Brown et al. [134] concluded that both fasting and postprandial blood glucose concentrations in pregnant women involved in exercise programs were reduced compared with the control groups. Shepherd et al. [135] based in a review of 23 RCT concluded that moderate-quality evidence suggests reduced risks of GDM and caesarean section with combined diet and exercise interventions during pregnancy as well as reductions in gestational weight gain, compared with standard care. However, both authors concluded that current evidence is confounded by the large variety of exercise (and diet) interventions [134, 135]. Davenport et al. [136] reviewed 106 RCT and concluded that exercise-only interventions were effective at lowering the odds of developing GDM, as well as gestational hypertension and pre-eclampsia. Moreover, their meta-analysis point that to achieve at least a 25% reduction in the odds of developing GDM (and also gestational hypertension and pre-eclampsia), pregnant women need to accumulate at least 600 MET-min/week of moderate-intensity exercise (i.e., approximately 140 min) [136]. Recently, the integrative review of Ribeiro et al. [137] supported that exercise in pregnancy is safe for both mother and fetus, contributing to prevent pregnancy-related disorders, such as GDM.

8.7.2 Excess Weight and Obesity

Gestational weight gain (GWG) has often been identified in the literature as a critical modifier of maternal and fetal health. In a systematic review and meta-analysis of randomized controlled trials performed by Choi et al. [138], the authors suggest that supervised physical activity plus diet programs were most effective in managing weight among overweight and obese pregnant and postpartum women. The American College of Obstetricians and Gynecologists reaffirmed in 2017 [139], that "in pregnancy, physical inactivity and excessive weight gain have been recognized as independent risk factors for maternal obesity and related pregnancy complications, including gestational diabetes mellitus" (p. 136). The same experts' advice that obese pregnant women should be encouraged to engage in healthy lifestyle modification in pregnancy that includes physical activities and judicious diets [139]. This special population should start with low-intensity, shorts periods of exercise and gradually increase as able [16, 18]. The effect of exercise among pregnant, obese women in systematic review studies has been demonstrated modest reductions in weight gain and no adverse outcomes among those who were assigned to exercise [140, 141]. More recently, a review of 36 RCT [142] concluded that diet and physical activity-based interventions during pregnancy reduce gestational weight gain and lower the odds of caesarean section. Ruchat et al. [143] reviewed 86 RCT and concluded that prenatal exercise reduced the odds of excessive GWG (and postpartum weight gain) but increased the risk of inadequate GWG (based in 5 RCT). Recently, the integrative review of Ribeiro et al. [137] supported that exercise in pregnancy is safe for both mother and fetus, contributing to prevent pregnancy-related disorders, such as excessive weight gain and postpartum weight retention.

8.7.3 Hypertension and Preeclampsia

Hypertensive disorders in pregnancy may produce adverse perinatal outcomes for both, mother and the fetus or newborn. Preeclampsia is an exclusive pathology in pregnancy and postpartum period due to an abnormal development of uterine spiral arteries that, furthermore, produces an alteration in the placental exchange, leading to oxidative stress and producing antiangiogenic factors in the maternal body that can reach target organs such as the liver or kidney. There are also other pathologies related to hypertensive disorders in pregnancy, such as chronic hypertension, which can produce important complications when associated with preeclampsia. Thus, prevention of these complications is critically important. Despite the scientific advances related to the determination of risk factors associated with preeclampsia, and the introduction of preventive measures to try to prevent its appearance, it remains the second most prevalent cause of global maternal mortality, reaching 14% [144]. And these preventive measures do not provide sufficient evidence to be able to reduce it, so that the only treatment known nowadays is the termination of gestation [145, 146].

At present, most research to try to prevent this disease focuses on improving the development of uterine spiral arteries, determining factors related to genetic predisposition, and improving the low immunological response of most pregnant women that develop this pathology [147]. This is why exercise has played a leading role in this pathology because it promotes the improvement of maternal circulation, increasing placental vascularity thanks to the release with the exercise of an anti-inflammatory component and stimulates the immune system of women at risk of preeclampsia [148]. Chawla and Anim-Nyame [149] advise that exercise in pregnancy seems to be beneficial in pregnancies complicated by hypertension. In the systematic review by Magro-Malosso et al. [38] aerobic exercise for about 30–60 min, two to seven times per week during pregnancy, as compared with being more sedentary, is associated with a significantly reduced risk of gestational hypertensive disorders overall, gestational hypertension. However, the intensity of the exercise to be recommended for specific types of these conditions remains unclear. More recently, the meta-analysis of Davenport et al. [136] point that to achieve at least a 25% reduction in the odds of developing gestational hypertension and preeclampsia (and also GDM), pregnant women need to accumulate at least 600 MET-min/week of moderate-intensity exercise (i.e., approximately 140 min). The integrative review of Ribeiro et al. [137] also supported that exercise in pregnancy is safe for both mother and fetus, contributing to prevent pregnancy-related disorders, such as gestational hypertensive disorders.

8.7.4 Low Back Pain

The majority of pregnant women experience low back pain and pelvic girdle during their pregnancy. These circumstances worsen as pregnancy progresses and interferes with their daily routine. In the last few years various studies showed the effectiveness of exercise in reducing back pain [150–152]. Based on the meta-analysis of 11 randomized controlled trials with 2.347 pregnant women, Shiri et al. [153] concluded that exercise reduced the risk of low back pain in pregnancy by 9% and prevented new episodes of sick leave due to lumbopelvic pain. Evidence from single studies suggests that acupuncture [154] or craniosacral therapy improves pregnancy-related pelvic pain, and osteomanipulative therapy or a multi-modal intervention (manual therapy, exercise and education) may also be of benefit [155].

Further evidence is very likely to have an important impact on our confidence in the estimates of effect and change the estimates. Studies would benefit from the introduction of an agreed classification system that can be used to categorize women according to their presenting symptoms, so that treatment can be tailored accordingly. The meta-analysis of Davenport et al. [156] conclude that, compared with not exercising, prenatal exercise decreased the severity of low back, pelvic girdle, and lumbopelvic pain during and following pregnancy but did not decrease the odds of any of these conditions at any time point. Shiri et al. [153] concluded that exercise appears to reduce the risk of low back pain in pregnant women, but there is no clear evidence for an effect on pelvic girdle pain. The integrative review of Ribeiro et al. [137] also supported that exercise in pregnancy may contribute to prevent lumbopelvic pain. However, exercise interventions varied on type, frequency, intensity, and duration, hindering a possible association of specific types of exercise interventions with these outcomes.

8.7.5 Depression and Mental Disorders

Ohman et al. [157] reported that among the most common concerns raised by pregnant women were: fear of labor pain, fear of perinatal complications, fetal health problems, or the possibility of miscarriage. The prevalence of depression during the first trimester of pregnancy was reported as 7.4–11%; in the second trimester reaches 12.8%; and in the third trimester from 8.5% to 12%. The prevalence of depression at 40 weeks of pregnancy was 18.4% [158, 159].

Physical exercise practice is included in the guidelines as a therapeutic recommendation for the treatment of depression and there is sufficient scientific evidence to support it as a complement to pharmacological treatment even in major depression cases [160]. Padmapriya et al. [161] observed that in Asian women sufficient physical activity was associated with a reduced likelihood of probable antenatal depression and trait anxiety symptoms. A meta-analysis by McCurdy et al. [162] has shown that light-to-moderate intensity aerobic exercise improves mild-to-moderate depressive symptoms and increases the likelihood that mild-to-moderate depression will resolve in the postpartum period. The meta-analysis by Davenport et al. [163] concluded that prenatal exercise reduced the odds and severity of prenatal depression. More recently, Ribeiro et al. [137] also supported that exercise in pregnancy may contribute to prevent perinatal depression and anxiety.

To be noted that during the COVID-19 pandemic, a substantial worsening of the mental condition of future mothers has been observed [164], which results, among others, from changes in previous physical activity [165]. Thus, it is necessary to popularize pro-health exercises in pregnant women from various social groups, especially those with a low degree of involvement in physical activity before the pandemic [166].

8.8 Specific Considerations and Safety Issues Regarding Exercise During Pregnancy

There are several special considerations that should be taken into account to maximize the effective development and ensure the safety of an exercise program for pregnant women, including the following.

8.8.1 Weight Gain and Caloric Intake

- During pregnancy, the metabolic demand increases by 300 kcal/day. Caloric intake should increase to meet the caloric costs of pregnancy and exercise. Intake above or below recommended levels with concomitant changes in weight gain during pregnancy may be associated with adverse maternal and fetal outcomes [2]. Chapters 13 [167] and Chap. 14 [168] provide further information on this topic.
- In order to avoid excessive weight gain during pregnancy, the weight gain guidelines based on prepregnancy BMI, available from the Institute of Medicine (US) and the National Research Council (US) [169], should be consulted [2].
- High-intensity or prolonged exercise in excess of 45 min can lead to hypoglycemia; therefore, adequate caloric intake before exercise, or limiting the exercise session, is essential to minimize this risk [18].

- Since competitive athletes tend to maintain a more strenuous training schedule throughout pregnancy as compared to other pregnant women, they require frequent and closer supervision [18]. Such athletes should pay particular attention to avoiding hyperthermia, maintaining proper hydration, and sustaining adequate caloric intake to prevent weight loss, which may adversely affect fetal growth [18].

8.8.2 Hydration and Urinary Incontinence

- Pelvic floor muscle dysfunctions can lead to urinary incontinence, a condition which often affects women both during pregnancy and after childbirth. Urinary incontinence (UI) is prevalent in antenatal and postnatal women, and pelvic floor muscle training (PFMT) is the first-line treatment for UI [170].
- A recent systematic review by Woodley et al. [171] concluded that structured pelvic floor muscle training in early pregnancy for continent women may prevent the onset of UI in late pregnancy and postpartum. However, Yang et al. [170] concluded that evidence of weak quality supports the effectiveness of undertaking group-based PFMT in pregnancy to prevent UI during pregnancy and the postnatal period.
- PFMT (e.g., Kegel exercises) may be performed on a daily basis to reduce the odds of urinary incontinence [6, 16, 21, 22].
- Targeted exercises to strengthen the pelvic floor muscles are recommended by RANZCOG guidelines [12]. AGDH guidelines [17] advises that pelvic floor exercises help strengthen and tone the pelvic floor muscles and other tissues. Moreover, a strong pelvic floor can reduce the chance of having problems (such as UI) after giving birth and later in life, so it is important to learn how to do these correctly. If symptoms are present, assessment and training by a gynecologist/women's health physiotherapist is indicated [20].
- There are recommendations to increase hydration during pregnancy [6, 13, 16–18], and while and after exercising [172]. Pregnant women should drink water before, during and after exercise. However, pregnant women experience UI during exercise because of mechanical and anatomical changes. Thus, there are considerations to take into account to minimize urinary incontinence related to exercise, such as: voiding before activity; avoiding breath holding and use of Valsalva maneuver during exercise; practicing pelvic muscle-strengthening exercises; minimizing high-impact activities when incontinence symptoms appeared, and using an external pad during exercise [48].
- Moreover, pregnant women feel better when there is a bathroom available in the (indoor or outdoor) area where the exercise session is taken place.
- According to RANZCOG guidelines [12], activities that involve jumping or bouncing may add extra load to the pelvic floor muscles and are probably best avoided. However, there is some evidence that women participating in high-low impact exercise program (containing jumps and runs) supplemented it with pelvic floor muscle training, maintained urinary continence and improved neuromuscular activity of pelvic floor muscles [73].

8.8.3 Falls and Injury

- Pregnant women should avoid contact sports and sports or activities that may cause loss of balance or trauma to the mother and fetus (e.g., soccer, basketball, ice hockey, rollerblading, horseback riding, skiing, snowboarding, scuba diving, and vigorous intensity racquet sports) [2, 4, 6, 16, 20]. However, in the absence of medical contraindications, the decision to stop or continue particular sports activities should be based on the assessment of woman's individual abilities, skills, previous experience and her sense of security and comfort related with performing sports activities.
- The increase in body weight as pregnancy progresses is associated with increased loading at the joints [12, 63, 65, 173]. Thus, weight-supported activities such as water-based exercise or stationary cycling may be more comfortable compared with weight-bearing exercises such as walking in the later stages of pregnancy [12].
- During pregnancy an increase in the laxity of the musculoskeletal system is a natural adaptive process. So far, there is a very little scientific data on this subject. Schauberger et al. [173] found a significant increase in joint laxity in five of seven peripheral joints over the course of the pregnancy and postpartum. In the study by Dumas [174], the exercise program employing minimal to moderate weight-bearing did not result in any measurable increases in knee laxity and, therefore, appears to be appropriate with regard to knee stability.
- According to RANZOG guidelines [12], the increase in ligament laxity associated with pregnancy may have implications for the risk of injury. However, there is no scientific evidence that the prevalence of joint injury related to physical activity increases in pregnant women. For this reason, until more data is available, activities that require jumping movements and quick changes in direction (e.g., court sports, aerobic dancing, etc.) which can stress joints should be done with caution, and adapted to skill level, to minimize the risk of joint injury [7, 12].
- According to SMA guidelines [19], stretching exercises are also useful but should be done gently due to the increased joint laxity during pregnancy. Flexibility exercises should be individualized to reduce susceptibility to joint injury. Because of increased relaxation of ligaments in pregnancy, joints are supported less effectively, especially in women with poor muscle mass. Activities that may result in excessive joint stress should be discontinued, modified, or include cautionary advice, with consideration of individual abilities [7].
- The altered center of gravity resulting from the change in weight distribution as pregnancy progresses may influence balance [12, 63]. Thus, precaution should be taken to modify the exercise routine to minimize or avoid fast changes in direction, if necessary [12].
- Balance exercises can improve the ability to resist forces within or outside of the body that cause falls while a person is stationary or moving [4]. Strengthening muscles of the back, abdomen, and legs also improves balance [4].

8.8.4 Nausea and Dizziness

- In any activity, using the Valsalva maneuver, prolonged isometric contraction, and motionless standing should be avoided [2].
- For some women it may be necessary to avoid physical activity in the supine position or to modify this position after Week 16 of pregnancy [16, 18]. Due to the weight of the growing fetus, exertion or prolonged periods in the supine position may reduce venous return and cardiac output [2].
- Fast modifications of the movement plan (e.g., from lying or sitting to standing; fast stand to sit and sit to stand) may cause dizziness and imbalance, associated with a reduction in blood pressure.
- Exercise should always be completed with a slow and sustained a cool-down and never stopped suddenly [12].

8.8.5 Heat, Humidity, and Environment

- According to Ebi et al. [175], hot ambient conditions and associated heat stress can increase mortality and morbidity, as well as increase adverse pregnancy outcomes and negatively affect mental health.
- A scoping review by Dervis et al. [176] concluded that evidence suggest that during exercise, evaporative (sweating) and dry (skin blood flow and temperature) heat loss responses increase from early to late pregnancy in addition to greater cardiac output, blood volume and reduced vascular resistance.
- Pregnant women should avoid exercising in a hot humid environment, be well hydrated at all times, and dress appropriately to avoid heat stress [6, 16–18, 21]. Further information on this topic is available by ACSM [2, 172].
- Prolonged exercise should be performed in a thermoneutral environment or in controlled environmental conditions (air conditioning) with close attention paid to proper hydration and caloric intake [16, 18].
- Pregnant women are quite sensitive to smell. Exercise should be performed in a clean environment, avoiding air pollution and bad smell settings.
- When running or cycling, rocky terrains or unstable grounds should be avoided, since the joints are more lax in pregnancy, and ankle sprains and other injuries may occur.

8.8.6 Sportswear and Shoes

- Endocrine changes occurring during pregnancy result in increased laxity of the ligaments of the foot, and several gait adaptations may occur [65, 177].
- AGDH guidelines [17] advise that pregnant women should always wear appropriate shoes, non-restrictive clothing, and a supportive pregnancy-safe bra, and, if it is hot, to wear loose clothing made from "breathable" fabric.

- Pregnant women should wear comfortable and proper exercise footwear that gives strong ankle and arch support, and provides impact absorbing features and better balance, especially during weight-bearing activities and outdoor activities.
- Appropriate shoes that provide shock absorption and stability are particularly important for pregnant women. Shoe specialists can provide recommendations or appropriate shoes to meet individual biomechanical profiles.
- Special footwear designed for pregnant women [178] may increase comfort and safety.
- The breasts became more sensitive and will grow. A good sports bra helps to control breast movement during physical activities such as walking and running. Sometimes a sports bra is not enough to provide support during exercise. A proper pregnancy bra should provide comfort and support during exercise.
- Sportswear should be light, comfortable and allow perspiration. Moreover, it should be seamless, due to the increased sensitivity of the skin.

8.9 Exercise Supervision and Multidisciplinary Teams

During pregnancy women need to feel safe and professionally framed while exercising [179]. It is important to understand why it is not enough for pregnant women just to join general, non-specific classes in fitness clubs and why well-trained and qualified exercise professionals are required to conduct pre- and postnatal classes, in order to increase participation rates amongst pre- and postnatal clients and ensure safety and effectiveness. Supervision is recommended to ensure proper technique, provide confidence, and ensure the progression of appropriate levels of intensity and complexity. The exercise professional should provide regular feedback, positive reinforcement, and behavioral strategies to enhance adherence [14].

ACSM [21, 22] recommends that physical activity programs should be individualized for each woman based on situation, experience, and current health status. These guidelines also state that while it's not required, working with an exercise professional can help to reach fitness goals, tailor exercises to abilities and most importantly, minimize the risk of injury [21]. Moreover, an exercise professional can help with strength training, pelvic floor muscle training or yoga [22]. NHS guidelines [13] advise pregnant women going to exercise classes or water exercise classes to make sure the exercise professional is properly qualified and knows that they are pregnant (and how many weeks of gestation). The SMA guidelines [19] advise pregnant women that the doctor may recommend her to see a physiotherapist or exercise physiologist for an individually prescribed exercise program. The Canadian [16] and the RANZCOG [12] guidelines refer that among the target users of their evidence-based guidelines are fitness professionals and exercise physiologists who provide guidance on the impact of prenatal physical activity on maternal, fetal and neonatal health outcomes. The Physical Activity Guidelines for Americans by USDHHS [4] state that physical activity specialists can help people attain and maintain regular physical activity by providing advice on appropriate types of activities and ways to progress at a safe and steady pace. Moreover, they advise that people with chronic conditions and symptoms can consult a healthcare professional or physical activity specialist about the types and amounts of activity appropriate for them [4]. These references in the official position documents regarding physical activity during pregnancy, shows the increasing importance of the exercise professional in promoting and implementing effective and safe exercise programs.

The purpose of the Pregnancy and Postnatal Exercise Specialist is to build exercise participation for beginners and already active women at all stages of pregnancy and during the postpartum period. This could be done through group or individual exercise programs that meet their needs and objectives. In addition, the Pregnancy and Postnatal Exercise Specialist will be expected to assess overall physical fitness, to develop proper exercise programmes, to review participants' progress and to be able to report on adherence and outcomes to relevant stakeholders [14].

Exercise specialists should consider the multifaceted determinants and outcomes of prenatal physical activity and intervene to promote physical activity before, during, and after pregnancy, helping women to overcome any identified barriers. When working with pre- and postnatal clients specialized knowledge is needed in the following areas, amongst others: the official and updated guidelines for exercising during pregnancy; the absolute and relative contraindications to exercise; the symptoms indicating the need for the interruption of exercise; the methods for planning and delivering adapted exercise programs for this target group [14]. Further development of exercise selection and delivering methods is provided in Chap. 9 [112].

An exercise professional should also provide the safest possible training and testing environment, as well as preventing exercise-related emergencies, and be familiar with the safety and emergency procedures available at the fitness setting where the exercise program is delivered. Further development of this topic can be found in ACSM [2, 47, 48].

8.10 Further Research

The body of knowledge on prenatal exercise is increasing. Growing evidence has been supporting that several types of moderate exercise is safe for the mother [8, 18, 34, 35, 137, 180, 181] and fetus [34, 37, 39, 180, 181]. However, the information about the dose-response of exercise and its effects on the cardiovascular and musculoskeletal systems of the pregnant body are still relatively limited. More knowledge of the physiologic, biochemical, and musculoskeletal changes that result from various patterns of physical activity in pregnant women, i.e., short- and long-term, sustained and intermittent, isotonic and isometric, low to moderate, moderate to high intensity, high intensity, minimum-intensity threshold required for benefit, is needed. Harrison et al. [180] highlighted the need for large, high-quality studies to clarify the optimal type, frequency, duration, and intensity of physical activity required for beneficial health outcomes during preconception, pregnancy and postpartum.

Research on better and more effective physical activity and exercise interventions that improve long-term compliance with a physically active lifestyle is also needed. Future studies should focus not only on the benefits of physical activity and exercise, but also on exercise adherence strategies and the methods used to facilitate dissemination of present and future knowledge to pregnant women, healthcare providers, and exercise professionals.

Healthy women and female athletes can usually maintain their regular training regime once they become pregnant, however, as suggested by Kehler and Heinrich [182], research is needed to determine the upper limits of exercise frequency and intensity for pregnant women who are already trained.

Exercise interventions are complex interventions because they contain several interacting components [183, 184]. Applying the Criteria for Reporting the development and Evaluation of Complex Interventions in healthcare (CREDECI2) [184], as well as the Consensus on Exercise Reporting Template (CERT) [185] would allow a better understanding of the prenatal exercise program itself and the dose-response impact. Our study "development and validation of a complex intervention: ACTIVE PREGNANCY—a physical exercise program aimed at promoting health and fitness during pregnancy" [186] was the first validation study using this methodology. So far, there are no other validation studies regarding exercise interventions tailored to pregnant women. In addition, there is a lack of standardizing physical activity measurement during pregnancy, as well as specific fitness assessment batteries [67], allowing to quantify the effectiveness of exercise interventions for pregnant women in the physical fitness parameters, such as maternal cardiorespiratory fitness [35–37, 181].

Other focus would be the best types of exercise that could be beneficial for reducing the prevalence of symptoms, pain, and musculoskeletal disorders commonly associated to pregnancy, improving fitness and balance performance, decreasing fear of falling and incidence of falls, as well as to reduce sedentary behavior [4, 6].

Regarding clinical conditions, results from recent systematic reviews and meta-analysis suggest that structured moderate physical exercise programs during pregnancy may be used as adjunct treatment and provides protective effect against the development of gestational diabetes mellitus [8, 37, 40, 126–129, 132–137], excessive maternal weight gain [8, 37, 105, 132, 137, 138, 143, 181], low back and pelvic girdle pain [99, 136, 153, 155, 156], urinary incontinence [36, 78, 84, 170, 171], hypertensive disorders [8, 37, 38, 136, 145], and anxiety and depressive symptoms [8, 41, 42, 162, 163]. Physical exercise programs during pregnancy also impact on maternal health and perinatal outcomes [8, 35, 37, 39, 134, 137, 181], bone health [82, 83], and also a positive impact on offspring health in adulthood is observed [37, 43]. Moreover, diet and physical activity-based interventions during pregnancy reduce gestational weight gain and lower the odds of cesarean section [38, 143]. Nevertheless, current evidence is confounded by the large variety of exercise interventions [134]. Thus, further studies evaluating type, intensity, duration, and compliance of physical activity and exercise routines are needed to establish recommendations for exercise practice and best inform obstetric guidelines, as well as to provide advice for pregnant women with such clinical conditions or disabilities. Moreover, as suggested by Brown et al. [134], further research is required comparing different types of exercise interventions with another exercise intervention that reports on both the short- and long-term outcomes for mother and baby. Other field of study that lacks evidence-based knowledge is the quality, feasibility, engagement and effectiveness of maternal health and exercise mobile apps [187].

Overall, we suggest that future research should be focused on the dose-response of exercise and in comparing different types of exercise programs, either presential or online, rather than with no exercise control groups, which, based on current knowledge, might be considered as unethical and unnecessary procedure. Hopefully, texts like this will increase the recognition of the need for further research on the above-mentioned topics.

8.11 Conclusions

Exercise testing and prescription in pregnancy is the plan of exercise and fitness-related activities designed to meet the health and fitness goals and motivations of the pregnant woman, addressing the health-related fitness components and the pregnancy-specific conditions, based on previous health and exercise assessments, and taking into account the body adaptations and the pregnancy-related symptoms of each stage of pregnancy and postpartum, as well as fitness level, motivations and experience, in order to provide safe and effective exercise.

In this Chapter, we have reviewed the guidelines for exercise testing and prescription in pregnant women. Moreover, we proposed a sequential order for exercise prescription and planning. There is increasing evidence on the benefits of physical activity and exercise during pregnancy. The first step before planning to start or continuing an exercise program during pregnancy is the health screening of the woman by a healthcare provider. The second step is the appropriate pre-exercise evaluation, followed by the testing of determined fitness and postural components. Appropriate exercise prescription is then developed to tailor effective and safe exercise programs. When planning an exercise intervention, exercise professionals should bear in mind that for each type of exercise, i.e., aerobic, resistance, flexibility, or neuromotor, there is a frame of intensity, frequency, and duration, which will provide a metabolic, mechanical, and psychological stimulus. In addition, pelvic floor training and preparation for birth exercises are specific interventions for this special stage of life. Supervision of exercise programs by qualified exercise professionals is of particular importance to provide safe and effective exercise meeting women's goals and motivations. The synthesis of this information can be found in the infographic of the present Chapter (Fig. 8.7).

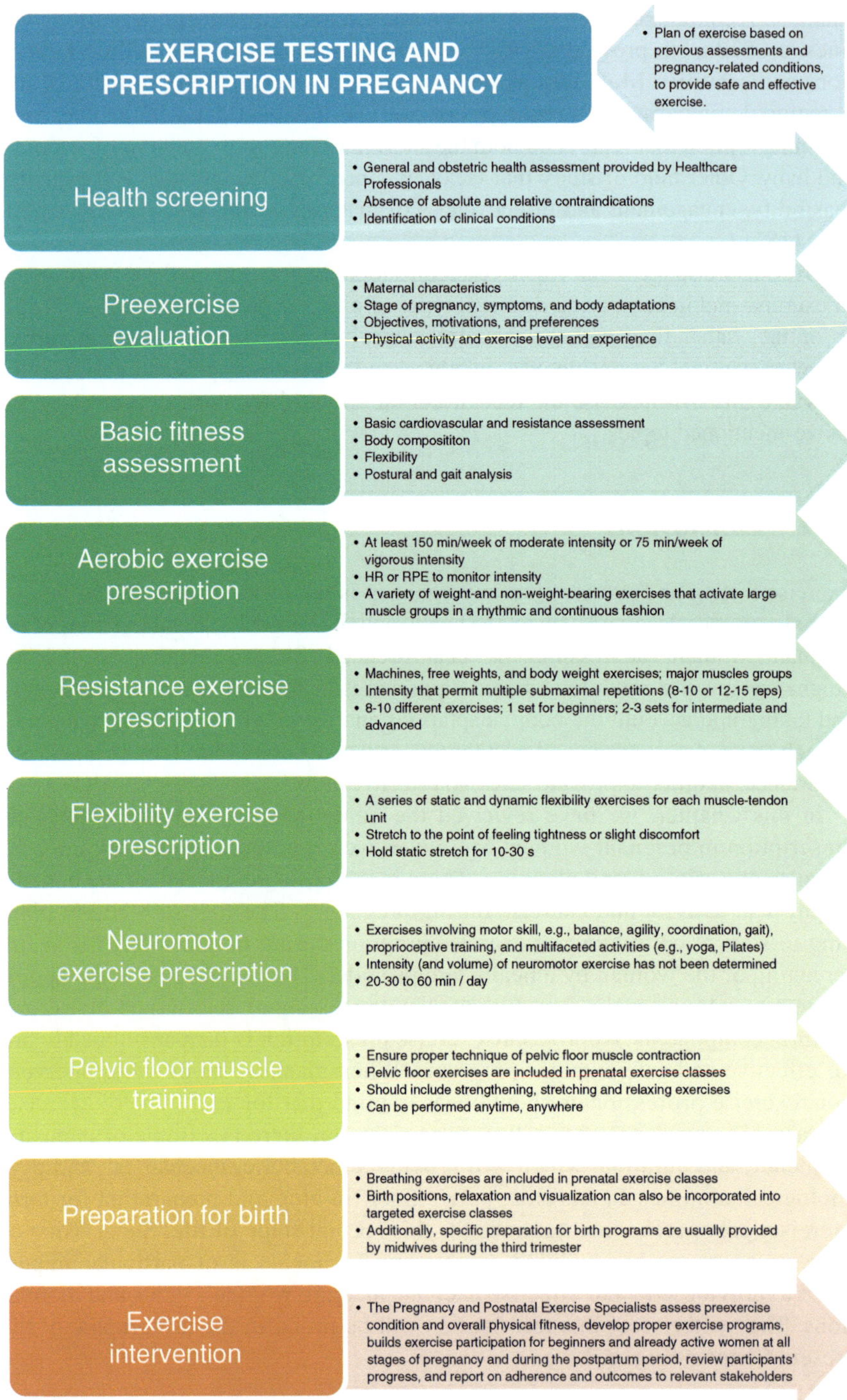

Fig. 8.7 Infographic of the chapter "Exercise Testing and Prescription in Pregnancy"

References

1. Suleman A, Heffner KD. Exercise prescription. Medscape, 2016. https://emedicine.medscape.com/article/88648-overview#a1. Accessed 3 Sep 2021.
2. ACSM - American College of Sports Medicine. ACSM's guidelines for exercise testing and prescription. 11th ed. Philadelphia, PA: Wolters Kluwer Health; 2021.
3. Caspersen CJ, Powell KE, Christenson GM. Physical activity, exercise, and physical fitness: definitions and distinctions for health-related research. Public Health Rep. 1985;100(2):126–31.
4. USDHHS - U.S. Department of Health and Human Services. Physical activity guidelines for Americans. 2nd ed. Washington, DC: U.S. Department of Health and Human Services; 2018.
5. Szumilewicz A, Worska A, Santos-Rocha R, Oviedo-Caro MA. Evidence-based and practice-oriented guidelines for exercising during pregnancy. In: Santos-Rocha R, editor. Exercise and physical activity during pregnancy and postpartum. evidence-based guidelines. 2nd ed. Cham: Springer International Publishing; 2022. Chapter 7.
6. WHO - World Health Organization. WHO guidelines on physical activity and sedentary behaviour. Geneva: World Health Organization; 2020.
7. Artal R. Exercise during pregnancy and the postpartum period. UpToDate®. Philadelphia, PA: Wolters Kluwer; 2021. www.uptodate.com. Accessed 3 Sep 2021.
8. Dipietro L, Evenson KR, Bloodgood B, Sprow K, Troiano RP, Piercy KL, Vaux-Bjerke A, Powell KE, 2018 Physical Activity Guidelines Advisory Committee*. Benefits of physical activity during pregnancy and postpartum: an umbrella review. Med Sci Sports Exerc. 2019;51(6):1292–302.
9. Borodulin K, Evenson KR, Herring AH. Physical activity patterns during pregnancy through postpartum. BMC Womens Health. 2009;9:32.
10. Sjögren Forss K, Stjernberg L. Physical activity patterns among women and men during pregnancy and 8 months postpartum compared to pre-pregnancy: a longitudinal study. Front Public Health. 2019;7:294.
11. Krans EE, Gearhart JG, Dubbert PM, Klar PM, Miller AL, Replogle WH. Pregnant women's beliefs and influences regarding exercise during pregnancy. J Miss State Med Assoc. 2005;46(3):67–73.
12. RANZCOG - The Royal Australian and New Zealand College of Obstetricians and Gynaecologists. Exercise in pregnancy. Melbourne, VIC: RANZCOG; 2020.
13. NHS - National Health Service. Exercise in pregnancy exercise in pregnancy. London: National Health Service; 2020. www.nhs.uk.
14. EuropeActive. EuropeActive standards - European qualification framework level 5 - pregnancy and postnatal exercise specialist. 2016. http://www.ehfa-standards.eu/es-standards. Accessed 30 Dec 2017. Updated in 2022: https://www.europeactive-standards.eu/sites/europeactive-standards.eu/files/EuropeActive_Summary_Pregnancy-Postpartum-2022_0.pdf.
15. Atkinson L, Teychenne M. Psychological, social and behavioural changes during pregnancy: implications for physical activity and exercise. In: Santos-Rocha R, editor. Exercise and physical activity during pregnancy and postpartum. Evidence-based guidelines. 2nd ed. Cham: Springer International Publishing; 2022. Chapter 2.
16. Mottola MF, Davenport MH, Ruchat S-M, Davies GA, Poitras VJ, Gray CE, et al. 2019 Canadian guideline for physical activity throughout pregnancy. Br J Sports Med. 2018;52(21):1339–46.
17. AGDH - Australian Government. Department of Health. Guidelines for physical activity during pregnancy. Guidelines for physical activity during pregnancy (health.gov.au). Indianapolis, IN: Australian Government. Department of Health; 2021.
18. ACOG - American College of Obstetricians and Gynecologists. ACOG Committee opinion no. 804: Physical activity and exercise during pregnancy and the postpartum period. Obstet Gynecol. 2020;135(4):e178–e88.

19. SMA. Pregnancy and exercise. Women in sport. Sydney Olympic Park, NSW: SMA. SMA_AWiS_Pregnancy_Exercise.pdf. Sport Medicine Australia. Accessed 13 Jul 2021.
20. Bø K, Artal R, Barakat R, Brown WJ, Davies GAL, Dooley M, et al. Exercise and pregnancy in recreational and elite athletes: 2016/2017 evidence summary from the IOC expert group meeting, Lausanne. Part 5. Recommendations for health professionals and active women. Br J Sports Med. 2018;52(17):1080–5.
21. ACSM - American College of Sport Medicine. ACSM information on pregnancy physical activity. Indianapolis, IN: American College of Sports Medicine; 2020. https://www.acsm.org/docs/currentcomments/exerciseduringpregnancy.pdf. Accessed 3 Sep 2021.
22. EIM/ACSM. Being active during pregnancy. Indianapolis, IN: Exercise is Medicine/American College of Sports Medicine; 2019.
23. ACOG - American College of Obstetricians and Gynecologists. Exercise during pregnancy and the postnatal period. Washington DC: American College of Obstetricians and Gynecologists; 1985.
24. ACOG - American College of Obstetricians and Gynecologists. Exercise during pregnancy and the postpartum period. ACOG Technical Bulletin, Number 189--February 1994. Int J Gynaecol Obstet. 1994;45(1):65–70.
25. ACOG - American College of Obstetricians and Gynecologists. ACOG Committee Opinion. Exercise during pregnancy and the postpartum period. Number 267, January 2002. American College of Obstetricians and Gynecologists. Int J Gynaecol Obstet. 2002;77(1):79–81.
26. Evenson KR, Barakat R, Brown WJ, et al. Guidelines for physical activity during pregnancy: comparisons from around the world. Am J Lifestyle Med. 2013;XX(X):1–20.
27. Szumilewicz A, Worska A, Rajkowska N, Santos-Rocha R. Summary of guidelines for exercise in pregnancy – are they comprehensive enough for designing the contents of a prenatal exercise program? Curr Women's Health Rev. 2015;11(1):3–12.
28. ACOG - American College of Obstetricians and Gynecologists. Physical activity and exercise during pregnancy and the postpartum period. Committee Opinion No. 650. American College of Obstetricians and Gynecologists. Obstet Gynecol. 2015;126:e135–42.
29. Bø K, Artal R, Barakat R, Brown W, Davies GA, Dooley M, Evenson KR, Haakstad LA, Henriksson-Larsen K, Kayser B, Kinnunen TI, Mottola MF, Nygaard I, van Poppel M, Stuge B, Khan KM. Exercise and pregnancy in recreational and elite athletes: 2016 evidence summary from the IOC expert group meeting, Lausanne. Part 1-exercise in women planning pregnancy and those who are pregnant. Br J Sports Med. 2016;50(10):571–89.
30. Bø K, Artal R, Barakat R, Brown W, Dooley M, Evenson KR, Haakstad LA, Larsen K, Kayser B, Kinnunen TI, Mottola MF, Nygaard I, van Poppel M, Stuge B, Davies GA. IOC Medical Commission. Exercise and pregnancy in recreational and elite athletes: 2016 evidence summary from the IOC expert group meeting, Lausanne. Part 2-the effect of exercise on the fetus, labour and birth. Br J Sports Med. 2016;50:1297.
31. Bø K, Artal R, Barakat R, Brown WJ, Davies GAL, Dooley M, Evenson KR, Haakstad LAH, Kayser B, Kinnunen TI, Larsén K, Mottola MF, Nygaard I, van Poppel M, Stuge B, Khan KM. IOC Medical Commission. Exercise and pregnancy in recreational and elite athletes: 2016/17 evidence summary from the IOC Expert Group Meeting, Lausanne. Part 3-exercise in the postpartum period. Br J Sports Med. 2017;51(21):1516–25.
32. Bø K, Artal R, Barakat R, Brown WJ, Davies GAL, Dooley M, Evenson KR, Haakstad LAH, Kayser B, Kinnunen TI, Larsén K, Mottola MF, Nygaard I, van Poppel M, Stuge B, Khan KM. Exercise and pregnancy in recreational and elite athletes: 2016/17 evidence summary from the IOC expert group meeting, Lausanne. Part 4-Recommendations for future research. Br J Sports Med. 2017;51:1724.
33. Kilpatrick SJ, Papile LA, Macones GA. Guidelines for perinatal care. 8th ed. Elk Grove Village, IL; Washington, DC: AAP Committee on Fetus and Newborn and ACOG Committee on Obstetric Practice; 2017. https://ebooks.aappublications.org/content/guidelines-for-perinatal-care-8th-edition.tab-info.
34. Barakat R, Perales M, Bacchi M, Coteron J, Refoyo I. A program of exercise throughout pregnancy. Is it safe to mother and newborn? Am J Health Promot. 2013;29(1):2–8.

35. Perales M, Santos-Lozano A, Ruiz JR, Lucia A, Barakat R. Benefits of aerobic or resistance training during pregnancy on maternal health and perinatal outcomes: a systematic review. Early Hum Dev. 2016;94:43–8.
36. Davenport MH, Skow RJ, Steinback CD. Maternal responses to aerobic exercise in pregnancy. Clin Obstet Gynecol. 2016;59(3):541–51.
37. Morales-Suárez-Varela M, Clemente-Bosch E, Peraita-Costa I, Llopis-Morales A, Martínez I, Llopis-González A. Maternal physical activity during pregnancy and the effect on the mother and newborn: a systematic review. J Phys Act Health. 2020;18(1):130–47.
38. Magro-Malosso ER, Saccone G, Di Tommaso M, Roman A, Berghella V. Exercise during pregnancy and risk of gestational hypertensive disorders: a systematic review and meta-analysis. Acta Obstet Gynecol Scand. 2017;96(8):921–31.
39. Magro-Malosso ER, Saccone G, Di Mascio D, Di Tommaso M, Berghella V. Exercise during pregnancy and risk of preterm birth in overweight and obese women: a systematic review and meta-analysis of randomized controlled trials. Acta Obstet Gynecol Scand. 2017;96(3):263–73.
40. Harrison AL, Shields N, Taylor NF, Frawley HC. Exercise improves glycaemic control in women diagnosed with gestational diabetes mellitus: a systematic review. J Physiother. 2016;62(4):188–96.
41. Daley AJ, Foster L, Long G, Palmer C, Robinson O, Walmsley H, Ward R. The effectiveness of exercise for the prevention and treatment of antenatal depression: systematic review with meta-analysis. BJOG. 2015;122(1):57–62.
42. Nakamura A, van der Waerden J, Melchior M, Bolze C, El-Khoury F, Pryor L. Physical activity during pregnancy and postpartum depression: systematic review and meta-analysis. J Affect Disord. 2019;246:29–41.
43. Blaize AN, Pearson KJ, Newcomer SC. Impact of maternal exercise during pregnancy on offspring chronic disease susceptibility. Exerc Sport Sci Rev. 2015;43(4):198–203.
44. SMA - Sport Medicine Australia. SMA statement the benefits and risks of exercise during pregnancy. J Sci Med Sport. 2002;5(1):11–9.
45. CSEP - Canadian Society for Exercise Physiology. Get Active Questionnaire for PREGNANCY. Ottawa, ON: Canadian Society for Exercise Physiology; 2021. https://csep.ca/2021/01/20/pre-screening-forphysical-activity/#. Accessed 6 Aug 2022.
46. PAR-Q+ Collaboration. Physical activity readiness questionnaire for everyone (PAR-Q+). 2017. http://eparmedx.com/. Accessed 9 Mar 2021.
47. ACSM - American College of Sports Medicine. ACSM's resources for the exercise physiologist. 2nd ed. Philadelphia, PA: Wolters Kluwer; 2018, 472 p.
48. ACSM - American College of Sports Medicine. ACSM's resources manual for guidelines for exercise testing and prescription. 7th ed. Philadelphia, PA: Wolters Kluwer, Lippincott Williams & Wilkins; 2014, 862 p.
49. ACSM - American College of Sports Medicine. ACSM's health status & health history questionnaire. Indianapolis, IN: ACSM. http://www.wm.edu/offices/wellness/campusrec/documents/fitnessquestionnaire.pdf. Accessed 3 Sep 2021.
50. Kavanagh JJ, Menz HB. Accelerometry: a technique for quantifying movement patterns during walking. Gait Posture. 2008;28(1):1–15.
51. Braakhuis HEM, Berger MAM, Bussmann JBJ. Effectiveness of healthcare interventions using objective feedback on physical activity: a systematic review and meta-analysis. J Rehabil Med. 2019;51(3):151–9.
52. Tang MSS, Moore K, McGavigan A, Clark RA, Ganesan AN. Effectiveness of wearable trackers on physical activity in healthy adults: systematic review and meta-analysis of randomized controlled trials. JMIR Mhealth Uhealth. 2020;8(7):e15576.
53. Sallis JF, Haskell WL, Wood PD, Fortmann SP, Rogers T, Blair SN. Physical activity assessment methodology in the Five-City Project. Am J Epidemiol. 1985;121:91–106.
54. Craig CL, Marshall AL, Sjostrom M, Bauman AE, Booth ML, Ainsworth BE. International physical activity questionnaire: 12-country reliability and validity. Med Sci Sports Exerc. 2003;35:1381–95.

55. Chasan-Taber L, Schmidt MD, Roberts DE, Hosmer D, Markenson G, Freedson PS. Development and validation of a pregnancy physical activity questionnaire. Med Sci Sports Exerc. 2004;36(10):1750–60.
56. Foxcroft KF, Callaway LK, Byrne NM, Webster J. Development and validation of a pregnancy symptoms inventory. BMC Pregnan Childb. 2013;13:3.
57. Barakat R, Pelaez M, Montejo R, Luaces M, Zakynthinaki M. Exercise during pregnancy improves maternal health perception: a randomized controlled trial. Am J Obstet Gynecol. 2011;204(5):402.e401–7.
58. Smith R, Reid H, Matthews A, Calderwood C, Knight M, Foster C, CMO Physical Activity Expert Committee for Physical Activity and Pregnancy. Infographic: physical activity for pregnant women. Br J Sports Med. 2017;52:532. https://www.gov.uk/government/uploads/system/uploads/attachment_data/file/622335/CMO_physical_activity_pregnant_women_infographic.pdf. Accessed 3 Sep 2021.
59. Kendall-Raynor P. Physical activity for pregnant women. Nurs Stand. 2017;31(46):15.
60. ACOG - American College of Obstetricians and Gynecologists. Your pregnancy and childbirth. 7th ed. Washington, DC: American College of Obstetricians and Gynecologists; 2021.
61. Perales M, Nagpal TS, Barakat R. Physiological changes during pregnancy. Main adaptations and discomforts and implications for physical activity and exercise. In: Santos-Rocha R, editor. Exercise and physical activity during pregnancy and postpartum. Evidence-based guidelines. 2nd ed. Cham: Springer International Publishing; 2022. Chapter 3.
62. Pimenta N, van Poppel M. Body composition changes during pregnancy and effects of physical exercise. In: Santos-Rocha R, editor. Exercise and physical activity during pregnancy and postpartum. Evidence-based guidelines. 2nd ed. Cham: Springer International Publishing; 2022. Chapter 4.
63. Bø K, Stuge B, Hilde G. Specific musculoskeletal adaptations in pregnancy: pelvic floor, pelvic girdle and low back pain. Implications for physical activity and exercise. In: Santos-Rocha R, editor. Exercise and physical activity during pregnancy and postpartum. Evidence-based guidelines. 2nd ed. Cham: Springer International Publishing; 2022. Chapter 6.
64. Fitzgerald CM, Segal NA. Musculoskeletal health in pregnancy and postpartum. Cham: Springer International Publishing; 2015.
65. Branco M, Santos-Rocha R, Aguiar L, Vieira F, Veloso AP. Biomechanical adaptations of gait in pregnancy. Implications for physical activity and exercise. In: Santos-Rocha R, editor. Exercise and physical activity during pregnancy and postpartum. Evidence-based guidelines. 2nd ed. Cham: Springer International Publishing; 2022. Chapter 5.
66. Dennis AT, Salman M, Paxton E, Flint M, Leeton L, Roodt F, Yentis S, Dyer RA. Resting hemodynamics and response to exercise using the 6-minute walk test in late pregnancy: an international prospective multicentre study. Anesth Analg. 2019;129(2):450–7.
67. Wowdzia JB, Davenport MH. Cardiopulmonary exercise testing during pregnancy. Birth Defects Res. 2021;113(3):248–64.
68. O'Toole ML, Artal R. Clinical exercise testing during pregnancy and the postpartum period. In: Weisman IM, Zeballos RJ, editors. Clinical exercise testing (Progress in respiratory research), vol. 32. Basel: Karger; 2002. p. 273–81.
69. Wolfe LA. Pregnancy. In: Skinner JS, editor. Exercise testing and exercise prescription for special cases: theoretical basis and clinical application. 3rd ed. Baltimore, MD: Lippincott Williams & Wilkins; 2005. p. 377–91.
70. Jędrzejko M, Nowosielski K, Poręba R, Ulman-Włodarz I, Bobiński R. Physical efficiency and activity energy expenditure in term pregnancy females measured during cardiopulmonary exercise tests with a supine cycle ergometer. J Matern Fetal Neonatal Med. 2016;29(23):3800–5.
71. Mottola MF, Davenport MH, Brun CR, Inglis SD, Charlesworth S, Stopper MM. VO2peak prediction and exercise prescription for pregnant women. Med Sci Sports Exerc. 2006;38(8):1389–95.
72. Tinius RA, Blankenship M, Maples JM, Pitts BC, Furgal K, Norris ES, Hoover DL, Olenick A, Lambert J, Cade WT. Validity of the 6-minute walk test and YMCA submaximal cycle test during midpregnancy. J Strength Cond Res. 2021;35(11):3236–42.

73. Szumilewicz A, Dornowski M, Piernicka M, Worska A, Kuchta A, Kortas J, Błudnicka M, Radzimiński Ł, Jastrzębski Z. High-low impact exercise program including pelvic floor muscle exercises improves pelvic floor muscle function in healthy pregnant women – a randomized control trial. Front Physiol. 2019;9:1867.
74. Melzer K, Schutz Y, Boulvain M, Kayser B. Physical activity and pregnancy: cardiovascular adaptations, recommendations and pregnancy outcomes. Sports Med. 2010;40(6):493–507.
75. Rikli RE, Jones CJ. Senior fitness test manual. 2nd ed. Champaign, IL: Human Kinetics; 2013.
76. Rose DJ. Fallproof!: a comprehensive balance and mobility training program. 2nd ed. Champaign, IL: Human Kinetics; 2015.
77. Garber CE, Blissmer B, Deschenes MR, Franklin BA, Lamonte MJ, Lee IM, Nieman DC, Swain DP, American College of Sports Medicine. American College of Sports Medicine position stand. Quantity and quality of exercise for developing and maintaining cardiorespiratory, musculoskeletal, and neuromotor fitness in apparently healthy adults: guidance for prescribing exercise. Med Sci Sports Exerc. 2011;43(7):1334–59.
78. Mørkved S, Bø K. Effect of pelvic floor muscle training during pregnancy and after childbirth on prevention and treatment of urinary incontinence: a systematic review. Br J Sports Med. 2014;48(4):299–310.
79. Miquelutti MA, Cecatti JG, Makuch MY. Developing strategies to be added to the protocol for antenatal care: an exercise and birth preparation program. Clinics. 2015;70(4):231–6.
80. Akca A, Corbacioglu Esmer A, Ozyurek ES, Aydin A, Korkmaz N, Gorgen H, Akbayir O. The influence of the systematic birth preparation program on childbirth satisfaction. Arch Gynecol Obstet. 2017;295(5):1127–33.
81. van Poppel M, Owe KM, Santos-Rocha R, Dias H. Physical activity, exercise and health promotion for the pregnant exerciser and the pregnant athlete. In: Santos-Rocha R, editor. Exercise and physical activity during pregnancy and postpartum. Evidence-based guidelines. 2nd ed. Cham: Springer International Publishing; 2022. Chapter 1.
82. Troy KL, Mancuso ME, Butler TA, Johnson JE. Exercise early and often: effects of physical activity and exercise on women's bone health. Int J Environ Res Public Health. 2018;15(5):878.
83. Sañudo B, de Hoyo M, Del Pozo-Cruz J, Carrasco L, Del Pozo-Cruz B, Tejero S, Firth E. A systematic review of the exercise effect on bone health: the importance of assessing mechanical loading in perimenopausal and postmenopausal women. Menopause. 2017;24(10):1208–16.
84. Boyle R, Hay-Smith EJ, Cody JD, Mørkved S. Pelvic floor muscle training for prevention and treatment of urinary and fecal incontinence in antenatal and postnatal women: a short version Cochrane review. Neurourol Urodyn. 2014;33(3):269–76.
85. Guelfi KJ, Ong MJ, Crisp NA, Fournier PA, Wallman KE, Grove JR, Doherty DA, Newnham JP. Regular exercise to prevent the recurrence of gestational diabetes mellitus: a randomized controlled trial. Obstet Gynecol. 2016;128(4):819–27.
86. Wang C, Wei Y, Zhang X, Zhang Y, Xu Q, Sun Y, Su S, Zhang L, Liu C, Feng Y, Shou C, Guelfi KJ, Newnham JP, Yang H. A randomized clinical trial of exercise during pregnancy to prevent gestational diabetes mellitus and improve pregnancy outcome in overweight and obese pregnant women. Am J Obstet Gynecol. 2017;216(4):340–51.
87. Andersen MB, Ovesen PG, Daugaard M, Ostenfeld EB, Fuglsang J. Cycling reduces blood glucose excursions after an oral glucose tolerance test in pregnant women: a randomized crossover trial. Appl Physiol Nutr Metab. 2020;45(11):1247–52.
88. Petrov Fieril K, Glantz A, Fagevik Olsen M. The efficacy of moderate-to-vigorous resistance exercise during pregnancy: a randomized controlled trial. Acta Obstet Gynecol Scand. 2015;94(1):35–42.
89. Barakat R, Perales M. Resistance exercise in pregnancy and outcome. Clin Obstet Gynecol. 2016;59(3):591–9.
90. Keskin Y, Kilic G, Taspinar O, Posul SO, Halac G, Eren F, Erol E, Urkmez B, Aydin T. Effectiveness of home exercise in pregnant women with carpal tunnel syndrome: randomized control trial. J Pak Med Assoc. 2020;70(2):202–7.

91. Mazzarino M, Kerr D, Wajswelner H, Morris ME. Pilates method for women's health: systematic review of randomized controlled trials. Arch Phys Med Rehabil. 2015;96(12):2231–42.
92. Rodríguez-Díaz L, Ruiz-Frutos C, Vázquez-Lara JM, Ramírez-Rodrigo J, Villaverde-Gutiérrez C, Torres-Luque G. Effectiveness of a physical activity programme based on the Pilates method in pregnancy and labour. Enferm Clin. 2017;27(5):271–7. English, Spanish.
93. Hagen S, Glazener C, McClurg D, Macarthur C, Elders A, Herbison P, Wilson D, Toozs-Hobson P, Hemming C, Hay-Smith J, Collins M, Dickson S, Logan J. Pelvic floor muscle training for secondary prevention of pelvic organ prolapse (PREVPROL): a multicentre randomised controlled trial. Lancet. 2017;389(10067):393–402.
94. Sonmezer E, Özköslü MA, Yosmaoğlu HB. The effects of clinical pilates exercises on functional disability, pain, quality of life and lumbopelvic stabilization in pregnant women with low back pain: a randomized controlled study. J Back Musculoskelet Rehabil. 2021;34(1):69–76.
95. Gong H, Ni C, Shen X, Wu T, Jiang C. Yoga for prenatal depression: a systematic review and meta-analysis. BMC Psychiatry. 2015;15:14.
96. Sheffield KM, Woods-Giscombé CL. Efficacy, feasibility, and acceptability of perinatal yoga on women's mental health and well-being: a systematic literature review. J Holist Nurs. 2016;34(1):64–79.
97. Kwon R, Kasper K, London S, Haas DM. A systematic review: the effects of yoga on pregnancy. Eur J Obstet Gynecol Reprod Biol. 2020;250:171–7.
98. Katz VL. Water exercise in pregnancy. Semin Perinatol. 1996;20(4):285–91.
99. Waller B, Lambeck J, Daly D. Therapeutic aquatic exercise in the treatment of low back pain: a systematic review. Clin Rehabil. 2009;23(1):3–14.
100. Rodríguez-Blanque R, Aguilar-Cordero MJ, Marín-Jiménez AE, Menor-Rodríguez MJ, Montiel-Troya M, Sánchez-García JC. Water exercise and quality of life in pregnancy: a randomised clinical trial. Int J Environ Res Public Health. 2020;17(4):1288.
101. Jarski RW, Trippett DL. The risks and benefits of exercise during pregnancy. J Fam Pract. 1990;30(2):185–9.
102. DeMaio M, Magann EF. Exercise and pregnancy. J Am Acad Orthop Surg. 2009;17(8):504–14.
103. Juhl M, Kogevinas M, Andersen PK, Andersen AM, Olsen J. Is swimming during pregnancy a safe exercise? Epidemiology. 2010;21(2):253–8.
104. Kramer MS, McDonald SW. Aerobic exercise for women during pregnancy. Cochrane Database Syst Rev. 2006;(3):CD000180.
105. Lamina S, Agbanusi E. Effect of aerobic exercise training on maternal weight gain in pregnancy: a meta-analysis of randomized controlled trials. Ethiop J Health Sci. 2013;23(1):59–64.
106. Sanders SG. Dancing through pregnancy: activity guidelines for professional and recreational dancers. J Dance Med Sci. 2008;12(1):17–22.
107. Haakstad LA, Bø K. Exercise in pregnant women and birth weight: a randomized controlled trial. BMC Pregnan Childb. 2011;11:66.
108. Jorge C, Santos-Rocha R, Bento T. Can group exercise programs improve health outcomes in pregnant women? A systematic review. Curr Women's Health Rev. 2015;11(1):75–87.
109. ASC - Australian Sports Commission. Pregnancy and sport: guidelines for the Australian sporting industry. Bruce, ACT: ASC; 2002.
110. Szymanski LM, Satin AJ. Strenuous exercise during pregnancy: is there a limit? Am J Obstet Gynecol. 2012;207(3):179.e1–6.
111. Pivarnik JM, Szymanski LM, Conway MR. The elite athlete and strenuous exercise in pregnancy. Clin Obstet Gynecol. 2016;59(3):613–9.
112. Szumilewicz A, Santos-Rocha R. Exercise selection during pregnancy. In: Santos-Rocha R, editor. Exercise and physical activity during pregnancy and postpartum. Evidence-based guidelines. 2nd ed. Cham: Springer International Publishing; 2022. Chapter 9.
113. Gellish RL, Goslin BR, Olson RE, McDonald A, Russi GD, Moudgil VK. Longitudinal modeling of the relationship between age and maximal heart rate. Med Sci Sports Exerc. 2007;39(5):822–9.
114. Centers for Disease Control and Prevention. Perceived exertion (Borg rating of perceived exertion scale). Atlanta, GA: CDC. http://www.cdc.gov/physicalactivity/basics/measuring/exertion.htm. Accessed 3 Sep 2021.

115. Persinger R, Foster C, Gibson M, Fater DC, Porcari JP. Consistency of the talk test for exercise prescription. Med Sci Sports Exerc. 2004;36(9):1632–6.
116. Tudor-Locke C, Hatano Y, Pangrazi RP, Kang M. Revisiting "how many steps are enough?". Med Sci Sports Exerc. 2008;40(7 Suppl):S537–43.
117. Mottola MF. Physical activity and maternal obesity: cardiovascular adaptations, exercise recommendations, and pregnancy outcomes. Nutr Rev. 2013;71(Suppl 1):S31–6.
118. Santos-Rocha R. Ativo em Casa / Active at Home. YouTube Channel. https://www.youtube.com/channel/UCEUWdoBeh5rgfM0kZOn9Xtg/videos.
119. Santos-Rocha R, Fernandes de Carvalho M, Prior de Freitas J. Gravidez Ativa - Active Pregnancy. YouTube Channel. https://www.youtube.com/channel/UC0VyookwcOmcQ5T70imtoNA/playlists.
120. Miquelutti MA, Cecatti JG, Makuch MY. Evaluation of a birth preparation program on lumbopelvic pain, urinary incontinence, anxiety and exercise: a randomized controlled trial. BMC Pregnan Childb. 2013;13:154.
121. Sichani LE, Bahadoran P, Fahami F, Esfahani PS. The investigation of effects of static immersion and calming in water on pregnant women's stress participating in preparation classes for childbirth. J Educ Health Promot. 2019;8:238.
122. Sivan E, Homko CJ, Chen XH, Reece EA, Boden G. Effect of insulin on fat metabolism during and after normal pregnancy. Diabetes. 1999;48(4):834–8.
123. Zhang CL, Ning Y. Effect of dietary and lifestyle factors on the risk of gestational diabetes: review of epidemiologic evidence. Am J Clin Nutr. 2011;94(6):1975S–9S.
124. Association AD. Standards of medical care in diabetes—2016. Diabetes Care. 2016;39(Suppl 1):S1–S106.
125. IDF. Diabetes atlas. 7th ed. Brussels: IDF; 2015.
126. Carolan-Olah MC. Educational and intervention programmes for gestational diabetes mellitus (GDM) management: an integrative review. Collegian. 2016;23:103–14.
127. Pettit D, Bennett PH, Knowler WC, et al. Gestational diabetes mellitus and impaired glucose tolerance during pregnancy: long-term effects on obesity and glucose intolerance in the offspring. Diabetes Care. 1985;34:119–22.
128. Horvath K, Koch K, Jeitler K, et al. Effects of treatment in women with gestational diabetes mellitus: systematic review and meta-analysis. BMJ. 2010;340:1395.
129. Russo LM, Nobles C, Ertel KA, et al. Physical activity interventions in pregnancy and risk of gestational diabetes mellitus: a systematic review and meta-analysis. Obstet Gynecol. 2015;125:576–82.
130. Brankston GN, Mitchell BF, Ryan EA, Okun NB. Resistance exercise decreases the need for insulin in overweight women with gestational diabetes mellitus. Am J Obstet Gynecol. 2004;190(1):188–93.
131. Barakat R, Cordero Y, Coteron J, Luaces M, Montejo R. Exercise during pregnancy improves maternal glucose screen at 24-28 weeks: a randomised controlled trial. Br J Sports Med. 2012;46(9):656–61.
132. Sanabria-Martínez G, García-Hermoso A, Poyatos-León R, Álvarez-Bueno C, Sánchez-López M, Martínez-Vizcaíno V. Effectiveness of physical activity interventions on preventing gestational diabetes mellitus and excessive maternal weight gain: a meta-analysis. BJOG. 2015;122(9):1167–74.
133. Bgeginski R, Ribeiro PAB, Mottola MF, Ramos JGL. Effects of weekly supervised exercise or physical activity counseling on fasting blood glucose in women diagnosed with gestational diabetes mellitus: a systematic review and meta-analysis of randomized trials. J Diabetes. 2017;9:1023–32.
134. Brown J, Ceysens G, Boulvain M. Exercise for pregnant women with gestational diabetes for improving maternal and fetal outcomes. Cochrane Database Syst Rev. 2017;6(6):CD012202.
135. Shepherd E, Gomersall JC, Tieu J, Han S, Crowther CA, Middleton P. Combined diet and exercise interventions for preventing gestational diabetes mellitus. Cochrane Database Syst Rev. 2017;11(11):CD010443.

136. Davenport MH, Ruchat SM, Poitras VJ, Jaramillo Garcia A, Gray CE, Barrowman N, Skow RJ, Meah VL, Riske L, Sobierajski F, James M, Kathol AJ, Nuspl M, Marchand AA, Nagpal TS, Slater LG, Weeks A, Adamo KB, Davies GA, Barakat R, Mottola MF. Prenatal exercise for the prevention of gestational diabetes mellitus and hypertensive disorders of pregnancy: a systematic review and meta-analysis. Br J Sports Med. 2018;52(21):1367–75.
137. Ribeiro MM, Andrade A, Nunes I. Physical exercise in pregnancy: benefits, risks and prescription. J Perinat Med. 2021;50:4.
138. Choi J, Fukuoka Y, Lee JH. The effects of physical activity and physical activity plus diet interventions on body weight in overweight or obese women who are pregnant or in postpartum: a systematic review and meta analysis of randomized controlled trials. Prev Med. 2013;56(6):351–64.
139. ACOG - American College of Obstetricians and Gynecologists. Obesity and pregnancy. ACOG Committee opinion No. 549. American College of Obstetricians and Gynecologists. Obstet Gynecol. 2013;121:213–7.
140. Mottola MF, Giroux I, Gratton R, et al. Nutrition and exercise prevent excess weight gain in overweight pregnant women. Med Sci Sports Exerc. 2010;42(2):265–72.
141. Renault KM, Norgaard K, Nilas L, Carlsen EM, Cortes D, Pryds O, et al. The treatment of Obese Pregnant women (TOP) study: a randomized controlled trial of the effect of physical activity intervention assessed by pedometer with or without dietary intervention in obese pregnant women. Am J Obstet Gynecol. 2014;210:134.e1–9.
142. International Weight Management in Pregnancy (i-WIP) Collaborative Group. Effect of diet and physical activity based interventions in pregnancy on gestational weight gain and pregnancy outcomes: meta-analysis of individual participant data from randomised trials. BMJ. 2017;358:j3119.
143. Ruchat SM, Mottola MF, Skow RJ, Nagpal TS, Meah VL, James M, Riske L, Sobierajski F, Kathol AJ, Marchand AA, Nuspl M, Weeks A, Gray CE, Poitras VJ, Jaramillo Garcia A, Barrowman N, Slater LG, Adamo KB, Davies GA, Barakat R, Davenport MH. Effectiveness of exercise interventions in the prevention of excessive gestational weight gain and postpartum weight retention: a systematic review and meta-analysis. Br J Sports Med. 2018;52(21):1347–56.
144. Say L, Chou D, Gemmill A, et al. Global causes of maternal death: a WHO systematic analysis. Lancet Glob Health. 2014;2(6):e323–33.
145. Gillon TE, Pels A, von Dadelszen P, et al. Hypertensive disorders of pregnancy: a systematic review of international clinical practice guidelines. PLoS One. 2014;9(12):e113715.
146. Berzan E, Doyle R, Brown CM. Treatment of preeclampsia: current approach and future perspectives. Curr Hypertens Rep. 2014;16(9):473.
147. Djurisic S, Hviid TV. HLA class Ib molecules and immune cells in pregnancy and preeclampsia. Front Immunol. 2014;5:652.
148. Mparmpakas D, Goumenou A, Zachariades E, et al. Immune system function, stress, exercise and nutrition profile can affect pregnancy outcome: lessons from a Mediterranean cohort. Exp Ther Med. 2013;5(2):411–8.
149. Chawla S, Anim-Nyame N. Advice on exercise for pregnant women with hypertensive disorders of pregnancy. Int J Gynaecol Obstet. 2015;128(3):275–9.
150. Abu MA, Abdul Ghani NA, Lim Pei S, Sulaiman AS, Omar MH, Muhamad Ariffin MH, et al. Do exercises improve back pain in pregnancy? Horm Mol Biol Clin Invest. 2017;32(3):1–7.
151. Watelain E, Pinti A, Doya R, Garnier C, Toumi H, Boudet S. Benefits of physical activities centered on the trunk for pregnant women. Phys Sportsmed. 2017;45(3):293–302.
152. Sklempe Kokic I, Ivanisevic M, Uremovic M, Kokic T, Pisot R, Simunic B. Effect of therapeutic exercises on pregnancy-related low back pain and pelvic girdle pain: secondary analysis of a randomized controlled trial. J Rehabil Med. 2017;49(3):251–7.
153. Shiri R, Coggon D, Falah-Hassani K. Exercise for the prevention of low back and pelvic girdle pain in pregnancy: a meta-analysis of randomized controlled trials. Eur J Pain. 2018;22(1):19–27.

154. Bishop A, Holden MA, Ogollah RO, Foster NE. Current management of pregnancy-related low back pain: a national cross-sectional survey of U.K. physiotherapists. Physiotherapy. 2016;102(1):78–85.
155. Liddle SD, Pennick V. Interventions for preventing and treating low-back and pelvic pain during pregnancy. Cochrane Database Syst Rev. 2015;(9):CD001139.
156. Davenport MH, Marchand AA, Mottola MF, Poitras VJ, Gray CE, Jaramillo Garcia A, Barrowman N, Sobierajski F, James M, Meah VL, Skow RJ, Riske L, Nuspl M, Nagpal TS, Courbalay A, Slater LG, Adamo KB, Davies GA, Barakat R, Ruchat SM. Exercise for the prevention and treatment of low back, pelvic girdle and lumbopelvic pain during pregnancy: a systematic review and meta-analysis. Br J Sports Med. 2019;53(2):90–8.
157. Ohman SG, Grunewald C, Waldenstrom U. Women's worries during pregnancy: testing the Cambridge Worry Scale on 200 Swedish women. Scand J Caring Sci. 2003;17(2):148–52.
158. Gavin N, Gaynes BN, Lohr KN, Meltzer-Brody S. Perinatal depression: a systematic review of prevalence and incidence. Obstet Gynecol. 2005;106(5):1071–83.
159. Bennett HA, Einarsson A, Taddio A. Prevalence of depression during pregnancy: systematic review. Obstet Gynecol. 2006;103(4):698–709.
160. Trivedi MH, Greer TL, Grannemann BD, Chambliss HO, Jordan AN. Exercise as an augmentation strategy for treatment of major depression. J Psychiatr Pract. 2006;12:205–13.
161. Padmapriya N, Bernard J, Liang S, Loy S, Shen Z, Kwek K, et al. Association of physical activity and sedentary behavior with depression and anxiety symptoms during pregnancy in a multiethnic cohort of Asian women. Archiv Women's Ment Health. 2016;19(6):1119–28.
162. McCurdy AP, Boulé NG, Sivak A, Davenport MH. Effects of exercise on mild-to-moderate depressive symptoms in the postpartum period: a meta-analysis. Obstet Gynecol. 2017;129:1087.
163. Davenport MH, McCurdy AP, Mottola MF, Skow RJ, Meah VL, Poitras VJ, Jaramillo Garcia A, Gray CE, Barrowman N, Riske L, Sobierajski F, James M, Nagpal T, Marchand AA, Nuspl M, Slater LG, Barakat R, Adamo KB, Davies GA, Ruchat SM. Impact of prenatal exercise on both prenatal and postnatal anxiety and depressive symptoms: a systematic review and meta-analysis. Br J Sports Med. 2018;52(21):1376–85.
164. Davenport MH, Meyer S, Meah VL, Strynadka MC, Khurana R. Moms are not OK. COVID-19 and maternal mental health. Front Glob Women's Health. 2020;1:1.
165. Gildner TE, Laugier EJ, Thayer ZM. Exercise routine change is associated with prenatal depression scores during the COVID-19 pandemic among pregnant women across the United States. PLoS One. 2020;15(12):1–15.
166. Atkinson L, De Vivo M, Hayes L, Hesketh KR, Mills H, Newham JJ, et al. Encouraging physical activity during and after pregnancy in the COVID-19 era, and beyond. Int J Environ Res Public Health. 2020;17(19):7304.
167. Silva MRG, Rodriguez Doñate B, Che Carballo KN. Nutritional requirements for the pregnant exerciser and athlete. In: Santos-Rocha R, editor. Exercise and physical activity during pregnancy and postpartum. Evidence-based guidelines. 2nd ed. Cham: Springer International Publishing; 2022. Chapter 13.
168. Jorge R, Teixeira D, Ferreira I, Alvarez-Fálcon AL. Diet recommendations for the pregnant exerciser and athlete. In: Santos-Rocha R, editor. Exercise and physical activity during pregnancy and postpartum. Evidence-based guidelines. 2nd ed. Cham: Springer International Publishing; 2022. Chapter 14.
169. Institute of Medicine (US) and National Research Council (US) Committee to reexamine IOM pregnancy weight guidelines, Rasmussen KM, Yaktine AL. Weight gain during pregnancy: reexamining the guidelines. Washington, DC: National Academies Press; 2009. https://www.ncbi.nlm.nih.gov/books/NBK32813/. Accessed 15 Sep 2021.
170. Yang X, Zhang A, Sayer L, Bassett S, Woodward S. The effectiveness of group-based pelvic floor muscle training in preventing and treating urinary incontinence for antenatal and postnatal women: a systematic review. Int Urogynecol J. 2021;33:1407.

171. Woodley SJ, Lawrenson P, Boyle R, Cody JD, Mørkved S, Kernohan A, Hay-Smith EJC. Pelvic floor muscle training for preventing and treating urinary and faecal incontinence in antenatal and postnatal women. Cochrane Database Syst Rev. 2020;5(5):CD007471.
172. American College of Sports Medicine, Sawka MN, Burke LM, et al. American College of Sports Medicine position stand. Exercise and fluid replacement. Med Sci Sports Exerc. 2007;39(2):377–90.
173. Schauberger CW, Rooney BL, Goldsmith L, Shenton D, Silva PD, Schaper A. Peripheral joint laxity increases in pregnancy but does not correlate with serum relaxin levels. Am J Obstet Gynecol. 1996;174(2):667–71.
174. Dumas GA, Reid JG. Laxity of knee cruciate ligaments during pregnancy. J Orthop Sports Phys Therapy. 1997;26(1):2–6.
175. Ebi KL, Capon A, Berry P, Broderick C, de Dear R, Havenith G, Honda Y, Kovats RS, Ma W, Malik A, Morris NB, Nybo L, Seneviratne SI, Vanos J, Jay O. Hot weather and heat extremes: health risks. Lancet. 2021;398(10301):698–708.
176. Dervis S, Dobson KL, Nagpal TS, Geurts C, Haman F, Adamo KB. Heat loss responses at rest and during exercise in pregnancy: a scoping review. J Therm Biol. 2021;99:103011.
177. Branco M, Santos-Rocha R, Vieira F. Biomechanics of gait during pregnancy. Sci World J. 2014;2014:527940.
178. Gimunová M, Zvonař M, Sebera M, Turčínek P, Kolářová K. Special footwear designed for pregnant women and its effect on kinematic gait parameters during pregnancy and postpartum period. PLoS One. 2020;15(5):e0232901.
179. Petrov Fieril K, Fagevik Olsén M, Glantz A, Larsson M. Experiences of exercise during pregnancy among women who perform regular resistance training: a qualitative study. Phys Ther. 2014;94(8):1135–43.
180. Harrison CL, Brown WJ, Hayman M, Moran LJ, Redman LM. The role of physical activity in preconception, pregnancy and postpartum health. Semin Reprod Med. 2016;34(2):e28–37.
181. Díaz-Burrueco JR, Cano-Ibáñez N, Martín-Peláez S, Khan KS, Amezcua-Prieto C. Effects on the maternal-fetal health outcomes of various physical activity types in healthy pregnant women. A systematic review and meta-analysis. Eur J Obstet Gynecol Reprod Biol. 2021;262:203–15.
182. Kehler AK, Heinrich KM. A selective review of prenatal exercise guidelines since the 1950s until present: written for women, health care professionals, and female athletes. Women Birth. 2015;28(4):e93–8.
183. Craig P, Dieppe P, Macintyre S, Michie S, Nazareth I, Petticrew M. Developing and evaluating complex interventions: the new Medical Research Council guidance. Int J Nurs Stud. 2013;50(5):587–92.
184. Möhler R, Köpke S, Meyer G. Criteria for reporting the development and evaluation of complex interventions in healthcare: revised guideline (CReDECI 2). Trials. 2015;16:204.
185. Slade SC, Dionne CE, Underwood M, Buchbinder R. Consensus on exercise reporting template (CERT): explanation and elaboration statement. Br J Sports Med. 2016;50:1428–37.
186. Santos-Rocha R, Fernandes de Carvalho M, Szumilewicz A. Active pregnancy - a physical exercise program aimed at promoting health and fitness during pregnancy. Development and validation of a complex intervention. Int J Environ Res Public Health. 2022;19:4902.
187. Biviji R, Williams KS, Vest JR, Dixon BE, Cullen T, Harle CA. Consumer perspectives on maternal and infant health apps: qualitative content analysis. J Med Internet Res. 2021;23(9):e27403.

Exercise Selection and Adaptations During Pregnancy

9

Anna Szumilewicz and Rita Santos-Rocha

Abstract

There are several guidelines supporting the benefits of exercising during pregnancy. Those documents contain very general recommendations on physical activity and exercise during pregnancy, such as general guidelines for health screening and prescription of aerobic exercise and strength training. They also include examples of safe physical activities during pregnancy, such as walking, running, swimming, stationary cycling, aerobics, modified yoga, and Pilates. However, those guidelines contain little information that exercise professionals could use when programming the contents of targeted exercise classes for pregnant women. This chapter addresses the steps for planning, conducting, and monitoring prenatal exercise classes, and explains how to select and adapt the exercises making them safe physical activities during pregnancy.

Keywords

Pregnancy · Exercise · Physical activity · Aerobics · Resistance · Flexibility
Functional · Neuromotor · Balance · Posture · Pelvic floor muscle training
Breathing · Fitness · Exercise planning

A. Szumilewicz (✉)
Gdansk University of Physical Education and Sport, Gdańsk, Poland
e-mail: anna.szumilewicz@awfis.gda.pl

R. Santos-Rocha
Sport Sciences School of Rio Maior - ESDRM, Polytechnic Institute of Santarém, Rio Maior, Portugal

Laboratory of Biomechanics and Functional Morphology, Interdisciplinary Centre for the Study of Human Performance - CIPER, Faculty of Human Kinetics - FMH, University of Lisbon, Lisbon, Portugal
e-mail: ritasantosrocha@esdrm.ipsantarem.pt

R. Santos-Rocha (ed.), *Exercise and Physical Activity During Pregnancy and Postpartum*, https://doi.org/10.1007/978-3-031-06137-0_9

9.1 Introduction

Scientific research conducted in the last decades has markedly changed the perception of prenatal physical activity. The conservative approach presented in the 1990s, which could significantly limit exercise during pregnancy [1], now appears to be detrimental to the health of women and their children. In current recommendations, prenatal physical activity is considered a necessary condition for normal pregnancy and fetal development. What is more, physical inactivity in pregnancy is a risky behavior [2, 3]. Exercise in pregnancy is not so much a luxury for the few women, but the responsibility of every future mother.

In the light of available research, the current question is not "if," but "how" a woman should exercise in pregnancy. A literature review from a few years ago [4] indicated that publicly available recommendations on prenatal physical activity did not provide answers on which exercises to choose and how they should be performed. Divergent, often unfounded information undermined the safety of certain exercises or modes of physical activity, higher intensities, and training loads. While the guidelines published in the last 5 years are far more progressive, there are still conflicting views in society about exercise in pregnancy. In addition, misguided social pressure may be a reason why pregnant women ill-advisedly reduce their physical activity because of the fear of the child's health [5, 6]. It should be noted that there is no clear scientific evidence that some sports activities or particular exercises are indeed dangerous for pregnancy and fetal development. The classification of the modes of physical activity as "not recommended for pregnant women" is rather due to the excessively cautious attitude. Medical experts who took part in the National Forum on Pregnancy and Sport in 2001 in Sydney advised that "damage to the womb of the kind that could injure an unborn child is usually associated with forces equivalent to those occurring in a car accident. All medical experts agreed that falls and direct contact of the kinds that occur during contact sports were unlikely to cause damage to the womb or the unborn child" [7].

Considering the above, there is no reason for a woman to give up a mode of physical activity or a particular exercise just because she has become pregnant. Certainly, one should minimize the risk of injury, bearing in mind that in pregnancy medical interventions, including the use of certain medications are limited. "Common sense" suggests that pregnancy is not the time to take part in new activities, especially if they are technically difficult. However, if a woman believes that her technical skills provide a sense of security and comfort and she has no medical contraindications, she may continue her current physical activity. An excellent example is a top tennis player Serena Williams who revealed in April 2017 that she was 20 weeks pregnant when she won the Australian Open [8].

The updated guidelines for physical activity are addressed in Chap. 7 by Szumilewicz et al. [9]. Chapter 8 by Santos-Rocha et al. [10] addresses and discusses the current knowledge on exercise testing and prescription for pregnant women. In this chapter, we present the general principles of planning and implementation of prenatal physical activity and suggestions for exercise adaptation. Exercise in pregnancy not only should be safe but also potentially effective for preventing and relieving typical pregnancy ailments and preparing a woman for childbirth and maternity [4]. We emphasize that the following suggestions do not exhaust the extensive list of exercises that pregnant women can perform. Guidelines for planning and implementing an exercise program for women with pregnancies at risk require a separate evidence-based description.

9.2 Planning, Conducting, and Monitoring of the Prenatal Exercise Sessions

According to the recommendations of World Health Organization [11] and the U.S. Department of Human and Health Services [12], the beneficial effects of exercise in most adults, including special populations and people with chronic conditions are indisputable and the benefits far outweigh the risks. Due to the health benefits of regular physical activity, it is best if it is taken continuously for several months before becoming pregnant, and then throughout pregnancy, postpartum and early motherhood, to smoothly go into lifelong activity until late age.

Unfortunately, after becoming pregnant by the end of the first trimester, many women stop exercising or significantly reduce the training load for fear of miscarriage. In the first trimester, the risk of spontaneous abortion is about 10% [13]. According to the available data, neither the continuation of recreational exercise will increase the risk of miscarriage nor its interruption will lower it [14]. Research indicates that there are no significant differences in the early miscarriage rate between recreational runners, aerobics participants, and physically active, fit controls [15]. It is scientifically justified to think that bounces associated with running or jumping can hinder implantation. Therefore, inter alia due to the alleviation of pregnancy symptoms, prenatal physical activity should be undertaken from the day of conception.

Before starting the exercises, obstetrician–gynecologists and other obstetric care providers should carefully evaluate women with medical or obstetric complications. If no such complications exist [16], both active and inactive women should be encouraged by the medical staff to take up the prenatal exercises. According to current guidelines, women with complicated pregnancies also should continue their normal everyday activity and modify their exercise programs, where necessary (see Chaps. 7 and 9). Close cooperation with qualified prenatal exercise specialists is recommended here. They will plan the right type, intensity, frequency, and duration of exercise (see Chaps. 8 and 10). Both professional groups should educate women and do their best to refute myths limiting prenatal physical activity. By participating in various forms of activity, women should be convinced of their safety and positive impact on the course of pregnancy and child development.

In working with pregnant women, it should be taken into account that the body is additionally burdened by the development of pregnancy, which significantly determines its response to exercise, manifested, among others, in larger fluctuations in heart rate and respiratory rate [17–20]. It significantly alters the management of the intensity of each training session, which sometimes requires extended warm-up. It should also be considered that owing to weight gain, the woman performing at the same exercise has greater training load in the same unit of time compared to the preconception period [21]. Therefore, reducing the time for physical activity or number of exercise repetition is not always associated with limiting physical effort.

In exercise planning, the exercise positions should be properly selected. An exercise specialist should consider both exercise purpose, external conditions (e.g., outdoor activities, available equipment in the rooms), and, most importantly, the well-being of the woman. To ensure the versatility of muscle work, good blood flow in the woman's body and the attractiveness of exercises, it is good practice to use frequent changes of position. When planning exercises for women in the second and third trimesters, it is worth taking into account that changing positions alone is associated with physical effort and sometimes requires slightly longer time than in non-pregnant women. We have described selected positions for pregnant women in Appendix 1. Nevertheless, a pregnant woman does not have to limit herself to them.

Pregnant women should be informed, not only what is the correct technique of each exercise, but also how to modify it in case of discomfort during its execution. It is good practice to propose various versions of the exercises, considering trimester of pregnancy and its progress, the level of skills and abilities of a woman. Due to continuous morphological, biomechanical, and physiological changes in the woman's body, the same exercises on different days may be differently received in terms of comfort. In exercising, women should take into account both the suggestions of an exercise specialist and signals from their bodies. Especially they should be sensitive to the warning signs that indicate the need to immediately stop exercising (see Chaps. 8, 10, and 16).

To participate in prenatal physical activity, a woman should be well nourished and hydrated according to recommendations for proper nutrition during pregnancy [22]. In each exercise session, one should plan rest breaks, inter alia to refill the fluids, depending on the volume and intensity of the exercise (e.g., 3–4 breaks during a 60-min session). If necessary, a woman should rest more often, according to her own well-being. If she exercises under the supervision of an exercise specialist, she should report any discomfort to this professional, thus enabling proper selection and modification of the physical activity program. A woman should also follow the norms of nighttime sleep and proper rest after the exercise session. The general recommendation is to have rest time during the day equal to the duration of the exercise session [23].

Women should use training clothing and footwear and sports equipment appropriate for the given form of physical activity, the temperature of the environment of the exercise, and its intensity. In addition to paying attention to the increasing abdominal circumference, the same rules apply as for the general adult population. In the case of beginners, in the selection of clothing and equipment, it is recommended to consult a specialist in a given form of physical activity. At the end of pregnancy, an abdominal support and an extra bra may be useful to ensure the greatest possible stabilization for the growing abdomen and sore tender breasts.

The appropriate level of the individual training components should be regularly monitored and evaluated according to the observed progress [23]. The most

Table 9.1 Exercise monitoring card

Exercise monitoring card								
Name and surname:					Date of the first classes			
Date	Form of physical activity*	The duration of exercise	Subjective intensity perception at RPE scale**		Rest time after exercise***	Well-being during or after classes /comments	The reason for absence	Participant's signature
			Aerobic part	Resistance part				
Example	Total body condition class	60–min	7	6	60–min	Good or e.g., backpain after exercise		

[a]You should enter all forms of physical activity, also individually taken, e.g., walking, cycling
[b]A women should use the RPE scale from 0–10 or 6–20, according to exercise specialist's instructions
[c]Rest time after exercises (entered at the next class)

significant effects are typically observed during the first 6–8 weeks of an exercise program [24]. The following is a useful tool to monitor and record a pregnant woman's well-being during and after exercise session (Table 9.1).

9.3 The Structure of the Exercise Session for Pregnant Women

The important purpose of prenatal physical activity is to stimulate the positive development of pregnancy, provide the greatest possible well-being for the future mother, and prepare her for childbirth and postpartum. Therefore, each training session should include several elements. A combination of aerobic and resistance exercises during pregnancy seems to induce the most favorable effect on maternal health during pregnancy [25, 26]. A pregnant woman should also perform flexibility, body posture, neuromotor, and pelvic-floor muscle exercises. Preparation for birth part, including breathing exercises, relaxation, birth visualization and birth position is recommended, as well [27–31].

Prenatal exercise sessions are usually scheduled for 45 to 90 min, depending on the capacity of the women. The recommended structure of the 60–90 min class is as follows:

1. Warm-up (7–10 min).
2. Aerobic exercise, e.g., low or high–low impact aerobics, walking or jogging on a treadmill, stationary cycling (15–20 min).
3. Resistance exercises (including abdominals exercises), postural and neuromotor (e.g., body balance) exercises (10–15 min).
4. Stretching exercises (5–10 min).
5. Pelvic floor exercises (5–10 min).

6. Cool down and preparation for birth exercises, e.g., birth position and breathing exercises (5–10 min) and also relaxation and visualization of pregnancy and childbirth (5–15 min).

Aerobic exercise may be substituted by anaerobic exercise, e.g., in a form of High-Intensity Interval Training (HIIT). Resistance exercises, involving large muscle groups, are usually used in the high-intensity exercise intervals. The prenatal HIIT classes usually are scheduled for 30–60 min. The structure of the prenatal HIIT classes may be as follows:

1. Warm-up (5–7 min).
2. High-intensity exercise intervals alternate with rest breaks (15–20 min).
3. Postural, neuromotor (e.g., body balance) and stretching exercises (5–10 min). These exercises can be performed during the rest break after high-intensity exercise intervals.
4. Pelvic floor exercises (5–10 min).
5. Cool down and preparation for birth exercises, e.g., birth position and breathing exercises (5–10 min) and also relaxation and visualization of pregnancy and childbirth (5–15 min).

9.3.1 Warm-Up

The main task of the warm-up part for prenatal activities is, as in any other activity, psychophysical preparation for the more rigorous demands of the cardiorespiratory and muscular and conditioning parts of the exercise session. The recommended time is 7–10 min. In warm-up, pregnant woman should pay attention to several elements:

1. Before each activity, the woman should make a self-assessment of her well-being. Even in normal pregnancies, there are occasional discomforts (e.g., dizziness, abdominal pain, and any other pain), which may indicate, for example, fatigue or a beginning of an infection. On such days, it is worthwhile to extend the warm-up, lower the intensity of exercise, or maybe even give up exercises. Observations, however, suggest that moderate physical activity improves the well-being of pregnant women [32, 33]. Therefore, the decision to give up exercise on a given day should not be taken too hastily.
2. It is good to start with the correction of body posture so as not to fix the posture defects in the course of further exercise [34]. Posture exercises improve body awareness [35] and it is likely that women will be more sensitive to signals from their body. This, in turn, can affect the effectiveness and safety of exercise.
3. During warm-up, simple, rehearsal moves should dominate, engaging all large muscle groups. These can be marches or runs, supplemented by arm swings or circulations. Aerobics moves can be used too. When music is used in the warm-up, the recommended tempo is 120–136 beats per minute [36].
4. Already during the warm-up, a woman should consciously activate the pelvic-floor muscles to practice how to prevent the urinary leakage in more intensive exercise in the main part of the exercise class.

5. In the warm-up, pregnant women should perform breathing exercises. First, as in general population, these exercises should help to supply more oxygen during increased muscle work. Secondly, the diaphragm, the major muscle involved in breathing, is like any muscle group and needs time to speed up its work. It is particularly important in the second and third trimesters, when the growing womb hinders the lowering of the diaphragm during inhalation. Thirdly, breathing exercises help a woman reduce discomfort associated with a feeling of breathlessness appearing at the beginning of physical exertion. This feeling is the result of elevated levels of progesterone, which initiates "overbreathing" by increasing the sensitivity of the central chemoreflex control of breathing to carbon dioxide [37]. Although this is often not pleasant for pregnant women, it increases the efficiency of oxygen uptake from the lungs and the elimination of carbon dioxide from the blood of mother and baby [23].
6. Due to continuous changes in the circulatory system throughout the pregnancy, the increase in intensity during warm-up should be gradual. Especially at the very beginning of pregnancy, when the vessels are already relaxed and dilated and the volume of blood has not yet caught up, the heart rate may be extremely high at one's usual intensity [23].
7. At the end of the warm-up, the woman should re-evaluate her well-being and readiness for greater physical effort in the main part of the class. It is also time to consume the fluids.
8. If the class is performed by an exercise professional, it is a good time to present to the participants the target of the main part of the exercise session, as well as provide important training tips, such as the importance of maintaining proper posture, proper breathing, monitoring exercise intensity and well-being, and fluid refills. Exercise professional also reminds women of the warning signs for immediate discontinuation of exercises and customization of exercises to individual capabilities.

Examples of warm-up section:

https://youtu.be/h11NnFDPlfs
https://youtu.be/tq5PwcTBuVE
https://youtu.be/Ca0uL5f2zQ8
https://youtu.be/VlEVuBD1LTk
https://youtu.be/_Hg6Trdhn0M
https://youtu.be/0Vvlojbxmag
https://youtu.be/aR7hJp9MhcI

9.3.2 Aerobic Exercise

According to the current guidelines [3, 11, 12, 38–41], healthy pregnant women should perform at least 150 min per week of moderate-intensity aerobic activity (i.e., equivalent to brisk walking). This activity should be spread throughout the week and adjusted as medically indicated. The guidelines advise that "the pregnant women who habitually engage in vigorous-intensity aerobic activity (i.e., the equivalent of running or jogging) or who are highly active can continue physical activity during pregnancy and the postpartum period, provided that they remain healthy and discuss with their health care provider how and when activity should be adjusted over time" [3, 11, 42]. Women who did not exercise before pregnancy should be encouraged to do physical activity at least three times a week starting from 15-min sessions, gradually lengthening them [16]. Aerobic exercise for pregnant women can be implemented in various forms, depending on the skills and abilities of women.

Typically, aerobic exercises are those that involve the use of large muscle groups in a repetitive or rhythmic fashion. Examples of aerobic activities include walking, jogging, running, cycling, swimming, and using aerobic-based machines, e.g., stair climber, elliptical machines [34]. Some activities are weight-dependent, meaning that body weight is moved during the exercise (e.g., walking, running). In other activities, body weight is not a factor because the body is supported (e.g., cycling, swimming). These activities are referred to as weight-bearing and non-weight-bearing exercises, respectively. The use of non-weight-bearing exercises may be particularly useful for women at the end of gestation due to the increasing body weight.

According to ACSM, endurance activities have been classified into four groups. Group A includes endurance activities that require minimal skill or fitness to perform, e.g., walking. These activities can easily accommodate individual fitness levels and thus are recommended for all adults, especially for beginners. Based on the review of guidelines on exercise in pregnancy [4], walking was the most frequently recommended form of physical activity for pregnant women (see Chaps. 7 and 9). Group B activities are those that require minimal skill but, in contrast to Group A activities, are typically performed at a more vigorous intensity, like jogging and running. Group B activities are appropriate for those who exercise regularly and who have at least an average level of fitness. Although in some countries jogging and running are considered as appropriate forms of physical activity for women during pregnancy, in other countries, the sight of a running pregnant woman is controversial. It should be emphasized that fears of miscarriage resulting from repetitive bounces typical for more vigorous exercises have not been confirmed in scientific research. Already in the 1980s, Clapp [15] observed that the rate of early pregnancy loss in recreational runners was even lower, although not statistically significant, than in controls (17 vs. 23%, respectively).

Examples of Group C activities are swimming and cross-country skiing. This group reflects activities that have a high relationship between skill and energy expenditure. For example, an experienced swimmer may be able to easily swim at a constant intensity, whereas a person with poor swimming skill would be very inefficient and would struggle to swim at an appropriate and constant intensity to gain cardiorespiratory benefits [34]. Swimming was the second, most frequently proposed exercise in pregnancy [4], mainly due to its non-weight-bearing form. However, due to the risk of genital tract infections in public swimming pools, not all women can participate in water activities. Other forms of movement from group C should be popularized for those pregnant women who regularly took part in them before conception.

Recreational sports like basketball, soccer, tennis, and other racquet sports are classified as Group D activities. These activities are typically vigorous and intermittent. The nature of these activities does not lend themselves to constant, controlled intensity levels. This is even more true when competition is involved. Activities from group D usually are on the list of "not recommended" forms of exercise for pregnant women (see Chaps. 7 and 9), although not much data is available on their potential risk.

We presented the most popular aerobic forms of prenatal physical activity below.

9.3.2.1 Aerobics

In an aerobics class, participants perform movements that work the large muscle groups to promote cardiorespiratory fitness and its benefits. These movements are traditionally dancelike and can be executed while keeping 1 ft on the floor at all times (low impact) or while jumping (high impact). Classes mixing high- and low-impact movements are labeled as high–low (or hi-lo) aerobics. A skilled exercise specialist is able to teach low- or high-impact options of movements in one choreography so that even in group classes, it is possible to adjust the intensity of exercise to the individual needs of the participants [36]. Music sets the cadence and rhythm of the moves [43]. Official guidelines on exercise in pregnancy from different countries advice women aerobics as a form of cardio exercise; however, several older guidelines limited this recommendation to low-impact aerobics [4].

Several authors have observed that low-impact aerobics is safe [44, 45] and beneficial for pregnant women, both for various conditions and parameters of the course of pregnancy [46, 47], and for labor and delivery [48, 49]. Nevertheless, too low intensity in low-impact aerobics may not be sufficient to stimulate the cardiopulmonary system [45] and not produce the desired health effects. Using high-impact movements during group classes gives the opportunity to increase quickly the intensity of exercise. It is especially important for women with high levels of exercise capacity and accustomed to participate in high-intensity classes before pregnancy. Adding jumps or runs during an aerobics class may be an option for such women [50].

There is some scientific evidence that the participation of pregnant women in hi-lo aerobics can lead to health benefits, with no adverse effects on the course of pregnancy or on birth outcomes [50, 51]. It is unsubstantiated belief that runs or jumps can cause miscarriage or premature labor. However, with the development of pregnancy and the growing womb, it may be necessary to limit high-impact movements. Potentially, they can cause an unpleasant bounce of pregnant belly or growing breasts, intensify urinary incontinence or lower back pain. However, the decision to eliminate high-impact movements should be based on the assessment of the well-being of a woman and not be a general rule for exercising during pregnancy.

The recommended music tempo for hi-low aerobics classes is 134–150 BPM (beats per minute) depending on the group's abilities [36]. With the progression of pregnancy and gaining weight, the training workload of a pregnant woman increases, so it may be necessary to use slower music in the third trimester. To get aerobic exercise, during the entire choreography, the woman should be able to breathe freely and maintain an exercise intensity of 14–16 on the RPE scale from 6 to 20, or 6–8 on the RPE scale from 1 to 10 (see Chaps. 8 and 10). Concerning the level of expertise, Laukkanen et al. [52] reported that intensity management during aerobics classes is generally successful regardless of the participants' prior participation in aerobics. However, in their study, some individuals who were older and/or had less prior participation tended to exceed the targeted heart rate.

The technique of performing aerobics moves does not differ significantly from the technique for the general population. Special attention should be paid to the correct body posture, not to deepen its defects. Perhaps at the end of pregnancy, due to the falling belly, it will be uncomfortable for a pregnant woman to perform the *front knee up* move, which can be replaced by *side knee up* move (see Appendix 2). It is certainly worthwhile to include conscious pelvic-floor muscle contractions at the end of each exercise (e.g., when attaching legs in *step touch* move or before jump or run). To prevent urine leakage during exercise, Bourcier [53] proposed to use "the knack" - a quick, strong, well-timed pelvic-floor muscle contraction before and during physical stress increasing intra-abdominal pressure. Using pelvic floor precontractions in high–low impact classes allowed pregnant women not only to maintain a good quality of life in terms of urinary incontinence but also to improve the electromyographic parameters of the pelvic floor muscles [50].

In aerobics, one should also incorporate upper-body moves to activate the whole body, increase the exercise intensity and improve coordination. The arms can move bilaterally (right and left sides perform the same movement simultaneously) or unilaterally (right and left sides move individually or perform different movements simultaneously) [36]. Some women are afraid to raise their arms above their heads, for fear of miscarriage. This is an unfounded opinion, which unnecessarily limits the range of exercises during the classes. Likewise, there is no justification for avoiding in pregnancy frequent changes in direction or any turns during choreography. Although the center of gravity, balance and coordination are changing in pregnancy, there is no scientific evidence that these changes increase the risk of collapse or collision during aerobics, compared to the general population. As mentioned above, the inclusion of changes in direction and turns in a choreography as well as cadence will depend on participants' level of expertise. However, there should always be an "easier" and "more challenging" option included in the session plan for the cases where there are participants with different levels of fitness and experience in the same group class. We presented examples of aerobics movements for pregnant women in Appendix 2.

9.3.2.2 Step Aerobics

Step aerobics is a classic cardio workout that uses a 10, 15, 20, or 25 cm height bench of approximately 102 cm (length) × 38.5 cm (width) (Fig. 9.1) to step up and down, around the step forward, sideways, and backward, and over the platform, usually combined in choreography. Different patterns of steps can be used to boost heart rate and breathing, as well as lower limb muscles resistance. Core muscles stabilize the trunk. Upper limb movements can also be added. Upbeat music sets the cadence, the number of moves, the rhythm and provides motivation. Exercise

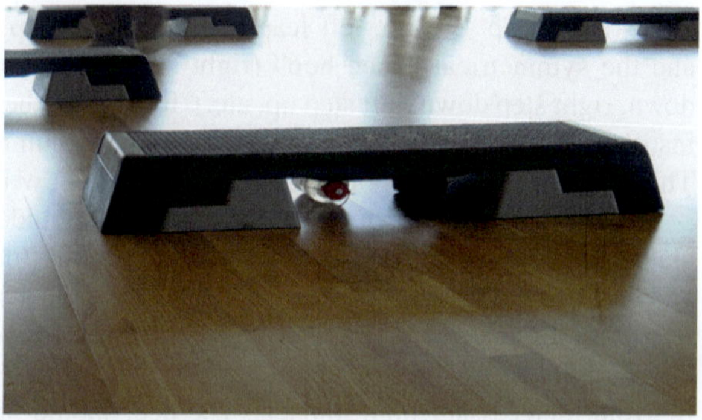

Fig. 9.1 Image of a 15-cm height Step Reebok™ bench

specialists show the moves, appropriate technique, and the progression of choreography. Moves' sequence building is important in order for participants to feel successful. Usually, participants are in a gym, in front of a mirror. However, this equipment can be used at home to follow video classes and exercise to music. If used outdoors, precautions should be taken regarding the type of floor: it must be flat and not slippery. Moreover, if the participant feels tired or she is a complete beginner, she can perform the moves on the floor, i.e., without a bench step (e.g., draw a rectangle on the floor with duct tape). A step aerobics class typically lasts 45–60 min.

The *Step Reebok*™ program was originally introduced as a low-impact activity (with a medium impact version called Power Step Reebok) since its proponents claimed that ground reaction forces were similar to those of walking [54, 55]. Step classes currently include propulsive movements that have changed the nature of impact of the activity [56]. The objectives of this group exercise are based on the improvement of cardiovascular and muscle efficiency, as well as motor coordination, balance, spatial orientation, body composition, and fun. One important characteristic of Step exercise is the repetition of exercises (or techniques, called "steps") that induce forces of low magnitude (around 1 to 2 BW—body weight) and of high frequency (around 3750 to 4050 times on a 30 min session, using music speed of 125 to 135 beats per minute) [56, 57].

Step aerobics moves range from simple to advanced depending on low- or high-impact, coordination, balance, change in position, speed and combination of choreographed steps. Regarding impact loading, this being a weight-bearing exercise, low-impact moves mean that there is always 1 ft on the bench or ground (e.g., basic step, knee lift, knee repeater, marching, mambo). High-impact moves mean that for a moment both feet are off the ground (e.g., run step, knee hop, jump step, knee leap). Regarding leading leg loading, step moves can be symmetrical or asymmetrical, i.e., the sequence of moves always start with the same leading leg followed by the impulsion leg, or the sequence of moves always starts with alternated leading legs. The Step aerobics low-impact basic moves are the asymmetrical "basic step" (right step up, left step up, right step down, left step down, etc.) and the symmetrical "knee lift" (right step up, left knee lift, left step down, right step down, left step up, etc.). The step aerobics medium-impact basic moves are the asymmetrical "run step" (right leap step up, left leap step up, right step down, left step down, etc.) and the symmetrical "knee hop" (right step up, left knee lift with hop, left step down, right step down, left step up, etc.). Regarding the dominant leg of each move, instructors must plan a session with a balanced number of asymmetrical moves. This is a very important point of the session since it will influence mechanical load.

Regarding technique, the head should be up, shoulders down and back, chest up, abdominals lightly contracted, and buttocks gently tucked under the hips. Knees and back should never hyperextend at any time. When stepping up, the body should lean from the ankles and not the waist to avoid excessive stress on the lumbar spine. The entire sole of the foot should contact the bench, stepping softly and quietly to avoid unnecessary high impacts. The heel should not land over the edge of the bench to avoid Achilles tendon injury. When stepping down, the step should be close to the bench (no more than one shoe length away) and the heel should contact the floor to help to absorb shock [54].

The class starts with a warm-up, followed by choreographed routines on the step, and a cool down at the end. The intensity can vary from low and medium to high, depending on the type of moves (impact, repeaters, amplitude, overhead upper limb moves, etc.), cadence, choreography, and bench height. This means that a session can be planned with the following objectives of meeting different fitness and skill levels: 1) low to medium intensity, low to medium impact, and easy to follow (i.e., pregnant women, older adults, children, some clinical populations and beginners); 2) medium to high intensity, impact, and complexity (i.e., skilled participants, including pregnant women); and 3) medium to high intensity and impact, but easy to follow (i.e., cross-training for athletes). There are no advantages of adding weights while stepping. The use of ankle and hand weights failed to enhance training adaptations [58]. After the cardio part, the set bench can also be used to perform strength training and stretching exercises. The only contraindications for step aerobics are the conditions of hip, foot, ankle, or knee pain, or recent back and knee injury.

Step aerobics is one of the main trends of activity undertaken by pregnant women [59]. Unfortunately, to our knowledge, only one prospective randomized controlled trial designed to assess the benefits and possible risks of aerobic exercise during pregnancy used step aerobics in the exercise intervention [60]. With a general population of pregnant women, the program should include low to medium impact moves, benches of 10–15 cm height, without too many changes of direction and jumps over the platform, in order to prevent falling or loss of balance. Pregnant women should always maintain visual contact with the platform. On the other hand, each woman feels safer on her own bench and space around it, compared to an aerobics class. It does not require much space and equipment and provides a good cardiovascular, resistance, and neuromotor exercise. Thus, it is a safe and effective exercise to start or continue during pregnancy, as long as intensity (e.g., slower cadence, lower bench) and complexity can be adjusted to fitness and skill level as pregnancy progresses. Important precautions include lowering the bench as the belly grows and the center of gravity changes, drinking water before and during exercise and not overheating. We presented examples of step aerobics movements for pregnant women in Appendix 3 of the present chapter.

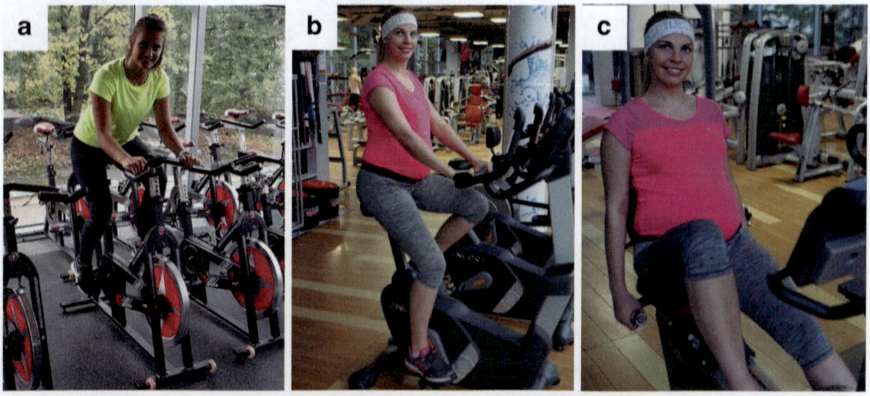

Fig. 9.2 Indoor cycling is a non-weight-bearing activity to be performed on: (**a**) a spinning bike; (**b**) a stationary bike; (**c**) a reclined bike

9.3.2.3 Indoor and Outdoor Cycling

Indoor cycling is a non-weight-bearing cardiovascular and lower body resistance exercise. An indoor cycling class typically lasts 45–60 min. Indoor cycling requires a stationary or "spinning" bike (Fig. 9.2a). The position of the saddle must be adjusted to participants' measurements (i.e., when standing beside the bike, the saddle must be at the same plane as the hips; when seated in the saddle, with foot on the pedal at the bottom of the stroke, the knee must be slightly bent; when seated, with the crank arms parallel to the ground, the horizontal distance from the handlebars to the saddle must be set when the knee line intersects the leading edge of the forward crank arm). Intensity depends on the speed, load on the bike, time (duration of the session), and change in position (sit or stand). Other options include a stationary bike (Fig. 9.2b) or a reclined bike (Fig. 9.2c) at a gym or at home.

Outdoor cycling is non-weight-bearing cardiovascular, lower body resistance, and neuromotor exercise. The findings by Skreden et al. [61] indicate that so-called active transportation, including cycling, is one possible approach to prevent excessive weight gain in pregnancy. An outdoor cycling session may last from a very short period to several hours depending on fitness level and comfort. Outdoor cycling requires a regular bike, usually, specific to the road, mountain or urban/fitness (Fig. 9.3a–c). However, there are other types available, such as tandem, touring, tricycle, hybrid, electric, etc., and bikes designed around female anatomy and dimensions. The frame, weight, and dimensions of the bike must be adjusted to participants' size, fitness level, comfort, and training objectives.

The characteristics of the bike will, of course, influence its price. However, the main question to have in mind is technique and a correct fit. Being a repetitive movement, sustained up to several hours, appropriate technique is of particular importance in order to perform effective and safe training, avoiding falls and preventing injuries.

Pregnant women that are regular or competitive cyclists will have very light and expensive bikes. It is very likely that competition and training for racing will need

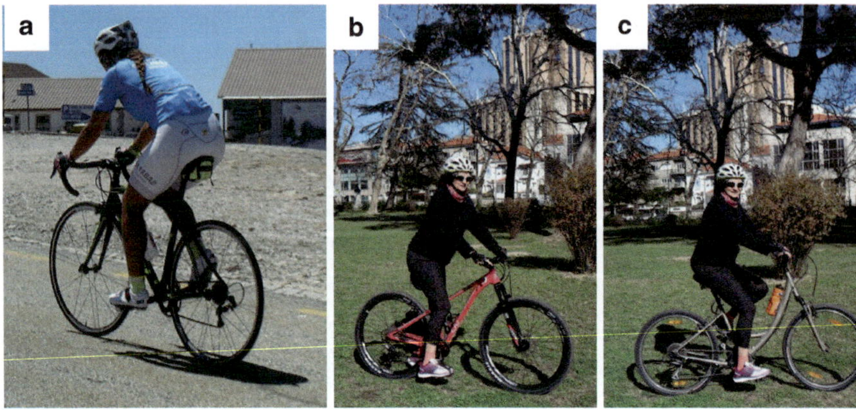

Fig. 9.3 Outdoor cycling requires: (**a**) a road bike; (**b**) a mountain bike; (**c**) an urban/fitness bike, among other types

to be suspended during pregnancy but athletes may wish to continue to train until the abdomen expands to the point that it is no longer comfortable to cycle, especially if the woman is a road bike athlete. In these cases, switching to a mountain or fitness bike, indoor cycling or using a more comfortable bike that allows a more upright position can be good options, taking into account that most of the body weight shifts onto the saddle, compressing intervertebral disks. Those who are recreational bikers, or use the bike for active commuting, may wish to continue as long as pregnancy progresses. In these cases, mountain bikes and urban/fitness bikes can offer very comfortable equipment regarding size, feminine geometry, suspension, woman's saddle, number of gears, and lightweight equipment. There are many brands on offer from very affordable to very expensive bikes. For those who do not know how to use a bike, starting this activity after the childbearing period may be a better option, unless using a stationary bike or a tricycle. Learning how to use the bike is a very demanding activity regarding balance skills. Pregnant women should avoid falling and trauma situations.

When cycling outdoors, several precautions should be taken:

1. To ensure proper technique: to use proper bike and ensure correct bike fit; feet should be properly placed on the pedals, with or without cycling shoes with a strapless pedal binding system (this system must be fitted to the cyclist' experience level).
2. To adjust the trunk position and the handlebar of the bike (in height and width) as belly grows.
3. To be sure of the condition and maintenance of the tires, brakes, and gears.
4. To know how to fix or replace a flat tire, and how to pump.
5. Always use a helmet.
6. To use a women's saddle, no matter the type of bike.
7. To avoid bad weather (too cold or too hot) and slippery ground.
8. To know the conditions of the weather and ground in advance.

9. To drink water before, during and after exercising (and carry light snacks).
10. To avoid air pollution and car traffic.
11. To be aware of traffic rules and hazards.
12. To use sun protection for skin (lotion) and eyes (glasses). Glasses also protect from dust and bugs.
13. To use cycling routes, lanes, and parks; preferably engage in a cycling group or ride with a partner (either on two bikes or using a tandem).
14. To use proper sportswear: bike or cross-training shoes, breathable shirt and jackets, supportive and comfortable bra, breathable underwear, shorts or leggings with saddle pads (or extra comfortable women's saddle).
15. To use fingerless or full cycling gloves to prevent blisters and to protect skin if the hands contact the ground in case of falling.
16. To avoid riding in the dark and to know how to deal with dogs (e.g., carrying some cookies, shouting back or dismounting and placing the bike between the body and the dog).

Some modifications may occur in accordance with common pregnancy-related symptoms and discomforts. If the pregnant woman has pelvic girdle pain, hemorrhoids, varicose veins in legs, varicose veins in the vulvar area, or vaginal yeast infection, just sitting in the saddle or sitting in the saddle for a long time will be uncomfortable. In some cases, there might be temporary vision changes due to hormonal effects and glasses may not be enough to ensure safety while riding outdoors. Other safety concerns are related to changes in the sense of balance and dizziness (in those cases indoor cycling is the best option).

An indoor or outdoor cycling training includes a warm-up, cardiovascular exercise, lower limb resistance exercises, and a cooldown part with stretching exercises. Any change in the bike will affect muscle activity and pedaling form, which in turn, will affect intensity. Cycling also allows monitoring heart rate, using a heart rate monitor, a GPS (global positioning system), or a smart phone.

Example of warm-up before a cycling session:

https://youtu.be/S6bDBWA7QAE

9.3.2.4 Walking, Jogging, or Running

Walking provides a good cardiovascular and lower limb resistance and core exercise to be performed outdoors (with or without poles) or using a treadmill (Fig. 9.4). Walking briskly requires attention to posture and technique: keeping the head up and looking forward; keeping head straight with chin parallel to the ground; properly blended arms swing with loose shoulders (arm counterbalance leg movements); hip aligned with shoulders avoiding sway back; and proper leg swing and stride length [62].

Walking is the most commonly reported form of exercise during pregnancy [63]. Walking is an affordable exercise that requires no special equipment or facility, and it is very good for beginners and for active women. There is no contraindication from its practice during pregnancy, except recent lower limb injury or pain. Several

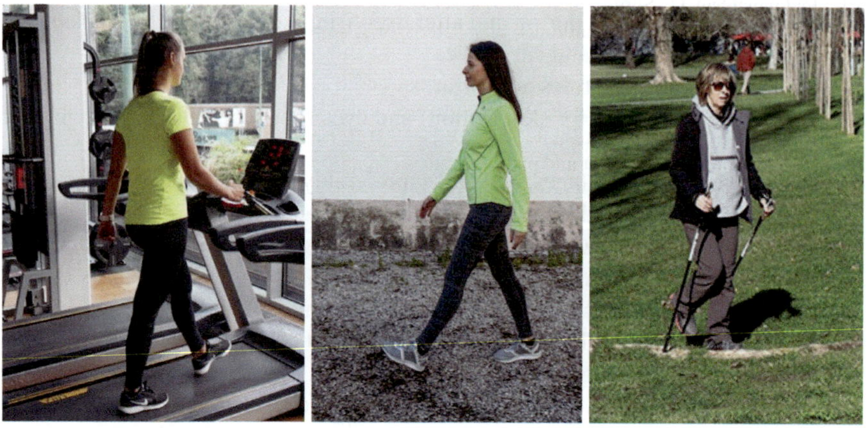

Fig. 9.4 Walking can be performed either outdoors (with or without poles) or using a treadmill

clinical trials have used walking as an intervention to assess the effects of exercise on maternal and perinatal outcomes and have found it to be an effective intervention [44, 64–66]. Running is a time-efficient aerobic activity [62], and is a good option for those who were recreational or competitive runners before pregnancy. Those athletes may wish to continue their training, although some adaptations may be needed, regarding intensity and impact. There have been several experimental trials [15, 67, 68] on the influence of regular running on maternal and/or fetal health, and no adverse effects were observed.

One important characteristic of walking and running is the repetition of strides (loading cycles) of low impact (inducing ground reaction forces of low magnitude, i.e., 1–2 BW) or medium impact (i.e., 2–4 BW), with high frequency (around 3570–5710 steps) during a 30-min session, at speeds of 5 km/h (~83 m/min) to 8 km/h (~133 m/min), respectively (assuming that the mean stride length of a woman is ~70 cm). There may be some changes needed as the belly grows, regarding the speed, balance, and gait pattern. Moreover, there are factors that may lead to cease running and substitute it for walking or other activities. These include joints and ligaments more vulnerable to strains or sprains, augmented pelvic pressure and urinary frequency, especially during the third trimester.

Proper stretching exercises both before and after a walking or running session are helpful to prevent injuries. When walking, hiking, or running outdoors, several precautions should be taken:

1. To ensure proper posture, technique (arm and leg swing), and breathing.
2. To avoid bad weather (too cold or too hot) and slippery ground.
3. To get familiar in advance with the conditions of the weather, trails, and ground, as well as bathroom facilities.
4. To avoid steep ascent or descent.
5. To drink water before, during, and after exercising.
6. To avoid air pollution and car traffic.

7. To avoid hiking at high altitudes due to reduced oxygen levels.
8. To use sun protection for skin (lotion), head (cap), and eyes (glasses).
9. To use eyes protection (glasses) against dust and bugs.
10. To use walking lanes and parks.
11. Preferably to engage in a walking/running group.
12. To use proper sports shoes: walking, running or cross-training shoes that provide comfort, ankle support, cushioning, and shock absorbing features.
13. To use comfortable socks with extra padding to prevent friction and blisters.
14. To use proper sportswear (and underwear): breathable shirt and jacket, pregnancy supportive bra, seamless and breathable underwear, shorts or leggings.
15. To ensure frequent rest and water breaks if exercising for a long time.

9.3.2.5 Water Exercise and Swimming

Water exercise is also a commonly reported form of exercise during pregnancy [63], very good for beginners and for active women (Fig. 9.5). Water exercise and swimming take the weight off the joints while exercising. It has been shown that water exercise is safe [69, 70] and beneficial for pregnant women [46]. In the study by Vallim et al. [71], a great majority of pregnant women considered that the practice of water aerobics had benefitted them in some way.

Most water workouts are done in the shallow end of the swimming pool and participants stand in chest-deep water. They can also stand in shoulder-deep water to perform other upper body exercises keeping the arms under water. It is a low-impact exercise, and the buoyancy of the water is supporting the body weight. Different patterns of lower limbs and upper limbs moves performed in the water can be used to boost heart rate and breathing, as well as muscular resistance and flexibility. Core exercises (abdominals and back muscles) may include lunges, side leg lifts,

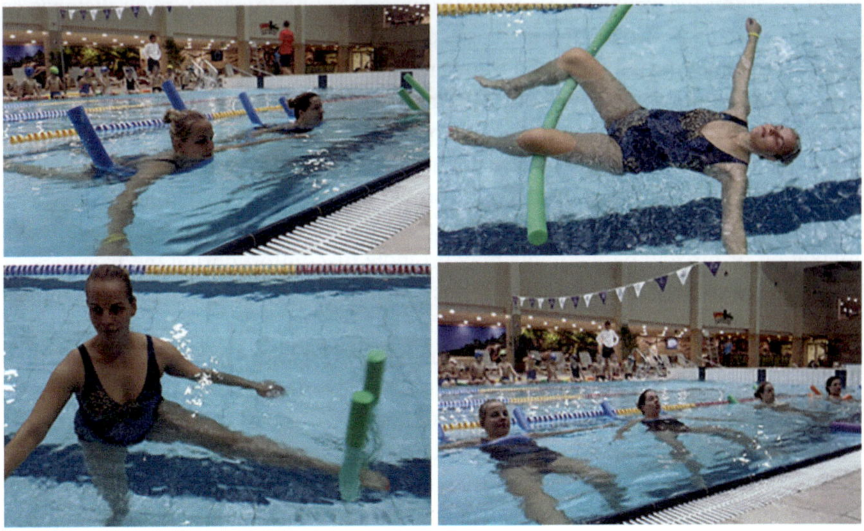

Fig. 9.5 Water exercise is a popular activity among pregnant women

etc., or exercising with legs and arms at the same time. Upper limb moves may include underwater bicep curls, etc. Lower limbs exercises may include water walking, water jogging, jumping jacks, squats, high knee kicks, and underwater kicks and jumps. Pelvic floor exercises can be performed by incorporating them in other stretching or strengthening exercises. Pool noodles, paddles, barbells, balls, kickboards, aqua joggers, foam weights and other specific equipment can also be used for added resistance.

Upbeat music sets the cadence, the number of moves, the rhythm, and provides motivation. Workout intensity can be increased by doing more repetitions of each move, increasing speed, or using some equipment to increase resistance. An advanced class might include underwater interval training. Classes also are performed in outdoor pools where and when the weather allows. Usually the exercise specialist, placed in the dock of the swimming pool, shows the exercises putting emphasis on technique and breathing. A water exercise class typically lasts 45–60 min.

Swimming is also a popular exercise among pregnant women, recommended in several guidelines (see Chaps. 7 and 9). A swimming class may include adaptation to water environment exercises, arms' exercises, legs' exercises, technique exercises, assisted or resisted exercises, breathing exercises, and backstroke, freestyle (crawl), breaststroke and butterfly styles of swimming (including flip turns). Some small equipment can also be used to focus the exercise only on the arms or lower limbs (kickboard, pull buoys or another flotation device), increase resistance (hand paddles) or propulsion (swim fins) of the swimming exercises. The selection of exercises for each session will depend on the level of experience, skill, and fitness. Butterfly stroke is the most demanding regarding technique and effort. Each swimming stroke has a specific arm and movements' technique and performance, but general aspects of swimming include efficient movement of the body through the water, keeping the strokes long and relaxed, and trying to get as much distance as possible with each stroke (and increase speed).

As pregnancy progresses, some lower back movements will probably become difficult or painful (butterfly and breaststroke) and the expanded abdomen will create more resistance (drag) in the water (butterfly, breaststroke, and freestyle) making body alignment in water more difficult as well. The same reason applies to flip turns. Thus, the speed work usually performed by competition swimmers should be postponed until after the childbirth. Moreover, the hormonal changes provoking the relaxation of hip and pelvic joints may promote discomfort during the frog kick of breaststroke. For the same reason, the neck movements of the breaststroke and freestyle (assuming that the participant breathes alternately to the right and left sides or every three-arm strokes) may also become uncomfortable. The alterations of spine alignment may also interfere with backstroke. Nevertheless, the best technique is the one that the pregnant woman is able to perform correctly and without pain and discomfort, and is more motivated to practice.

A swimming session can last 30–60 min. However, a short interval of 10–15 min can be added to a regular water exercise session, especially when the pregnant women are able to swim backstroke.

A water aerobics class or a swimming training includes a warm-up, cardiovascular exercise, muscular resistance exercises and a cooldown with stretching exercises. When swimming or practicing water exercise, several precautions should be taken:

1. To ensure proper posture, technique, and breathing regarding water exercises and swimming strokes.
2. To avoid too cold or too hot water.
3. To ensure the hygienic conditions of the pool.
4. To ensure that the swimming pool is supervised regarding safety and emergency conditions.
5. To drink water before, during, and after exercising.
6. To use skin (lotion) and eyes (glasses) sun protection when exercising in outdoor pools.
7. To avoid jumping into the pool or diving activities.
8. To use proper and comfortable maternity swimwear.
9. To use proper water goggles (to protect from irritation), swim cap (to protect hair from damage), and maternity swimwear with bra support included.
10. To ensure the availability of bathroom facilities.
11. To avoid sharing a lane with other swimmers (because of potential shocks).
12. To avoid swimming alone when exercising outdoors in a lake, river, or sea.

9.3.3 High-Intensity Interval Training (HIIT)

High-intensity interval training (HIIT) has become the second most popular mode of exercise in the European fitness trends [72]. There is a variety of HIIT protocols: they are based on short work intervals (<60 s to 8 min) of vigorous (70%–90% maximal heart rate or 14–16 of the 6–20 RPE Borg's scale) to high intensity (≥90% maximal heart rate or ≥17 of the 6–20 RPE Borg's scale) interspersed with active (40%–70% maximal heart rate or 8–13 of the 6–20 RPE Borg's scale) or passive (cessation of movement) recovery periods (of 1–5 min) [73].

The effectiveness of HIIT programs on a number of health indicators has been proven in various populations, including populations with cardiac or metabolic disorders [74], elderly people with dementia [75] and cancer patients [76]. Given the significant benefits of HIIT programs, both in terms of the impact on metabolic changes and the impact on the psyche of participants, they should also be implemented for women in the perinatal period. To date, only trace data on the benefits of HIIT in pregnancy have been published [77, 78].

Studies in rats by Songstad et al. [18] showed that females responded well to HIIT throughout pregnancy. The program consisted of performing five training sessions per week, consisting of ten 4-min intervals with an intensity of 85–90% of the VO_{2max}. The authors did not record the side effects of such an HIIT program on pregnancy and fetal development. Interestingly, the HIIT program modified some of the genes associated with oxidative stress in fetal livers and hearts. This indicates that adaptive mechanisms to intense physical exertion can be activated already in the fetal period.

Based on the research conducted on athletes, it is known that performing three to five submaximal running intervals, with an intensity of up to 90% VO_{2max}, did not adversely affect the fetal heart rate [19]. Temporary bradycardia appeared when their mother exceeded 90% VO_{2max} exercise intensity. Fetal parameters quickly normalized after the mother stopped exercise. Ong et al. [20] analyzed the effectiveness of a one-time interval session in a group of women in the third trimester, with an average level of activity before and during pregnancy. They observed that adding six 15-s intervals of subjectively maximum intensity to traditional moderate-intensity continuous training increased its energy expenditure by 28%. In addition, based on the PACES scale [21], the authors found that intensive intervals increased women's satisfaction with doing exercises. The studies by Salvesen et al. [14] have shown that high-class athletes performing near-maximum physical exercise in pregnancy gave birth to healthy newborns.

Nagpal et al. [79] noted, that due to the popularity of HIIT in general women population and the lack of evidence-based information and guidelines, pregnant women may inquire about HIIT on their own through online searches. The purpose of the study by Nagpal et al. was to systematically search and critically evaluate online resources that women may access when seeking guidance on how to participate in HIIT during pregnancy. Based on this study outcomes, publicly accessible online information on HIIT during pregnancy has been shown not to adhere routinely to evidence-based safety recommendations for prenatal exercise. The authors concluded that further research on HIIT during pregnancy and public dissemination of findings is required. There are a few projects already on the HIIT during pregnancy registered in the ClinicalTrials registration [80–82], but the study outcomes have not been yet published. Therefore, for now, women can participate in HIIT on the same terms as other special populations, taking into account the recent guidelines on physical activity during pregnancy.

The current recommendations do not set an upper limit for the intensity of physical effort in the perinatal period [3]. Women who regularly do intensive exercise can continue their physical activity during pregnancy and after delivery, provided that they remain healthy and that the pregnancy or delivery is normal. Although there is no scientific evidence, HIIT programs appear to be more appropriate for women who were active before pregnancy, as they are more likely to tolerate high-intensity exercise well during pregnancy. As any other exercise program, prenatal HIIT should be implemented gradually, starting with lower intensity. After a HIIT class, pregnant women should feel well and be motivated to train again.

An example of a prenatal HIIT can be a program of 3 sessions a week, in a duration of each session of 60 min. High-intensity intervals (approx. 85–90% of the maximum exercise capacity) should be planned as the main part of the training (15–20 min), e.g., 4 exercises, 3–4 series each. The high-intensity exercises will be performed for 30–60 s, alternating with a 30–60 s rest break, in the ratio of exercise time to rest 1:2, 1:1 or 2:1, according to the individual capabilities of the participant and taking into account the training progression and stage of pregnancy [82].

9.3.4 Resistance, Postural, and Neuromotor Exercises

9.3.4.1 Resistance Exercises

So far, there is sparse knowledge on strenuous strength training in the general pregnant population and there have been no studies on its effects in pregnant elite athletes [83]. According to Bø and coauthors [83], women who are considering heavy strength training in pregnancy should understand that the Valsalva maneuver used during weight training precipitates a rapid increase in blood pressure and intra-abdominal pressure [84–86] and therefore potentially may temporarily decrease blood flow to the fetus. The consequences of this process for the fetus development remain unknown. Heavy-strength training potentially may lead to pelvic floor disorders. Therefore, IOC experts [86] advised, the pelvic floor muscles should be contracted before and during heavy lifting to counteract the impact on the pelvic floor from increased intra-abdominal pressure. Research is needed to explain the above issues.

Nevertheless, in pro-health resistance training with a light-to-moderate load of free weights or weight machines (Fig. 9.6a–d), researchers have observed no adverse health

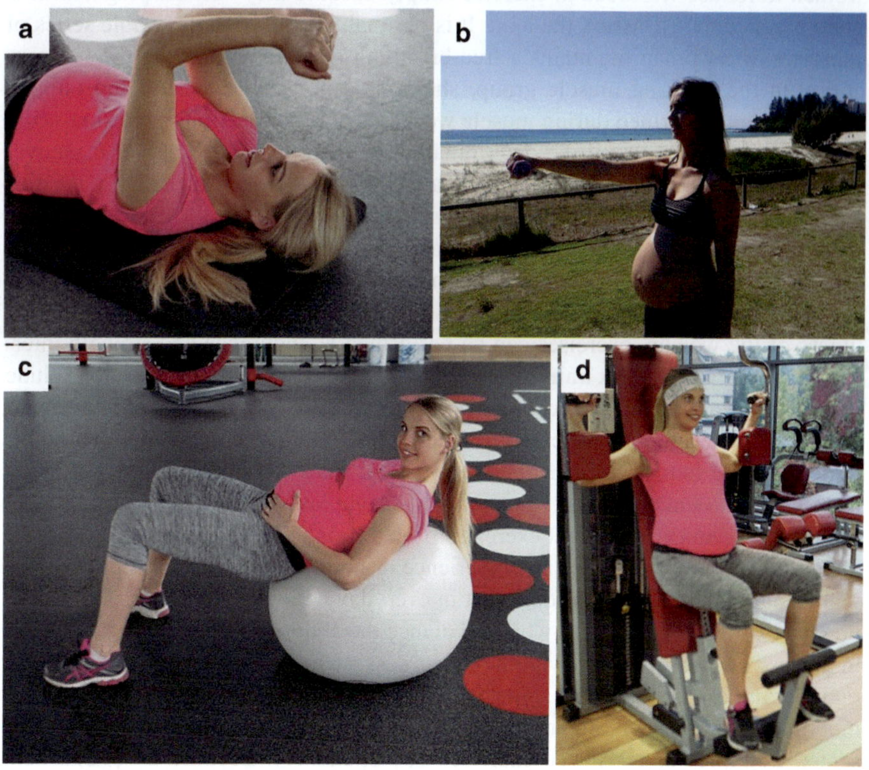

Fig. 9.6 Resistance training can be performed: (**a**) with body weight; (**b**) with load of free weights; (**c**) with stability ball; or (**d**) with weight machines

effects during pregnancy [26, 67, 87, 88]. Prenatal exercises strengthening particular body parts can improve both their appearance and functionality specific to pregnancy and motherhood. The fear of adverse effects of resistance training such as inadequate blood flow to the fetus during exercise was not supported by scientific research [26].

Resistance exercises for pregnant women follow the same training rules as for the general adult population. When applying the principle of training progression, one should consider the increase in body weight (at the end of pregnancy, it may be over a dozen kilograms). Additional body weight should be considered in exercises with body resistance. For example, it will be important in doing squats, but it will not matter in straightening the legs with the resistance of the machine in supine position. Keeping the same number of repetitions in exercises with body resistance until the end of pregnancy should be treated as training progress.

In the selection of the training load (also external load in the form of e.g., dumbbells, resistance bands, medicine balls, the resistance of machines), the individual level of fitness of the woman and her well-being during and after the exercises must be taken into consideration. There is no (and probably will not be) a maximum load allowed during pregnancy either in absolute values, e.g., in kilograms, or relative, e.g., in the percentage of maximum capabilities. There is no scientific basis for women to reduce workload in exercise simply because they became pregnant. It is good practice to self-assess the load. It is optimal when during the whole series of exercises, the woman maintains a free breathing rhythm, and during the last repetition in the working muscle group, she feels a noticeable tension and fatigue. Exhalation is performed during muscle work / muscle contraction, inhalation while muscles are relaxed. Until the determination of the impact of Valsalva maneuver (increased exhalation against closed airways) on the course of pregnancy, it is rational to limit it in both exercises and daily activities.

In 60-min sessions, after 30 min of aerobic exercise, the organization of 8–9 exercises strengthening main muscle groups in 2–3 sets of 12–24 repetitions fits very well. This is of course only a suggestion. Depending on the training goals and fitness of the woman, exercises can be performed at endurance and strength intervals, in the form of circuit training and others. There is no scientific basis to exclude specific training methods or techniques due to pregnancy. Special attention should be paid to the technique of exercise, including body posture, in order not to increase lordosis in the lumbar region. There are typical rules for teaching new exercises, from known to unknown and from simple to complex. There is no scientific basis to exclude technically difficult exercises from a training session if a woman is able to do them properly and does not experience discomfort while performing them.

It should be taken into account that in everyday activities the back muscles of a pregnant woman do intensive work to balance the abdominal mass [89]. Therefore, in the last weeks of pregnancy, it may be necessary to modify, exclude, or limit the range of the exercises for the spinal erectors. Leg muscles also work hard in locomotion. One must keep this in mind when planning an exercise program. We presented examples of resistance exercises in Appendix 4. Because abdominal and pelvic floor muscles are of particular importance for the course of pregnancy, we described them separately.

9.3.4.2 Pilates Mat

Pilates is an exercise technique which focuses on body–mind balance, muscle strengthening, flexibility, muscle control, posture, breathing, and the power center of stabilization [90]. The equipment required for a Pilates class may vary from a single mat, small and big balls, to specific machines called "reformer." The exercises are usually done in a specific order, one right after another, starting from a standing position, to other positions such as knees and hands, seating and laying positions. The movements have names, like the "100," the "Swan," the "Criss-Cross," the "Elephant," etc. Regarding intensity, Pilates can be very easy or very demanding, depending on the difficulty of the movements. The movements are usually performed in slow motion requiring precision and control to enhance muscle resistance and flexibility. This resistance and neuromotor exercise are a great addition to an aerobic program. Usually, the exercise specialist shows the exercises putting a strong emphasis on technique and breathing. Due to precision and control of movements, the supervision of movements by a qualified exercise professional is helpful even with experienced participants.

It is a safe and effective exercise to start or continue during pregnancy, as long as intensity (e.g., the amplitude of movements, repetitions, sustained time and position, lying positions) and complexity (muscles involved, resistance and flexibility required) can be adjusted to fitness and skill level as pregnancy progresses. However, pregnant women may need to avoid certain Pilates moves if they do not feel comfortable (i.e., head down, lying backward, etc.). Usually, participants are in a gym, in front of a mirror. However, a mat can be used at home to follow video classes if the participant is experienced and is able to use the appropriate technique. If the mat is used outdoors, precautions should be taken regarding the type of floor: it must be flat and not slippery. Although these exercises could have interesting intersections with pregnancy musculoskeletal adaptations, there are insufficient data in the literature to assess the effect on pregnant women.

A Pilates class typically lasts 45–60 min. However, short periods of 10–15 min of Pilates exercises can be included in a complete prenatal exercise session. A recent back or knee injury may be contraindications for Pilates exercise program. However, Pilates would be a good choice if the pregnant woman has low back pain.

9.3.4.3 Abdominals Exercises

Owing to, inter alia, the growing uterus, changes in the curvature of the spine and the effect of pregnancy hormones, abdominal muscles are heavily stretched [91]. As a result, almost 70% of all pregnant women experience lower back pain [92]. To minimize this risk, the ACOG [16] recommends the strengthening of abdominal and back muscles. Strong abdominal muscles also play an important role in the pushing process necessary during natural delivery. Although this still requires scientific evidence support, abdominal muscles maintained in good condition throughout pregnancy are more likely to recover quickly after delivery.

Despite the many obvious advantages of abdominal muscle exercises, this is a controversial topic. The reason for this phenomenon may be opinions appearing in the society that the abdominal muscles exercises during pregnancy can lead to miscarriage or a more painful childbirth [93]. Even a significant part of exercise professionals are convinced that women should not exercise abdominal muscles in pregnancy [94]. It should be emphasized that so far, no studies have been published that could confirm the allegedly negative impact of abdominal muscle exercises on the course of pregnancy, childbirth, or development of a child.

The most important principles recommended for the implementation of abdominal muscle exercises during pregnancy are as follows:

1. When selecting the exercises for abdominal muscles, the stage of pregnancy should be taken into account. A large uterus will certainly hinder the abdominal muscle shortening during contraction. A growing fetus takes up space in the abdominal cavity. Therefore, in the high pregnancy, it is rational to limit the movements which additionally will reduce it, like in crunches. Nevertheless, it is the uncomfortable feeling of a woman in a given exercise that should be an indicator for its elimination or modification. Creating the so-called list of abdominal muscle exercises forbidden in pregnancy seems to have no scientific justification.
2. During exercise, one must remember to breathe properly; exhalation should be performed with muscle contraction, inhalation - when relaxing.
3. After a series of exercises to strengthen the abdominal muscles, it is recommended to relax them by conscious abdominal breathing (the abdomen protrudes as the diaphragm is lowered). The ability to move quickly from the state of tension to the relaxation of the abdominal muscles seems to be useful during delivery.
4. Due to the increase in lumbar lordosis during pregnancy, special attention should be paid to lay down on the back with the legs straightened as a starting position for exercise, e.g., in raising straight legs. In such exercises, the lumbar spine should be stabilized by shortening the abdominal muscles throughout the entire period of motion.
5. The supine position should be individually considered for a woman. Jeffreys et al. [95] observed that in women after 28 weeks of gestation, performing 60- to 90-s periods of abdominal crunches and leg exercise at moderate/high intensity (Borg's rating of perceived exertion 14 ± 1) in supine position, uterine blood flow decreased. However, the uterine blood flow decrease in those women was twice larger during 5-min rest in the supine position. There is still no scientific evidence that such temporary decrease in uterine blood flow has any negative influence on the course of pregnancy, fetus development, and its well-being. Based on systematic review by Mottola et al. [96], there was insufficient evidence to ascertain whether maternal exercise in the supine position is safe or should be avoided during pregnancy.
6. Exercises from the front or side plank positions are recommended mainly for advanced women. For women who are trying to perform planks for the first time in advanced pregnancy, there may be a problem with the correct technique and the risk of excessive deepening of the lumbar lordosis. It is then recommended to perform the exercise in a more upright version with the support on the forearms on a chair.

7. It is recommended to activate pelvic floor muscles in abdominal muscle exercises. This may prevent unwanted urine leakage during increasing intra-abdominal pressure.
8. Owing to the permanent stretching of the abdominal muscles by the growing uterus, it seems justified to limit the exercises stretching this muscle group. An alternative in this regard is to perform abdominal breathing.
9. Attention should be paid to the occurrence of prodromal uterine contractions (Braxton-Hicks contractions). Although they are not dangerous, if they are intense, they can cause tension in the abdominal area [97]. The Braxton–Hicks contractions may make women anxious and discourage them from being physically active [6]. Although it has not been proven scientifically, when prodromal uterine contractions strongly interfere with the pregnant woman, it is rational on the given day to limit the contraction stimuli by giving up exercises strengthening the abdominal muscles and replacing them with breathing and relaxing exercises.
10. Bearing in mind the fact that in some societies strengthening abdominal muscle exercises are unfoundedly labeled dangerous [94], exercise professionals and obstetrics care providers should pay special attention to educating women in this area.

Both before and during the exercise program, pregnant women should control the condition of their abdomen in terms of diastasis recti abdominis (DRA). It is a separation of the two rectus abdominis muscles along the *linea alba*, which appears in 66 to 100% of women in the third trimester [91]. The etiology of this condition is not clear. In the light of the available scientific evidence, there are no grounds to argue that intense exercises to strengthen abdominal muscles before conception or during pregnancy increase the risk of abdominal muscle separation. On the other hand, no reliable data are available, confirming whether diastasis recti abdominis can be prevented or treated with abdominal or other exercises during pregnancy. In one study, the researchers found that the acute response on inter-rectus distance (IRD) produced by drawing-in exercise was a widening of the IRD in postpartum, while the abdominal crunch exercise induced an acute narrowing response of the IRD in pregnancy and in postpartum [98].

Diastasis recti abdominis test should be performed as follows: lying back, legs bent, head and shoulder blades raised (as in abdominal crunch). One should check along the *linea alba* if there is no space between the abdominal muscles. The test is positive (diastasis recti abdominis is diagnosed) with palpation of$\geq$ 2 finger-breadths 4.5 cm above, at, or 4.5 cm below the umbilicus [99, 100]. A woman with a positive test requires consultation with a doctor or physiotherapist. To date, there is no consensus on whether to measure the distance along the *linea alba*, or on the cut-point for diagnosing the condition [91]. According to the study [101], evaluating the normal width of the *linea alba* in first-time pregnant women, the researchers found: during pregnancy at the 35–41 week of gestation, the 20th and the 80th percentile corresponded to 49–79 mm below the umbilicus, 54–86 mm at 2 cm above the umbilicus and 44–79 mm at 5 cm above the umbilicus. At 6 months postpartum, the 20th and the 80th percentile corresponded to 9–21 mm at 2 cm below the umbilicus, from 17 to 28 mm at 2 cm above the umbilicus and from 12 to 24 mm at 5 cm above the umbilicus.

Although there is not much evidence on preventive or therapeutic exercises of DRA for pregnant women, there are some small experimental studies performed in postpartum women.

It is worth taking a look at an interesting, though small, study conducted in the USA by Walton et al. [7]. Two groups of women after giving birth followed one of the two training programs for 6 weeks. One program, the so-called traditional, included: abdominal crunches, posterior pelvic tilts, pelvic floor muscle contractions (Kegels), and Russian twists. In the second experimental program, the abdominal crunches were replaced with planks. Additionally, both groups used abdominal bracing, which was defined as using a large towel or sheet secured around the abdominal section for each patient. A statistically significant reduction in DRA was observed in both groups: 2.01 cm through the "abdominal crunch program" and 1.65 cm through the "plank program." Therefore, in this study, crunches were slightly more effective. What is more, both programs significantly reduced back pain problems reflected by a lower ODI score—Oswestry Disability Index (but not statistically significant, which could have resulted from the small study group).

The high effectiveness of both exercise programs carried out by Walton et al. [102] could result, inter alia, from the use of external "abdominal bracing." Confirmation of this assumption can be a randomized controlled trial (RCT) in postpartum women, published in 2019 by the international team Thabet et al. [103] from Egypt, Saudi Arabia, and Australia. For 8 weeks, one group of postpartum women performed traditional abdominal muscle training included: static abdominal contractions, posterior pelvic tilts, reverse sit-up exercises, trunk twists, and reverse trunk twists. Their DRA decreased by an average of 2.5 cm. The experimental group performed the same exercises, and additionally: mechanical support by abdominal bracing, abdominal breathing, pelvic floor muscle contractions, planks, and isometric abdominal muscle contractions. In this group, the DRA decreased by an average of 8.30 cm. Both programs were significantly effective in reducing the DRA, but the experimental one statistically significantly more ($p = 0.0001$). Once again, the effectiveness of the comprehensive impact has been proven.

There is no reason not to use the abdominal exercises mentioned above also during pregnancy. Before the results of high-quality research are available, for abdominal muscle exercises in pregnant women diagnosed with abdominal muscle separation, it is worth introducing rules based on movement biomechanics analysis:

1. Limit or completely eliminate exercise positions, in which the trunk is parallel to the floor and the uterus rests on the front wall of the abdomen as in a hammock, for example, front plank, supported kneeling.
2. Limit the range of trunk rotation and lateral flexion not to intensify mechanically the separation of the abdominal muscles.
3. Shorten the range of motion or eliminate exercises in which a bulge appears along *linea alba*.

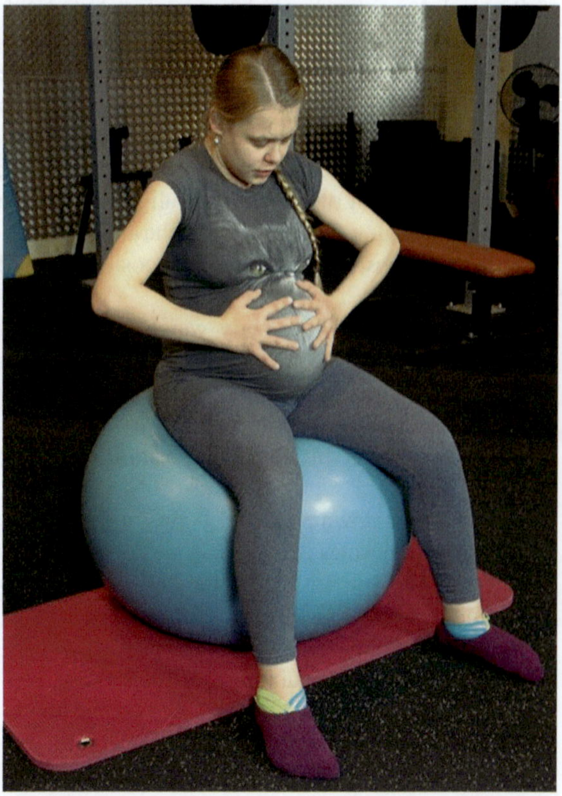

Fig. 9.7 Using hands in the abdominal exercises in the prevention of the diastasis recti abdominis

4. Pay particular attention to exhalation during the abdominal muscle contraction to minimize intra-abdominal pressure.
5. Utilize the work of the hands to mechanically bring the abdominal muscles toward the *linea alba* (Fig. 9.7), especially in places where their separation has been observed. One can use a towel or a sweatshirt, as well.

The validity of the above recommendations should be confirmed by experimental research. We presented examples of abdominal exercises, also in the presence of diastasis recti abdominis in Appendix 5. See Chaps. 6 and 12 for further explanation on this topic.

9.3.4.4 Postural Exercises

Proper posture can alleviate many of the muscular and skeletal discomforts, especially back pain [104]; improve breathing efficiency [105, 106] as well as improve one's self-confidence [106]. In pregnancy, postural exercises are particularly important due to various biomechanical changes in the musculoskeletal system [107]. The growing uterus and breasts intensify women's tendency to protrude the belly and pull the shoulders forward.

Postural exercises should be a regular element of prenatal classes. It is recommended to perform them at the beginning of each exercise session and to repeat them a few times throughout the session, especially before those exercises, in which incorrect technique could consolidate postural defects. Postural exercises can be performed in standing, sitting, kneeling, and lying positions. In addition to the immediate effect of the posture correction, they should increase the body awareness and promote a habit of proper body alignment in everyday activities. A mirror is a good tool for giving feedback for postural exercises.

The correct posture in the standing position should be performed as follows:

- Feet slightly apart, the body weight rests in the middle of the feet, avoiding excessive heel load.
- Legs straightened in the hip and knee joints (avoiding hyperextension), knees are over the feet, hips over the knees.
- The pelvis is set in a neutral position, avoiding excessive tilts backward or forward.
- Arms straight down along the body.
- Abdominal muscles activated.
- Chest "open," but not too far forward.
- Shoulder blades pulled back, without causing non-physiological backward movement of the shoulders.
- Shoulders lowered, maintained at the same level.
- Spine elongated.
- The head in the extension of the torso, not tilted back, the chin should not be extended forward.
- The back of the head, shoulder blades, and buttocks should be in one plane.

We present examples of flexibility exercises for pregnant women in Appendix 6.

9.3.4.5 Neuromotor Exercise

A special place should be occupied by neuromotor exercises, e.g., balance and coordination exercises [34] (Fig. 9.8). Although the center of gravity changes during pregnancy, women who continue previously practiced form of activity are able to perform exercises requiring a high level of balance. Coordination exercises are typically included, e.g., in a step aerobics or dance session. Balance exercises can be included as a part of other sessions, e.g., Pilates session, aerobics, and resistance training session.

The balance-enhancing activities are those, which include:

- Narrowing the base of support.
- Perturbation of the ground support.
- Decrease in proprioceptive sensation.
- Diminished or misleading visual inputs.
- Disturbed vestibular system input.
- Increased compliance of the support surface.

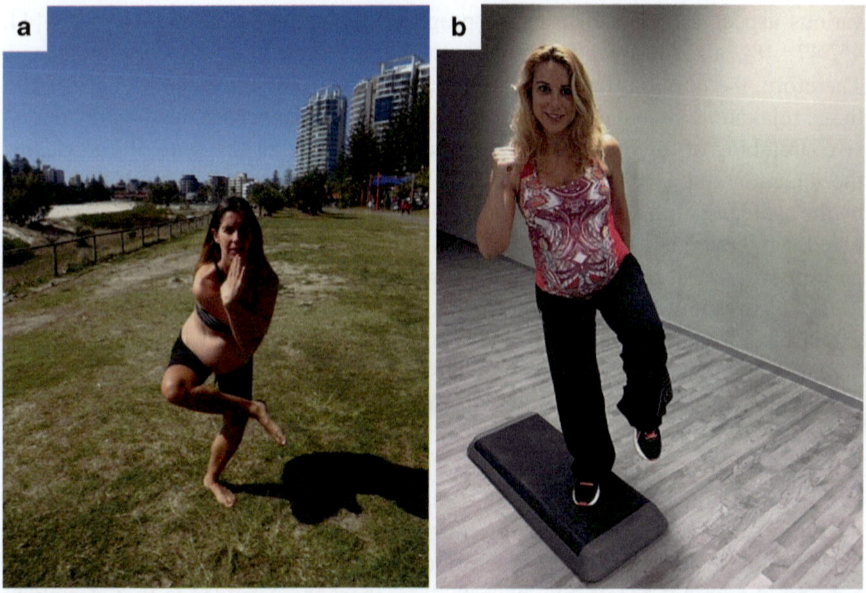

Fig. 9.8 Exercises requiring balance (**a**) and coordination (**b**) skills are examples of neuromotor exercises

- Movement of the center of mass of the body away from the vertical.

General techniques for neuromotor exercise can include following elements:

- Narrowing the base of support for the body.
- Displacing the center of mass to the limits of tolerance.
- Removing or minimizing contributions of visual, vestibular, and proprioceptive pathways to balance.

The validity of the above recommendations should be confirmed by experimental research. We presented examples of balance exercises for pregnant women in Appendix 7.

9.3.5 Flexibility Exercises

Flexibility (stretching) exercises should be part of a comprehensive exercise program, inter allia to reduce muscle tension and soreness, increase relaxation, improve range and ease of moves, and prevent injury [34, 108]. There are negligible scientific data on changes in the level of flexibility during pregnancy. Price et al [60]. observed that the sit-and-reach flexibility scores did not vary significantly between exercising pregnant women and sedentary control group. Their intervention circuit sessions ended with 5 min of hamstring, quadriceps, and calf stretching. No study participants reported injuries related to the exercise regimen. In studies analyzing various aspects of prenatal exercise programs including stretching exercises [44, 45, 47, 48], also no negative impact on musculoskeletal system was indicated. Therefore, the opinion that due to the action of pregnancy hormones that increase tissue relaxation, prenatal stretching exercises can be dangerous, leading to "excessive stretching of the muscles" is unfounded. With the current state of knowledge, the selection and execution of stretching exercises in pregnancy should be guided by the same principles as for the general adult population. It should only be remembered that the large belly will limit the trunk flexion. Stretching exercises should be performed in positions recommended for pregnant women (see Appendix 1). Due to the large weight load in standing positions, it is advisable to perform stretching exercises in the sitting, kneeling, and lying positions.

An interesting research issue is the use of abdominal stretching exercises during pregnancy. As the fetus grows, the abdominal muscles remain in permanent stretching until the day of delivery. The negative effect of this may be the separation of the abdominal muscles (see Chap. 12). Therefore, approaching it logically, one should concentrate on the stimuli compensating the effect of pregnancy development, i.e., limiting the stretching of the abdominal muscles by the proper selection of position and intensification of exercises that relax this muscle group, e.g., by abdominal breathing. Nevertheless, there is no evidence that stretching exercises for abdominal muscles during pregnancy may intensify or reduce the feeling of unpleasant tightness or expansion of the abdomen or predispose to the diastasis recti abdominis.

Stretching exercises are a good tool to regulate the intensity of activities. Their performance in the main part immediately after exercises strengthening a given muscle group effectively reduces the intensity and extends the break time. Therefore, this solution is proposed for beginners with a lower level of performance. In turn, for advanced women, it will be more reasonable to perform strengthening exercises directly after each other and to leave stretching for the final part. Before performing a stretching exercise, one must remember to relax the whole body, especially the muscle group being stretched and to breathe deeply and calmly [34].

During pregnancy, it is worth paying special attention to stretching:

1. The anterior (hip flexors) and medial (hip adductors) compartments of thigh muscles in preparation for a natural birth.
2. The hamstrings and hip abductors, in the prevention of the piriformis syndrome (pain and/or numbness in the area of the buttock radiating down the buttock and the leg, resulting from the compression of the sciatic nerve around the piriformis muscle).
3. The back muscles to lower their excessive tension and soreness caused by balancing the posture with the growing belly.
4. The muscles of the chest and the anterior shoulder girdle that have a tendency to shorten during pregnancy.

We present examples of flexibility exercises for pregnant women in Appendix 8.

9.3.6 Pelvic Floor Muscle Exercises

Pelvic floor muscles stabilize the body, support pelvic organs, and determine the quality of sexual life [109, 110]. Systematic reviews have shown that pelvic-floor exercises should be recommended for prevention and treatment of urinary incontinence [111–113], a chronic health complaint occurring in 14 to 69% of European women [114]. Pregnancy and vaginal birth are the causal factors for pelvic floor disorders [115], which relate to symptoms of urinary or anal incontinence, pelvic organ prolapse, sensory or emptying abnormalities of the lower urinary tract, defecation dysfunction, sexual dysfunction, and pelvic floor pain syndromes. Although adults of all ages should exercise pelvic floor muscles, it is particularly important in pregnancy.

Correct contraction of pelvic floor muscles in exercise training is described as contracting and inward lifting of the muscles around pelvic openings while keeping outer abdominal, gluteal, and hip adductor muscles relaxed [116–119]. In recent studies, the proportion of women who were unable to correctly activate the pelvic floor on initial exam varied from 14 to 53% [119–122]. Only two-thirds are confident that they were doing pelvic-floor exercises correctly [123] while at least one in five may have had misplaced their confidence [121]. That is why good instructions how to exercise pelvic floor muscles are essential [120–122]. Some authors recommend biofeedback sessions to learn the technique of contracting pelvic floor muscles [124–126].

Various pelvic floor muscle exercises and training protocols [127, 128] have been published, but none of them has been considered a gold standard. However, in the implementation of pelvic floor muscle exercises, it is worth taking into account the following principles:

1. The first stage is the location of the pelvic floor muscles. A woman must be convinced that she is operating the right muscles. A typical mistake is to activate synergistic muscles (e.g., abdomen, buttocks, and thighs) or pushing (strain) of the pelvic floor muscles by increasing intra-abdominal pressure, often while inhaling [129]. Examples of exercises on the location of pelvic floor muscles and the ability to isolate them in a conscious contracting are presented in Appendix 9. When specialized equipment is available to assess the activation of pelvic floor and synergistic muscles, the use of a 1–4 score scale (Table 9.2) to evaluate the technique of pelvic floor muscle contraction is recommended [119].
2. In order to properly locate it, it is worth using specialist equipment providing biofeedback [126] and visualization (e.g., imagining the feeling of tightening a vaginal

Table 9.2 Technique scores for pelvic floor contractions [119]

Score	Score description	Pelvic floor muscles	Synergistic muscles
4	Correct technique	Activated	Not activated
3	Incorrect technique	Activated first in order	Activated after pelvic floor
2	Incorrect technique	Activated but not first in order	Activated before pelvic floor
1	Incorrect technique	Not activated	Activated

tampon or a small balloon). The so-called pee-stop exercise is controversial. Undoubtedly, it gives excellent feedback on both the location of the pelvic floor muscles and on their strength (e.g., the urinary stream can be weakened of completely stopped). On the other hand, there are not scientifically proven views that such an action may cause a urinary retreat from the lower urinary tract contributing to infections and it may interfere with the micturition mechanism. In fact, there is one study by Chesnel et al. [130] who reported that the urine stream interruption during a single micturition increases the post-void residual volume and translates into less efficient micturition. However, to date, there are no studies confirming the harmful, long-term effects of this exercise in healthy women. Until reliable data are available on the subject, it seems rational to use "pee-stop" exercise sporadically as a kind of self-assessment but not as a basis for regular training.

3. A complex training for pelvic-floor muscles should be focused both on their contraction and relaxation [116]. Contractions are to improve, among others, supporting functions for pelvic organs and continence. Relaxing exercises are helpful for the correct process of micturition, defecation, and delivery.
4. In the pelvic floor muscle exercises, the proper breathing technique should be maintained – the same as in the case of exercises of other muscle groups: exhalation is performed during contraction and inhalation during relaxation [34].
5. One should start from simple exercises (e.g., short contractions, the so-called quick flicks), gradually moving to more complex tasks (e.g., several-second holds at different rates) [131].
6. It is important to have a comprehensive impact on the motor skills of pelvic floor muscles, improving their speed, strength, endurance, and muscular coordination, and engaging both fast and slow twitch muscle fibers [132].
7. Exercises should start with an isolated form, i.e., when the pelvic floor is taut the rest of the body should be relaxed. According to Bø and Mørkved [129], the simultaneous activation of large synergistic muscles may mask the awareness and strength of pelvic floor muscle contraction.
8. Due to the low intensity of the isolated pelvic floor muscles exercises, they should be planned for the end of the exercise sessions.
9. Gradually, it is useful to incorporate pelvic floor muscle exercises in exercises that condition other muscle groups, e.g., abdomen, buttocks, and thighs. Thanks to this, in one exercise session, one can get more training stimuli for pelvic floor muscles [129, 132].
10. Conscious activation of pelvic floor in marching, running, or aerobics movements is a more difficult stage, but may be helpful to prevent urine leakage during these activities [50, 51].
11. An important task is to implement a conscious habit of contracting the pelvic floor muscles in daily activities, against the increase of the intra-abdominal pressure, e.g., before lifting heavy objects, before coughing, laughing, sneezing, etc. [131].

See Chaps. 6 and 12 for further explanation on this topic.

9.3.7 Cool-Down

The cool-down should be a part of every exercise session [36], also for pregnant women. Its main role is to calm the body systems after intense physical effort. It is good when after this part the respiratory rhythm and the heart rate return to the level close to pre-exercise values [34]. In the cool-down, the woman should assess her well-being and the intensity and difficulty of the exercises. If they were conducted by an exercise professional, there should be a summary and motivation for the next exercise sessions. It is also time to ask questions and provide professional information to build women's beliefs about the safety and benefits of prenatal exercise. In the cool-down, it is recommended to perform stretching exercises, according to the exercises carried out in the main part. It is also a great time to do exercises to prepare women for natural labor and delivery.

Natural birth, i.e., a birth without any medical intervention, is the best end of the pregnancy for the mother and the baby, both from the psychophysical and the social point of view [133]. Methods of childbirth other than physiological should be used only when justified [134]. Preparation for natural birth should be one of main goals of the future mothers, their families, and the healthcare system during antenatal education course [31]. Regular participation in the prenatal exercise program can significantly support this goal.

The onset and course of delivery are significantly influenced by the interaction of hormones, including an appropriate production of oxytocin. Its secretion can be affected by too high catecholamine levels, specific to the state of threat [133]. Russell et al. [135] observed among strenuous exercising athletes that catecholamines elevated by exercise may interact with female hormones. Magann et al. [136] found that heavy physical exercise in military training during pregnancy significantly increased the risk of induction or augmentation of labor with oxytocin and longer first stages of labor resulting in total longer labors. It is likely that the direction of women's mind to the aggressive, non-maternity tasks, reduced their psychological and physical readiness for the birth, manifested in disorders in its initiation and progression. Research by Magann et al. [136] may be evidence that not only the quantity but also the quality of prenatal exercise are important in order to get their positive impact on pregnancy and childbirth.

Both for hormonal balance, as well as for mental and physical preparation of women for childbirth and motherhood there are proposed, inter alia, birth positions, breathing exercises, relaxation, and visualization [27–31]. The cool-down part usually takes 5–10 min, but when planning visualization, it is worth prolonging it for an additional 15–20 min.

9.3.7.1 Birth Positions

According to the global trend of promoting natural birth, it is important to prepare a woman for the so-called use of birth positions. There is not one universal, most convenient birth position. The choice of position by the woman, the way of breathing or movement should be completely intuitive and may change with the progress of labor [137, 138].

Many women thinking about childbirth have a picture of childbearing in the so-called classic position or lithotomy position, i.e., lying on your back with legs gaping, raised up. However, this position is the least favorable from the point of view of labor physiology and biomechanics of movement, because a woman has to push the child against the force of gravity [137, 138]. In vertical (or up-right) positions, the force of gravity supports the maternal effort of pushing, facilitates proper descent of the child into the birth canal and cervical dilation. Thanks to this, the time of delivery may be shortened and the necessity of using labor augmentation is reduced. In turn, the kneeling positions with the flexed trunk and the lying positions reduce the pressure of fetal head on the perineum area. They are particularly helpful in the first stage of delivery, when the laboring woman should not push because the cervix is incompletely opened, and also in long deliveries when the woman lacks the strength to maintain her vertical position. The use of different birth positions decreases perineal injury. In addition, it positively affects the psyche of the woman giving birth: it reduces the sense of anxiety, encourages active participation in childbirth, and increases the satisfaction with its course [139, 140].

To fully take advantage of the various birth positions, physical preparation for them is necessary. Some require strengthening or stretching of specific muscle parts. When planning prenatal physical activity, birth positions should be treated as one of the functional exercises and performed in each session, in accordance with generally accepted principles of teaching movement and training progression. The educational aspect is also important here. It is likely that a woman who has learned various birth positions during pregnancy, both theoretically and practically, will try to use them during the delivery. The study by Miquelutti et al. [30] showed that women who during antenatal education received instructions to adopt the vertical positions, comparing to controls, spent significantly more time in the upright positions and considered them more comfortable than the horizontal positions.

Recommended principles of performing birth positions in prenatal classes are as follows:

1. Exercises of birth positions can be performed as cool-down exercises at the end of the training session. They can also be included as relaxation or stretching exercises between a series of exercises strengthening various muscle groups.
2. In all birth positions, the coccyx bone should be maximally bent backward and pelvis tilted anteriorly to increase pelvic dimensions.
3. The whole body of a woman, and in particular the pelvic floor muscles, abdominals, thighs and buttocks, should be maximally relaxed, which is to build the ability to relax during painful contractions.
4. It is good to do breathing exercises in the birth positions, which helps to build the ability to breathe properly during delivery.

5. Birth position exercise may be accompanied by rhythmic pelvis movements to the front and back or up and down, which during the delivery may reduce the pain. This technique is particularly effective when it is combined with a rapid respiratory rhythm (e.g., pant breathing).
6. It is recommended to maintain birth positions by min. 20–30 s to get the right training stimulus (e.g., for muscle stretching).

We present examples of birth position exercises in Appendix 10.

9.3.7.2 Breathing Exercises

Breathing exercises bring many health benefits, including a reduction in the level of stress [141] and in the muscle fatigue [142] and an improvement in function of the circulatory system [143]. They are particularly recommended for pregnant women as, among others they may compensate for physiological and biomechanical changes in breathing pattern induced by pregnancy and increase the amount of oxygen transported to the fetus [144]. Owing to breathing exercises, a woman can reduce discomfort associated with a feeling of breathlessness appearing at the beginning of physical exertion. Breathing exercises are particularly important in the second and third trimesters, when the growing womb hinders the lowering of the diaphragm during inhalation.

Breathing exercises are an important element of preparation for delivery [29, 30]. Boaviagem et al. [145] observed that 6-week stress management program including relaxation breathing and progressive muscle relaxation twice a day contributed to the reduction of perceived stress and increased the sense of control in pregnant women. Abdominal breathing or the so-called belly breathing technique is advocated to improve the excursion of the diaphragm [146]. In the study by Amola et al. [147], 4-week training of diaphragmatic breathing exercises relieved dyspnea and improved pulmonary functions and capacity during third trimester of pregnancy. In addition, appropriate breathing techniques help to cope with pain during delivery [148] and protect against perineal damage during labor [149]. It may increase the efficiency of child displacement during childbirth.

Research indicates that the occasional use of breathing exercises does not bring the desired effect. In the study by Bergström et al. [150], four 2-h sessions with training in breathing and relaxation techniques during natural childbirth preparation did not decrease the use of epidural analgesia during labor, nor did it improve the birth experience or affect parental stress in early parenthood in nulliparous women, compared with a standard form of antenatal education. Boaviagem et al. [145] in turn have shown that breathing techniques offered to women during the first period of labor were not effective to control anxiety, pain, fatigue, and maternal satisfaction.

The above studies suggest that in order to achieve the effectiveness of breathing exercises and the possibility of their use during labor, it is necessary to perform them systematically throughout pregnancy [151]. Breathing exercises perfectly blend in prenatal exercises, both in the cool-down part and in rest breaks between the series of strengthening exercises. The easiest way to do it is in a sitting position, which provides space in the chest and abdominal cavity, and facilitates relaxation of the abdominal muscles and observation of their work. One can treat breathing exercises performed in other positions, for example lying on the back or side, as a functional exercise. In most exercises, inhaling is done through the nose, exhaling through mouth and nose. We present examples of breathing exercises in Appendix 11.

9.3.7.3 Visualization of Pregnancy and Birth

In mental visualization training, one uses imagination to program the mind to perform in a particular situation in the best possible manner. Such exercises performed systematically and repeatedly lead to the development of neuronal connections between muscles and the central nervous system. Mental visualization training is commonly used in elite sports training and rehabilitation [152]. Visualization is increasingly becoming an important element of preparation for childbirth [31, 151]. The randomized control study by Rakhshani et al. [153] on yoga-based visualization and relaxation in high-risk pregnancy has shown significantly better uteroplacental and fetoplacental blood flow velocity in the yoga group compared to the control group. Ricchi et al. proved that women who had practiced visualization in their antenatal classes had a higher likelihood of taking advantage of the visualization exercises during the labor [151].

During visualization, a woman can imagine the proper development of a child during pregnancy and/or the delivery process. These ideas have a positive effect on the hormonal balance, reduce the level of anxiety, and build a positive attitude to delivery, including faith in their own strength to give birth to a child. Although the impact of visualization has not yet been well researched, certainly exercises of this type are a good form of rest after physical exercise. Women should take a comfortable position, preferably lying on their side or on the back, if in this position the pressure of the uterus does not cause discomfort. It will be useful to cover the body, due to the significant reduction in body temperature after intense physical exercise in the main part. They can use ready-made materials with a recorded voice or create pictures themselves. It is important that they evoke positive emotions and do not perpetuate fear. Depending on the organizational possibilities, the visualization may last from several to between 10 and 20 min.

9.4 Further Research

Owing to the fact that many unjustified ideas limit prenatal physical activity (like the need to wait up to 12–13 weeks of gestation to start exercising, the need to avoid raising hands above shoulder level or abdominal exercises, etc.), it is necessary to conduct research in this area and disseminate the findings. It seems reasonable to classify the forms of physical activity as safe for pregnancy or not on the basis of multidimensional research analysis, not just on implied opinions. Certainly, there is a lack of scientific data on how strenuous, high impact and/or technically complex activities can influence the course of pregnancy, labor and delivery, and child development and how one can reduce their potential risks.

Insufficient information is available on flexibility exercises for pregnant women. A particularly interesting issue is whether the stretching exercises of the abdominal muscles predispose pregnant women to the diastasis recti abdominis or reduce its prevalence. It is also worth investigating whether any prenatal exercise program (including or excluding specific exercises) can have a preventive or therapeutic effect on the separation of the abdominal muscles in pregnancy. The validity of the recommendations for DRA prevention presented in this chapter should be confirmed by experimental research, as well. It is also interesting to evaluate the possibility of alleviating other pregnancy and puerperal symptoms and complications through specific exercise programs.

No information is available on neuromotor exercises for pregnant women. A particularly interesting issue is whether balance and coordination exercises included in a prenatal program would be effective in preventing falls.

There is a need for more experimental studies confirming the effectiveness of exercises preparing for birth (including various breathing techniques, birth position exercises, relaxation, and visualization) in improving the delivery outcomes.

We also notice a heterogeneous way of reporting exercise programs and a lack of information regarding the validity of experimental studies using "prenatal exercise programs" described as a complex intervention in the context of healthcare [154]. A particularly interesting issue is validating such programs before a pilot, feasibility, or a protocol study is performed. It would be helpful in understanding whether or not, which and how the exercise program was effective.

9.5 Conclusion

This chapter addresses the steps for planning, conducting, and monitoring prenatal exercise classes, and explains how to select and adapt different forms of exercises to achieve their maximum safety and efficiency. With the current state of knowledge and scientific rejection of the existing myths associated with the alleged harmful effects of physical activity on the course of pregnancy, birth, and fetal development, prenatal exercises can be more and more diverse and available to women with different needs.

Appendix 1: Exercise Positions for Pregnant Women

Standing Position (Fig. 9.9)

Execution: feet apart to the width of the hips, buttocks slightly contracted, abdominal muscles activated (shortened), pelvis in neutral position, relaxed knees, straight back, shoulders blades depressed and retracted, head in the spine extension. The modification is standing upright with various foot settings (e.g., parallel, outside).

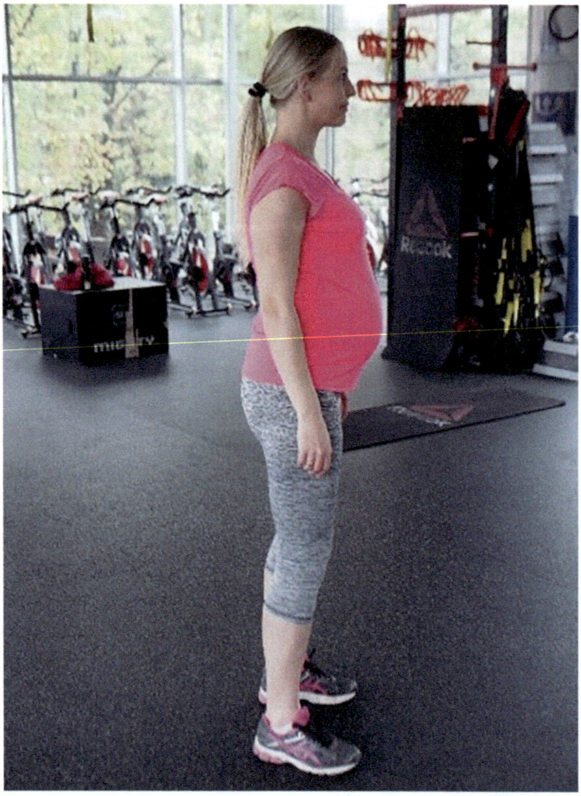

Fig. 9.9 Standing position

Recommendations: The best position for body posture correction. Half-squats, squats, and lunges are performed from this position. Exercises for other muscle groups with equipment (e.g., dumbbells) or without may be performed. Standing position should be used in such activities, where it is impossible or contraindicated to sit or lie down (e.g., in outdoor exercises or directly after aerobic classes when the heart rate is still high).

Contraindications and remarks: In some guidelines, there is the recommendation to avoid motionless standing [155]. Carvalho et al. [156] noted that maintaining the **standing** position for a long time worsened low back pain in 27.2% of pregnant women in the third trimester. Although there is no clear scientific evidence, it seems that owing to the force of gravity. The standing position is inappropriate for women with pubic symphysis [157].

Sitting Positions (Figs. 9.10 and 9.11)

Execution: Sit-downs can be done in different versions: with straight legs or bent legs, with legs in parallel or in a straddle. The back is straight, the shoulders blades depressed and retracted, the head is in the extension of the spine.

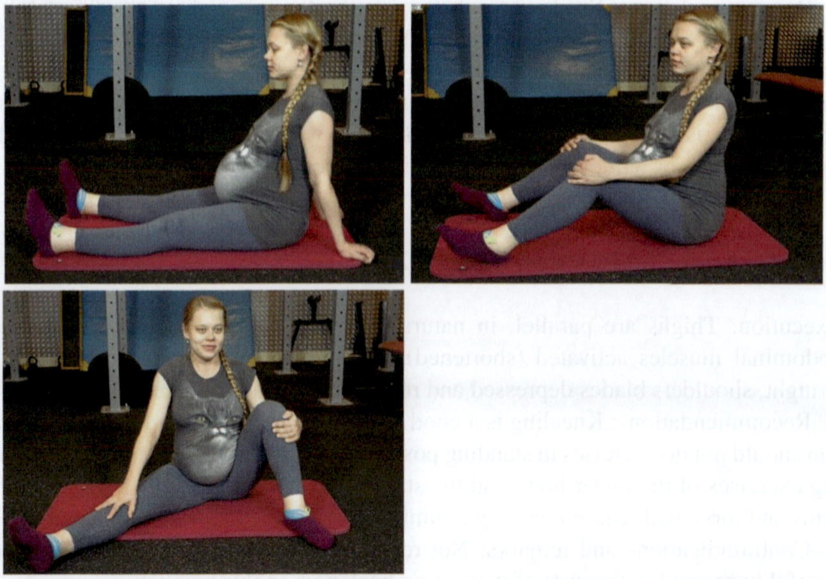

Fig. 9.10 Sitting positions on the ground

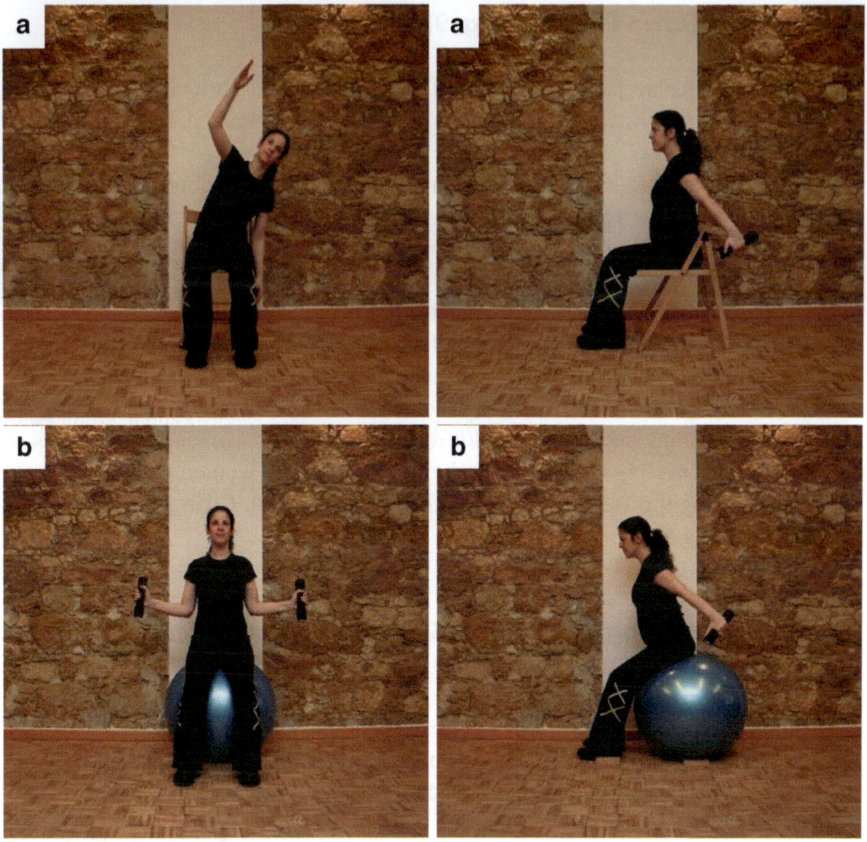

Fig. 9.11 Sitting positions: (**a**) on the chair; (**b**) on the stability ball

Recommendations: Sit-downs, whether on the floor in a chair or on a stability ball are a very good alternative for women who for some reason should not do exercises in standing positions. Due to the fact that the torso is still upright, they are suitable for the posturing exercises of the upper body. They are a good starting position for exercising arm muscles, torso, front legs, with equipment (e.g., dumbbells, exercise bands) or without, and for breathing exercises.

Vertical Kneeling Position (Fig. 9.12a)

Execution: Thighs are parallel, in natural spacing, buttocks slightly contracted, abdominal muscles activated (shortened), pelvis in neutral position, the back is straight, shoulders blades depressed and retracted, head in spine extension.

Recommendations: Kneeling is a good alternative for women who for some reason should not do exercises in standing positions. It is a good position for the posturing exercises of the upper body and the starting position for muscle training of the arms and torso with equipment (e.g., dumbbells) or without.

Contraindications and remarks: Not recommended for people with injuries or painful knees and in the case of worsening back pain in this position.

Kneeling Sit-Down Position (Fig. 9.12b)

Execution: Thighs are parallel, in natural spacing or apart, buttocks resting on the feet, the back is straight, shoulders blades depressed and retracted, the head is in the extension of the spine.

Recommendations: Kneeling sit-down position is a very good alternative for women who for some reason should not do exercises in standing positions, especially for those with back pain (the hip flexion reduces lumbar lordosis). Due to the fact that the torso is still upright, they are suitable for the posturing exercises of the upper body. They are a good starting position for exercising the muscles of the arms and torso with equipment (e.g., dumbbells) or without and for breathing exercises. The performance of kneeling alone is an exercise stretching the quadriceps muscles, anterior muscle group of the lower leg and foot.

Contraindications and remarks: Not recommended for women with injuries or painful knees. Kneeling sit-downs can be problematic for women with excessively shortened and tight quadriceps and / or flexors of the foot. Change position if leg numbness occurs.

Supported Kneeling Position (So-Called On All Fours) On Forearms or Hands (Fig. 9.12c)

Execution: The weight of the body rests evenly on the knees and hands, thighs, and arms are arranged in parallel, in natural spacing, hips over the knees, shoulders over the hands, active elbow joints, straight back, back and abdominal muscles activated, head in the spine extension.

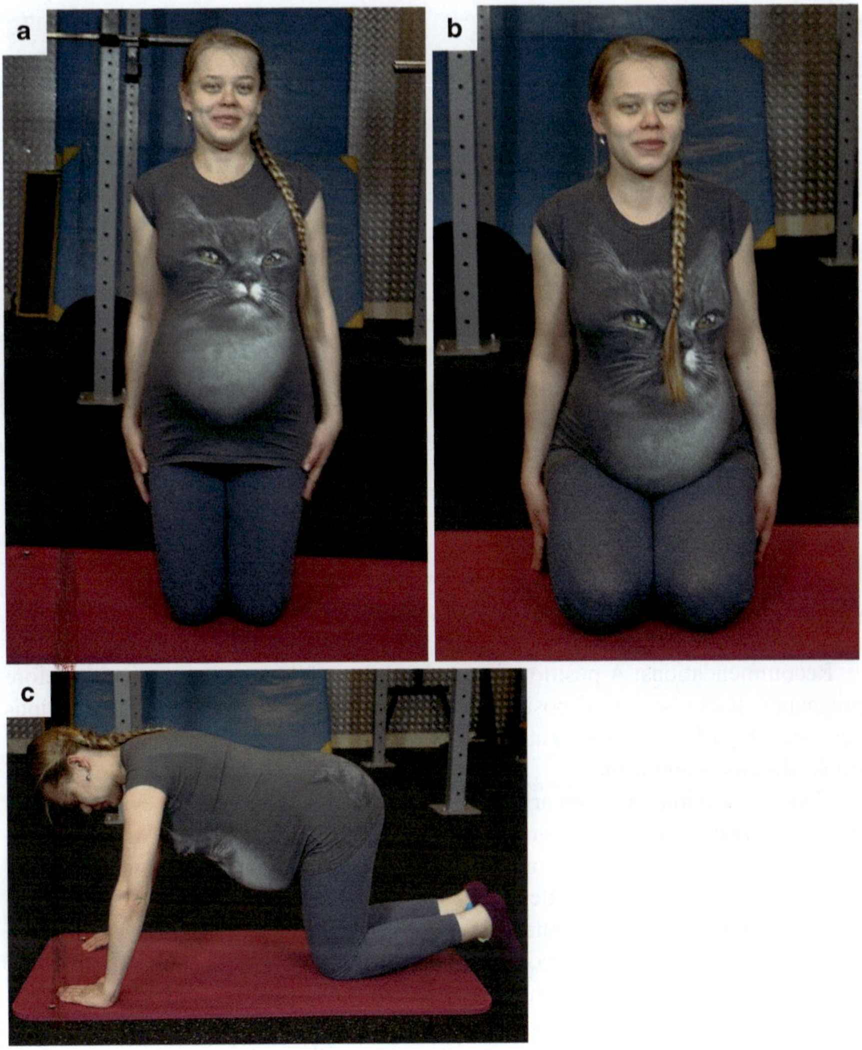

Fig. 9.12 Kneeling positions: (**a**) vertical kneeling position; (**b**) kneeling sit-down position; (**c**) supported kneeling position

Recommendations: When the abdominal and back muscles are properly activated, the position of the supported kneeling may be a good position for the exercise of the hamstrings and gluteus muscles, posterior muscles of the trunk, shoulders, and neck and also chest muscles (various versions of push-ups).

Contraindications and remarks: Although there is no scientific evidence, taking into account the force of gravity, this position may deepen the diastasis recti abdominis (heavy uterus rests on the abdominal muscles as in a hammock, weakened abdominal tissue due to uterine pressure may be further separated). Therefore, the position in the supported kneeling should be used in moderation in asymptomatic

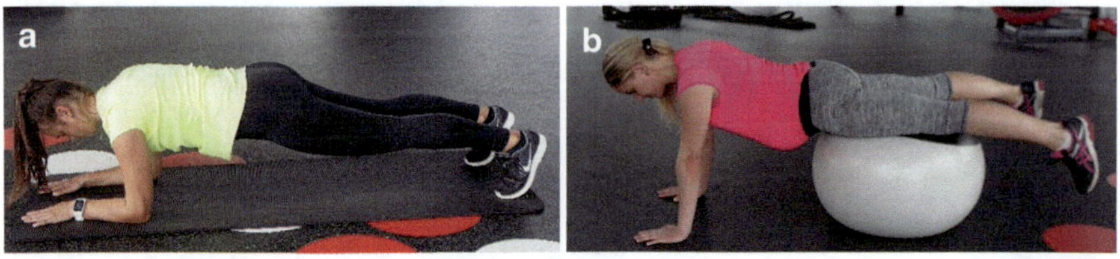

Fig. 9.13 Frontal plank position: (**a**) on the forearms; (**b**) with legs supported on the stability ball

women. In women with confirmed separation of the rectus abdominis muscles, it seems reasonable to completely exclude this position. For a wider use of the supported kneeling for prenatal exercises, one can support the abdomen on a stability ball or big bean bags.

Frontal Plank Position (Fig. 9.13)

Execution: The weight of the body rests evenly on the feet and hands (or forearms), and the arms are parallel, in natural spacing, the shoulders over the hands, active elbow joints, straight back, trunk muscles activated, head in spine extension.

Recommendations: A position directed to advanced women who used it before pregnancy. It can be a good position for the exercise of the chest muscles (various versions of push-ups), hamstrings and gluteus muscles, posterior muscles of the trunk, shoulders and neck.

Contraindications and remarks: Although there is no scientific evidence, taking into account the force of gravity, this position may deepen the diastasis recti abdominis (heavy uterus rests on the abdominal muscles as in a hammock, weakened abdominal tissue due to uterine pressure may be further separated). Therefore, the position in the supported kneeling should be used in moderation in asymptomatic women. In women with confirmed separation of the rectus abdominis muscles, it seems reasonable to completely exclude this position. Increasing weight of the uterus can hinder proper maintenance of the spine and abdominal contraction; therefore, it is necessary to systematically evaluate the technique of exercises performed in this position.

Supine Position (Fig. 9.14)

Execution: The back of the body lies on the floor, the legs can be straight or bent, the arms along the body, sideways or up.

Recommendations: Excellent relaxation position, relieving the spine, good position for pelvic floor muscle exercises, breathing exercises, and visualization.

Contraindications and remarks: Majority of guidelines on exercise in pregnancy recommended avoiding or limiting the supine position after the first

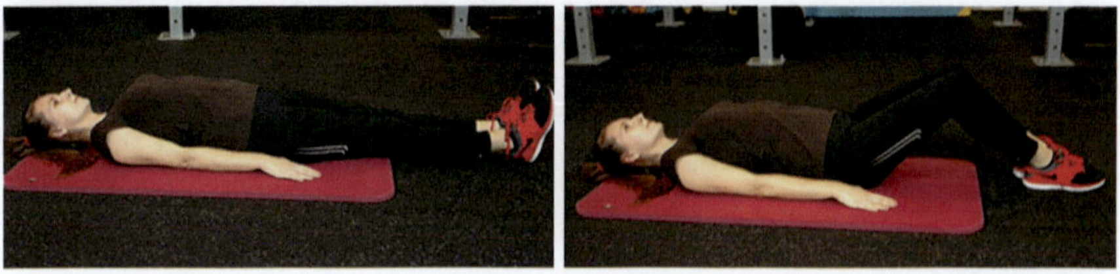

Fig. 9.14 Supine positions

Fig. 9.15 Supine position with the support of the back

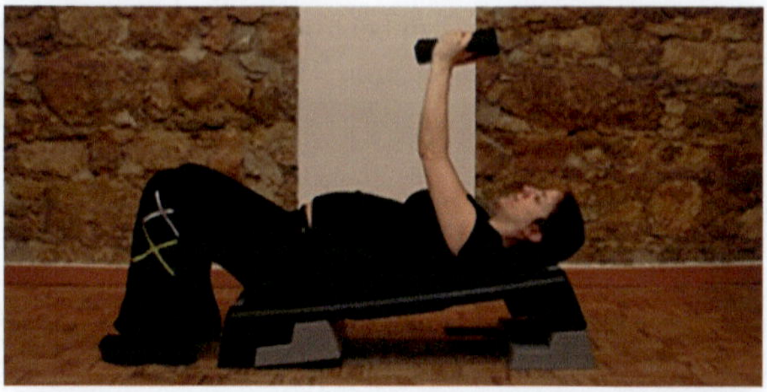

trimester, or after 16 weeks of gestation, or after the fourth month of gestation (see Chaps. 7 and 9). In this position, the heavy uterus presses on the inferior vena cava and decreases the uterine blood flow [95], which may result in discomfort, dizziness, or anxiety in a pregnant woman. The observation, however, shows that not all women experience a worsening of well-being in this position [158]. Therefore, the complete elimination of exercises in supine positions is not justified and should be supported by an individual assessment of the woman's well-being. An alternative solution is to put a pillow or towel underneath one hip [159], change the position for lying on the side, or support the back to get a less horizontal body position (Fig. 9.15).

Lying on the Side (Fig. 9.16)

Execution: The weight of the body rests on one side, evenly from the legs to the shoulders, the head rests on the lower arm stretched along the torso, the trunk muscles can be relaxed. For balance, you can support the front on the palm of the upper hand and / or bend the legs in the hip joints and / or knee joints (according to the purpose of the exercise being performed).

Recommendations: Perfect relaxation position, relieving the spine, good position for pelvic floor muscle exercises, breathing exercises, visualization. It is a good alternative to changing positions for women who feel discomfort in lying on their backs. For longer lying, a left-sided position is more desirable [160], facilitating the free flow of venous blood to the heart. A comfortable way to change the side of lying down seems to be going through lying on the back.

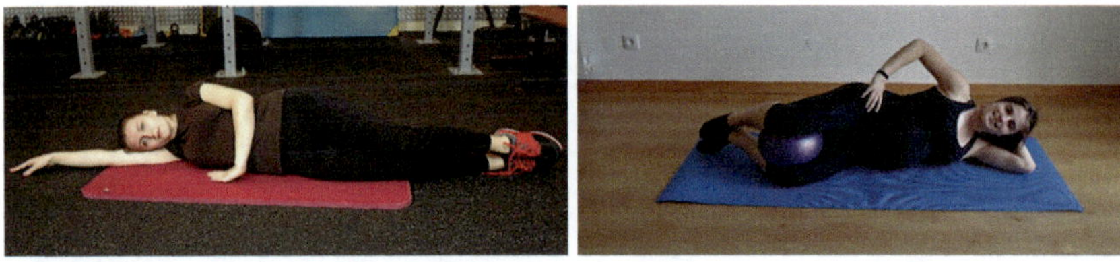

Fig. 9.16 Lying on the side

Contraindications and remarks: A frequent mistake is supporting the head on the hand of the lower arm bent in the elbow or lifting the torso through support on the forearm of the lower arm. This position unnecessarily affects one side of the neck spine.

Prone Position (Lying on the Front)

Due to the growing uterus, lying on the front is a very uncomfortable position for pregnant women, especially in the second and third trimesters. Until more information becomes available, ACSM suggests avoiding prone position [161]. So far, however, there is no scientific evidence that the prone position is dangerous to the course of pregnancy.

Recommendations: Before the belly protrudes, a good position for the hamstrings, gluteus muscles, and posterior muscles of the trunk, shoulders, and neck.

Contraindications and remarks: As the pregnancy progresses, a woman may feel both physical and psychological discomfort associated with the pressure on the abdomen.

Appendix 2: Examples of Aerobics Movements for Pregnant Women

1. Step touch—from the basic standing position step side to side transferring the body weight with the leading leg and putting a foot to the foot (Fig. 9.17). The movement to the side should be extensive to involve the adductors and abductors of the thigh as much as possible. When the body weight is completely transferred, the pelvic floor should be contracted. Modification of the step touch is performed in various spatial variants, e.g., double step touch, L-step, square step (step touch in a square), step touch traveling diagonally (zigzag).
2. Step out (or side to side)—standing with feet apart by a slight bent of both knees (count of 1), the weight of the body is transferred toward the movement being performed, the other leg rests with the toes on the ground (count of 2). When the body weight is completely transferred, the pelvic floor should be contracted. The step is performed alternately in both directions. The torso is in a straight line, the foot of the stepping leg is fully attached to the ground, while

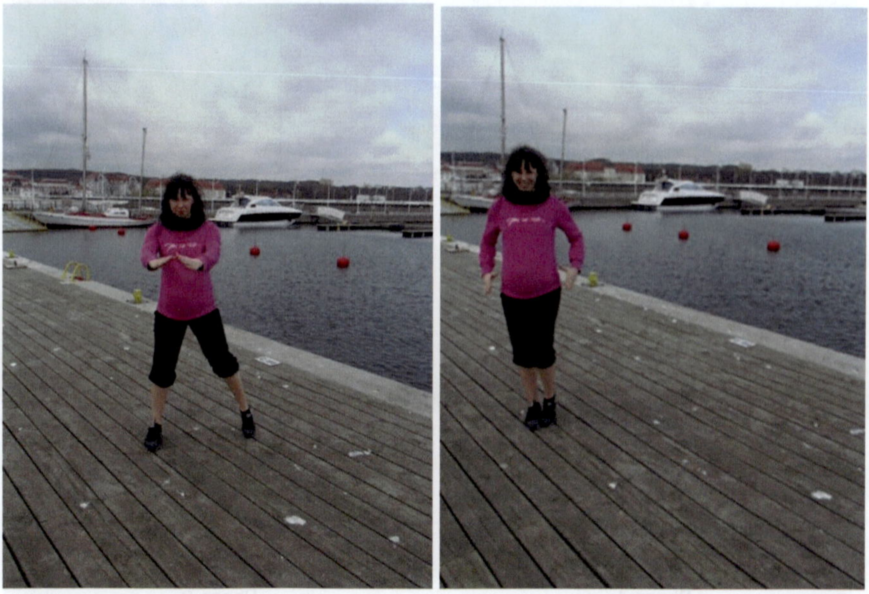

Phase 1 Phase 2

Fig. 9.17 Step touch

the second foot emphasizes the movement with the toes only. Both feet are in one line (Fig. 9.18).

3. Heel back. The step is performed as a step-out step, but in the last phase the second leg is detached from the ground, bent at the knee joint to about 90 degrees, the heel pointing toward the buttock (count of 2). When the body weight is completely transferred, the pelvic floor should be contracted. It is necessary to eliminate the forward movement of the hips in the final stage of the step that increases the lumbar lordosis (Fig. 9.19).
4. Knee up or knee lift. The knee can be raised forward (front knee up – Fig. 9.20a) or sideways (side knee up – Fig. 9.20b). The step is performed as a step-out step, but in the final stage, the second leg is detached from the ground, bent at the knee joint to about 90 degrees, with the knee pointing forward or sideways at the thigh (count of 2). When the weight is completely transferred to the side and the knee is lifted up, the pelvic floor should be stretched. It is necessary to eliminate the forward movement of the hips in the final stage of the step that increases the lumbar lordosis. When detaching the lower limb from the ground and lifting the knee, focus on maintaining the balance of the body. In women with advanced pregnancy, it may be necessary to shorten the lift of the leg so as not to cause the abdomen to be hit from the bottom by the thigh.

    The knee up step can be made in repetitions, e.g., twice or four times (four knee-up repeats). Done four times it is a step changing the leading leg in choreography.

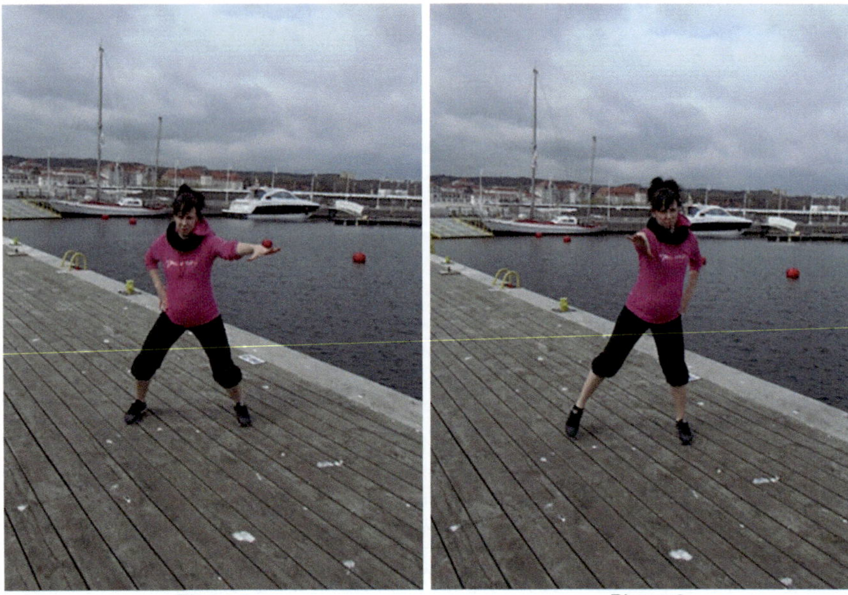

Phase 1 Phase 2

Fig. 9.18 Step out

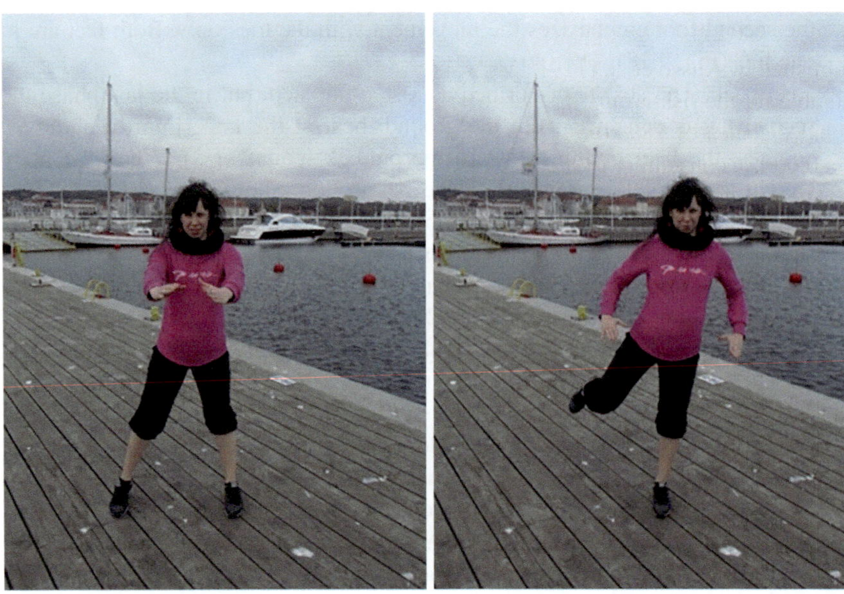

Phase 1 Phase 2

Fig. 9.19 Heel back

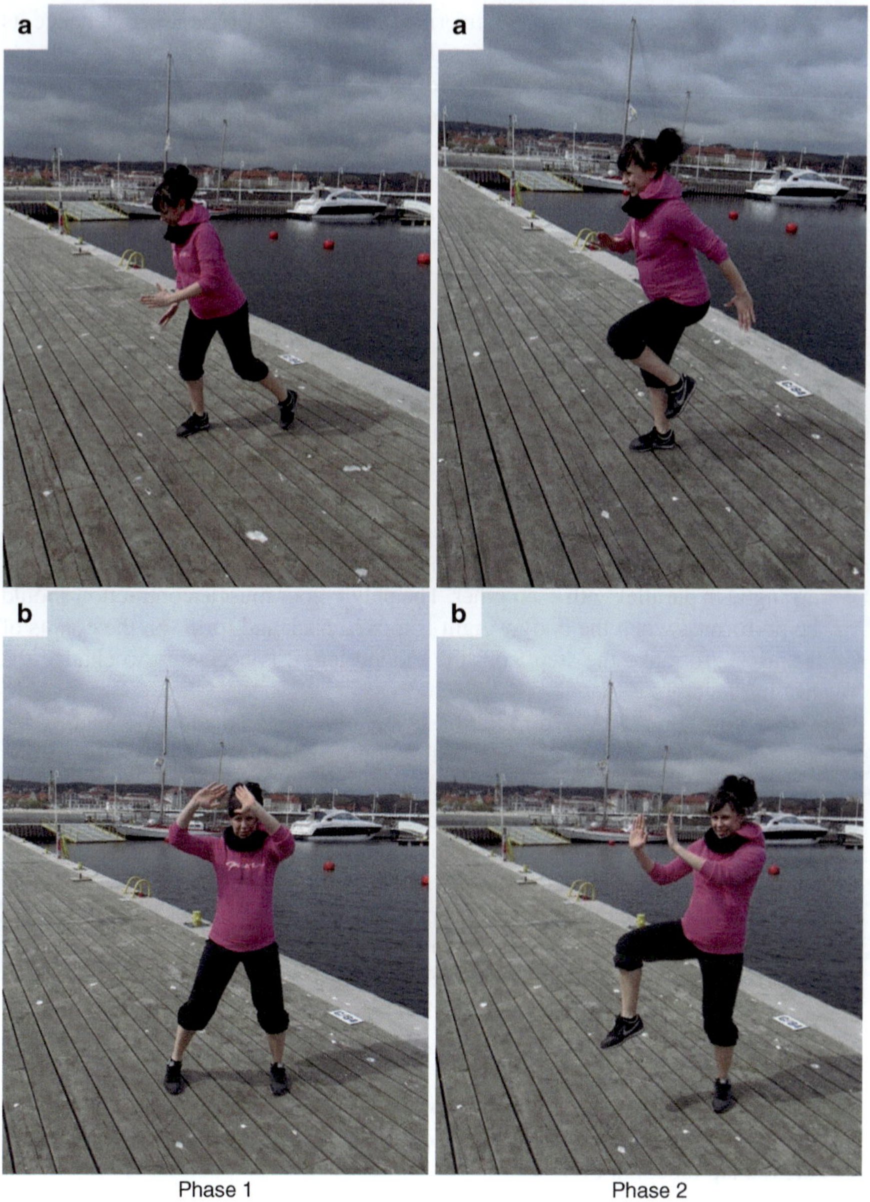

Fig. 9.20 Knee up (**a**—to the front; **b**—to the side)

5. V-step (Fig. 9.21). The step is performed in the shape of the letter V, hence its name. From the basic standing position, step 1 ft diagonally forward, outside (count of 1), then step the second leg diagonally forward, outside to the position of feet apart (count of 2), return of the first leg to the starting position (count of 3), return of the second leg to the starting position (count of 4).

   The forward movement is carried out naturally from the heel, and the feet are directed toward the outside. When returning to the back, the feet are in a parallel position, the entire sole attached to the ground. When the feet are joining in the final stage of the step, the pelvic floor should be contracted. The center of gravity should be as far as possible at the same level, without raising it or lowering it too much. The step is performed alternately in both directions. When the movement starts from the backward direction, the step is called A step.
6. Mambo forward and backward (Fig. 9.22)—from the basic standing position, moving the leading leg forward with the body weight (count of 1), returning the weight of the body onto the second stationary leg (count of 2), moving the leading leg back together with the weight of the body (count of 3), the return of the weight of the body to the stationary leg (count of 4). The stationary leg is always in contact with the ground and remains at the same place, and the feet are arranged in parallel with each other. The pelvic floor muscle contraction should be performed when the body weight is moved back and forth (on the counts of 1 and 3). To make the step from the second leg, it is necessary to change the leading leg.
7. Grape vine (Fig. 9.23). From the basic standing position, step the leading leg sideways with the body-weight transfer (count of 1), the crossing of the second leg at the back (count of 2), another step with the leading leg sideways with the weight transfer (count of 3) and bringing the second leg to (count of 4). The feet are directed slightly to the outside, all the time in one line. To increase the work of the abductor and adductor muscles, the feet are set far to the sides. The pelvic floor muscle contraction should be performed at the moment of crossing the legs (on the count of 2) and with joining the legs in the final step (on the count of 4). The step is performed alternately in both directions.
8. Marching forward/backward (Fig. 9.24)—is a modification of the march. The march forward is performed on 1, 2, 3, attaching legs, the so-called tap on 4 (can be made with knee up or a kick). Return to the starting position by moving backwards to 1, 2, 3, attaching legs to 4. Both legs should be loaded evenly. The pelvic floor muscle contraction should be performed at the moment of performing the tap (at count of 4).

   In order to increase the intensity of exercises, it is possible to perform high impact movements. Adding jumps and hops most often takes place in the final phase of the exercise, e.g., in step touch at the moment of joining the legs (on

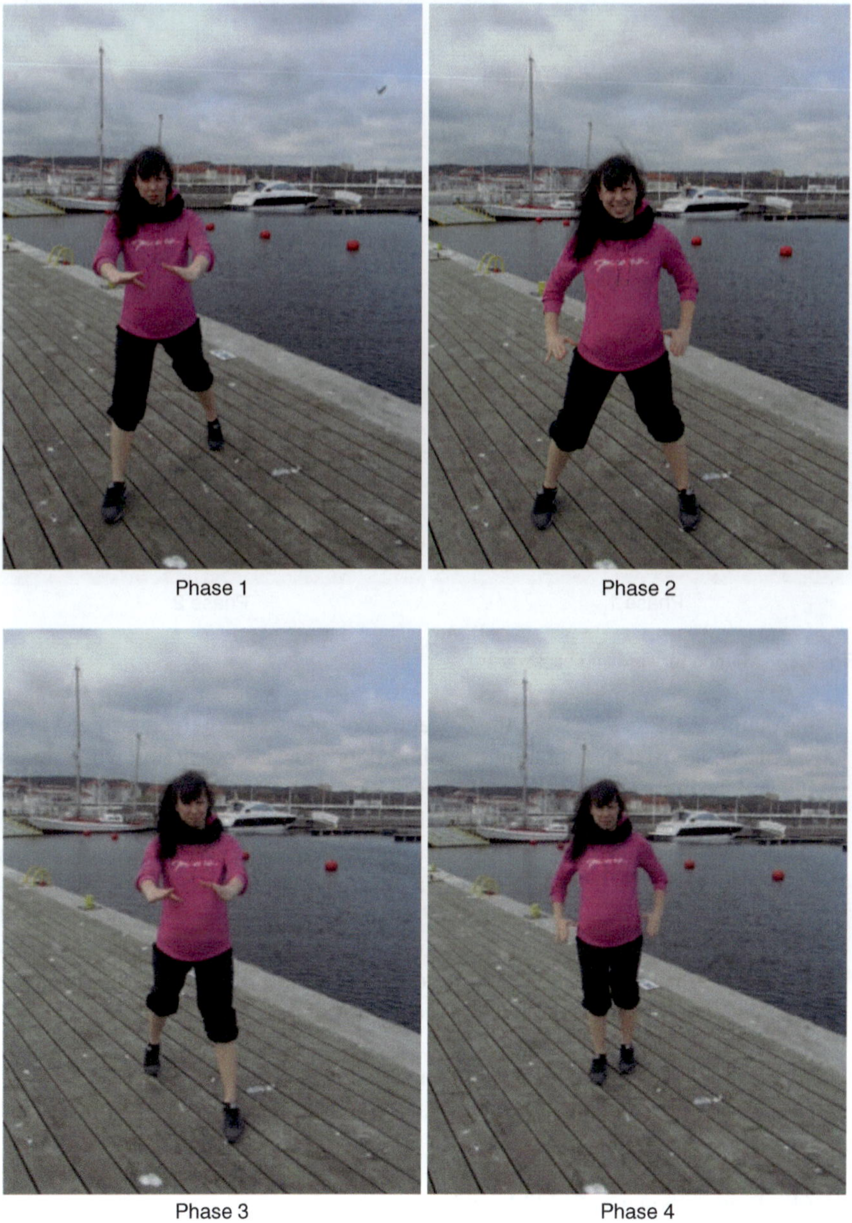

Fig. 9.21 V-step

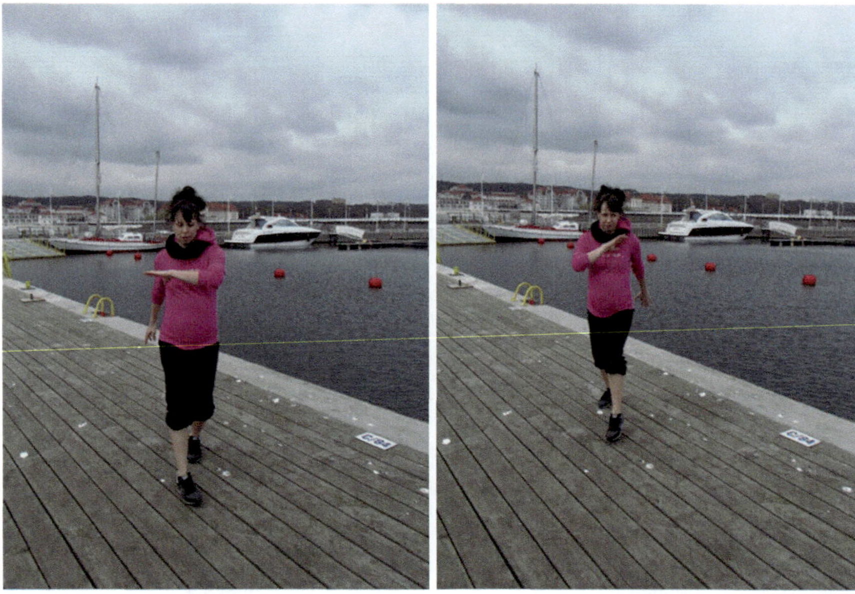

Phase 1 Phase 2

Fig. 9.22 Mambo forward and backward

the count of 2, Fig. 9.25). For the prevention of urinary incontinence, the woman should be advised to maintain the pelvic floor muscle contraction when jumping and the intra-abdominal pressure is at its greatest. It is easier to maintain the pelvic floor muscle activation and the continence in movements where the thighs are together. It is likely that urine leakage may occur in movements where thighs are apart at an increase in intra-abdominal pressure, e.g., in jumping jacks. Although there is a lack of scientific research on the relationship of the frequency and intensity of stress urinary incontinence in high-impact aerobics in pregnant women, it is common sense not to recommend high-impact aerobics for those who already experience this discomfort.

9. Examples of combinations:
   (a) Step touch right (2 beats) + step touch left (2 beats) x 8 times [32 beats].
   (b) Double step touch right (4 beats) + double step touch left (4 beats) x 4 times [32 beats].
   (c) Repeat sequence 1) [32 beats].
   (d) Repeat sequence 2) [32 beats].
   (e) Step touch right (2 beats) + step touch left (2 beats) x 8 times [32 beats].
   (f) Grapevine right (4 beats) + grapevine left (4 beats) x 4 times [32 beats].
   (g) Repeat sequence 5) [32 beats].

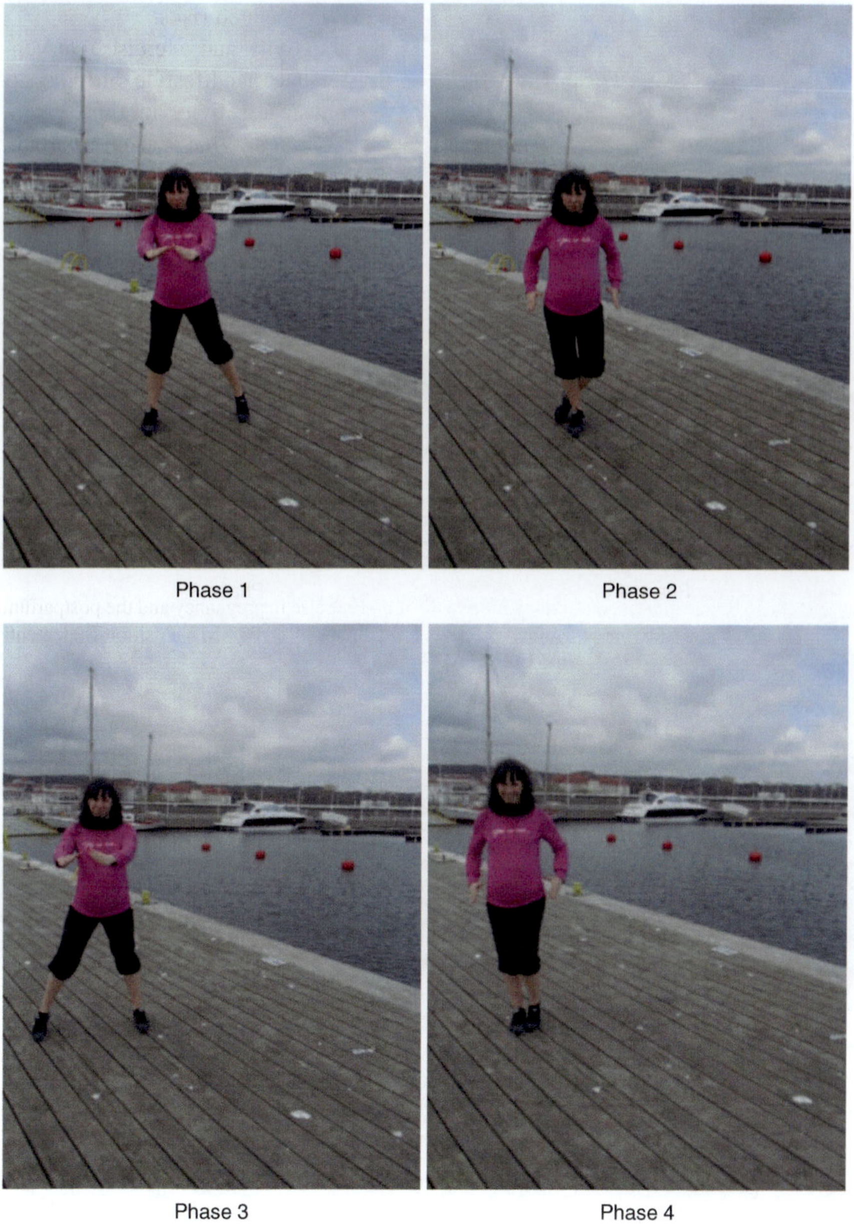

Fig. 9.23 Grape vine

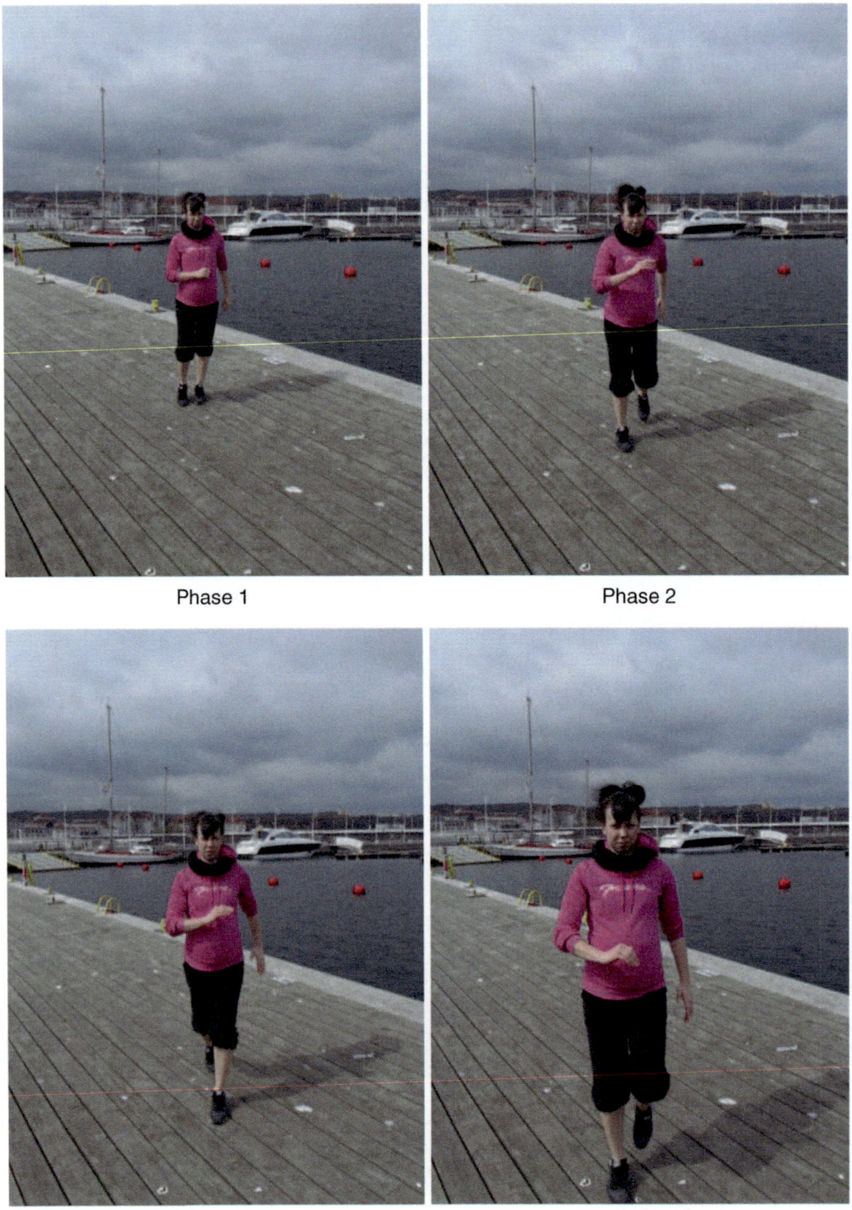

Phase 1 Phase 2 Phase 3 Phase 4

Fig. 9.24 Marching forward/backward

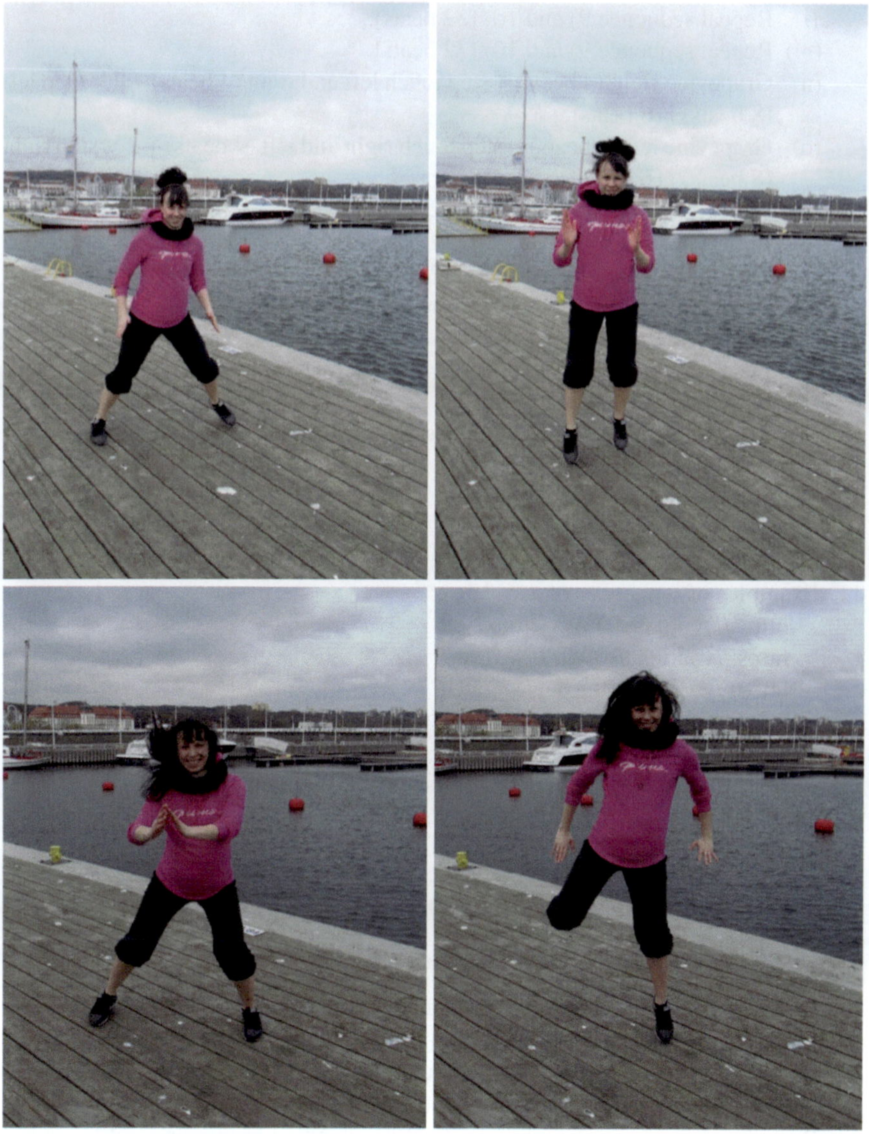

Fig. 9.25 Adding high impact elements to the aerobics movements

(h) Repeat sequence 6) [32 beats].
(i) Grapevine right (4 beats) + 3 step touch left and right (12 beats) [16 beats].
(j) Grapevine left (4 beats) + 3 step touch right and left (12 beats) [16 beats].
(k) Repeat sequence 9) and 10) [32 beats].

(l) Repeat sequence 9) and 10) [32 beats].
(m) Repeat sequence 9) and 10) [32 beats].
(n) Grapevine right (4 beats) + step touch left and right (4 beats) + 2 V step left (8 beats) [16 beats].
(o) Grapevine left (4 beats) + step touch right and left (4 beats) + 2 V step right (8 beats) [16 beats].
(p) Repeat sequence 14) and 15) [32 beats].
(q) Repeat sequence 14) and 15) [32 beats].
(r) Repeat sequence 14) and 15) [32 beats].
(s) Progression: replace 2 V step with 2 mambo (or 1 mambo +1 mambo with pivot).
(t) Progression: replace 2 V step with 3 steps forward +1 knee lift +3 steps backwards +1 leg curl.
(u) Intensity: adding jumps and hops, adding arm moves, increasing cadence.

10. Examples of sequences of aerobics:
    https://youtu.be/42cPuwrcR1g
    https://youtu.be/fxvu5nWiQjg
    https://youtu.be/dcn4yFbmbd4
11. Examples of sequences of aerodance:
    https://youtu.be/TCWvVionxEM
    https://youtu.be/NOdhY2Ve19c
    https://youtu.be/BCUDyLwgwUg
    https://youtu.be/s1fNIWg2oB4
12. Examples of workouts:
    https://youtu.be/w27AHbkfC2Y [aerobics; Portuguese].

Appendix 3: Examples of Basic Step Aerobics Exercises for Pregnant Women

Technique considerations: Head up, shoulders down and back, chest up, abdominals lightly contracted and buttocks gently tucked under the hips. Knees and back should never hyperextend at any time. When stepping up the body should lean from the ankles. The entire sole of the foot should contact the bench, stepping softly and quietly to avoid unnecessary high impacts. When hopping or jumping, softly contact the bench or the floor. The heel should not land over the edge of the bench to avoid Achilles tendon injury. When "touching" the bench, the toes should be used. During knee lift, leg curl, and leg abduction, avoid hyperextending the other knee and the back. When stepping down, the step should be close to the bench (no more than one shoe length away) and the heel should contact the floor. Keep a comfortable distance between the body and the bench (neither too close nor too far).

1. March: Walk/steps in the same place.
2. Basic step: Moves up and down facing the step (Fig. 9.26).

3. Step Touch: Step from side to side, on the step (Fig. 9.27).
4. Step Knee: Step from side to side, lifting your knee, each side on the step (Fig. 9.28).
5. Leg Curl: Step from side to side, kicking your heel back, each side on the step (Fig. 9.29).
6. V Step: Move forward by stepping out wide in front of you with one leg at a time. Then step backward with one leg at a time closing the distance between your feet. Imagine you are making a V shape on the floor with your steps (Fig. 9.30).
7. Tap: Tap 1 ft up on the step and then the other foot (Fig. 9.31).

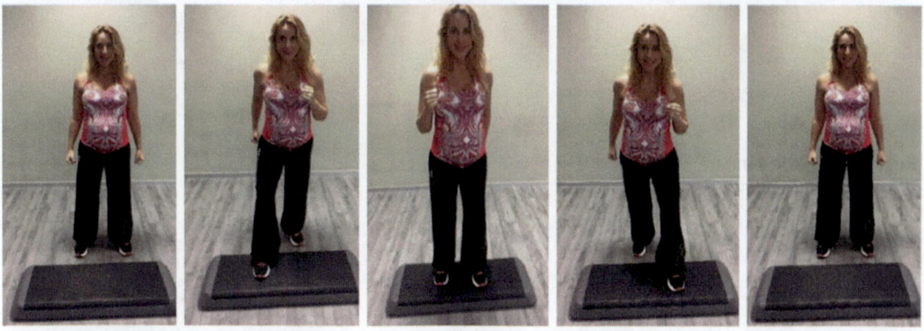

Fig. 9.26 Basic step

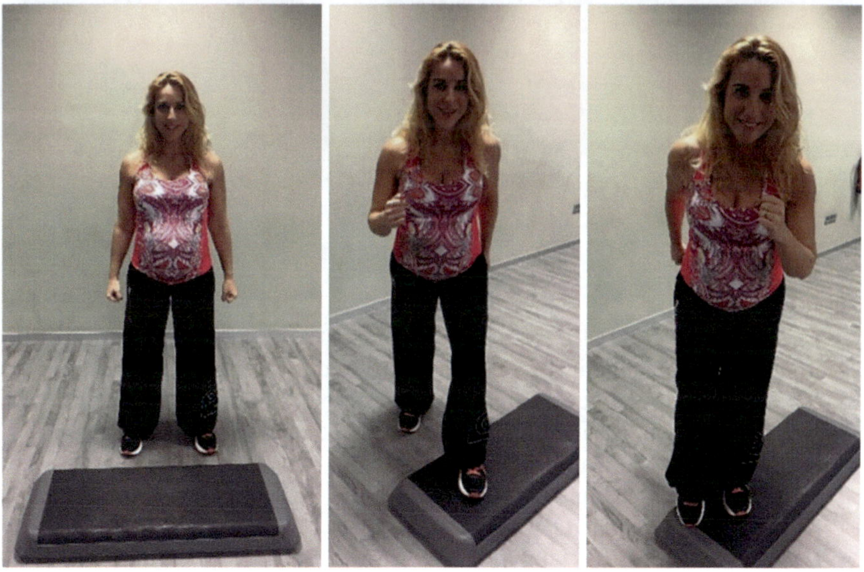

Fig. 9.27 Step Touch with step bench

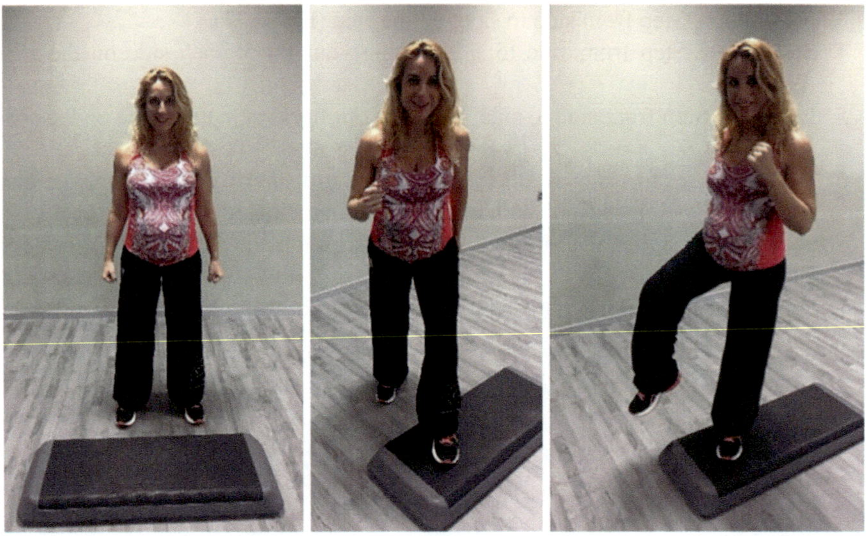

Fig. 9.28 Step Knee

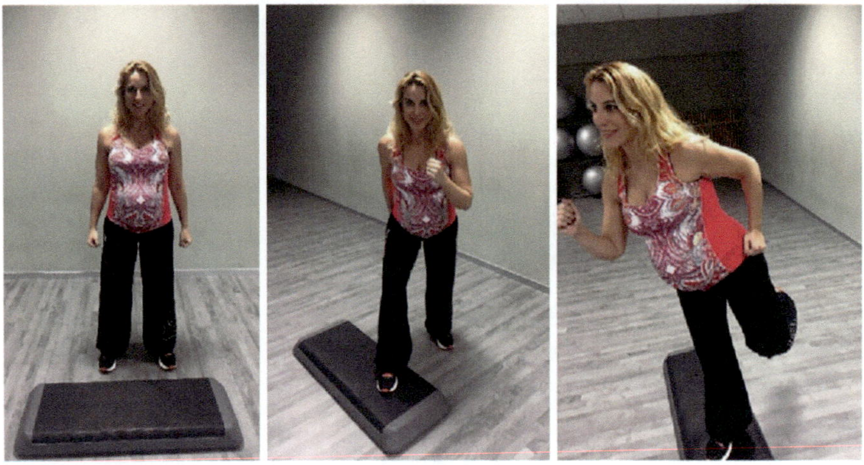

Fig. 9.29 Leg Curl

8. Mambo: The mambo involves stepping forward the step and then backward in the floor (or in the bench), repeatedly with the same foot while shifting the weight between the supporting, static foot and the moving foot (Fig. 9.32).
9. Examples of Combinations
   (a) Front tap right and left (4 beats) × 8 times [32 beats].
   (b) Cross tap right and left (4 beats) × 8 times [32 beats].
   (c) Repeat sequence 1) [32 beats].
   (d) Repeat sequence 2) [32 beats].

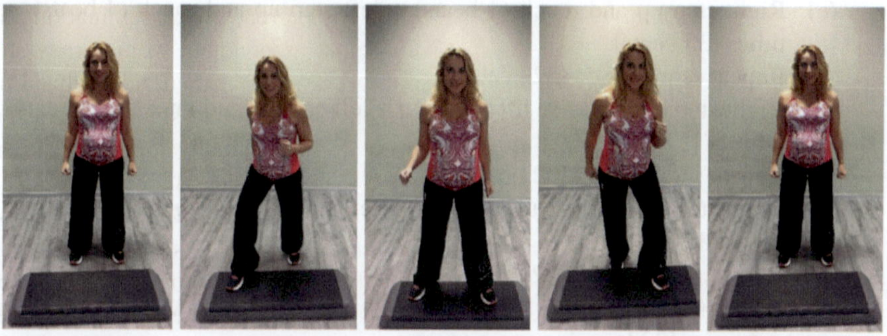

Fig. 9.30 V Step

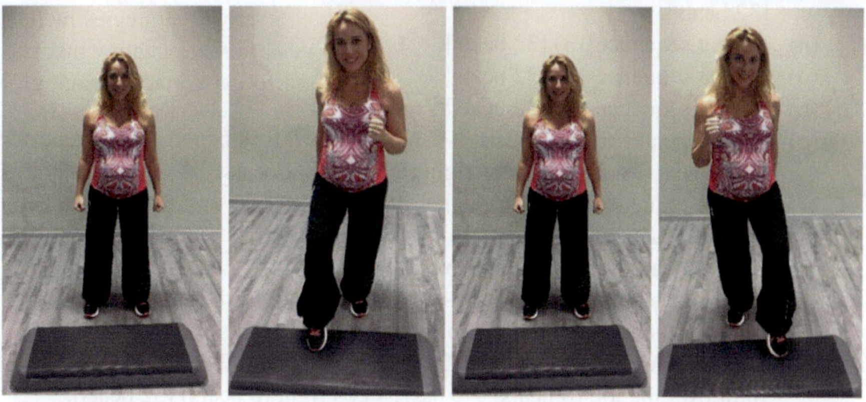

Fig. 9.31 Tap

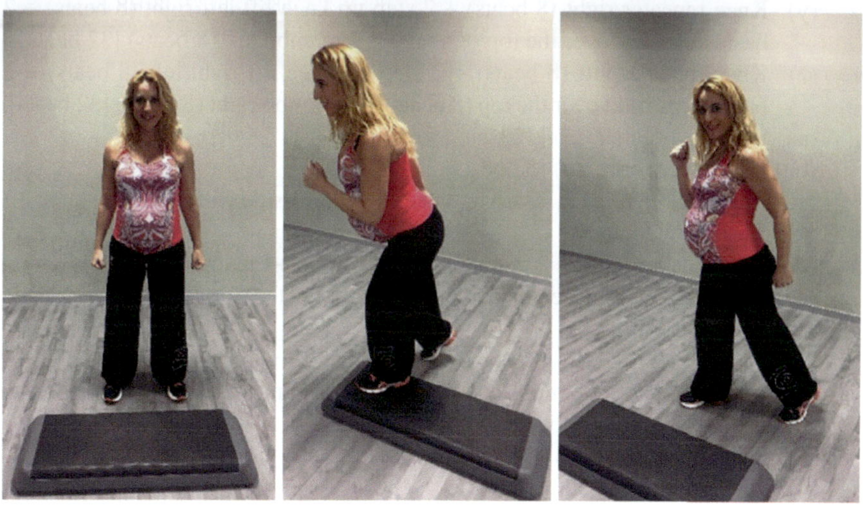

Fig. 9.32 Mambo

(e) Right step up and touch (4 beats) + left step up and touch (4 beats) × 4 times [32 beats].
(f) Repeat sequence 5) [32 beats].
(g) Right step up and knee lift (4 beats) + left step up and knee lift (4 beats) × 4 times [32 beats].
(h) Repeat sequence 7) [32 beats].
(i) Right step up and leg curl (4 beats) + left step up and leg curl (4 beats) × 4 times [32 beats].
(j) Repeat sequence 9) [32 beats].
(k) Right step up and knee hop (4 beats) + left step up and knee hop (4 beats) × 4 times [32 beats].
(l) Repeat sequence 11) [32 beats].
(m) Knee repeater right (8 beats) + knee repeater left (8 beats) × 2 times [32 beats].
(n) Repeat sequence 13) [32 beats].
(o) Repeat sequence 13) [32 beats].
(p) Repeat sequence 13) [32 beats].
(q) Knee repeater right (8 beats) + 2 basic steps left (8 beats) + knee repeater left (8 beats) + 2 basic steps right (8 beats) [32 beats].
(r) Repeat sequence 17) [32 beats].
(s) Knee repeater right (8 beats) + 6 basic steps left (24 beats) [32 beats].
(t) Knee repeater left (8 beats) + 6 basic steps right (24 beats) [32 beats].
(u) Knee repeater right (8 beats) + 2 basic steps left (8 beats) + 2 basic steps left over the top (8 beats) + 2 basic steps left (8 beats) [32 beats].
(v) Knee repeater left (8 beats) + 2 basic steps right (8 beats) + 2 basic steps right over the top (8 beats) + 2 basic steps right (8 beats) [32 beats].
(w) Repeat sequence 21) [32 beats].
(x) Repeat sequence 22) [32 beats].
(y) Knee repeater right (8 beats) + 2 step up knee lift left/right (8 beats) + 2 basic steps left over the top (8 beats) + 2 mambo left (8 beats) [32 beats].
(z) Knee repeater left (8 beats) + 2 step up knee lift right/left (8 beats) + 2 basic steps right over the top (8 beats) + 2 mambo right (8 beats) [32 beats].
(aa) Repeat sequence 25) [32 beats].
(bb) Repeat sequence 26) [32 beats].
(cc) Progression: replace 4 step up knee lift side-to-side with 4 step up knee lift "around the world".
(dd) Progression: replace 2 mambo with 1 mambo +1 mambo with pivot.
(ee) Progression: replace knee repeater with L step forward-side + L step side-backward.
(ff) Progression/intensity: replace step up knee lift with step knee hop.
(gg) Intensity: adding jumps and hops, adding arm moves, increasing cadence, using different approaches to the bench.

10. Examples of sequences of step exercise:
    https://youtu.be/pPvX_tpI-dI
    https://youtu.be/aR3XYAnz2y8

11. Examples of sequences of "invisible step":
    - https://youtu.be/d3hB9B9n32Q
    - https://youtu.be/-uCqgy4IBi8

Appendix 4: Examples of Resistance Exercises for Pregnant Women

1. Squats—from a standing position with feet apart to the width of the hips, bend the legs in the ankles, knees and hips lowering the center of gravity, then return to the starting position. Throughout the exercise, the soles fully touch the ground; the weight of the body rests more on the heels and the outsides of the feet. The torso remains in the neutral position, the abdominal muscles are activated, and the head is in the extension of the torso. The arms are moving forward for the balance. Returning to the starting position should be done with exhalation and simultaneous contraction of the pelvic floor muscles.

   Working muscles: muscles of the lower extremities, trunk muscles

   Difficulty options: The intensity of the exercise can be adjusted by the range of movement; the simplest version is a quarter-squat, intermediate half-squat and advanced - full squat. For a balance exercise, you can add the raising of the bent leg to the front. Squats can be performed with a load, such as dumbbells in the hands or barbells on the shoulders. Arm work can be attached to squats, for example, elbow flexion to activate biceps brachii (Fig. 9.33).
2. So-called Sumo squats—squats performed in the straddle, feet directed outwards.

   Working muscles: as above and additionally, thigh adductor muscles are more engaged.
3. Backward, forward, or sideways lunges—from a standing position a large step backward, forwards or sideways, lowering the center of gravity, then return to

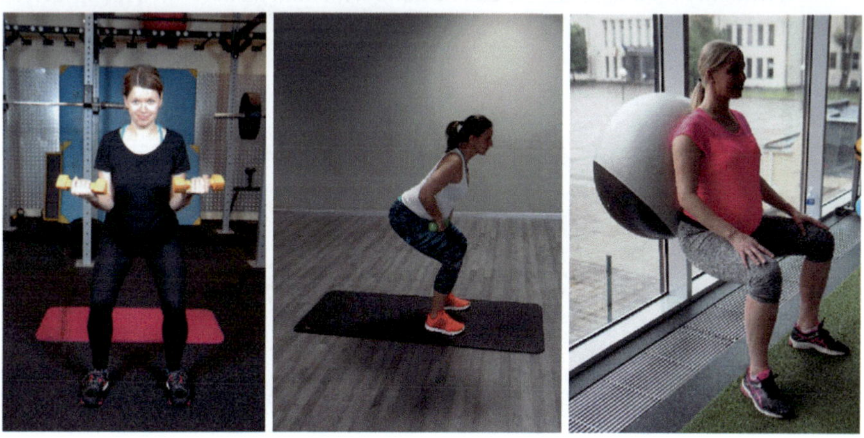

Fig. 9.33 Quarter-squat exercises

the starting position. The torso remains in the neutral position, the abdominal muscles are activated, and the head is in the extension of the torso. The arms are moving forward for the balance. Returning to the starting position should be done with exhalation and simultaneous contraction of the pelvic floor.

Working muscles: in backward and forward lunges, mainly flexors and extensors of the lower extremities, in sideways lunges additionally work the hip abductor and adductor muscles.

Difficulty options: The intensity of the exercise can be adjusted by the range of flexion in the joints of the legs, the smaller the flexion the easier the exercise option. For a balance exercise after backward or forward lunges, you can add the raise of the bent leg forward, with sideways lunges - raising a straight leg to the side. Lunges can be done with a load, such as dumbbells in the hands or barbell on the shoulders. Arms exercise can be added to lunges, for example, the raising of arms to the front or side (activation of the shoulder muscles, Fig. 9.34).

Exercises in high positions (various options of squats and lunges) are good functional exercises, preparing the body of a pregnant woman to move with the growing belly. Due to the fact that they engage several large muscle groups, they are more intensive compared to exercises performed in low positions (sitting, kneeling or lying). Nevertheless, in the case of worsening back pains, it is recommended to replace them with exercises performed while sitting, kneeling or lying down.

4. French press—from a sitting position with legs resting against the ground for stabilization, perform the elbow extension (Fig. 9.35).

   Main working muscles: triceps brachii.

   Difficulty options: the exercise can be done single-handed or with two-handed weight, e.g., a dumbbell or exercise band.

5. Modified unilateral behind the neck press (Fig. 9.36)—from sitting position on a stability ball, with legs resting against the ground for stabilization, shoulders lowered, arms bent in the elbow joints, straighten arm in the elbow joint upwards.

   Main working muscles: triceps brachii, shoulder, and upper back muscles.

   Difficulty options: exercise can be done with both hands with a load, such as a dumbbell.

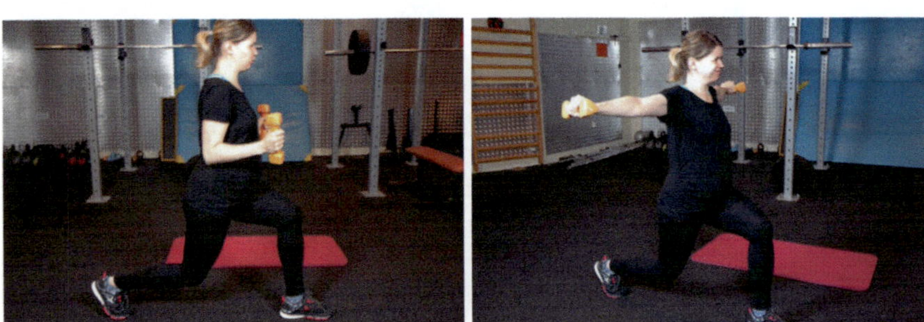

Fig. 9.34 Lunges with different arm moves

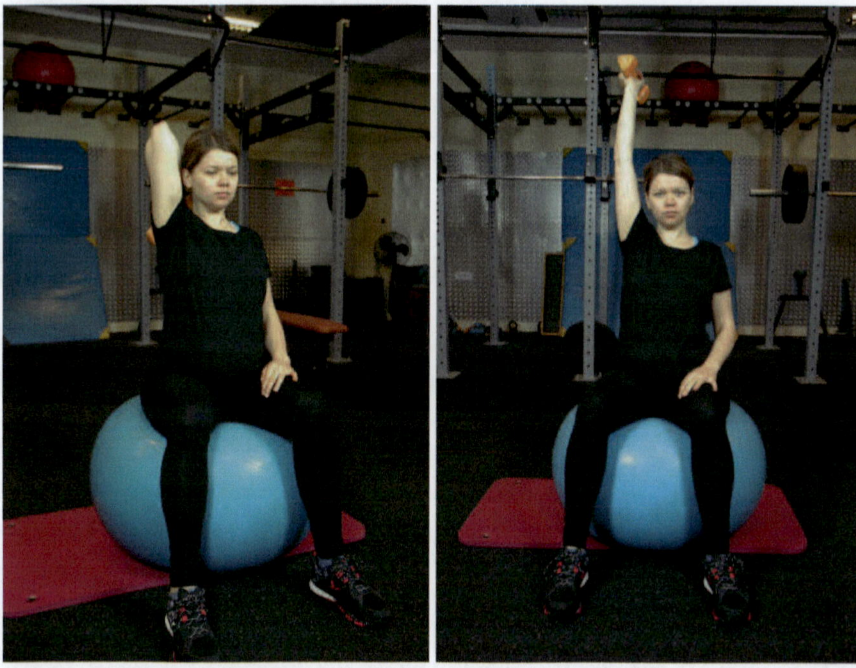

Starting position Exercise

Fig. 9.35 French press

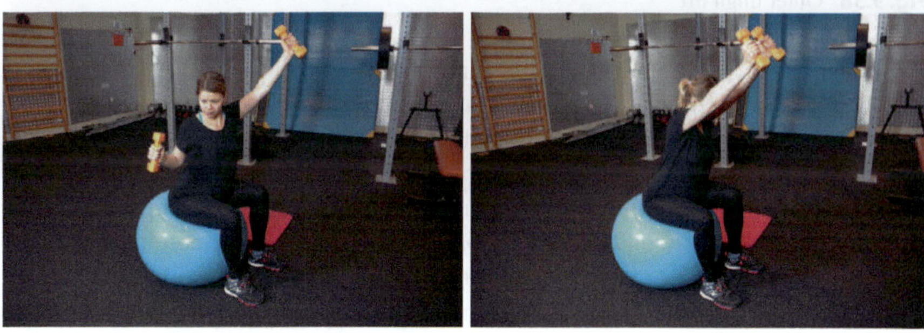

Starting position Exercise

Fig. 9.36 Modified unilateral behind the neck press

6. Pelvic bridging (Fig. 9.37)—from lying on the back, knees flexed, feet on the ground, lift hips together with hip joint extension, while feet, shoulders and head maintain contact with the ground. It is recommended to contract pelvic floor muscle together with lifting the hips.

   Main working muscles: hip extensor muscles.

   Difficulty options: The intensity and difficulty of the exercise can be increased by putting feet on a platform or a stability ball or by performing the exercise on one leg.

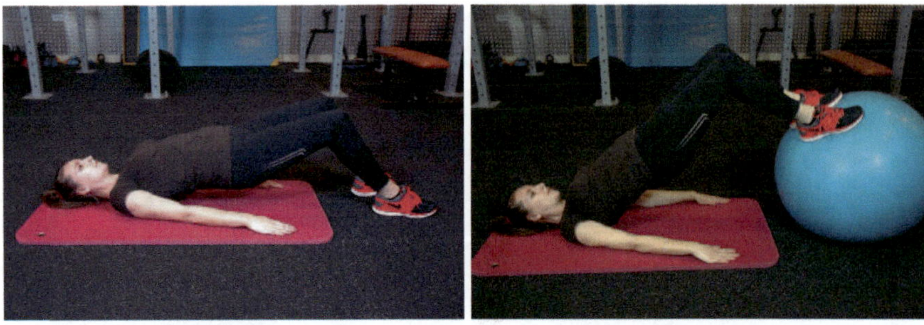

Easy option Advanced option

Fig. 9.37 Pelvic bridging

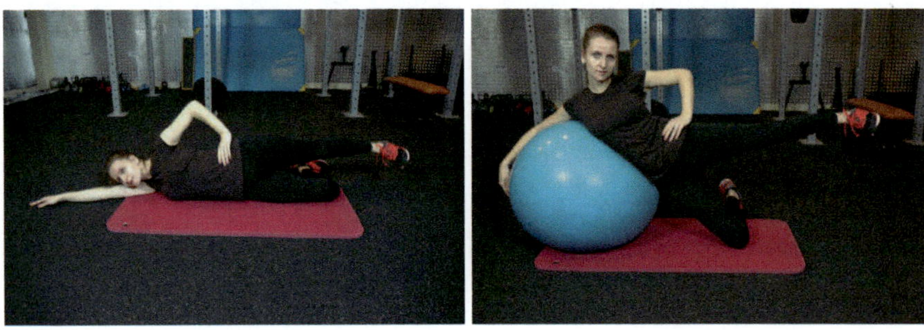

Easy option Advanced option

Fig. 9.38 Outer thigh lift

7. Outer thigh lift (Fig. 9.38)—from lying on the side, hip and knee of the lower leg flexed to stabilize the body, lift (abduct) the upper leg.

   Main working muscles: thigh abductors.

   Difficulty options: The intensity of the exercise can be adjusted by increasing the time of the abductor muscles contraction by keeping the upper leg up or by putting the body on the stability ball (which activates the core muscles).
8. Inner thigh lift (Fig. 9.39)—lying on the side, hip and knee of the upper leg flexed to about 90 degrees, placed in front of the body, lift (adduct) the lower leg. It is recommended to contract the pelvic floor muscle together with the leg lift.

   Main working muscles: thigh adductors.

   Difficulty options: The intensity of the exercise can be adjusted by increasing the time of the adductor muscle contraction by keeping the lower leg up.
9. Squeezing the ball with your knees and hands (Fig. 9.40)—from the seated position, knees flexed, feet on the ground, stability ball in the front between the thighs, hands on the upper part of the ball. At exhalation there is simultaneous pressure of thighs and hands on the ball, with inhalation—relaxation. It is recommended to contract abdominal and pelvic floor muscles together with the activation of the thigh and chest muscles.

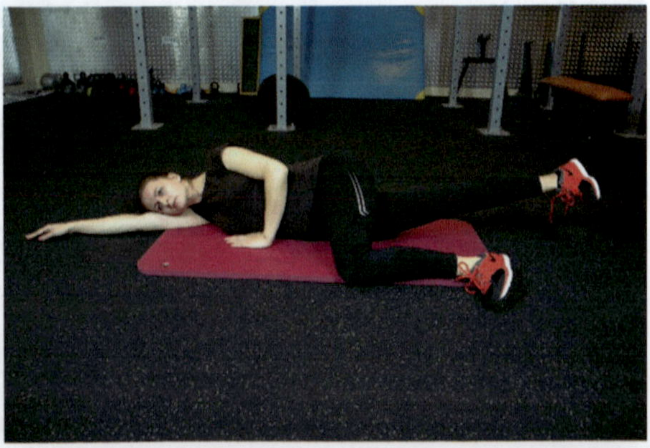

Fig. 9.39 Inner thigh lift

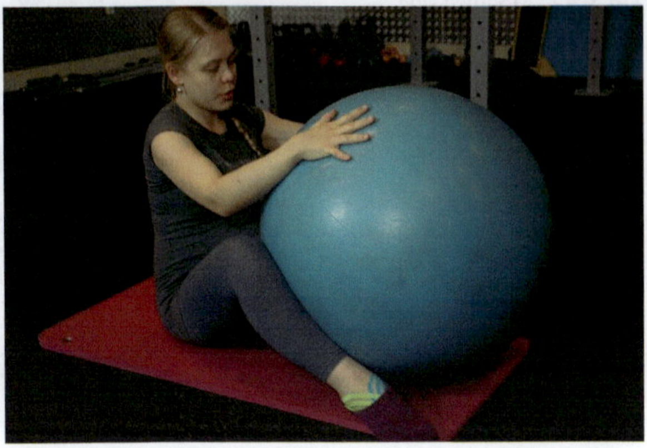

Fig. 9.40 Squeezing the ball with your knees and hands

Main working muscles: thigh adductors, chest muscles, optionally abdominal and pelvic floor muscles.

Difficulty options: The intensity of the exercise can be adjusted by increasing the time to maintain muscle contraction (squeezing the ball).

10. Sideways push-ups (Fig. 9.41)—in the position of lying on the side, hips and knees flexed to stabilize the body. The hand of the lower arm covers the abdomen, the hand of the upper arm on the ground at the chest level. Straighten the upper arm.

    Main working muscles: triceps brachii, unilateral trunk muscles.

    Difficulty options: advanced exercise, toward the end of pregnancy, it may be necessary to shorten the extension movement in the elbow joint (incomplete extension).

11. Modified side plank (Fig. 9.42)—in lying on the side position, in the position of lying on the side, hips, and knees flexed to stabilize the body, the forearm of the lower arm is a support for the trunk. Lift the hips laterally. It is recommended to contract pelvic floor muscles together with the hips lift.

    Main working muscles: unilateral trunk muscles, hips abductors.

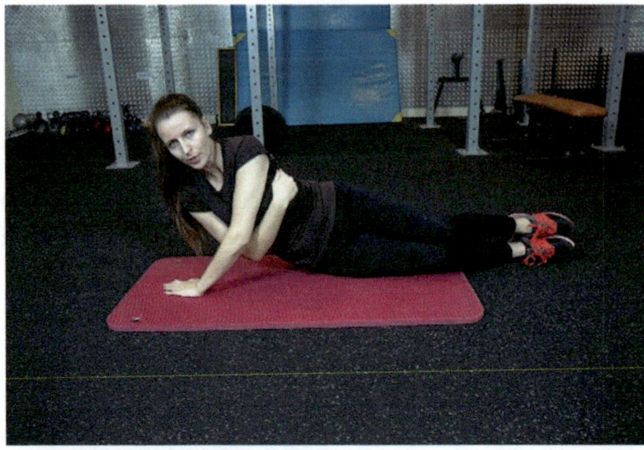

Fig. 9.41 Sideways push-ups

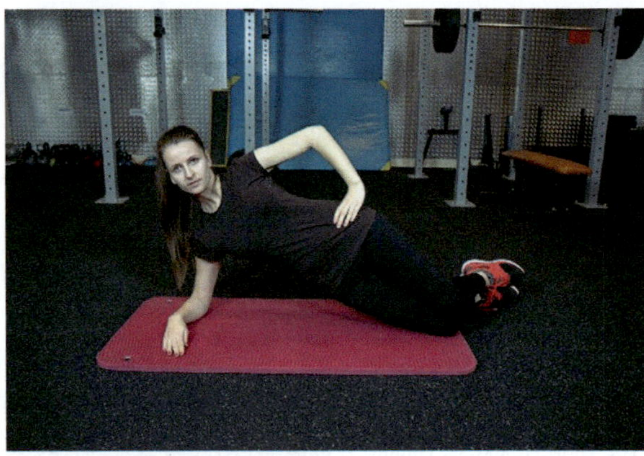

Fig. 9.42 Modified side plank

Difficulty options: advanced exercise, toward the end of pregnancy, additional support of the torso on the upper hand may be necessary.

12. Examples of sequences of resistance exercises (upper body):
    https://youtu.be/dRA-oA9_x7o (only arms).
    https://youtu.be/TxF_SO97qnE (bar).
    https://youtu.be/glqDhwxmz-0 (with bottle).
    https://youtu.be/ym6jkV_mx8Q (with bottle).
13. Examples of sequences of resistance exercises (lower body):
    https://youtu.be/5rlvSh46fLA (only legs).
    https://youtu.be/s1WYFR7fcb0 (squat, free weights).
    https://youtu.be/n7gaDSMKbYM (squat).
14. Examples of sequences of resistance exercises (core and back):
    https://youtu.be/O6O7IC5B7pA
15. Examples of workouts of resistance exercises:
    https://youtu.be/_yZVEoY1elM (free weights) [Portuguese].
    https://youtu.be/v8q55RtFPp4 (bar) [Portuguese].
    https://youtu.be/UybynJ0m_aQ (Pilates) [Portuguese].
    https://youtu.be/wtPBLgvKN5w (Pilates) [Portuguese].

Appendix 5: Examples of Abdominal Exercises for Pregnant Women Previously Inactive

1. Breathing abdominally, air pushing the belly forward, increasing the waist circumference (inhale through the nose, exhale through the mouth). Exercise can be performed in any position.
2. Sit on the ball, arms crossed on the chest, tilt the trunk back while rotating the pelvis forward and performing a full exhalation, return.
3. Sit on the ball, arms along the torso, bend the trunk to the right, return, and change sides. You can add a load in your hands (e.g., dumbbells, kettlebells).
4. Sit on the ball, arms to the side. Twist the trunk to the right, return to the starting position, change sides.
5. Sit on the ball, circular movements on the pelvis.
6. Sit on the ball, alternating the lift of the bent leg. A more difficult option of this exercise is the alternate lift of the bent leg from the semi-squat position, with the back resting against the wall (the ball may be under the back).
7. Sitting down with legs bent on the floor, hands are holding the back of the thigh. Tilting of the trunk back, back to the starting position. Exercise recommended for beginners. A more difficult version of this exercise is to keep your hands crossed on the chest. The more the trunk tilts back, the greater the activation of the abdominal muscles.
8. Sitting down with bent legs, torso twists. A more difficult version of the exercise is the twist of the torso with simultaneous tilting back. The more the torso tilts back, the greater the activation of the abdominal muscles.
9. A kneeling sit, a "cat's back" or emphasizing the thoracic and lumbar part of the spine, activating the abdominal muscles. In women with no diastasis recti abdominis, the exercise can be performed in the position of a supported kneeling (see exercise positions, p. 51).
10. Lying back, legs bent. Arms along the torso. Pelvic lift, return to starting position.
11. Lying on the side. Side-lying trunk lifts.

    Active women can continue their pre pregnancy abdominal exercises as long as the large abdomen does not interfere with the proper exercise technique (Fig. 9.43).
12. Example of sequence of core exercise:

    https://youtu.be/uwvYPWrIPcE

Suggestions for Exercises in the Presence of Diastasis Recti Abdominis

The following exercises are recommended for both pregnant and postpartum women with the separation of abdominal muscles.

1. While lying on the back, slowly perform an abdominal crunch lifting the head and shoulders, with a deep exhalation, pelvic floor contraction, and abdominal

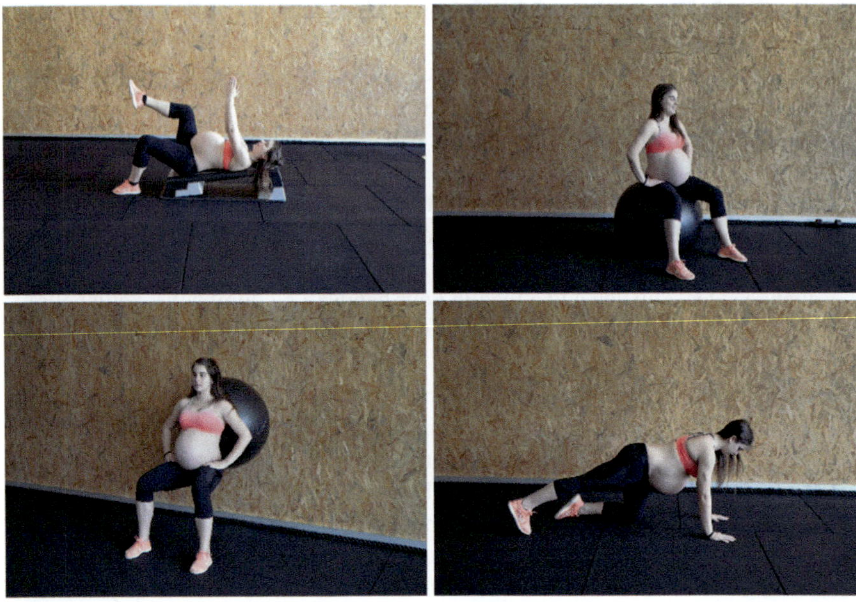

Fig. 9.43 Core exercises

bracing, using hands or a large towel or sheet secured around the abdominal section, so as to bring the two sides of the rectus abdominis muscle as close as possible. If you do not feel well in the supine position, sit in a chair or on the ball, tilt your torso back slightly to activate your abdominal muscles and bend your torso as if you are performing a crunch exercise with the same technique as described above.

2. Standing, back based on the wall (alternatively using a stability ball). Perform elongation of the spine with the simultaneous activation of the abdominal muscles. Try to make sure that your entire back is leaning against the wall. Make a slight flexion in the knee joints while trying to keep the spine straight.
3. Sit cross-legged or sit on the ball, hands on the abdomen. Inhale through the nose, abdomen forward. Exhaling with the mouth, direct the navel towards the spine. Imagine that you hug the baby with the outer part of the abdomen. (Exercise combined with visualization, activating the transversus abdominis muscles).
4. Straddle sit with legs bent. The ball in the front is held with the inner side of the thighs and palms, simultaneous pressure with the legs and hands on the ball with the exhalation and conscious abdominal contraction.
5. Sit on the ball, back straight, arms along the torso. Raise the right knee, or gently bend the lower limb in the hip joint. Lower, change sides. It is important that the back remains in the same position during the exercise.

Appendix 6: Examples of Posture Exercises for Pregnant Women

1. In a standing position balancing from the front to the back of the foot and back looking for the moment when the weight of the body rests exactly in the middle of the foot. Exercise can be done with eyes closed (Fig. 9.44).
2. Exercise as above balancing on both sides of the body.
3. In standing position, the head, shoulders, buttocks, and feet are touching the wall, the task is to touch the wall with the largest part of the back.
4. In standing, sitting or kneeling position, keeping your hands on the belly, conscious activation of the abdominal muscles by making a loud grunt or an energetic exhalation through the mouth. The back and head remain in an unchanging vertical position.
5. Maintaining the correct posture in march and / or aerobic movements.
6. In sitting position consciously "opening" the chest, making the maximum inhale, pushing out the chest and pulling the shoulders back.
7. In the standing, sitting, or kneeling position, performing the elongation of the spine, independently checking the position of the head, shoulders, shoulder blades, and activation of the abdominal muscles.
8. In supine position, arms to the side, shoulder blades touching the floor, the task is to touch the floor with the largest part of the back. Note: for some women, this position may be uncomfortable. The alternative is to practice this exercise in standing back to the wall.
9. Examples of sequences of posture exercises:
   https://youtu.be/qT0_-fRzpro (Yoga).
   https://youtu.be/a7eIvHa-s0Q (barre).
   https://youtu.be/ilcUBX1Gmn0 (barre).
   https://youtu.be/ztgZT6n9DwA (barre).
   https://youtu.be/bWqaSG4s0FA (barre).
   https://youtu.be/Gl1Udp38aPs (arms).
   https://youtu.be/WEyYXs3FOVc (back).

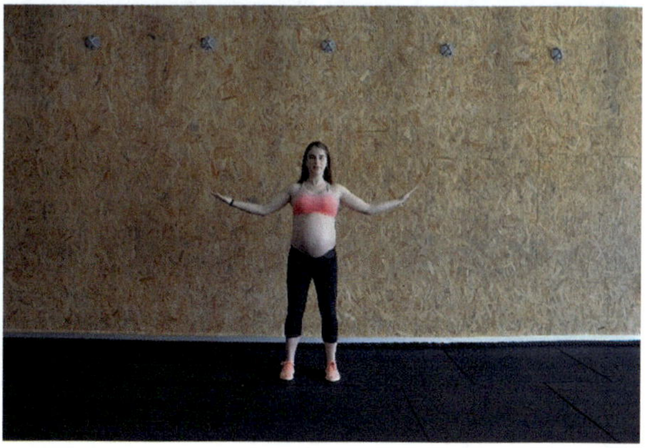

Fig. 9.44 Posture exercise

Appendix 7: Examples of Balance Exercises for Pregnant Women

1. In a standing position, maintain correct posture, checking the elongation of the spine, the position of the head, shoulders, shoulder blades, and activation of the abdominal muscles (Fig. 9.45).
2. Difficulty can be increased by adding arm moves, increasing the time of the exercise, or by performing the exercises with eyes closed.
3. Difficulty can be decreased by performing the exercises with support (wall, chair, etc.).
4. Example of sequence of balance exercises:
   https://youtu.be/CMkoEhCSqA4

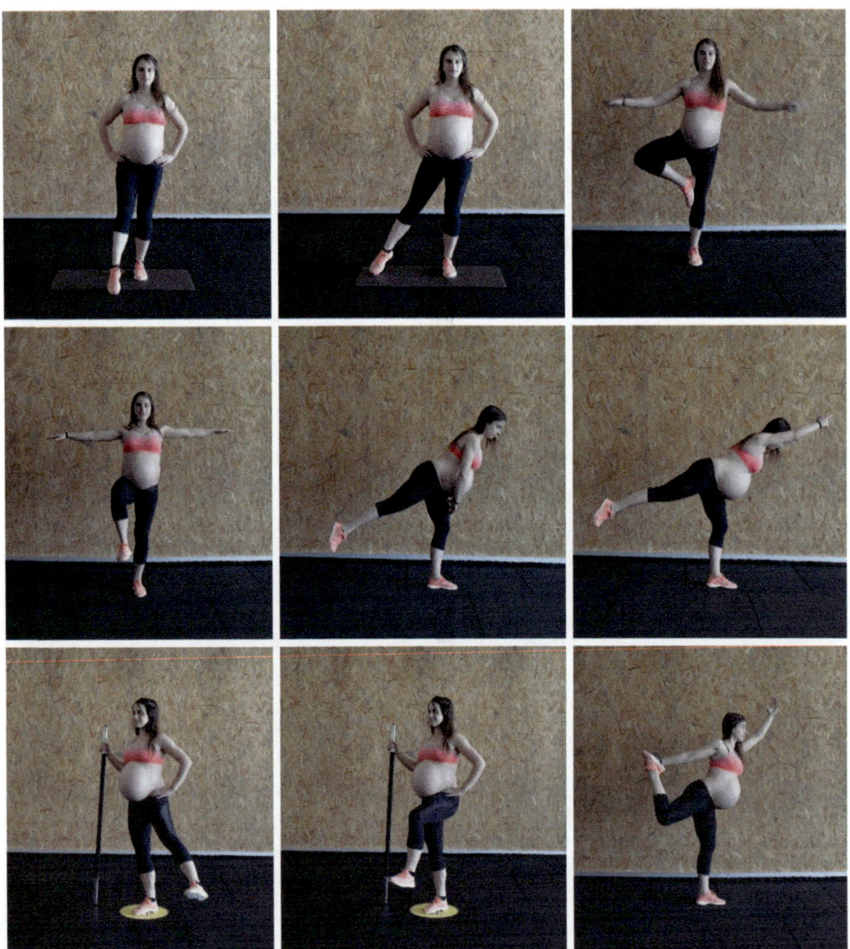

Fig. 9.45 Examples of balance exercises

https://youtu.be/isX_y7AiUpE
https://youtu.be/9JRawKd6N-I

5. Example of Workout of Balance Exercise
   https://youtu.be/jgyE3wj_6CY [Portuguese]

Appendix 8: Examples of Flexibility Exercises for Pregnant Women

1. Hip Flexor Stretch—from the kneeling position, the stability ball held on the side for balance, forward step, shifting the weight of the body on the forward leg with the maximum movement of the hips down and forward. Exercise is performed alternately, first on one, then on the other side (Fig. 9.46).
2. Inner thigh (thigh adductors) stretch with both legs bent—from the sitting position with the soles of the feet together, moving the knees maximally downwards. Optionally, one can gently press the inner parts of the thighs with a smooth motion (Fig. 9.47).
3. Inner thigh (thigh adductors) stretch with one leg bent - from the position of sitting with straight legs, bending of one leg and its maximum move outwards. A hand on the same side of the body can hold the leg and support the movement (Fig. 9.48).
4. Trunk muscle stretch in kneeling position—from the kneeling position, the trunk flexion with the maximum extension of the arms forward. Optionally, the exercise can be performed with a roller or a ball (Fig. 9.49).
5. Back muscle stretch in sitting position—from the sitting position with legs slightly bent, in a slight stride, the maximum rounding of the back with the chin pulled toward the sternum (stretching of the upper back muscles and posterior neck muscles). When the trunk flexion is deepened, the stretching of the lower part of the back muscles also intensifies. When performing this exercise

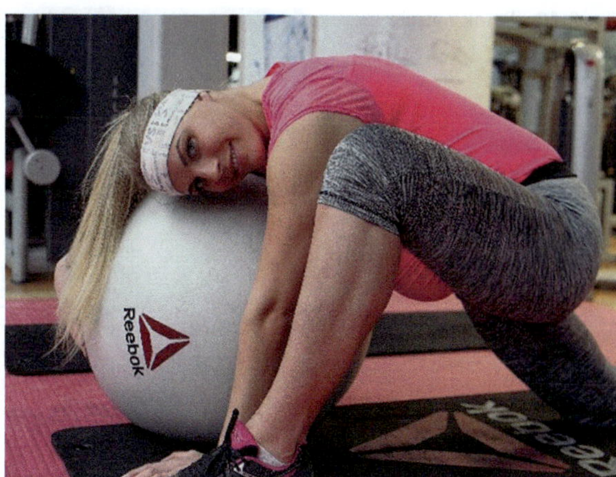

Fig. 9.46 Hip flexor stretch

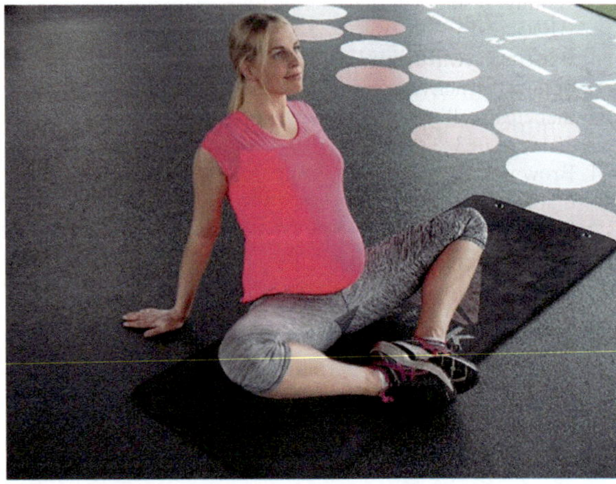

Fig. 9.47 Hip flexor stretch with both legs bent

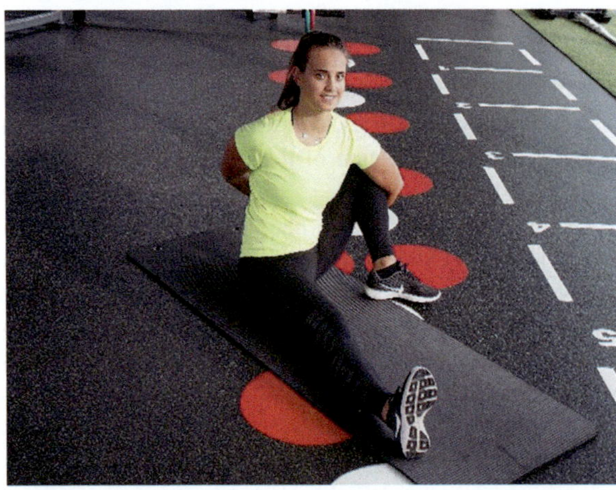

Fig. 9.48 Inner thigh stretch with one leg bent

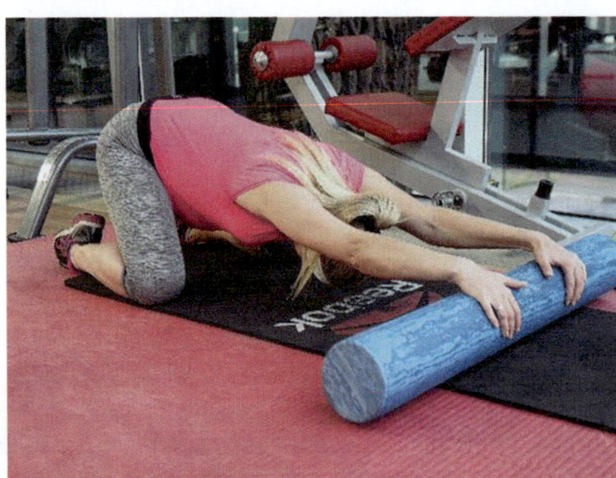

Fig. 9.49 Trunk muscle stretch

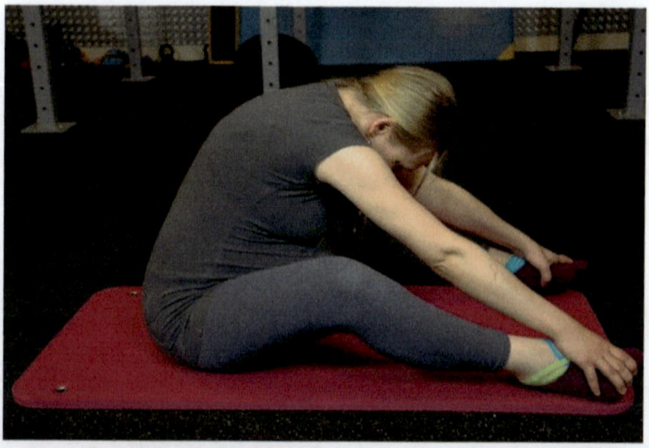

Fig. 9.50 Back muscle stretch in sitting position

in a sitting position with straight legs, the hamstrings will also be stretched (Fig. 9.50).

6. Chest muscle stretch—from the supine position, the roller under the chest, the arms to the side, the bulge of the chest up. Optionally, the exercise can be performed on a stability ball. Due to the lack of data on the potential impact of stretching exercises on the intensification of abdominal muscle separation, it is recommended to limit the stretching movement at abdominal level in this exercise (Fig. 9.51).
7. Trunk muscle and thigh abductors stretch in lying back position—from the supine position one-sided flexion in the hip and knee joints, and then performing internal rotation trying to put the inner part of the knee on the floor. Throughout the exercise, both shoulders should be in contact with the floor. This is a very good position for strengthening the diaphragm by abdominal breathing (Fig. 9.52).
8. Examples of sequences of stretching exercises:
   https://youtu.be/0xqoOWQtcb8 (sitting position)
   https://youtu.be/TF_bNAz5yTg (sitting position)
   https://youtu.be/AoUUzyZcjQI (standing position)
   https://youtu.be/wMs0zsfn308 (standing position)
   https://youtu.be/n3w1aejyn7k (standing position)
   https://youtu.be/wihJoAFLAZE (chair)
   https://youtu.be/DiID0v9uQ4o (neck stretch)
   https://youtu.be/4XQyxy38E1M (hands stretch)
9. Examples of workouts of stretching exercises:
   https://youtu.be/uAgJVlZ1t10 [Portuguese]

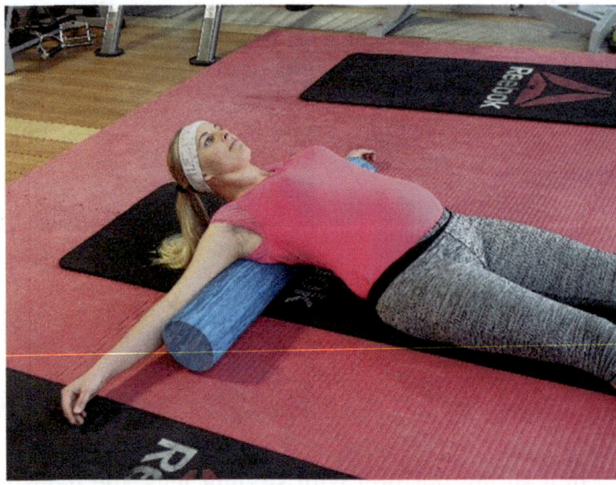

Fig. 9.51 Chest muscle stretch

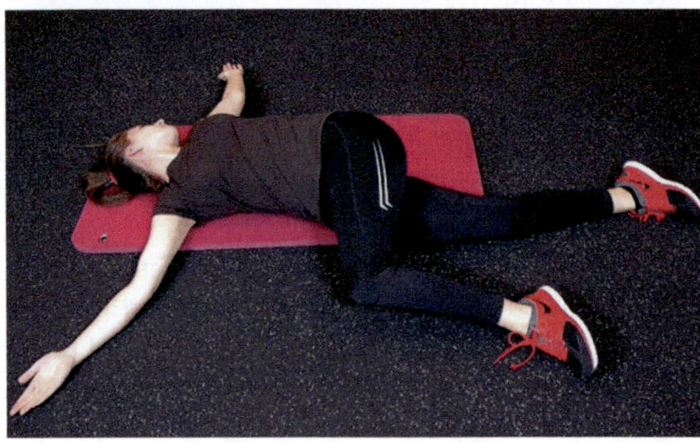

Fig. 9.52 Trunk muscle and thigh abductors stretch

Appendix 9: Examples of Exercises for Proper Pelvic Floor Muscle Contraction

1. It is best to perform the exercises lying on your back with bent knees and feet resting on the floor (alternatively lying sideways or sitting with your back leaning against the wall or stability ball) (Fig. 9.53).
2. Contract pelvic-floor muscles for 3–5 s, as if you were trying to stop a flow of urine or squeeze a tampon. Then relax these muscles. Try recognizing the difference between contracting and relaxing these areas.
3. Put your hands on your abdomen and contract abdominal muscles for 3–5 s as if you wanted to grunt or cough. Then relax those muscles. Try feeling the difference between contracting and relaxing abdominal muscles.
4. Put your hands on your buttocks and contract gluteal muscles for 3–5 s, lifting slightly your hips off the floor. Then relax those muscles. Try feeling the difference between contracting and relaxing gluteal muscles.

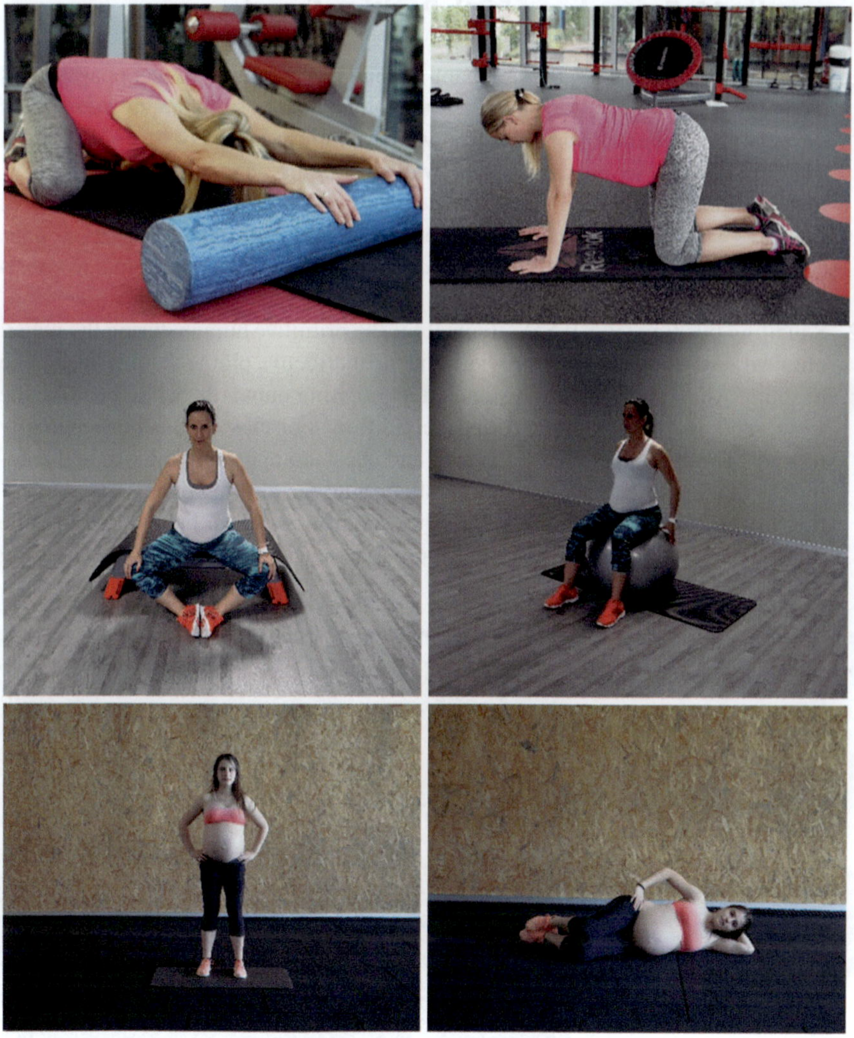

Fig. 9.53 Pelvic floor muscles exercises

5. Put your hands on the inner parts of thighs and contract thigh adductor muscles for 3–5 s pushing one knee into the other. Then relax those muscles. Try feeling the difference between contracting and relaxing the thigh adductor muscles.
6. Breathe deeply in and out relaxing all the above muscles.
7. Try keeping the abdominal, gluteal and thigh muscles relaxed and once again contract the pelvic-floor muscles for 3–5 s, as if you tried stopping urine flow or squeezing a tampon.

Appendix 10: Examples of Birth Position Exercises

1. Standing birth position—the pregnant woman is standing with feet apart; hands are based on thighs. In this position, the woman can perform any movements of the pelvis, circular, forward, and backward. Another version of this position is a standing position leaning against the wall or hanging on ladders.

   Recommendations and remarks: The position is proposed between a series of exercises strengthening the muscles of the legs in high positions, i.e., squats, half-squats, and lunges. Recommended for beginners as an alternative to squatting position (Fig. 9.54).
2. Squatting position (Fig. 9.55)—typical for the primitive human during the physiological, instinctive push. It provides the most effective biomechanics during the pushing. A full squat should be made, feet pointing outwards, while bending the torso. The abdomen, buttocks, and pelvic floor muscles should be maximally relaxed. Thighs can touch the stomach and chest, compressing the ribs and making the diaphragm's work easier, thus shortening the pushing phase. The inclination of the body forward along with the weight transfer on hands based on the floor ensures correct positioning of the pelvis and the coccyx bone, increasing

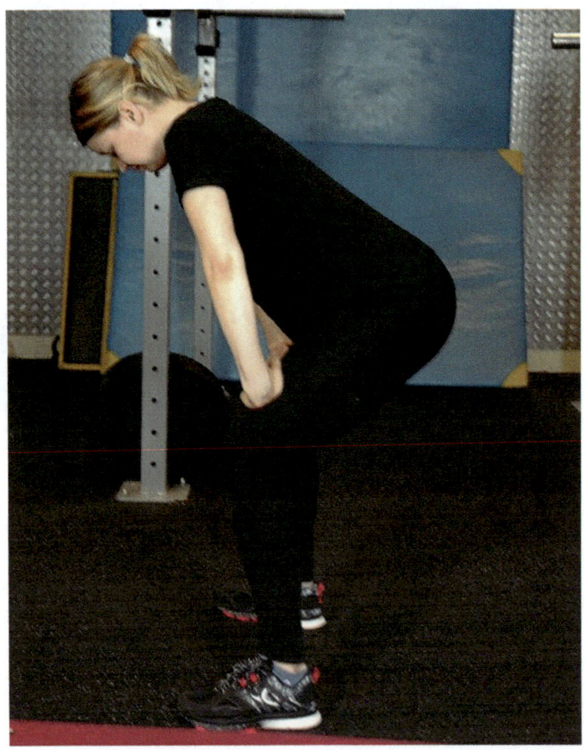

Fig. 9.54 Standing birth position

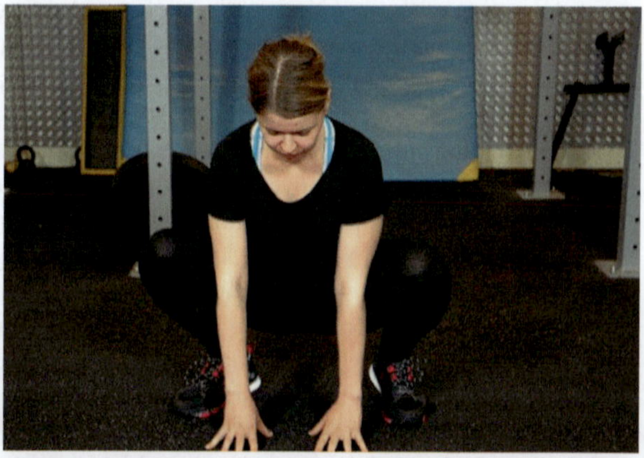

Fig. 9.55 Squatting position

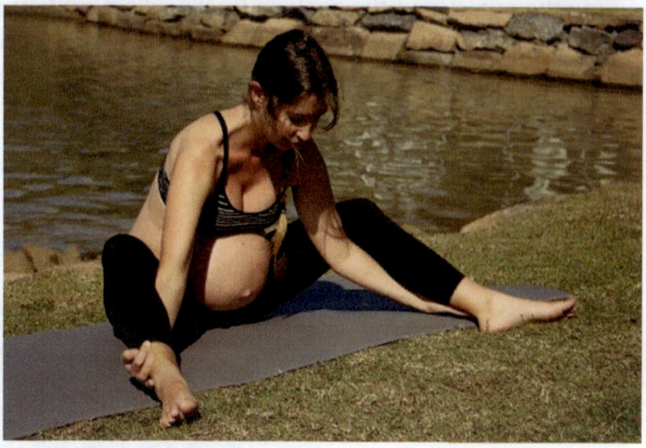

Fig. 9.56 Sitting birth position

the space of the birth canal. In addition, laying the body close to the ground responds to the instinctive need of the woman. The position allows the woman to give birth to a child on her own.

Recommendations and remarks: The position is proposed between a series of exercises strengthening the muscles of the legs in high positions, i.e., squats, half-squats, and lunges. Performing the above position requires strong leg muscles, as well as stretching of the anterior and inner thigh and shank muscles. As most Western adults find it difficult to squat with heels down, compromises are often made such as putting a support under the elevated heels or another person supporting the squatter. For beginners, it is recommended to start from a standing delivery position (Fig. 9.54), gradually increasing the flexion in the joints of lower extremities.

3. Sitting birth position (Fig. 9.56)—the pregnant woman is sitting with her legs apart, knees are bent, her hands can hold her thighs or lower legs, her torso is slightly bent forward. Recommendations and remarks: The position is proposed between a series of exercises strengthening the abdominal muscles from the sitting position.

An option of this position can be performed sitting on the ball with legs apart, hands resting on the women's thighs, her torso leaning slightly forward, her feet on the floor. One can add circular movement of the hips. The position is proposed between a series of exercises strengthening the various muscle groups made from the sitting position on the ball. The elasticity of the ball supports the rhythm of the up-down movement of the hips and facilitates relaxing of the pelvic muscles. Both sitting positions are a good alternative for women who for some reason cannot execute the standing or squatting positions.

4. Horizontal kneeling, or so-called child position (Fig. 9.57)—the pregnant woman is in the sit-on kneeling position (sitting on the heels) the torso maximally bent, arms forward, the forehead can be based on the hands.

   Recommendations and remarks: The position is proposed between a series of exercises strengthening various muscle groups from the position of kneeling or kneeling sit-down. It is a very good position for relaxation and exercise stretching the muscles of the back, buttocks, chest, and arms.

5. "All fours" position (Fig. 9.58)—kneeling supported on the straightened arms, thighs in a slight straddle, the coccyx high up. Birthing in this position requires the help of a third party.

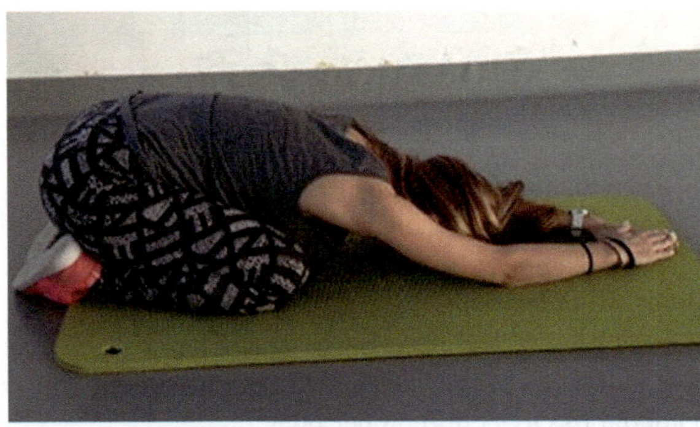

Fig. 9.57 Horizontal kneeling

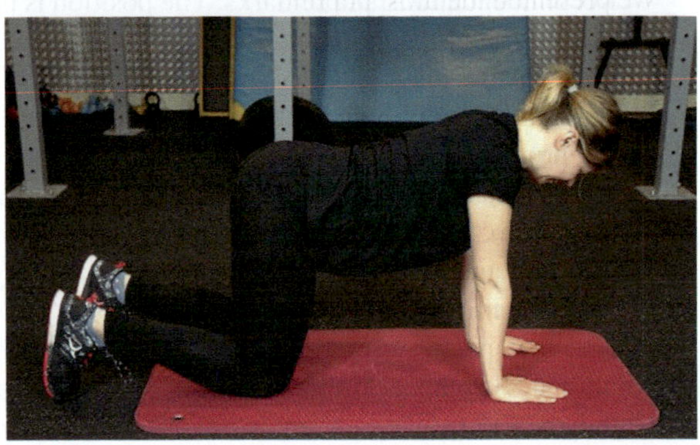

Fig. 9.58 "All fours" position

Recommendations and remarks: The position relieves the spine. Proposed between series of exercises strengthening different muscle groups from the position of kneeling or kneeling sit-down. It is not recommended for women with a diagnosed diastasis recti abdominis.

6. Knee-elbow position (Fig. 9.59)—it is a variation of a kneeling position, with the upper body resting on bent forearms. Thanks to this, it is possible to lift the pelvis higher up. Birthing in this position requires the help of a third party.

   Recommendations and remarks: The position relieves the spine. Proposed between series of exercises strengthening various muscle groups from the position of kneeling or kneeling sit-down. It is not recommended for women with a diagnosed diastasis recti abdominis. One should be cautious about using it for women with a tendency to a headache (blood flows to the head with gravity).

7. Side-lying with open legs (Fig. 9.60)—lying sideways, upper leg bent, moved apart, knee pointing up, the hand of the upper arm grabs the leg below the knee and pulls it towards the chest. Birthing in this position requires the help of a third party.

   Recommendations and remarks: The position relieves the spine. Proposed between a series of strengthening exercises performed from the position lying sideways. During labor, it is recommended to lie on the left side to ensure the proper flow of venous blood to the heart. However, during the exercise classes,

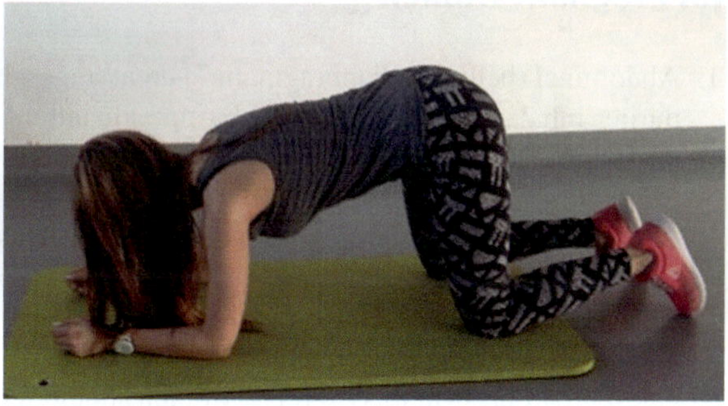

Fig. 9.59 Knee-elbow position

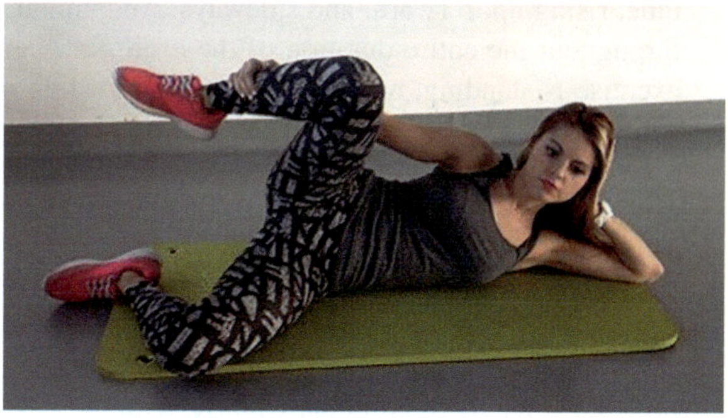

Fig. 9.60 Side-lying with open legs

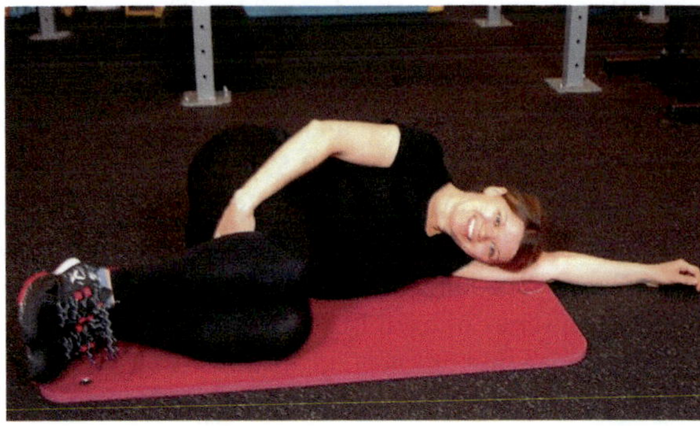

Fig. 9.61 Side-lying curled up

to ensure the bilateral balance of muscular work, one should change the sides of the exercises of this position.

8. Side lying curled up, or so-called fetal position (Fig. 9.61)—lying sideways, body curled up, legs bent and drawn toward the chest. Birthing in this position requires the help of a third party.

   Recommendations and remarks: As for the side lying with open legs position (see Fig. 9.60).

Appendix 11: Examples of Breathing Exercises for Pregnant Women

1. Abdominal (belly or "diaphragmatic") breathing—the abdominal cavity expands during inhalation and decreases during exhalation. During the exercise, take a deep breath, directing the air to the abdomen, and then perform a calm maximum exhalation. In this exercise, the diaphragm maximally drops into the abdomen, creating more space for optimal oxygen intake. This way of breathing improves blood flow to the abdominal region and helps to relax abdominal muscles. It also calms the nervous system and that is why it is recommended for relaxation and also during labor (Fig. 9.62).
2. Chest breathing—in this exercise, women should focus on working rib cage during breathing. At the time of inhalation, the chest should clearly increase in volume, rising up, forward, and sideways. Abdominal muscles should be activated throughout the entire duration of the exercise. A good position to perform this exercise is standing, requiring constant activation of the abdominal muscles to maintain the correct posture. They can be performed on a walk or during other exercises involving large muscle groups, e.g., during squats. Chest breathing is useful especially in the last weeks of pregnancy, when a large uterus makes it difficult to lower the diaphragm.
3. "Three-dimensional breathing"—both above exercises can be supported by an additional sensory stimulus. While breathing, the woman puts her hands in the front and on the side of the abdomen or chest and then on the back. With each breath, the hands should float slightly, with the exhalation slightly falling.

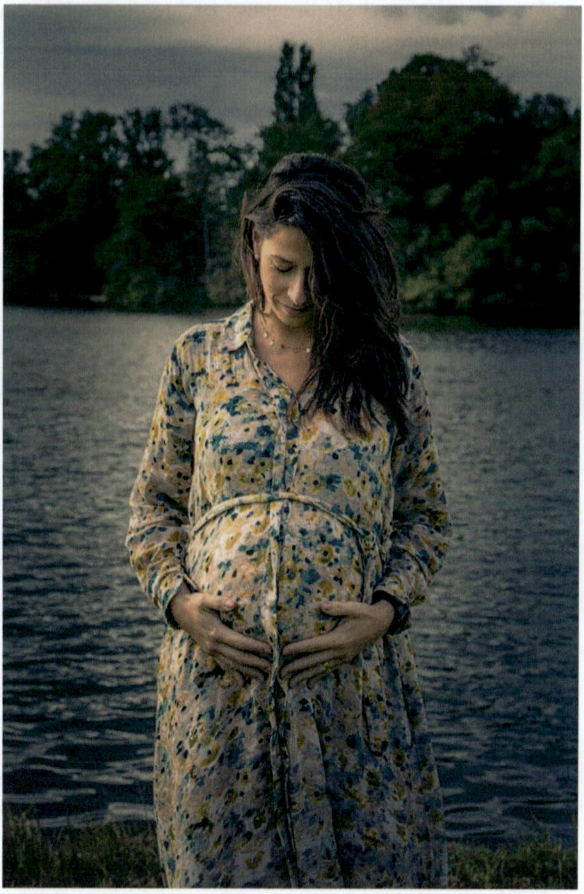

Fig. 9.62 Breathing exercises

4. Breath visualization—the effectiveness of the breath can be increased by visualization. For example, you can imagine your abdominal cavity or lungs as a large vase, which fills with water when you inhale and is emptied during exhalation. In another exercise, a woman can imagine that during the breath her child performs inhalation and exhalation together with her. Such exercises are to increase the awareness of breathing.
5. Diaphragm exercises in trunk lateral flexion and rotations. Deep abdominal breathing is an exercise for strengthening the diaphragm. It is difficult to breathe this way when the trunk is laterally inclined or twisted, which changes the biomechanical conditions for diaphragm operation.
6. Breathing exercises preparing for delivery. Painful uterine contractions during delivery disturb the respiratory rhythm and may lead an inexperienced woman to hold her breath. The task of the pregnancy exercise session is to prepare the woman's body for a quick and shallow breath, which can help her to overcome the pain of childbirth. The breathing resembles the panting or blowing out of a candle or feather flame, hence the name pant breathing or feather blowing.

Acceleration and shallowness of breath impede gas exchange and may cause hyperventilation in a beginner. Therefore, this exercise should start from 15–20 s, gradually extending to 60–90 s. Respiratory delivery exercises are good to perform in delivery positions, including visualization of labor and delivery pain. Each breathing sequence can be ended with a long, deep inhale through the nose followed by a long, deep exhale through the mouth, recommended for pushing. The exercise of the pushing itself is not recommended during pregnancy.

7. Example of breathing exercise sequences:
   https://youtu.be/z6UxFIsfQpE
   https://youtu.be/EKPsQAcKiT8
   https://youtu.be/DxqVr139-O0

References

1. Pivarnik JM, Mudd L. Oh baby! Exercise during pregnancy and the postpartum period. ACSMs Health Fit J. 2009;13(3):8–13.
2. ACOG. ACOG Committee Opinion No. 650. Physical activity and exercise during pregnancy and the postpartum period. In: Obstetrics and gynecology. Philadelphia: Lippincott Williams & Wilkins; 2015. p. e135–e42. Reaffirmed 2017.
3. ACOG. ACOG Committee Opinion No. 804. Physical activity and exercise during pregnancy and the postpartum period. Obstet Gynecol. 2020;135(4):e178–e88.
4. Szumilewicz A, Worska A, Rajkowska N, Santos-Rocha R. Summary of guidelines for exercise in pregnancy—are they comprehensive enough for designing the contents of a prenatal exercise program? Curr Women Health Rev. 2015;11(1):3–12.
5. Wojtyła A, Kapka-Skrzypczak L, Paprzycki P, Skrzypczak M, Biliński P. Epidemiological studies in Poland on effect of physical activity of pregnant women on the health of offspring and future generations—adaptation of the hypothesis development origin of health and diseases. Ann Agric Environ Med. 2012;19(2):315–26.
6. Hanghøj S. When it hurts I think: now the baby dies. Risk perceptions of physical activity during pregnancy. Women Birth. 2013;26(3):190–4.
7. ASC. Pregnancy in sport: guidelines for the Australian sporting industry. Bruce, ACT: Australian Sports Commission; 2002.
8. ASC. A new doubles partner: staying active during pregnancy—such as by hitting the court—can be beneficial to a woman's health. Tennis. 2017;53(5):14.
9. Szumilewicz A, Worska A, Santos-Rocha R, Oviedo-Caro M. Evidence-based and practice-oriented guidelines for exercising during pregnancy. In: Santos-Rocha R, editor. Exercise and physical activity during pregnancy and postpartum. Evidence-based guidelines. 2nd ed. Cham: Springer International; 2022, Ch.7.
10. Santos-Rocha R, Corrales-Gutierrez I, Szumilewicz A, Pajaujiene S. Exercise testing and prescription in pregnancy. In: Santos-Rocha R, editor. Exercise and physical activity during pregnancy and postpartum. Evidence-based guidelines. 2nd ed. Cham: Springer International; 2022, Ch.8.
11. WHO. WHO guidelines on physical activity and sedentary behaviour. Geneva: World Health Organization; 2020.
12. DHHS. Physical activity guidelines for Americans. 2nd ed. Washington, DC: U.S. Department of Health and Human Services; 2018.
13. ACOG. Early pregnancy loss. 2015. https://www.acog.org/-/media/Practice-Bulletins/Committee-on-Practice-Bulletins%2D%2D%2D%2DGynecology/Public/pb150.pdf. Accessed 6 Jan 2018.

14. Artal R. Exercise during pregnancy and the postpartum period. Wolters Kluwer; 2017. https://www.uptodate.com/contents/exercise-during-pregnancy-and-the-postpartum-period.
15. Clapp JF. The effects of maternal exercise on early pregnancy outcome. Am J Obstet Gynecol. 1989;161:1453–6.
16. ACOG. Physical activity and exercise during pregnancy and the postpartum period. The American College of Obstetricians and Gynecologists (ACOG). Committee Opinion No. 650; 2015.
17. Pivarnik JM. Cardiovascular responses to aerobic exercise during pregnancy and postpartum. Semin Perinatol. 1996;20(4):242–9.
18. Wolfe LA, Weissgerber TL. Clinical physiology of exercise in pregnancy: a literature review. J Obstet Gynaecol. 2003;25(6):473–83.
19. Wolfe LA, Kemp JG, Heenan AP, Preston RJ, Ohtake PJ. Acid-base regulation and control of ventilation in human pregnancy. Can J Physiol Pharmacol. 1998;76(9):815–27.
20. McAuley SE, Jensen D, McGrath MJ, Wolfe LA. Effects of human pregnancy and aerobic conditioning on alveolar gas exchange during exercise. Can J Physiol Pharmacol. 2005;83(7):625–33.
21. Pivarnik JM, Connolly CP, Marshall MR, Schlaff RA. Can pregnancy be an ergogenic aid to athletic performance?: a review. Women Sport Phys Activ J. 2017;25(2):111–7.
22. WHO. Nutritional interventions. In: WHO recommendations on antenatal care for a positive pregnancy experience [Internet]. Geneva: World Health Organization; 2016. p. 14–39. https://www.health.govt.nz/system/files/documents/publications/food-and-nutrition-guidelines-preg-and-bfeed.pdf. Accessed 6 Jan 2018.
23. Clapp JF, Cram C. Exercise through your pregnancy. 2nd ed. Omaha, NE: Addicus Books; 2012. p. 268.
24. Bryant CX, Franklin BA, S. N-M. ACE's guide to exercise testing and program design: a fitness professional's handbook. 2nd ed. Monterey: Healthy Learning; 2007.
25. Perales M, Santos-Lozano A, Ruiz JR, Lucia A, Barakat R. Benefits of aerobic or resistance training during pregnancy on maternal health and perinatal outcomes: a systematic review. Early Hum Dev. 2016;94:43–8.
26. White E, Pivarnik J, Pfeiffer K. Resistance training during Pregnancy and perinatal outcomes. J Phys Act Health. 2014;11(6):1141–8.
27. Karowicz-Bilińska A, Sikora A, Estemberg D, Brzozowska M, Berner-Trabska M, Kuś E, et al. Physiotherapy in obstetrics. Ginekol Pol. 2010;81(6):441–5.
28. Zwelling E. Overcoming the challenges: maternal movement and positioning to facilitate labor progress. Am J Matern Child Nurs. 2010;35(2):72–8.
29. Artieta-Pinedo I, Paz-Pascual C, Grandes G, Espinosa M. Framework for the establishment of a feasible, tailored and effective perinatal education programme. BMC Pregnancy Childbirth. 2017;17:1–10.
30. Miquelutti MA, Cecatti JG, Makuch MY. Antenatal education and the birthing experience of Brazilian women: a qualitative study. BMC Pregnancy Childbirth. 2013;13(1):1–8.
31. Levett KM, Smith CA, Bensoussan A, Dahlen HG. The complementary therapies for labour and birth study making sense of labour and birth - experiences of women, partners and midwives of a complementary medicine antenatal education course. Midwifery. 2016;40:124–31.
32. Gaston A, Prapavessis H. Tired, moody and pregnant? Exercise may be the answer. Psychol Health. 2013;28(12):1353–69.
33. Foxcroft KF, Rowlands IJ, Byrne NM, McIntyre HD, Callaway LK. Exercise in obese pregnant women: the role of social factors, lifestyle and pregnancy symptoms. BMC Pregnancy Childbirth. 2011;11(1):1–7.
34. ACSM. In: Thompson WR, editor. ACSM's resources for the personal trainer. 5th ed. Philadelphia: Wolters Kluwer Health; 2017. p. 632.
35. Eckmann T, Stoddart D. The power of posture: a program to encourage optimal posture. J Active Aging. 2015;14(4):54–68.

36. Kennedy-Armbruster C, Yoke MM. Methods of group exercise instruction. 3rd ed. Champaign, IL: Human Kinetics; 2014. p. 440.
37. Jensen D, Wolfe LA, Slatkovska L, Webb KA, Davies GAL, O'Donnell DE. Effects of human pregnancy on the ventilatory chemoreflex response to carbon dioxide. Am J Physiol Regul Integr Comp Physiol. 2005;288(5):R1369–R75.
38. SMA. Pregnancy and exercise. Women in sport. SMA_AWiS_Pregnancy_-_Exercise.Pdf: sport medicine Australia. Accessed 13 Jul 2021.
39. RANZCOG. Exercise in pregnancy. The Royal Australian and New Zealand College of Obsterticians and Gynaecologists; 2020.
40. Mottola MF, Davenport MH, Ruchat S-M, Davies GA, Poitras VJ, Gray CE, et al. 2019 Canadian guideline for physical activity throughout pregnancy. Br J Sports Med. 2018;52(21):1339–46.
41. ACSM. ACSM information on Pregnancy physical activity. Indianapolis, IN: American College of Sports Medicine; 2020.
42. DHHS US. 2008 Physical activity guidelines for Americans. U.S. Department of Human and Health Services; 2008. https://health.gov/paguidelines/pdf/paguide.pdf.
43. Santos-Rocha R, Pimenta N. Teaching group fitness to music. In: Santos Rocha R, Rieger T, Jimenez A, editors. EuropeActive's essentials for Fitness Instructors. Champaign, IL: Human Kinetics; 2015.
44. Haakstad LAH, Bø K. Exercise in pregnant women and birth weight: a randomized controlled trial. BMC Pregnancy Childbirth. 2011;11:66.
45. Halvorsen S, Haakstad LAH, Edvardsen E, Bø K. Effect of aerobic dance on cardiorespiratory fitness in pregnant women: a randomised controlled trial. Physiotherapy. 2013;99(1):42–8.
46. Barakat R, Cordero Y, Coteron J, Luaces M, Montejo R. Exercise during pregnancy improves maternal glucose screen at 24-28 weeks: a randomised controlled trial. Br J Sports Med. 2012;46(9):656–61.
47. Stafne SN, Salvesen K, Romundstad PR, Torjusen IH, Mørkved S. Does regular exercise including pelvic floor muscle training prevent urinary and anal incontinence during pregnancy? A randomised controlled trial. BJOG. 2012;119(10):1270–80.
48. Barakat R, Pelaez M, Montejo R, Refoyo I, Coteron J. Exercise throughout pregnancy does not cause preterm delivery: a randomized, controlled trial. J Phys Act Health. 2014;11(5):1012–7.
49. Barakat R, Pelaez M, Lopez C, Montejo R, Coteron J. Exercise during pregnancy reduces the rate of cesarean and instrumental deliveries: results of a randomized controlled trial. J Matern Fetal Neonatal Med. 2012;25(11):2372–6.
50. Szumilewicz A, Dornowski M, Piernicka M, Worska A, Kuchta A, Kortas J, et al. High-low impact exercise program including pelvic floor muscle exercises improves pelvic floor muscle function in healthy pregnant women—a randomized control trial. Front Physiol. 2019;9:1867.
51. Szumilewicz A, Kuchta A, Kranich M, Dornowski M, Jastrzębski Z. Prenatal high-low impact exercise program supported by pelvic floor muscle education and training decreases the life impact of postnatal urinary incontinence: a quasiexperimental trial. Medicine. 2020;99(6):e18874.
52. Laukkanen RM, Kalaja MK, Kalaja SP, Holmala EB, Paavolainen LM, Tummavuori M, et al. Heart rate during aerobics classes in women with different previous experience of aerobics. Eur J Appl Physiol. 2001;84(1–2):64–8.
53. Bourcier AP. Incontinence during sports and fitness activities. In: Baessler K, Schüssler K, Burgio KL, Moore K, Norton PA, Stanton SL, editors. Pelvic floor re-education principles and practice. 2nd ed. Berlin: Springer; 2008. p. 267–70.
54. Reebok University Press. Introduction to step reebok. Stoughton: Reebok International; 1994.
55. Reebok University Press. Power Step Reebok. Stoughton: Reebok International; 1994.
56. Santos-Rocha R, Veloso A, Machado ML. Analysis of ground reaction forces in step exercise depending on step pattern and stepping rate. J Strength Cond Res. 2009;23(1):209–24.
57. Santos-Rocha RA, Oliveira CS, Veloso AP. Osteogenic index of step exercise depending on choreographic movements, session duration, and stepping rate. Br J Sports Med. 2006;40(10):860–6.
58. Engels HJ, Currie JS, Lueck CC, Wirth JC. Bench/step training with and without extremity loading. Effects on muscular fitness, body composition profile, and psychological affect. J Sports Med Phys Fitness. 2002;42(1):71–8.

59. Forczek W, Curyło M, Forczek B. Physical activity assessment during gestation and its outcomes: a review. Obstet Gynecol Surv. 2017;72(7):425–44.
60. Price BB, Amini SB, Kappeler K. Exercise in pregnancy: effect on fitness and obstetric outcomes-a randomized trial. Med Sci Sports Exerc. 2012;44(12):2263–9.
61. Skreden M, Øverby NC, Sagedal LR, Vistad I, Torstveit MK, Lohne-Seiler H, et al. Change in active transportation and weight gain in pregnancy. Int J Behav Nutr Phys Activ. 2016;13:10.
62. Butler JM. Fit & pregnant. The pregnant women guide to exercise. 2nd ed. Montpelier: Vitesse Press; 2006. p. 192.
63. Nascimento SL, Surita FG, Godoy AC, Kasawara KT, Morais SS. Physical activity patterns and factors related to exercise during pregnancy: a cross sectional study. PLoS One. 2015;10(6):1–14.
64. Davenport MH, Mottola MF, McManus R, Gratton R. A walking intervention improves capillary glucose control in women with gestational diabetes mellitus: a pilot study. Appl Physiol Nutr Metab. 2008;33(3):511–7.
65. de Oliveria Melo AS, Silva JLP, Tavares JS, Barros VO, Leite DFB, Amorim MMR. Effect of a physical exercise program during pregnancy on uteroplacental and fetal blood flow and fetal growth: a randomized controlled trial. Obstet Gynecol. 2012;120(2 Pt 1):302–10.
66. Ruchat SM, Davenport MH, Giroux I, Hillier M, Batada A, Sopper MM, et al. Walking program of low or vigorous intensity during pregnancy confers an aerobic benefit. Int J Sports Med. 2012;33(8):661–6.
67. Garnæs KK, Nyrnes SA, Salvesen KÅ, Salvesen Ø, Mørkved S, Moholdt T. Effect of supervised exercise training during pregnancy on neonatal and maternal outcomes among overweight and obese women. Secondary analyses of the ETIP trial: a randomised controlled trial. PLoS One. 2017;12(3):1–15.
68. Garnæs KK, Mørkved S, Salvesen KÅ, Salvesen Ø, Moholdt T. Exercise training during pregnancy reduces circulating insulin levels in overweight/obese women postpartum: secondary analysis of a randomised controlled trial (the ETIP trial). BMC Pregnancy Childbirth. 2018;18:1–11.
69. Baciuk EP, Pereira RI, Cecatti JG, Braga AF, Cavalcante SR. Water aerobics in pregnancy: cardiovascular response, labor and neonatal outcomes. Reprod Health. 2008;5:10.
70. Cavalcante SR, Cecatti JG, Pereira RI, Baciuk EP, Bernardo AL, Silveira C. Water aerobics II: maternal body composition and perinatal outcomes after a program for low risk pregnant women. Reprod Health. 2009;6:1.
71. Vallim AL, Osis MJ, Cecatti JG, Baciuk ÉP, Silveira C, Cavalcante SR. Water exercises and quality of life during pregnancy. Reprod Health. 2011;8(1):14–20.
72. Batrakoulis A. European survey of fitness trends for 2020. ACSMs Health Fit J. 2019; 23(6):28–35.
73. Wood G, Murrell A, van der Touw T, Smart N. HIIT is not superior to MICT in altering blood lipids: a systematic review and meta-analysis. BMJ Open Sport Exerc Med. 2019;5(1):e000647.
74. Campbell WW, Kraus WE, Powell KE, Haskell WL, Janz KF, Jakicic JM, et al. High-intensity interval training for cardiometabolic disease prevention. Med Sci Sports Exerc. 2019;51(6):1220–6.
75. Yeh S-W, Lin L-F, Chen H-C, Huang L-K, Hu C-J, Tam K-W, et al. High-intensity functional exercise in older adults with dementia: a systematic review and meta-analysis. Clin Rehabil. 2021;35(2):169–81.
76. Lavín-Pérez AM, Collado-Mateo D, Mayo X, Humphreys L, Liguori G, James Copeland R, et al. High-intensity exercise to improve cardiorespiratory fitness in cancer patients and survivors: a systematic review and meta-analysis. Scand J Med Sci Sports. 2021;31(2): 265–94.
77. Songstad NT, Kaspersen K-HF, Hafstad AD, Basnet P, Ytrehus K, Acharya G. Effects of high intensity interval training on pregnant rats, and the placenta, heart and liver of their fetuses. PLoS One. 2015;10(10):1–15.
78. Ong MJ, Wallman KE, Fournier PA, Newnham JP, Guelfi KJ. Enhancing energy expenditure and enjoyment of exercise during pregnancy through the addition of brief higher intensity

intervals to traditional continuous moderate intensity cycling. BMC Pregnancy Childbirth. 2016;16(1):161.
79. Nagpal TS, Everest C, Goudreau AD, Manicks M, Adamo KB. To HIIT or not to HIIT? The question pregnant women may be searching for online: a descriptive observational study. Perspect Public Health. 2021:1757913920985898.
80. El Refaye G. Insulin sensitivity response to high-intensity training in insulin resistance during pregnancy. NCT04830995 ClinicalTrials.gov; 2021.
81. Moholdt T. Acute effects of high intensity training in pregnancy on fetal well-being and blood flow distribution. NCT04288479 ClinicalTrials.gov; 2021.
82. Szumilewicz A. HIIT vs MICT during pregnancy and health and birth outcomes in mothers and children (HIIT MAMA). ClinicalTrials.gov; 2021.
83. Bø K, Artal R, Barakat R, Brown W, Davies GAL, Dooley M, et al. Exercise and pregnancy in recreational and elite athletes: 2016 evidence summary from the IOC expert group meeting, Lausanne. Part 1-exercise in women planning pregnancy and those who are pregnant. Br J Sports Med. 2016;50(10):571–89.
84. Palatini P, Mos L, Munari L, Valle F, Del Torre M, Rossi A, et al. Blood pressure changes during heavy-resistance exercise. J Hypertens Suppl. 1989;7(6):S72–S3.
85. Harman EA, Frykman PN, Clagett ER, Kraemer WJ. Intra-abdominal and intra-thoracic pressures during lifting and jumping. Pressions intra-abdominales et intra-thoraciques lors de souleves de poids et de sauts. Med Sci Sports Exerc. 1988;20(2):195–201.
86. Bø K, Artal R, Barakat R, Brown WJ, Davies GAL, Dooley M, et al. Exercise and pregnancy in recreational and elite athletes: 2016/2017 evidence summary from the IOC expert group meeting, Lausanne. Part 5. Recommendations for health professionals and active women. Br J Sports Med. 2018;52(17):1080–5.
87. Avery ND, Stocking KD, Tranmer JE, Davies GA, Wolfe LA. Fetal responses to maternal strength conditioning exercises in late gestation. Can J Appl Physiol. 1999;24(4):362–76.
88. O'Connor PJ, Poudevigne MS, Cress ME, Moti RW, Clapp IIIJF. Safety and efficacy of supervised strength training adopted in Pregnancy. J Phys Act Health. 2011;8(3):309–20.
89. Dumas GA, Leger A, Plamondon A, Charpentier KM, Pinti A, McGrath M. Fatigability of back extensor muscles and low back pain during pregnancy. Clin Biomech. 2010;25(1):1–5.
90. Wells C, Kolt GS, Bialocerkowski A. Defining Pilates exercise: a systematic review. Complement Ther Med. 2012;20(4):253–62.
91. Benjamin DR, van de Water ATM, Peiris CL. Effects of exercise on diastasis of the rectus abdominis muscle in the antenatal and postnatal periods: a systematic review. Physiotherapy. 2014;100(1):1–8.
92. Shu-Ming W, Dezinno P, Maranets I, Berman MR, Caldwell-Andrews AA, Kain ZN. Low back pain during pregnancy: prevalence, risk factors, and outcomes. Obstet Gynecol. 2004;104(1):65–70.
93. Kwiecińska K. Aksjomaty nt. Prenatalnej aktywności fizycznej w świadomości przyszłych matek (the axioms about the prenatal physical activity in the awareness of expectant mothers). Gdansk: Gdansk University of Physical Education and Sport; 2013.
94. Worska A, Szumilewicz A. Aktywność fizyczna kobiet w ciąży w świadomości przyszłych instruktorów rekreacji ruchowej (physical activity of expecting mothers in the awareness of future exercise professionals). J Educ Health Sport. 2015;5(8):91–102.
95. Jeffreys RM, Stepanchak W, Lopez B, Hardis J, Clapp JF. 3rd. Uterine blood flow during supine rest and exercise after 28 weeks of gestation. BJOG. 2006;113(11):1239–47.
96. Mottola MF, Nagpal TS, Bgeginski R, Davenport MH, Poitras VJ, Gray CE, et al. Is supine exercise associated with adverse maternal and fetal outcomes? A systematic review. Br J Sports Med. 2019;53(2):82–9.
97. Raines DA, Whitten RA. Braxton Hicks Contactions. Treasure Island, FL: StatPearls; 2017.
98. Mota P, Pascoal AG, Vaz C, João F, Veloso A, Bø K. Diastasis recti during pregnancy and postpartum. In: Brandão S, DaRoza T, Ramos I, Mascarenhas T, editors. Women's health and biomechanics: where medicine and engineering meet. Lecture notes in computational vision and biomechanics, vol. 29. Cham: Springer; 2018. p. 121–32.

99. Bø K, Hilde G, Tennfjord MK, Sperstad JB, Engh ME. Pelvic floor muscle function, pelvic floor dysfunction and diastasis recti abdominis: prospective cohort study. NeurourolUrodyn. 2017;36(3):716–21.
100. Boissonnault JS, Blaschak MJ. Incidence of diastasis recti abdominis during the childbearing year. Phys Ther. 1988;68(7):1082–6.
101. Mota P, Pascoal AG, Carita AI, Bø K. Normal width of the inter-recti distance in pregnant and postpartum primiparous women. Musculoskelet Sci Pract. 2018;35:34–7.
102. Walton LM, Costa A, LaVanture D, McIlrath S, Stebbins B. The effects of a 6 week dynamic core stability plank exercise program compared to a traditional supine core stability strengthening program on diastasis recti abdominis closure, pain, oswestry disability index (ODI) and pelvic floor disability index scores (PFDI). Phys Ther Rehabil. 2016;3.
103. Thabet AA, Alshehri MA. Efficacy of deep core stability exercise program in postpartum women with diastasis recti abdominis: a randomised controlled trial. J Musculoskelet Neuronal Interact. 2019;19(1):62–8.
104. Maring-Klug R. Reducing low back pain during pregnancy. Nurse Pract. 1982;7(10):18.
105. Szczygieł E, Blaut J, Zielonka-Pycka K, Tomaszewski K, Golec J, Czechowska D, et al. The impact of deep muscle training on the quality of posture and breathing. J Mot Behav. 2017:1–9.
106. Bouisset S, Duchêne JL. Is body balance more perturbed by respiration in seating than in standing posture? Neuroreport. 1994;5(8):957–60.
107. Opala-Berdzik A, Bacik B, Kurkowska M. Biomechanical changes in pregnant women. Physiotherapy/Fizjoterapia. 2009;17(3):51–5.
108. Behm DG, Blazevich AJ, Kay AD, McHugh M. Acute effects of muscle stretching on physical performance, range of motion, and injury incidence in healthy active individuals: a systematic review. Appl Physiol Nutr Metab. 2016;41(1):1–11.
109. Bø K, Berghmans B, Mørkved S, Van Kampen M. Evidence-based physical therapy for the pelvic floor: bridging science and clinical practice. 1st ed. London: Churchill Livingstone/Elsevier; 2007. p. 456.
110. Wagg A, Bunn F. Unassisted pelvic floor exercises for postnatal women: a systematic review. J Adv Nurs. 2007;58(5):407–17.
111. Woodley SJ, Boyle R, Cody JD, Mørkved S, Hay-Smith EJC. Pelvic floor muscle training for prevention and treatment of urinary and faecal incontinence in antenatal and postnatal women. Cochrane Database Syst Rev. 2017;12:CD007471.
112. Davenport MH, Nagpal TS, Mottola MF, Skow RJ, Riske L, Poitras VJ, et al. Prenatal exercise (including but not limited to pelvic floor muscle training) and urinary incontinence during and following pregnancy: a systematic review and meta-analysis. Br J Sports Med. 2018;52(21):1397–404.
113. Woodley SJ, Lawrenson P, Boyle R, Cody JD, Mørkved S, Kernohan A, et al. Pelvic floor muscle training for preventing and treating urinary and faecal incontinence in antenatal and postnatal women. Cochrane Database Syst Rev. 2020;5:CD007471.
114. Cerruto MA, D'Elia C, Aloisi A, Fabrello M, Artibani W. Prevalence, incidence and obstetric factors' impact on female urinary incontinence in Europe: a systematic review. Urol Int. 2013;90(1):1–9.
115. Delancey JOL, Kane Low L, Miller JM, Patel DA, Tumbarello JA. Graphic integration of causal factors of pelvic floor disorders: an integrated life span model. Am J Obstet Gynecol. 2008;199(6):610.e1–5.
116. Newman DK. Pelvic floor muscle rehabilitation using biofeedback. Urol Nurs. 2014;34(4):193–202.
117. Bø KB, Mørkved S. Motor learning. Ability to contract the pelvic-floor muscles. In: Bø KB, Mørkved S, Van Kampen M, editors. Evidence-based physical therapy for the pelvic floor: bridging science and clinical practice. 1st ed. London: Churchill Livingstone; 2007. p. 113–9.
118. Miller JM. Graduated strength training: a pelvic muscle exercise program. The Regents of the University of Michigan; 2012. http://www.med.umich.edu/1libr/HealthyHealing/GraduatedStrengthTraining.pdf.

119. Szumilewicz A, Hopkins WG, Dornowski M, Piernicka M. Exercise professionals improve their poor skills in contracting pelvic-floor muscles: a randomized controlled trial. Res Q Exerc Sport. 2019;90(4):641.
120. Kandadai P, O'Dell K, Saini J. Correct performance of pelvic muscle exercises in women reporting prior knowledge. Female Pelvic Med Reconstr Surg. 2015;21(3):135–40.
121. Vermandel A, De Wachter S, Beyltjens T, D'Hondt D, Jacquemyn Y, Wyndaele JJ. Pelvic floor awareness and the positive effect of verbal instructions in 958 women early postdelivery. Int Urogynecol J. 2015;26(2):223–8.
122. Henderson JW, Wang S, Egger MJ, Masters M, Nygaard I. Can women correctly contract their pelvic floor muscles without formal instruction? Female Pelvic Med Reconstr Surg. 2013;19(1):8–12.
123. Chiarelli P, Murphy B, Cockburn J. Women's knowledge, practices, and intentions regarding correct pelvic floor exercises. NeurourolUrodyn. 2003;22(3):246–9.
124. Batista RLA, Franco MM, Naldoni LMV, Duarte G, Oliveira AS, Ferreira CHJ. Biofeedback and the electromyographic activity of pelvic floor muscles in pregnant women. biofeedback na atividade eletromiográfica dos músculos do assoalho pélvico em gestantes. Braz J Phys Ther. 2011;15(5):386–92.
125. Bump RC, Hurt GW, Fantl AJ, Wyman JF. Assessment of Kegel pelvic muscle exercise performance after brief verbal instruction. Am J Obstet Gynecol. 1991;165(2):322–9.
126. Bludnicka M, Piernicka M, Szumilewicz A. The characteristics of biofeedback techniques used in pelvic floor muscle training for healthy pregnant women. A narrative review. Baltic J Health Phys Activ. 2019;11(4):87–95.
127. Opara J, Socha T, Prajsner A, Poświata A, Opara J, Socha T, et al. Fizjoterapia w wysiłkowym nietrzymaniu moczu u kobiet Część I. Aktualne rekomendacje dotyczące ćwiczeń według Kegla / Physiotherapy in stress urinary incontinence in females. Part I. Contemporary recommendations for Kegel exercises (PFME). Physiotherapy. 2011;19(3):41–9.
128. Piernicka M, Duda-Biernacka B, Bludnicka M, Szumilewicz A. The characteristics of the pelvic floor muscle training programs used in experimental studies with surface electromyography in non-Pregnant women: a systematic review. Iran J Public Health. 2020;49(6):1022–32.
129. Bø K, Mørkved S. Motor learning. In: Bø K, Berghmans B, Mørkved S, Van Kampen M, editors. Evidence-based physical therapy for the pelvic floor: bridging science and clinical practice. 1st ed. London: Churchill Livingstone/Elsevier; 2007. p. 113–9.
130. Chesnel C, Charlanes A, Tan E, Turmel N, Breton FL, Ismael SS, et al. Influence of the urine stream interruption exercise on micturition. Int J Urol. 2019;26(11):1059–63.
131. Miller JM. On pelvic floor muscle function and stress urinary incontinence: effects of posture, parity and volitional control. Dissertation [Thesis]. University of Michigan, Horace H. Rackham School of Graduate Studies; 1996, pp. 145–157.
132. Carriere B. Fitness for the pelvic floor. Stuttgart, New York: Thieme; 2002. p. 112.
133. Odent M. New reasons and new ways to study birth physiology. Int J Gynaecol Obstet. 2001;75(Suppl 1):S39–45.
134. WHO. Care in normal birth: a practical guide. Geneva: World Health Organization; 1996. http://apps.who.int/iris/bitstream/10665/63167/1/WHO_FRH_MSM_96.24.pdf.
135. Russell JB, Mitchell D, Musey PI, Collins DC. The relationship of exercise to anovulatory cycles in female athletes: hormonal and physical characteristics. Obstet Gynecol. 1984;63(4):452–6.
136. Magann EF, Evans SF, Weitz B, Newnham J. Antepartum, intrapartum, and neonatal significance of exercise on healthy low-risk pregnant working women. Obstet Gynecol. 2002;99(3):466.
137. Desseauve D, Fradet L, Lacouture P, Pierre F. Position for labor and birth: state of knowledge and biomechanical perspectives. Eur J Obstet Gynecol Reprod Biol. 2017;208:46–54.
138. Blankfield A. The optimum position for childbirth. Med J Aust. 1965;2(16):666–8.

139. Jianfang W, Xuemei L, Chunhong W, Xuemei L. The effectiveness of delivery ball use versus conventional nursing care during delivery of primiparae. Pak J Med Sci. 2020;36(3):550–4.
140. Zang Y, Lu H, Zhao Y, Huang J, Ren L, Li X. Effects of flexible sacrum positions during the second stage of labour on maternal and neonatal outcomes: a systematic review and meta-analysis. J Clin Nurs. 2020;29(17/18):3154–69.
141. Panda S. Stress and health: symptoms and techniques of psychotherapeutic management. Indian J Posit Psychol. 2014;5(4):516–20.
142. Illi SK, Held U, Frank I, Spengler CM. Effect of respiratory muscle training on exercise performance in healthy individuals: a systematic review and meta-analysis. Sports Med. 2012;42(8):707–24.
143. Dominelli PB, Archiza B, Ramsook AH, Mitchell RA, Peters CM, Molgat-Seon Y, et al. Effects of respiratory muscle work on respiratory and locomotor blood flow during exercise. Exp Physiol. 2017;102(11):1535–47.
144. Berk B. Motherwell maternity fitness plan. Champaign, IL: Human Kinetics; 2005. p. 232.
145. Boaviagem A, Melo Junior E, Lubambo L, Sousa P, Aragão C, Albuquerque S, et al. The effectiveness of breathing patterns to control maternal anxiety during the first period of labor: a randomized controlled clinical trial. Complement Ther Clin Pract. 2017;26:30–5.
146. Lewis LK, Williams MT, Olds T. Short-term effects on outcomes related to the mechanism of intervention and physiological outcomes but insufficient evidence of clinical benefits for breathing control: a systematic review. Aust J Physiotherapy. 2007;53(4):219–27.
147. Amola M, Pawara S, Kalra S. Effect of inspiratory muscle training and diaphragmatic breathing exercises on dyspnea, pulmonary functions, fatigue and functional capacity in pregnancy during third trimester. J Clin Diagn Res. 2019;13(8):1–4.
148. Yildirim G, Sahin NH. The effect of breathing and skin stimulation techniques on labour pain perception of Turkish women. Pain Res Manag. 2004;9(4):183–7.
149. Ahmadi Z, Torkzahrani S, Roosta F, Shakeri N, Mhmoodi Z. Effect of breathing technique of blowing on the extent of damage to the perineum at the moment of delivery: a randomized clinical trial. Iran J Nurs Midwifery Res. 2017;22(1):62–6.
150. Bergström M, Kieler H, Waldenström U. Effects of natural childbirth preparation versus standard antenatal education on epidural rates, experience of childbirth and parental stress in mothers and fathers: a randomised controlled multicentre trial. BJOG. 2009;116(9):1167–76.
151. Ricchi A, La Corte S, Molinazzi MT, Messina MP, Banchelli F, Neri I. Study of childbirth education classes and evaluation of their effectiveness. Clin Ter. 2020;170(1):e78–86.
152. Munzert J, Lorey B, Zentgraf K. Cognitive motor processes: the role of motor imagery in the study of motor representations. Brain Res Rev. 2009;60(2):306–26.
153. Rakhshani A, Nagarathna R, Mhaskar R, Mhaskar A, Thomas A, Gunasheela S. Effects of yoga on utero-fetal-placental circulation in high-risk pregnancy: a randomized controlled trial. Adv Prev Med. 2015;2015:1–10.
154. Möhler R, Köpke S, Meyer G. Criteria for reporting the development and evaluation of complex interventions in healthcare: revised guideline (CReDECI 2). Trials. 2015;16:204.
155. Barsky E, Smith T, Patricios J, Collins R, Branfield A, Ramagole M. South African sports medicine association position statement on exercise in Pregnancy. S Afr J Sports Med. 2012;24(2):69–71.
156. Carvalho MECC, Lima LC, de Lira Terceiro CA, Pinto DRL, Silva MN, Cozer GA, et al. Low back pain during pregnancy. Rev Bras Anestesiol. 2017;67(3):266–70.
157. Stover MD, Edelstein AI, Matta JM. Chronic anterior pelvic instability: diagnosis and management. J Am Acad Orthop Surg. 2017;25(7):509–17.
158. Bartnikowska I. Ćwiczenia oddechowe i pozycje porodowe w subiektywnym odczuciu kobiet ciężarnych w prenatalnych ćwiczeniach fizycznych (breathing exercises and positions of childbirth in the perception of pregnant women in prenatal exercise programs). Gdansk: Gdansk University of Physical Education and Sport; 2016.
159. ACNM. Exercise in pregnancy. J Midwifery Womens Health. 2014;59(4):473–4.
160. Oz M, Roizen M. Sleep like a baby. Fit Preg. 2012:56.
161. ACSM. Current comment: exercise during pregnancy [press release].

Exercise Prescription and Adaptations in Early Postpartum

10

Rita Santos-Rocha and Anna Szumilewicz

Abstract

There are several guidelines supporting the benefits of exercising during pregnancy and postpartum. Scientific research conducted in the last decades has markedly changed the perception of prenatal physical activity, overlapping the conservative approach presented in the first publications. However, those guidelines contain very general recommendations on physical activity during the postpartum period and little information that exercise professionals could use when programming the contents of targeted exercise classes for early postpartum women. Regarding the physical adaptations that persist for several weeks after birth, the early postpartum period can be assumed as the "fourth trimester." This chapter addresses the steps for planning, conducting, and monitoring early postpartum exercise classes, aiming to help women to resume exercise and sports practice in a transition stage to "normal" life.

Keywords

Postpartum · Exercise · Physical activity · Fitness · Exercise planning

---

R. Santos-Rocha (✉)
Sport Sciences School of Rio Maior - ESDRM, Polytechnic Institute of Santarém, Rio Maior, Portugal

Laboratory of Biomechanics and Functional Morphology, Interdisciplinary Centre for the Study of Human Performance - CIPER, Faculty of Human Kinetics - FMH, University of Lisbon, Lisbon, Portugal
e-mail: ritasantosrocha@esdrm.ipsantarem.pt

A. Szumilewicz
Gdansk University of Physical Education and Sport, Gdańsk, Poland
e-mail: anna.szumilewicz@awf.gda.pl

R. Santos-Rocha (ed.), *Exercise and Physical Activity During Pregnancy and Postpartum*, https://doi.org/10.1007/978-3-031-06137-0_10

10.1 Introduction

The purpose of this chapter is to provide exercise and healthcare professionals an understanding about the planning of the several steps of health screening, pre-exercise evaluation, exercise testing, and exercise prescription during the early postpartum period, assumed as the "fourth trimester."

During pregnancy, moderate-intensity physical exercise can be considered safe and provides benefits for both the mother and the fetus and newborn, in general terms. As seen in the previous Chap. 7 [1], there are several international guidelines on exercise during pregnancy that support these claims. Less information can be found regarding the postpartum period. However, there are specific physiological, morphological, and musculoskeletal changes occurring during pregnancy that may persist for 4–6 weeks after birth. Postpartum women's recovery from birth can be assisted through increased physical activity [2] (Fig. 10.1).

In this line, health and exercise professionals must take into consideration different phases of the postpartum period, with specific objectives and exercise selection needs. Again, there is the need for a multidisciplinary approach regarding exercise and health professionals since there are different objectives regarding exercise in each period. The time periods can be divided into distinct but continuous phases [3]:

1. The initial or acute period involves the first 6–12 h postpartum. Usually, it is hospital-based (i.e., during a hospital stay after delivery). This is a time of rapid change with the potential for immediate crises, such as postpartum hemorrhage, uterine inversion, amniotic fluid embolism, and eclampsia.
2. Immediate postpartum (i.e., hospital discharge to 6 weeks postpartum, depending on the type of delivery). During this phase, the body is undergoing major changes in terms of hemodynamics, genitourinary recovery, metabolism, and emotional status. Nonetheless, the changes are less rapid than in the acute post-

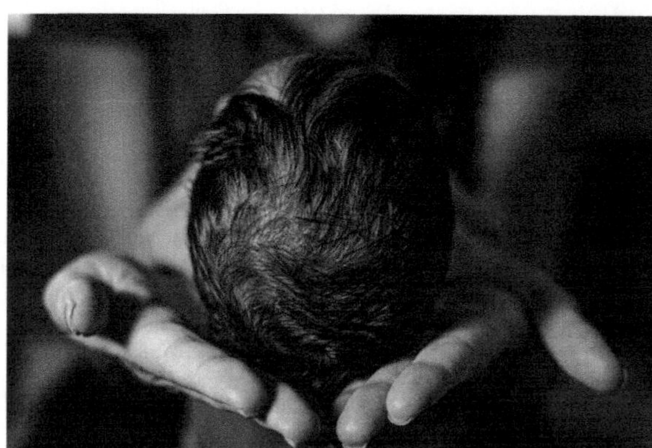

Fig. 10.1 Postpartum women's recovery from birth can be assisted through increased physical activity

partum phase and the patient is generally capable of self-identifying problems. These may run the gamut from ordinary concerns about perineal discomfort to peripartum cardiomyopathy or severe postpartum depression.

3. Later or delayed postpartum (i.e., 6 weeks to 1 year, corresponding to the cessation of breastfeeding). Changes during this phase are extremely gradual, and pathology is rare.

Thus, the postpartum period is defined as the time immediately after birth, but there is no clearly defined end to the postpartum period. Therefore, it is usually considered to be 6–26 weeks following the birth [4]. The hospital-based period is very limited regarding exercise, and women are very focused on the baby. However, simple exercises to stimulate the cardiorespiratory system and improve the blood flow in particular muscle groups can be performed while walking through the hospital corridors or laying in bed. Some postural and light stretching exercises are also possible. Pelvic floor training can be implemented anytime. It is important to stress the importance of performing pelvic floor exercises (also known as Kegel exercises) during pregnancy and in all postpartum periods, in order to strengthen the pelvic floor, reducing the number of episiotomies, improving perinatal results, and providing a much faster recovery [5]. Moreover, Kegel exercises and those that strengthen the pelvic floor are recommended to decrease the risk of urinary incontinence during and after pregnancy [6]. Further information on this topic can be found in Chaps. 6 [7] and 9 [8], as well as in Bø et al. [9]. The immediate postpartum period is focused on recovering from delivery and caring for the infant [10]. Many of the physical and physiological changes that occur during pregnancy will persist for 4–6 weeks after delivery [4]. The later postpartum, which duration can vary regarding breastfeeding and body recovery, is a transition stage to "normal" life.

Although the timing for recovery will be different for each woman, it will cover the immediate postpartum and, normally, until the first 6 weeks of the later postpartum. Regarding physical activity and exercise, we call this stage the "early postpartum" or the "fourth trimester," assuming that, between the third and the sixth months after delivery, the woman will be able to resume normal physical activity and exercise.

10.2 Physical Activity and Health in the Early Postpartum, the "Fourth Trimester"

The short-term benefits of postpartum physical activity and exercise include improvement in mood and cardiorespiratory fitness, promotion of weight loss, and a reduction in postpartum depression and anxiety [10, 11]. The improvement of other fitness components (i.e., muscular fitness) and posture, and the reduction of fatigue and urinary incontinence are other health issues related to physical activity and exercise during the early postpartum.

Postpartum **mood imbalance**, also called "baby blues" or serious mental disorders including postpartum depression can have detrimental effects on both a mother's physical and mental health and on her child's growth and emotional development [12].

A recent systematic review by Davenport et al. [13] concluded that prenatal exercise did not alter the odds of postpartum depression or the severity of depressive symptoms, nor anxiety or anxiety symptoms during or following pregnancy. On the contrary, Kołomańska-Bogucka et al. [14] concluded that physical activity during postpartum can be an essential factor in the prevention of depressive disorders in women in the postnatal period. Also, the systematic reviews by Pritchett et al. [15], Carter et al. [12], and Nakamura et al. [16] provide support for the effectiveness of exercise in reducing postpartum depressive symptoms.

There is good evidence that physical activity interventions initiated postpartum are effective in reducing weight retention [17, 18]. Saligheh et al. [17] state that studies identified as most likely to associate with postnatal depression and/or **weight loss** changes were those with supervision (one-to-one, and in group), structure (weekly frequency, scheduled durations, and moderate-intensity), which adhered to specific exercise or physical activity guidelines over an extended postpartum period (e.g., more than 12 weeks) and were supplemented by several psychosocial support strategies (e.g., educational information, exercise/physical activity advice, and counseling). Nascimento et al. [18] also reported that there is benefit from overall lifestyle interventions on **weight loss** in postpartum women and exercise plus intensive diet and objective targets are the most effective intervention strategies.

Fatigue is also a common adverse experience in pregnant and postpartum women and is associated with poor outcomes and can seriously affect maternal and infant health and quality of life [19]. The systematic review by Liu et al. [19] concluded that postpartum exercise in a supervised program lasting more than 8 weeks may be beneficial for reducing postpartum fatigue.

Pelvic Floor Muscle raining (PFMT) is often recommended to treat postpartum **Urinary Incontinence** (UI). The review by Woodley et al. [20] provides evidence that early, structured PFMT in early pregnancy for continent women may prevent the onset of UI in late pregnancy and postpartum. Wu et al. [21] concluded that postpartum PFMT likely reduces the risk of UI, particularly stress urinary incontinence symptoms. However, there is currently little evidence about postpartum PFMT and long-term pelvic floor function, mainly, the role of postpartum PFMT in Pelvic Organ Prolapse (POP), sexual function, and Anal Incontinence (AI) are still unclear.

In our previous study by Szumilewicz et al. [22], we analyzed postpartum quality of life-related to urinary incontinence symptoms. We observed substantially better outcomes in terms of UI in women who participated in prenatal exercise programs compared to a control group, both in the rate and in the severity of this dysfunction 2-months and 1-year postpartum. It is very likely that these positive results were related to better function of pelvic floor muscles gained in pregnancy and to higher awareness and better skills on how and when to perform pelvic floor muscles after birth in the training women. In the survey conducted by Moossdorff et al. [23], only 12% of women reported having pelvic floor muscle training 3-months postpartum.

In contradiction to these data, in our study, 83% of the training group started pelvic floor muscle training within the 8 weeks after childbirth. The worrying outcome is that almost half of the control women (48%) did not start pelvic floor muscle training during the year after delivery [22]. Above studies indicate an urgent need to educate women on the topic of pelvic floor muscle training during the perinatal period.

Nevertheless, several studies refer to substantial heterogeneity of trials and point that more available data from large-scale and high-quality trials are needed to demonstrate the effects of exercise on postpartum health issues [12, 19].

In conclusion, there is currently no specific guidance on the role of exercise in managing the main postpartum health issues, such as depression, fatigue, UI, and international guidance is inconsistent. Nevertheless, Pritchett et al. [15] showed that group exercise, participant-chosen exercise, and exercise with co-interventions all may be effective interventions. The postpartum period provides an opportunity for women to begin or reengage in an active lifestyle or a specific exercise program. At this stage, exercise professionals, having in mind possible situations related to the incomplete recovery of women after childbirth, have to understand the main facilitators and barriers to exercise during postpartum. There is some evidence that to increase physical activity levels in postpartum women educational interventions should be started already during pregnancy. In our previous study women who underwent prenatal exercise and educational program-initiated exercise substantially earlier postpartum than the controls [22].

10.3 Physical Activity Guidelines in the Early Postpartum

Scientific research conducted in the last decades has markedly changed the perception of prenatal physical activity, overlapping the conservative approach presented in the first publications. However, those guidelines contain very general recommendations on physical activity during the postpartum period and little information that exercise professionals could use when programming the contents of targeted exercise classes for early postpartum women.

Given its numerous health benefits for both pregnant women and their children, national and international guidelines have recommended regular PA for all healthy pregnant women since the 1980s [24]. In 1985, the ACOG issued the first guidelines for prenatal and postnatal physical activity [25]. In the last four decades several "official guidelines" or "position statements" have been published regarding the issue "Physical Activity and Exercise During Pregnancy and the Postpartum Period." Postpartum guidelines for physical activity should help women quickly achieve levels of physical activity that are commensurate with guidelines for all adults [26]. However, we noticed that these documents barely addressed the postpartum period. We also noticed the need for specific exercise guidelines for exercise professionals and sports trainers.

The World Health Organization's Guideline on Physical Activity [27] have been recommending that adults aged 18–64 years engage in at least 150 min of moderate-intensity aerobic activity throughout the week in bouts of at least 10 min, or at least 75 min of vigorous-intensity aerobic activity, or an equivalent combination of the two. Muscle strengthening should be done two or more days per week. The guideline states that postpartum women may need extra precaution and should seek medical advice before striving to achieve these recommendations. These guidelines have been updated recently regarding the pregnancy and postpartum periods [27].

Evenson et al. [10], provided a summary of international guidelines for physical activity following pregnancy, in 2013. This review included published guidelines on physical activity during the postpartum period, and peer-reviewed studies published between 1990 and 2013, as well. The authors highlight the importance of resuming physical activity during this time is often not made clear to women [10]. Moreover, women should return to prepregnancy exercise levels gradually, not resuming high impact too soon. The authors suggest that there should be country-specific postpartum physical activity guidelines that inform both healthcare providers and women about safe levels of physical activity during this unique period. Moreover, a qualitative study by Murray-Davis et al. [28] highlighted a lack of guidance and information about exercise in the postpartum period, as well as about healthy eating and weight management.

The Committee Opinion on "Physical Activity and Exercise During Pregnancy and the Postpartum Period" published by ACOG in 2015 [29] barely addressed the postpartum period. These ACOG 2015 guidelines stated that the postpartum period is an opportune time for reinforcing a healthy behavior lifestyle, since the level of participation in exercise programs diminishes after childbirth, frequently leading to overweight and obesity. Thus, resuming exercise activities after delivery is important in supporting lifelong healthy habits [29].

Three important guidelines were supported by ACOG, in 2015:

- *Exercise routines may be resumed gradually after pregnancy as soon as medically safe, depending on the mode of delivery, vaginal or cesarean, and the presence or absence of medical or surgical complications. In the absence of medical or surgical complications, rapid resumption of these activities has not been found to result in adverse effects. Some women are capable of resuming physical activities within days of delivery.*
- *Pelvic floor exercises could be initiated in the immediate postpartum period.*
- *Regular aerobic exercise in lactating women has been shown to improve maternal cardiovascular fitness without affecting milk production, composition, or infant growth* [30]. *Nursing women should consider feeding their infants before exercising in order to avoid exercise discomfort of the engorged breast.*

In the last years, from 2017 to 2021, several new and updated documents were published as "recommendations for physical activity during pregnancy and postpartum." Table 10.1 resumes the main recommendations addressing the postpartum period.

Table 10.1 Resume of the recommendations for physical activity focused on the postpartum period

Organization/authors and year of publication	Recommendations on returning to physical activity after birth
IOC Expert Group Meeting, 2017 [26]	• In the postpartum period, endurance training should start gradually. Low impact activities, such as cross-country skiing, fast walking, low impact aerobics, and step training put little pressure on the pelvic floor and can start soon after birth • Strength training in the postpartum period should start gradually with a 'pelvic floor muscle first' focus. Focus should also be on abdominal and back muscles • Strength training of the pelvic floor muscles can start directly after birth • Athletes may find exercise more comfortable after breastfeeding. Breastfeeding athletes may also find a fitted bra with features of greater breast elevation more comfortable than a standard encapsulation sports bra • Athletes presenting with low back and pelvic girdle pain at 6 weeks postpartum should be referred to a sport/women's health physiotherapist • To date, there is no evidence to guide elite athletes on which abdominal exercises are the most effective in reducing the distance between the two rectus muscles and strengthening the abdominals postpartum. If the condition persists postpartum and is affecting the athlete's performance, referral for physiotherapy and/or surgical correction is indicated
IOC Expert Group Meeting, 2017 [31]	• Postpartum resumption of physical activity is an individualized process. Prepregnancy exercise routines may be resumed gradually, as soon as it is physically and medically safe • It may be prudent for athletes whose delivery was complicated by a risk factor for levator ani muscle injury (anal sphincter tear, forceps delivery, long second stage, large baby) to minimize activities that generate large increases in intra-abdominal pressure and/or repetitive high impact for several months postpartum (…) however, that there is no evidence to support this recommendation • Most, but not all, women will be physically recovered to begin training 4–6 weeks after surgery (cesarean section). The decision when to recommence exercise after a cesarean section will be dependent on issues, such as blood pressure, anemia, fatigue, pain management, and wound healing • Once medically cleared, women may participate in both aerobic and strength training starting gradually and increasing exercise time, frequency, and intensity as tolerated by their body • Moderate exercise during lactation does not affect the quantity or composition of breast milk or impact infant growth • Nursing women should consider feeding their infants (or using a breast bra) before exercising to avoid the discomfort of engorged breasts during exercise • Athletes may benefit from wearing a personally fitted sports bra that offers support rather than compression • There is no consensus on which abdominal exercises to recommend correcting diastasis recti abdominis postdelivery • There is strong evidence that stabilization exercises generally are not more effective than any other form of active exercise in the long term, regarding low back pain and pelvic girdle pain • There is strong evidence for pelvic floor muscle training as a treatment of urinary incontinence in the general postpartum population

(continued)

Table 10.1 (continued)

Organization/ authors and year of publication	Recommendations on returning to physical activity after birth
Sports Medicine Australia, 2017 [4]	• Women should seek guidance from their healthcare provider before they begin or recommence their physical activity/exercise regime • In general, all healthy women should aim (through gradual progression) to accumulate 150–300 min of moderate-vigorous intensity aerobic exercise per week • Return to high impact activities or those that cause high gravitational load on the pelvic floor should occur gradually, and in consideration of recovery to any damage to the pelvic floor and abdominal muscles, which will vary according to the mode of delivery • Moderate to vigorous-intensity physical activity/exercise and sports will not negatively affect breast milk volume, as long as there is appropriate food and fluid intake (the caloric cost of breastfeeding is estimated to be about 600 kcal/day). This type of exercise or physical activity has also been shown not to affect the composition of breast milk or infant growth. However, if babies appear to be unsettled after feeding immediately after maternal exercise, mothers could feed their baby before exercise, postpone feeding to 1 h after physical activity/exercise, or express milk before exercising, so that it may be used after the activity
USDHHS, 2018 [32]	• Women should do at least 150 min (2 h and 30 min) of moderate-intensity aerobic activity a week during pregnancy and the postpartum period. Preferably, aerobic activity should be spread throughout the week • Women who habitually engaged in vigorous-intensity aerobic activity or who were physically active before pregnancy can continue these activities during pregnancy and the postpartum period. • Women who are pregnant can consult their healthcare provider about whether or how to adjust their physical activity during pregnancy and after the baby is born

Table 10.1 (continued)

Organization/authors and year of publication	Recommendations on returning to physical activity after birth
ACOG, 2019 [33]	• After having a baby, you should get at least 150 min of moderate-intensity aerobic activity every week. You can divide the 150 min into 30-min workouts on 5 days of the week or into smaller 10-min sessions throughout each day. For example, you could go for three 10-min walks each day • If you had a healthy pregnancy and a normal vaginal delivery, you should be able to start exercising again soon after the baby is born. Usually, it is safe to begin exercising a few days after giving birth—Or as soon as you feel ready. If you had a cesarean birth or other complications, ask your healthcare professional when it is safe to begin exercising again • Aim to stay active for 20–30 min a day. When you first start exercising after childbirth, try simple postpartum exercises that help strengthen major muscle groups, including abdominal and back muscles. Gradually add moderate-intensity exercise. Remember, even 10 min of exercise benefits your body. If you exercised vigorously before pregnancy or you are a competitive athlete, you can work up to vigorous-intensity activity. Stop exercising if you feel pain • When you are ready to start exercising, walking is a great way to get back in shape. Another good way to get daily exercise is by joining an exercise class • Check with your local fitness clubs or community centers for classes that interest you, such as yoga, Pilates, spinning, and dance. Some gyms offer special postpartum exercise classes and classes you can take with your baby. (...) if you want to exercise on your own, check out fitness videos and online exercise programs. Many are designed for women who have just had a baby • As you get ready for your workout, follow these steps: – Wear loose-fitting clothing that will help keep you cool – If you are breastfeeding, feed your baby or express your milk before your workout to avoid any discomfort that may come from engorged breasts – Wear a bra that fits well and gives plenty of support to protect your breasts – Have a bottle of water handy and take several sips during your workout
ACOG, 2020 [34]	• Exercise routines may be resumed gradually after pregnancy as soon as medically safe, depending on the mode of delivery (vaginal or cesarean birth) and the presence or absence of medical or surgical complications. Some women are capable of resuming physical activities within days of delivery • Pelvic floor exercises can be initiated in the immediate postpartum period • Abdominal strengthening exercises, including abdominal crunch exercises and the drawing-in exercise, a maneuver that increases abdominal pressure by pulling in the abdominal wall muscles, have been shown to decrease the incidence of diastasis recti abdominus and decrease the inter-rectus distance in women who gave birth vaginally or by cesarean birth • Regular aerobic exercise in lactating women has been shown to improve maternal cardiovascular fitness without affecting milk production, composition, or infant growth. Women who are lactating should consider feeding their infants or expressing milk before exercising to avoid discomfort of engorged breasts. They also should ensure adequate hydration before commencing physical activity

(continued)

Table 10.1 (continued)

Organization/authors and year of publication	Recommendations on returning to physical activity after birth
ACSM, 2020 [35]	• Prepregnancy physical activity routines can be resumed gradually as soon as physically and medically safe, which will vary depending on the mode of delivery, health status, and other individual factors • Mild physical activity with pelvic floor exercises and stretching should be able to be resumed immediately • Consult with a healthcare provider if there are any questions
Australian Government—Department of Health, 2021 [36]	• Women should do at least 150 min (2 h and 30 min) of moderate-intensity aerobic activity a week during pregnancy and the postpartum period. Preferably, aerobic activity should be spread throughout the week • Women who habitually engaged in a vigorous-intensity aerobic activity or who were physically active before pregnancy can continue these activities during pregnancy and the postpartum period • Women who are pregnant should be under the care of a healthcare provider who can monitor the progress of the pregnancy. Women who are pregnant can consult their healthcare provider about whether or how to adjust their physical activity during pregnancy and after the baby is born • The timing of resuming physical activity after childbirth is different for everyone. A gradual return to recommended levels of activity is generally considered safe after the 6-week postnatal check with a health professional, however, this may differ depending on individual circumstances • Try to do pelvic floor exercises every day before and during your pregnancy, and then start again as soon as possible after birth
WHO, 2020 [27]	It is recommended that all (pregnant and) postpartum women without contraindication should: • Undertake regular physical activity throughout (pregnancy and) postpartum • Do at least 150 min of moderate-intensity aerobic physical activity throughout the week for substantial health benefits • Incorporate a variety of aerobic and muscle-strengthening activities. Adding gentle stretching may also be beneficial • Return to physical activity gradually after delivery, and in consultation with a healthcare provider, in the case of delivery by cesarean section • If (pregnant and) postpartum women are not meeting the recommendations, doing some physical activity will benefit their health • (Pregnant and) postpartum women should start by doing small amounts of physical activity, and gradually increase frequency, intensity, and duration over time • (Pregnant and) postpartum women should limit the amount of time spent being sedentary • There was no reason to alter the amount or frequency of recommended moderate-intensity physical activity for (pregnant and) postpartum women compared with the general adult population

Table 10.1 (continued)

Organization/ authors and year of publication	Recommendations on returning to physical activity after birth
RAN-ZCOG, 2021 [37]	• Pelvic floor exercises can help prevent UI (at least 25 repetitions at various times of the day) • A balanced diet and gentle exercise will help improve the strength and tone of the stomach muscles • In case of diastasis recti, women should be referred to a physiotherapist who will advise of some postnatal exercises and support garments that will help bring these muscles back together • In general, women can start exercising 4 to 6 weeks after the birth. However, they should check with a doctor before starting exercising, especially if they had a cesarean section. Before this time though, women should try to get outside, take walks, or keep blood moving with a gentle workout
Brazilian Society of Cardiology, 2021 [38]	• The postpartum exercise routine should gradually return to normal as soon as it is safe, which depends on the type of delivery (vaginal or cesarean) and whether there were surgical complications • It is recommended that exercise begin again approximately 6 weeks after cesarean delivery and 4 weeks after vaginal delivery. Progression should be slower if there is discomfort or other relevant factors, such as anemia or wound infection • Patients who exercised regularly prior to delivery should reduce the intensity in the first few months postpartum and progress gradually • Breastfeeding women can perform mild- to moderate-intensity aerobic exercise without damaging milk production or the growth of the child. Ideally, exercise should be performed after breastfeeding to avoid the discomfort of engorged breasts and should include adequate support • Resistance exercises are allowed, but care should be taken not to involve trunk flexion (traditional abdominal exercises), due to the risk of increased diastasis in the rectus abdominis muscles • Pilates, a suitable option for training deep abdominal muscles and the pelvic floor, can help return the woman's body to its pre-gestational state • Pelvic muscle training should be initiated during pregnancy • Jumping exercises should be avoided in the postpartum period due to the fragility of the pelvic floor

10.4 Pre-Exercise Assessment in the Early Postpartum

The postpartum exercise routine it is an individual process. It should gradually return to normal as soon as it is safe, which depends on the type of delivery and whether there were surgical complications. Nevertheless, some women are capable of resuming physical activities within days of delivery. In the absence of medical or surgical complications, rapid resumption of exercise activities has not been found to result in adverse effects. However, despite the benefits, the majority of women do not resume their prepregnancy physical activity levels after birth. This situation sets up the risk of remaining inactive for many years [10].

Physical activity levels are lower in pregnant women compared to their nonpregnant counterparts [39], and longitudinal studies have shown a decline in physical activity levels as pregnancy progresses [40]. Thus, only a small proportion of women achieve the recommended levels of physical activity during pregnancy [41, 42]. So far, there are no data regarding the prevalence of physical activity during the postpartum period, but we suppose that it is lower than the pregnancy stage.

Thus, it is also of utmost importance to understand and implement the most effective strategies for promoting exercise during postpartum. Saligheh et al. [2] concluded that the provision of specifically tailored and appropriate exercise programs could potentially enable increased physical activity in postpartum women, thereby improving their health. During the postpartum period, there is a fundamental objective of losing weight (or recovering prepregnancy weight) and the education of the water retention that reaches its maximum levels in the third quarter. For this, the combination of physical exercise with a balanced diet allows reaching higher levels of success in achieving the described objective. This is attested by a systematic review carried out by Lim et al. [43] in which the combination of diet and physical exercise was much more effective in reducing weight than physical exercise alone.

According to Evenson et al. [10], promising strategies include increasing knowledge, regular counseling and support, self-monitoring with diaries and pedometers, increasing self-efficacy, addressing barriers, referral to community resources for physical activity, and use of walking groups. Saligheh et al. [2] concluded that encouraging the facilitation of exercise through mothers' groups, mothers' exercise clubs, or postnatal classes suggesting behavioral and social change is needed. Moreover, the interaction between individuals, communities, organizations, and policymakers are required.

The following topics must be taken into consideration when planning an exercise program during the early postpartum period:

- The stages of the postpartum period.
- The type of birth and its impacts on musculoskeletal health (e.g., UI, pelvic girdle pain, low back pain).
- The common pains and discomforts during postpartum, and its implications for exercise adaptation (e.g., running, water exercise, and cycling).
- Diastasis recti and exercise modalities requiring the intervention of a physiotherapist.
- Low back pain and exercise selection, which may require the intervention of a physiotherapist.
- Pelvic floor training, requires the intervention of a physiotherapist or an exercise physiologist.
- Lactation and exercise adaptation, may require the intervention of a midwife.
- The infant's mobility, sleeping, and feeding practices.

- Women's motivations.
- Perception of health and quality of life.
- Social support.

The RANZCOG [37] recommendations on when a postpartum woman should contact a doctor or midwife are the following:

Your doctor or midwife will want to see you for a postnatal checkup 2 to 6 weeks after the birth of your baby. Contact your doctor or midwife earlier, if you notice any of the following:

- Heavy clotting or bleeding.
- Offensive smell.
- High temperature or fever.
- Pain, tenderness. Or warmth in your calf or thigh, particularly when you flex your foot.
- A lump or hardened area in your breast.
- Redness, heat, or oozing from your stitches.
- Depression that affects your ability to cope and does not subside after a few days.

10.5 Exercise Prescription in the Early Postpartum

There is a lack of information on the specific guidelines and real strategies for adaptation of several recreational and sports activities that might be adapted to healthy pregnant women. In accordance with the guidelines above-mentioned, Table 10.2 resumes the main physical activity-related recommendations and Table 10.3 resumes the components of exercise prescription addressing the early postpartum period, so-called the fourth trimester.

Table 10.2 Physical activity-related recommendations for the early postpartum period

General physical activity
• Women should undertake regular physical activity throughout (pregnancy and) postpartum [27] • There was no reason to alter the amount or frequency of recommended moderate-intensity physical activity for (pregnant and) postpartum women compared with the general adult population [27] • Women should do at least 150 min of moderate-intensity aerobic physical activity throughout the week for substantial health benefits, incorporating a variety of aerobic and muscle-strengthening activities. Adding gentle stretching may also be beneficial [27] • (Pregnant and) postpartum women should start by doing small amounts of physical activity, and gradually increase frequency, intensity, and duration over time [27] • If (pregnant and) postpartum women are not meeting the recommendations, doing some physical activity will benefit their health [27]. Even 10 min of exercise benefits the body [33] • Women should stop exercising if they feel pain [33]

(continued)

Table 10.2 (continued)

Pre-exercise health screening
• Women should seek guidance from their healthcare provider before they begin or recommence their physical activity/exercise regime [4, 32, 35, 36] • Return to physical activity gradually after delivery, and in consultation with a healthcare provider, in the case of delivery by cesarean section and whether there were surgical complications [27, 33, 38] • Progression should be slower if there is discomfort or other relevant factors, such as anemia or wound infection [33, 34, 37, 38] • Postpartum resumption of physical activity is an individualized process [36]. Prepregnancy exercise routines may be resumed gradually, as soon as it is physically and medically safe [26, 33, 35, 36], which will vary depending on the mode of delivery, health status, and other individual factors [35] • The decision on when to recommence exercise after cesarean section will be dependent on issues, such as blood pressure, anemia, fatigue, pain management, and wound healing [26] • Before this time though, women should try to get outside, take walks, or keep blood moving with a gentle workout [37]. Mild exercises should be able to be resumed immediately [33, 35]
Breastfeeding
• Regular aerobic exercise in lactating women has been shown to improve maternal cardiovascular fitness [34] • Mild- to moderate-intensity exercise during lactation does not affect the quantity or composition of breast milk or impact infant growth [4, 26, 34, 38], as long as there is appropriate food and fluid intake (the caloric cost of breastfeeding is estimated to be about 600 kcal/day) [4] • Nursing women may find exercise more comfortable after breastfeeding, to avoid the discomfort of engorged breasts during exercise [4, 26, 31, 33, 34, 38] • Mothers could feed their baby before exercise, postpone feeding to 1 h after physical activity/exercise, or express milk before exercising, so that it may be used after the activity [4]
Bra and sportswear
• Women should wear a bra that fits well and gives plenty of support to protect the breasts [33, 38] • Breastfeeding women may find wearing a fitted bra with features of greater breast elevation more comfortable than a standard encapsulation sports bra (or compression) [26, 31] • Women should wear loose-fitting clothing that will help keep them cool [33]
Low back and pelvic girdle pain
• There is strong evidence that stabilization exercises generally are not more effective than any other form of active exercise in the long term, regarding low back pain and pelvic girdle pain [26] • Women presenting with low back and pelvic girdle pain at 6 weeks postpartum should be referred to a sport/women's health physiotherapist [31]
Diastasis recti
• To date, there is no evidence to guide women on which abdominal exercises are the most effective in reducing the distance between the two rectus muscles and strengthening the abdominals postpartum [26, 31]. If the condition persists postpartum, referral for physiotherapy and/or surgical correction is indicated [31] • In case of diastasis recti, women should be referred to a physiotherapist who will advise of some postnatal exercises and support garments that will help bring these muscles back together [37]
Other issues
• Women should ensure adequate hydration before commencing physical activity [34] • Women should have a bottle of water handy and take several sips during the workout [33] • Women should check with local fitness clubs or community centers for (group exercise) classes that interest them. Some gyms offer special postpartum exercise classes and classes that they can take with the baby. If women prefer to exercise on their own, they should check out fitness videos and online exercise programs designed for postpartum women [33] • Women should be referred to a nutritionist to prescribe an adequate diet for this period, taking into account breastfeeding and the volume of physical activity • (Pregnant and) postpartum women should limit the amount of time spent being sedentary [27]

Table 10.3 Exercise prescription components for the early postpartum period

Aerobic exercise
• Exercise routines should incorporate a variety of aerobic activities [27]; exercises that activate large muscle groups in a rhythmic and continuous fashion • A variety of weight-bearing activities are well tolerated during the postpartum period • Women who habitually engaged in a vigorous-intensity aerobic activity or who were physically active before pregnancy can continue these activities during pregnancy and the postpartum period [36] • Aerobic exercise should start gradually [26, 31, 33], and increase exercise time, frequency, and intensity as tolerated by the body [26] • In general, all healthy women should aim (through gradual progression) to accumulate 150–300 min of moderate-vigorous intensity aerobic exercise per week [4, 27, 32, 33, 36]. Moderate intensity exercise refers to 3–5.9 METs; RPE = 12–13; 40%–60% $VO_{2reserve}$ • Preferably, aerobic activity should be spread throughout the week [27, 32, 36]. The 150 min can be divided into 30-min workouts on 5 days of the week or into smaller 10-min sessions throughout each day (e.g., three 10-min walks each day) [33] • Women who habitually engaged in vigorous-intensity aerobic activity or who were physically active before pregnancy can continue these activities during pregnancy and the postpartum period [32]. If the woman exercised vigorously before pregnancy or she is a competitive athlete, she can work up to vigorous-intensity activity [33]. Low impact activities such as cross-country skiing, fast walking, low impact aerobics and step training put little pressure on the pelvic floor and can start soon after birth [31]. Walking and joining an exercise class (e.g., spinning and dance) are good ways to get daily exercise and get back in shape [33] • It may be prudent for women whose delivery was complicated by a risk factor for levator ani muscle injury (anal sphincter tear, forceps delivery, long second stage, large baby) to minimize activities that generate repetitive high impact for several months postpartum [26] • Return to high impact activities or those that cause high gravitational load on the pelvic floor should occur gradually, and in consideration of recovery to any damage to the pelvic floor and abdominal muscles, which will vary according to the mode of delivery [4] • Activities with risk of fall and trauma should be avoided. Activities that require jumping movements and quick changes in direction which can stress joints should be done with caution to—minimize the risk of joint injury
Resistance/strength exercise
• Exercise routines should incorporate a variety of muscle-strengthening activities [27] • A variety of machines, free weights, and body weight exercises are well tolerated during the postpartum period • Strength exercise should start gradually [26, 31], and increasing exercise time, frequency, and intensity as tolerated by their body [26] • Intensity that permits multiple submaximal repetitions (i.e., 8–10 or 12–15 repetitions) to be performed to the point of moderate fatigue (40%–60% of estimated one repetition maximum) • First focus should be on abdominal and back muscles [31, 33] • It may be prudent for women whose delivery was complicated by a risk factor for levator ani muscle injury (anal sphincter tear, forceps delivery, long second stage, large baby) to minimize activities that generate large increases in intra-abdominal pressure for several months postpartum [26] • Abdominal strengthening exercises, including abdominal crunch exercises and the drawing-in exercise, a maneuver that increases abdominal pressure by pulling in the abdominal wall muscles, have been shown to decrease the incidence of diastasis recti abdominus and decrease the inter-rectus distance in women who gave birth vaginally or by cesarean birth [34] • A balanced diet and gentle exercise will help improve the strength and tone of the stomach muscles [37] • Pilates, a suitable option for training deep abdominal muscles and the pelvic floor, can help return the woman's body to its pre-gestational state [38]

(continued)

Table 10.3 (continued)

Pelvic floor muscles training
• Complex training for pelvic-floor muscles should be focused both on their contraction and relaxation. Different exercises should be performed to improve pelvic floor muscle speed, strength, endurance and muscular coordination, and engaging both fast and slow twitch muscle fibers • Proper technique should be ensured • There is strong evidence for pelvic floor muscle training as prevention and treatment of urinary incontinence in the general postpartum population [26, 37] • Pelvic floor muscles training should be performed during pregnancy, and can start directly after birth [31, 34–36, 38], at least 25 repetitions at various times of the day [37] • An effective intensity (and volume) of pelvic floor muscles exercise has not been determined, but it can be performed 10–30 min/day, 1–7 days/week • Pelvic floor muscles training can be performed anywhere, anytime, every day • Jumping exercises should be avoided in the postpartum period due to the fragility of the pelvic floor [38]
Stretching exercise
• Adding gentle stretching to exercise routines may also be beneficial [27] • Stretching exercises should be able to be resumed immediately [35] • A series of active or passive static and dynamic flexibility exercises for each muscle-tendon unit should be performed • Stretch to the point of feeling tightness or slight discomfort, holding a static stretch for 10–30 s (up to 60 s); 2–4 repetitions of each exercise; at least 2–3 up to 7 days/week • Excessive joint stress should be avoided until more data is available
Balance and coordination exercise
• Exercises involving motor skills (e.g., balance, agility, coordination, gait), proprioceptive training, and multifaceted activities (e.g., Pilates, yoga, tai chi) are well tolerated during the postpartum period • Joining an exercise class (e.g., yoga, and Pilates) is a good way to get daily exercise and get back in shape [33] • Balance and/or coordination exercises can be included in daily activities (e.g., functional training) • Intensity in balance or coordination training refers to the degree of difficulty of the postures, movements, or routines practiced. An effective intensity (and volume) of neuromotor exercise has not been determined, but it can be performed 20–30 to 60 min/day, at least 2–3 up to 7 days/week • Positions and movements that are uncomfortable or likely to result in loss of balance and falling should be avoided

RPE rating of perceived exertion (6–20 scale), *METs* metabolic equivalents, $VO_{2reserve}$ oxygen uptake reserve ($VO_{2max} - VO_{2rest}$)

10.6 Exercise Selection and Adaptation in the Early Postpartum

10.6.1 Exercises to Be Implemented in the Early Postpartum

Figures 10.2, 10.3, 10.4, 10.5, 10.6, 10.7, 10.8 and 10.9 show examples of the main physical activities and exercises to be implemented progressively in the early postpartum period. All the following forms of exercise are recommended types of

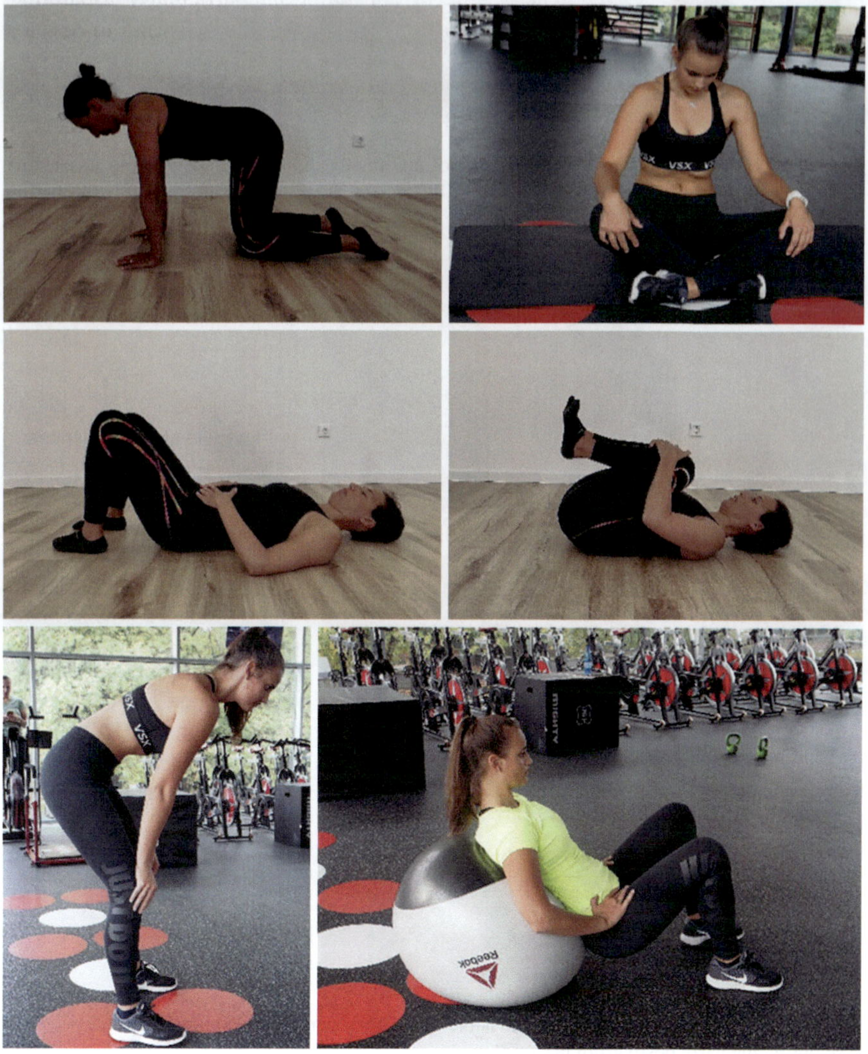

Fig. 10.2 Pelvic floor muscle training are among the recommended types of exercise during the early postpartum period

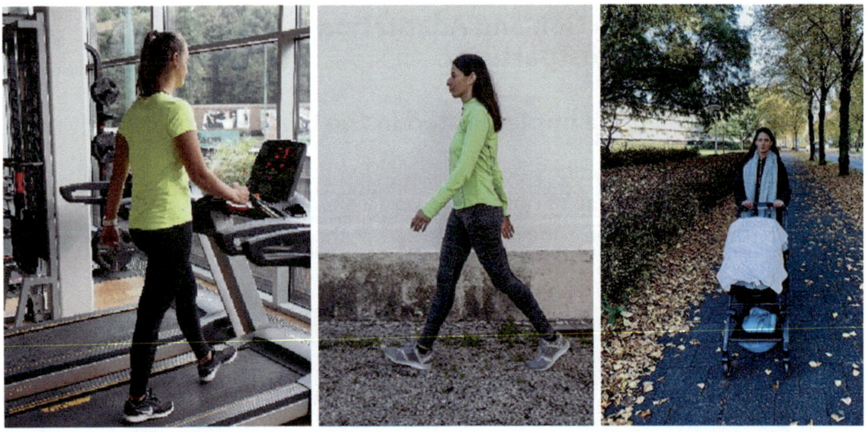

Fig. 10.3 Walking indoor and walking outdoor are among the recommended types of exercise during the early postpartum period

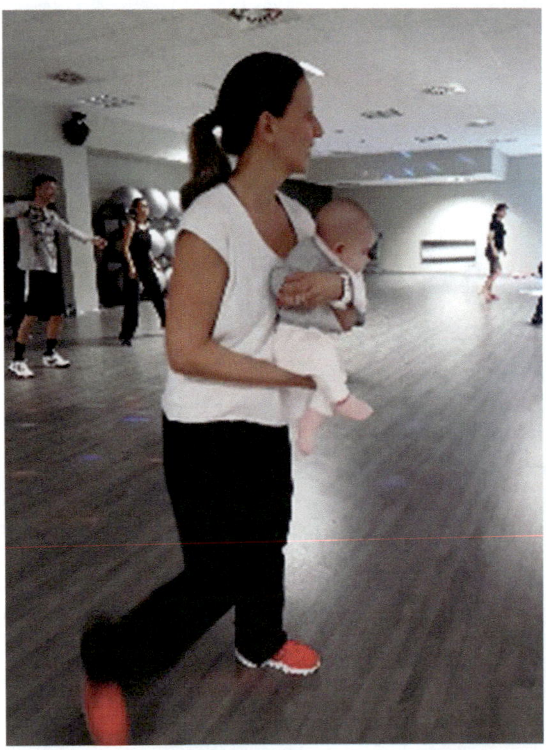

"Invisible step" sequences:
https://youtu.be/d3hB9B9n32Q
https://youtu.be/-uCqgy4IBi8

Step sequences:
https://youtu.be/pPvX_tpl-dl
https://youtu.be/aR3XYAnz2y8

Aerobics / dance sequences:
https://youtu.be/j-e261TkfaM
https://youtu.be/iUQQKJVIns4
https://youtu.be/8w5eOje6cmc
https://youtu.be/42cPuwrcR1g

Fig. 10.4 Aerobics, Dancing, Step, "Invisible Step" are among the recommended types of exercise during the early postpartum period

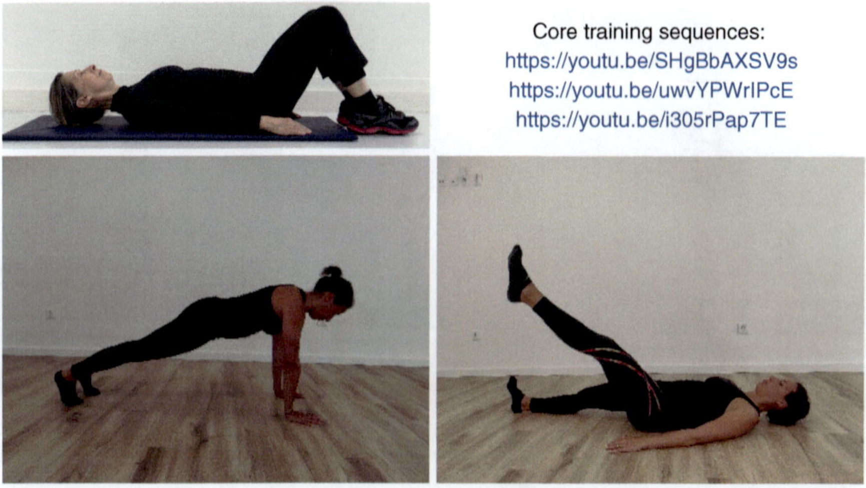
Core training sequences:
https://youtu.be/SHgBbAXSV9s
https://youtu.be/uwvYPWrlPcE
https://youtu.be/i305rPap7TE

Fig. 10.5 Pilates and Core training are among the recommended types of exercise during the early postpartum period

physical activity to be performed in postpartum period. The main question is when to start or to continue. Most, but not all, women will be physically recovered to exercise 4–6 weeks after a vaginal birth or surgery (i.e., cesarean section). Most women who have had a normal delivery and puerperium can start earlier, gradually increasing the load and intensity. The decision when to recommence exercise after cesarean section will be dependent on issues such as blood pressure, anemia, fatigue, pain management, and wound healing [26]. It means that some activities will be limited until musculoskeletal health issues are recovered.

10.6.2 Exercises to Be Implemented in the Early Postpartum, After Full Recovery of Pelvic Organs and Musculoskeletal Structures

Pregnancy and childbirth impact the maternal musculoskeletal system, and vaginal birth can be likened to the impact of an acute sports injury [31]. Thus, Figs. 10.10, 10.11, 10.12, and 10.13 shows examples of recommended types of exercise during the postpartum period, after full recovery of pelvic organs and musculoskeletal structures. It is necessary to be fully recovered from stitches after a cesarean section, tearing, or an episiotomy since it can cause discomfort when walking, dancing, running, seating on an exercise machine, or riding a bike. The same situation may occur due to swelling or pain around the opening of the vagina. The period-like bleeding as the uterus returns to its prepregnancy size will prevent women from exercising in the water (i.e., swimming a pool, river, or sea).

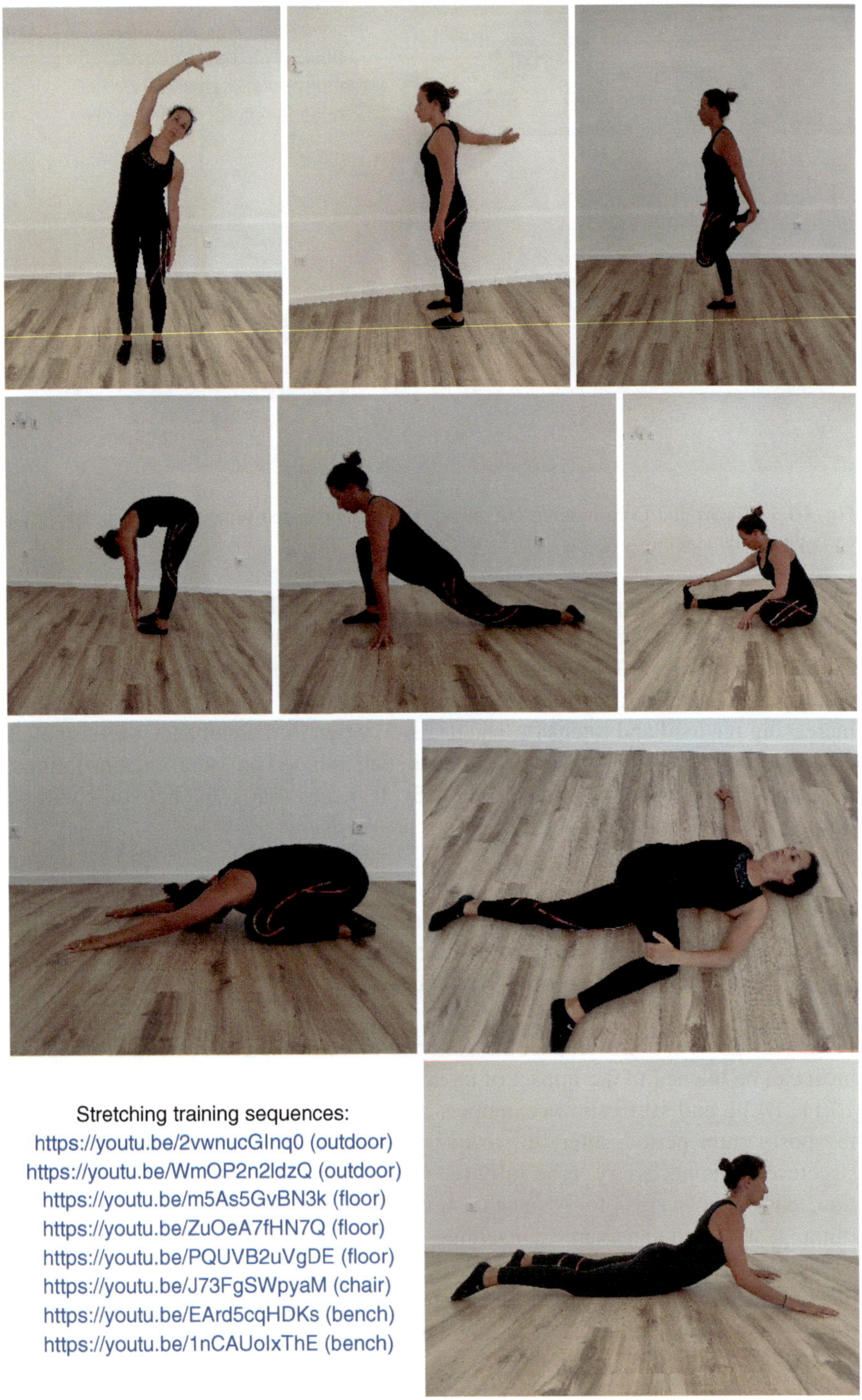

Fig. 10.6 Stretching exercises are among the recommended types of exercise during the early postpartum period

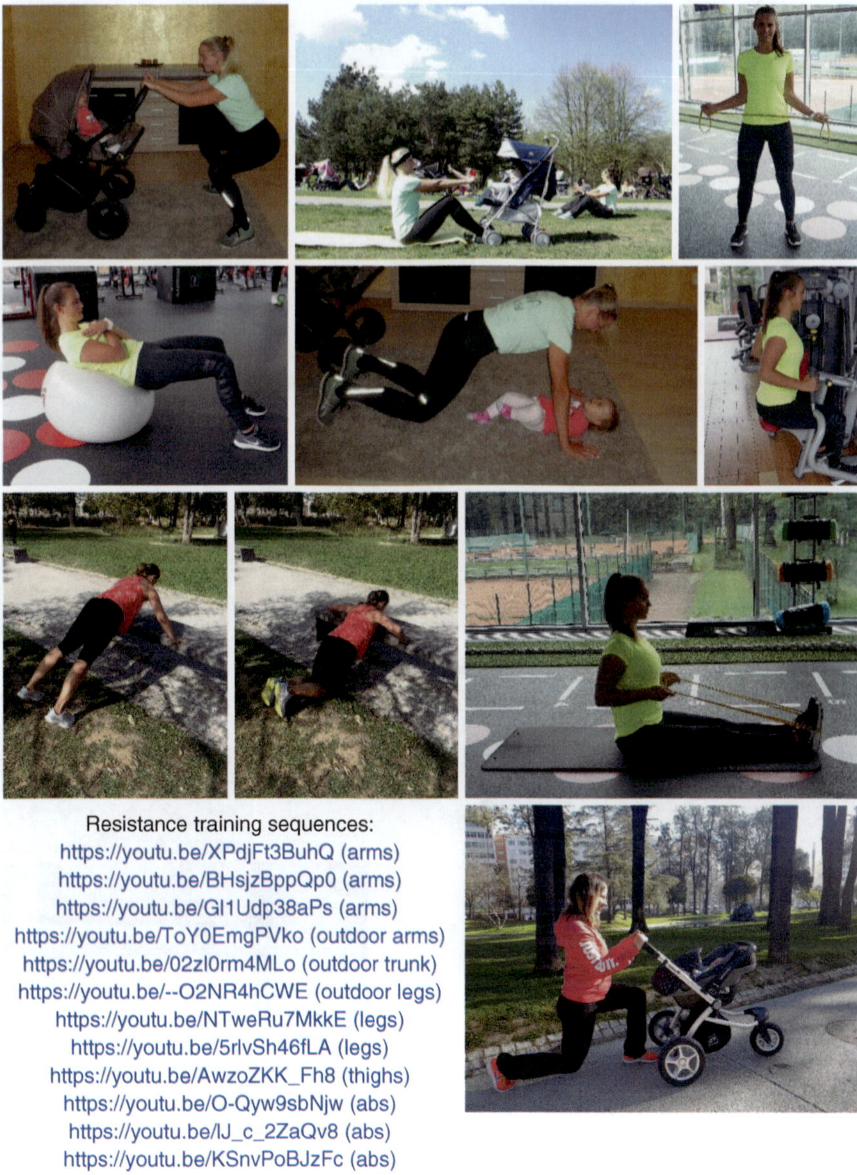

Fig. 10.7 Resistance training is among the recommended types of exercise during the early postpartum period

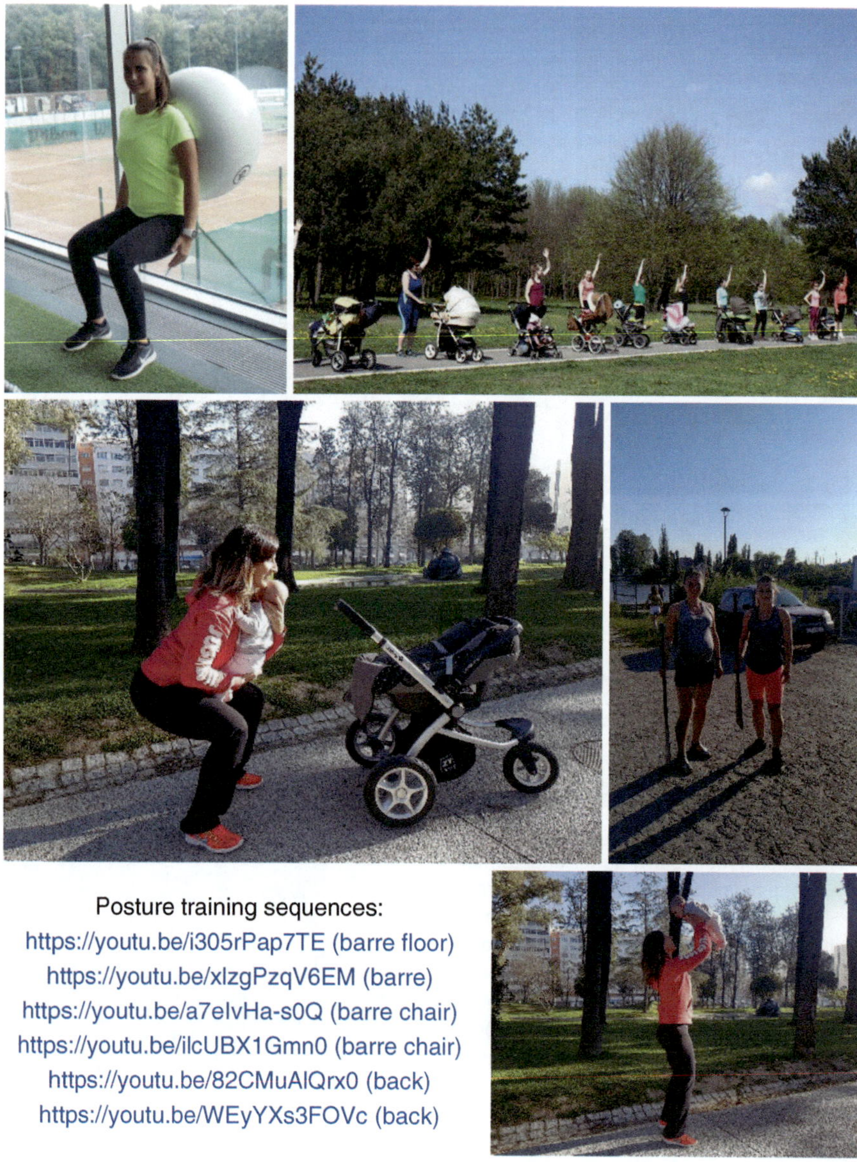

Fig. 10.8 Posture and functional training are among the recommended types of exercise during the early postpartum period

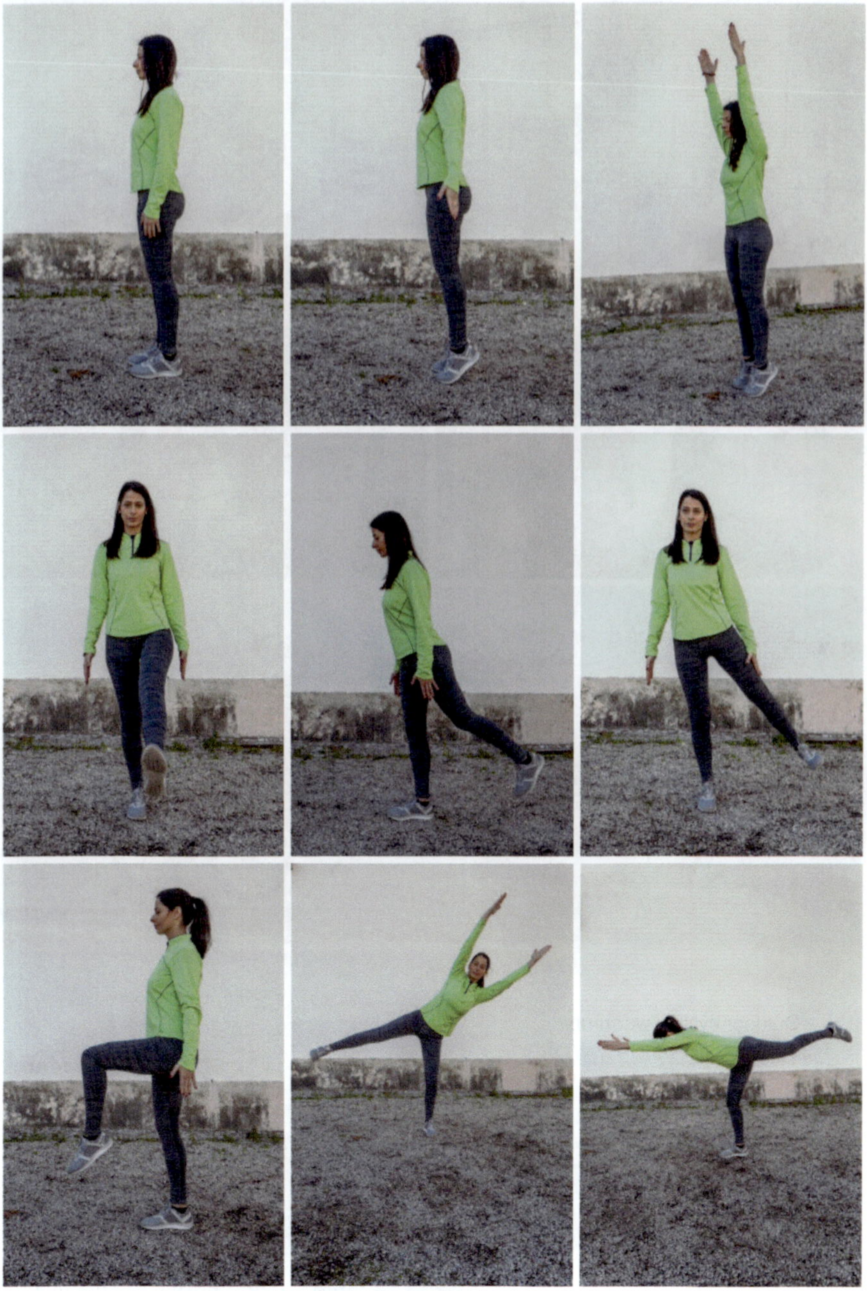

Balance training sequences:
https://youtu.be/isX_y7AiUpE
https://youtu.be/NUQ5oJlEHtQ (yoga balance)

Fig. 10.9 Balance training is among the recommended types of exercise during the early postpartum period

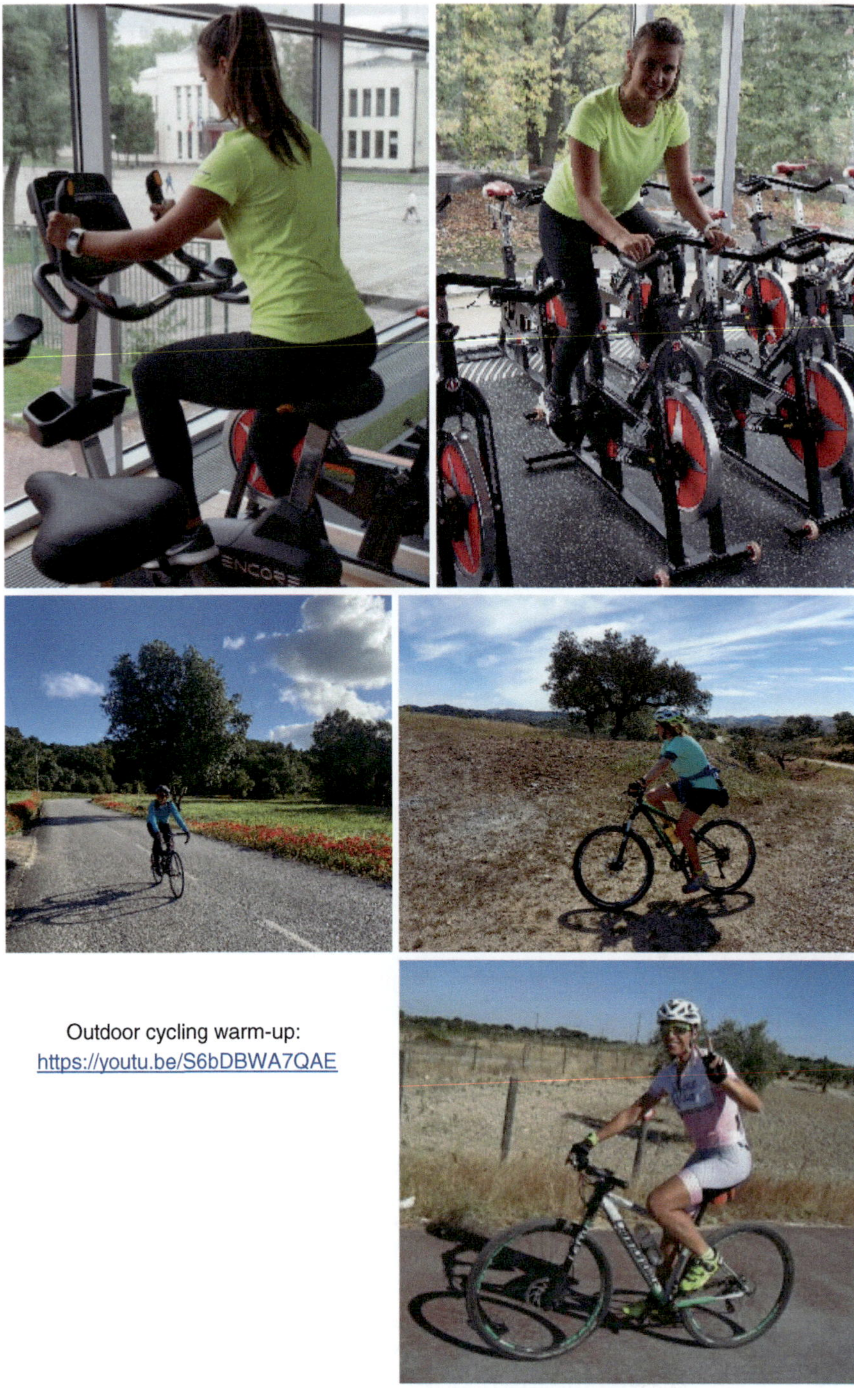

Fig. 10.10 Indoor and outdoor cycling are among the recommended types of exercise during the postpartum period, after full recovery of pelvic organs and musculoskeletal structures

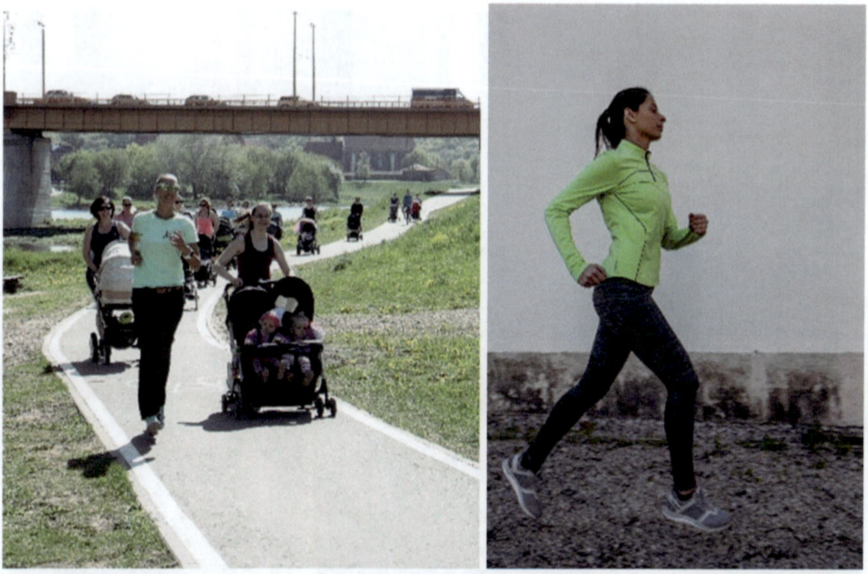

Fig. 10.11 Jogging or running are among the recommended types of exercise during the postpartum period, after full recovery of pelvic organs and musculoskeletal structures

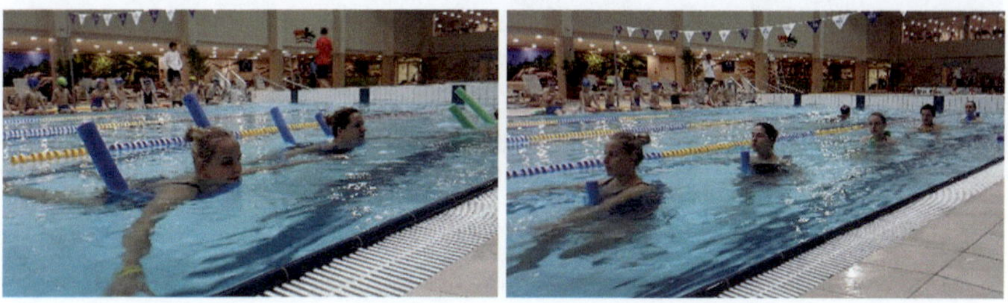

Fig. 10.12 Water exercise and swimming are among the recommended types of exercise during the postpartum period, after full recovery of pelvic organs and musculoskeletal structures

If the weather is appropriate in some countries, exercising outdoors, in the group, would be a very good option. Caution should be taken regarding the wind, the rain, and slipping pavement while running or cycling. Proper sportswear and shoes, as well as adequate diet and hydration, and sun and head protection (e.g., hat or bike helmet) are other recommendations for exercising outdoor or indoor. To manage any discomfort, nursing women should wear a well-fitted maternity bra for support during weight-bearing activities. In case of exercising indoors with or without (online) supervision, women should choose a place with adequate space and floor, ventilation, and temperature, as well as proper exercise equipment or common household materials. The keypoint is safety, i.e., if there is no bench step, it is preferable to perform the step exercise on the floor (i.e., "invisible step") rather than use an inadequate bench. Another example is to use a stable and not slippy chair if the exercise program is performed on a chair.

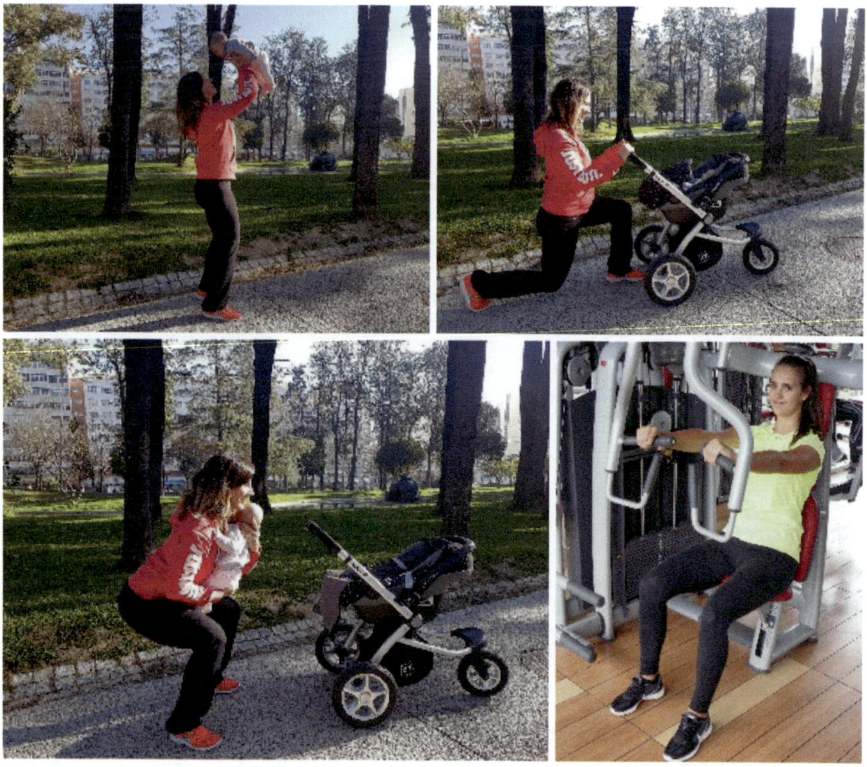

Fig. 10.13 More intense functional and strength training are among the recommended types of exercise during the postpartum period, after full recovery of pelvic organs and musculoskeletal structures

More examples of exercises and workouts of different activities can be found in our YouTube Channels: Active Pregnancy [44] and Active at home and outdoors [45], and in Chaps. 9 [8], and 8 [46].

Recently, a group of experts working under the affiliation of The Association of Chartered Physiotherapists in Sports and Exercise Medicine in the United Kingdom have developed guidelines on returning to postnatal running. The examples of exercise progression from the first week up to 12 weeks after giving birth proposed by this expert group are presented in Table 10.4. Similar progression can be used for returning to other sports activities in the postnatal period.

10.6.3 Other Forms of Increasing the Volume of Physicochemical Activity or Exercise

According to the WHO, for the general population, doing any physical activity is better than doing none [27]. If the postpartum woman does not do any physical activity, she should be advised to start by doing some, and gradually build up to the

Table 10.4 Guidelines on Returning to Postnatal Running [47]

Examples of exercise progression in the postnatal runner	
Weeks postnatal	Examples of exercise progression
Weeks 0–2	• Pelvic floor muscle strength and endurance • Basic core exercises, e.g., pelvic tilts • Walking for cardiovascular exercise
Weeks 2–4	• Progress walking/pelvic floor muscle/core rehab • Introduce squats, lunges and bridging in line with day-to-day requirements
Weeks 4–6	• Low impact exercise—static cycling • Low impact—cross trainer • Individualize according to postpartum recovery, mode of delivery, perineal trauma and saddle comfort
Weeks 6–8	• Scar mobilization (for either c-section or perineal scar) • Power walking • Increase low impact exercise • Add deadlifts • Add resistance to lower limb and core
Weeks 8–12	• Activity-dependent if lochia stopped and wound healing satisfactory • Introduce swimming • Spinning if comfortable sitting on a spinning saddle
Weeks 12 and beyond	• Goal-specific activity • Graded return to running • Consider risk factors • Monitor signs and symptoms and modify program appropriately or signpost to professional help to address postnatal issues

Source [47]: Goom T, Donnelly G, Brockwell E. Returning to running postnatal. Guidelines for medical, health, and fitness professionals menaging this population: The Association of Chartered Physiotherapists in Sports and Exercise Medicine; 2019

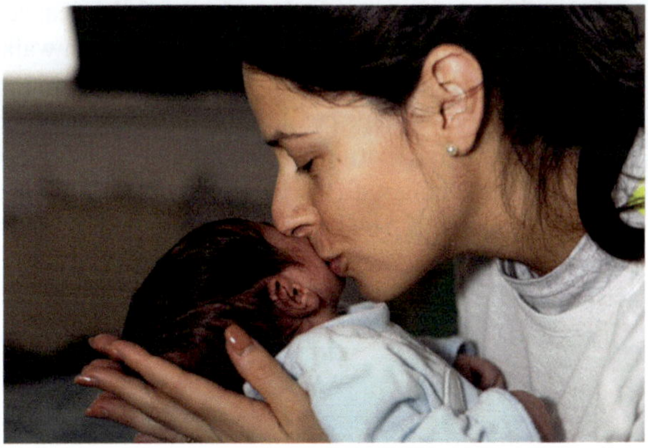

Fig. 10.14 During this very special period of life, the baby is the center of the world, but the mother also needs time for herself and physical activity

recommended amount. During this very special period of life, the baby is the center of the world (Fig. 10.14), but the mother also needs time for herself. Family support is quite important for the mother during this very special period of life, allowing her some time for physical activity (Fig. 10.15).

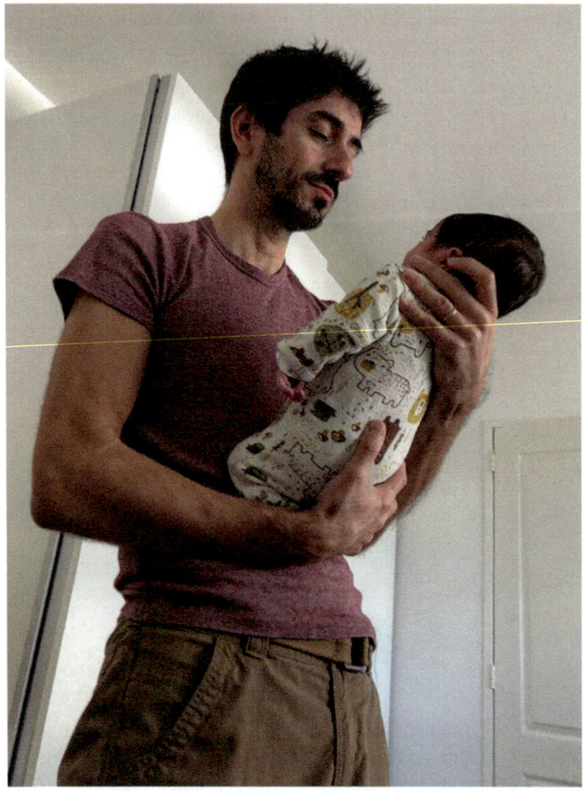

Fig. 10.15 Family support is quite important for the mother during this very special period of life, allowing her some time for physical activity

Other forms of increasing the volume of physical activity or exercise are by integrating it into daily activities, such as engaging in walking groups with other mothers and babies (Fig. 10.16), using a pedometer and increasing the walking time to a minimum of 10,000 steps per day, not standing in the same position for long periods of time, limiting the seating time and doing stretching pauses, playing with the baby (Fig. 10.17), dancing with the music at home, taking short bouts of exercise at home (e.g., by following YouTube videos [44, 45], or by using available apps that encourage physical activity), walking the dog, among other forms of physical activity.

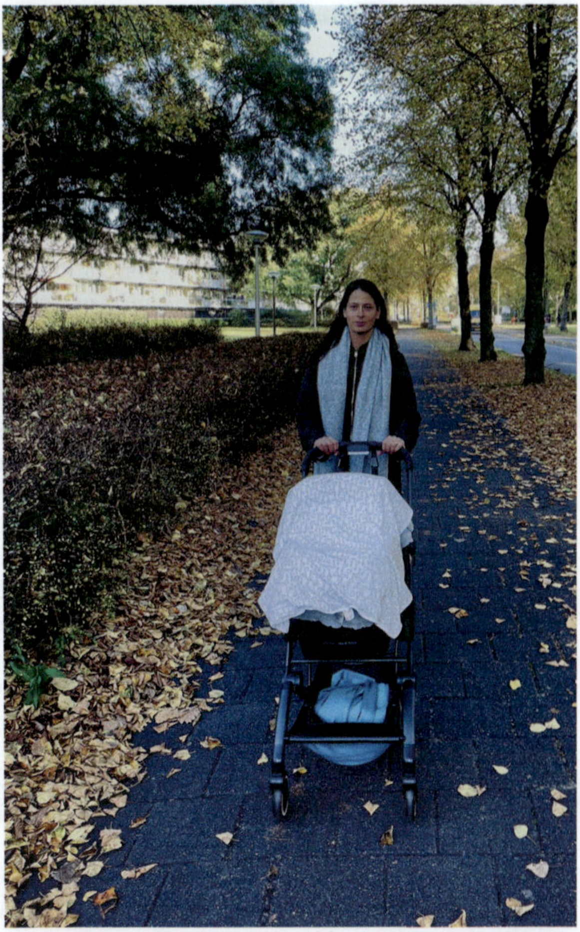

Fig. 10.16 Engaging in walking groups with other mothers and babies, or with family, is a very good form of increasing the daily volume of physical activity

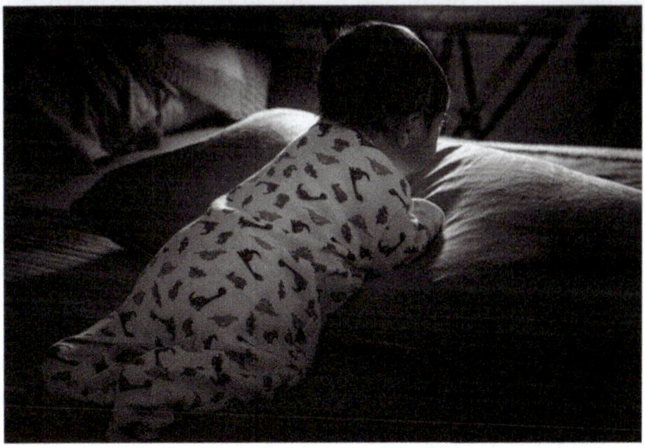

Fig. 10.17 Playing with the baby and stimulating the baby is a very good form of increasing the daily volume of physical activity

10.7 Further Research

Although beneficial effects of physical activity in postpartum on maternal health are established, some open questions remain. No consensus is reached on the type and intensity of physical activity required, especially for obese and unfit women. There is a gap in the literature regarding the dose-response for positive effects regarding recovery outcomes. Most studies in this field are from developed countries, and voluntary physical activity might have different effects on health outcomes than non-voluntary physical activity (e.g., at work or for transport). Whether this type of physical activity in postpartum has the same beneficial effect on maternal outcomes is grossly understudied.

Although there are international guidelines for physical activity during postpartum recommending regular physical activity for healthy postpartum women, little is known about the pattern of exercise and physical activity of postpartum women worldwide. Well-designed longitudinal investigations reporting postpartum-related changes in physical activity would help to fill this gap. Not only the various designs but also the various instruments used in the studies limit comparisons of studies on the practice of exercise. It would be of particular importance that researchers would use the same precise, reliable, acculturated, and validated instruments for physical activity and exercise measurement, which concerns quantity and quality.

Moreover, results indicate a need for more information and motivation for moderate exercise throughout the postpartum period. Promoting physical activity remains a priority in public health policy, and postpartum women should be encouraged to maintain an active lifestyle or to adopt a tailored exercise routine during postpartum in order to avoid sedentary- and obesity-associated risks.

Research on better and more effective physical activity and exercise interventions that improve long-term compliance to a physically active lifestyle during postpartum is needed. The methods of increasing physical activity in this special population must be developed, implemented, and evaluated. What is also important, special educational, evidence-based training for exercise professionals should be developed and promoted to enable them to properly conduct exercise programs for postpartum women.

References

1. Szumilewicz A, Worska A, Santos-Rocha R, Oviedo-Caro MA. Evidence-based and practice-oriented guidelines for exercising during pregnancy. In: Santos-Rocha R, editor. Exercise and physical activity during pregnancy and postpartum. Evidence-based guidelines. 2nd ed. Cham: Springer International; 2022, Ch.7.
2. Saligheh M, McNamara B, Rooney R. Perceived barriers and enablers of physical activity in postpartum women: a qualitative approach. BMC Pregnancy Childbirth. 2016;16(1):131.
3. Romano M, Cacciatore A, Giordano R, La Rosa B. Postpartum period: three distinct but continuous phases. J Prenatal Med. 2010;4(2):22–5.
4. SMA. Sports Medicine Australia Position Statement. Exercise in pregnancy and the postpartum period. 2017. http://sma.org.au/sma-site-content/uploads/2017/08/SMA-Position-Statement-Exercise-Pregnancy.pdf. Accessed 20 Aug 2021.

5. Leon-Larios F, Corrales-Gutierrez I, Casado-Mejía R, Suarez-Serrano C. Influence of a pelvic floor training programme to prevent perineal trauma: a quasi-randomised controlled trial. Midwifery. 2017;50:72–7.
6. Mottola MF. Exercise in the postpartum period: practical applications. Curr Sports Med Rep. 2002;1(6):362–8.
7. Bø K, Stuge B, Hilde G. Specific musculoskeletal adaptations in pregnancy: pelvic floor, pelvic girdle and low back pain. Implications for physical activity and exercise. In: Santos-Rocha R, editor. Exercise and physical activity during pregnancy and postpartum. Evidence-based guidelines. 2nd ed. Cham: Springer International; 2022, Ch. 6.
8. Szumilewicz A, Santos-Rocha R. Exercise selection and adaptations during pregnancy. In: Santos-Rocha R, editor. Exercise and physical activity during pregnancy and postpartum. Evidence-based guidelines. 2nd ed. Cham: Springer International; 2022, Ch. 9.
9. Bø K, Berghmans B, Mørkved S, van Kampen M. Evidence-based physical therapy for the pelvic floor. In: Bridging science and clinical practice. Amsterdam: Elsevier; 2007, 435 p.
10. Evenson KR, Mottola MF, Owe KM, Rousham EK, Brown WJ, P. Summary of International for physical activity following pregnancy. Obstet Gynecol Surv. 2014;69(7):407–14.
11. Zourladani A, Zafrakas M, Chatzigiannis B, Papasozomenou P, Vavilis D, Matziari C. The effect of physical exercise on postpartum fitness, hormone and lipid levels: a randomized controlled trial in primiparous, lactating women. Arch Gynecol Obstet. 2015;291(3):525–30.
12. Carter T, Bastounis A, Guo B, Jane MC. The effectiveness of exercise-based interventions for preventing or treating postpartum depression: a systematic review and meta-analysis. Arch Womens Ment Health. 2019;22(1):37–53.
13. Davenport MH, McCurdy AP, Mottola MF, Skow RJ, Meah VL, Poitras VJ, Jaramillo Garcia A, Gray CE, Barrowman N, Riske L, Sobierajski F, James M, Nagpal T, Marchand AA, Nuspl M, Slater LG, Barakat R, Adamo KB, Davies GA, Ruchat SM. Impact of prenatal exercise on both prenatal and postnatal anxiety and depressive symptoms: a systematic review and meta-analysis. Br J Sports Med. 2018;52(21):1376–85.
14. Kołomańska-Bogucka D, Mazur-Bialy AI. Physical activity and the occurrence of postnatal depression-a systematic review. Medicina (Kaunas). 2019;55(9):560.
15. Pritchett RV, Daley AJ, Jolly K. Does aerobic exercise reduce postpartum depressive symptoms? A systematic review and meta-analysis. Br J Gen Pract. 2017;67(663):e684–91.
16. Nakamura A, van der Waerden J, Melchior M, Bolze C, El-Khoury F, Pryor L. Physical activity during pregnancy and postpartum depression: systematic review and meta-analysis. J Affect Disord. 2019;246:29–41.
17. Saligheh M, Hackett D, Boyce P, Cobley S. Can exercise or physical activity help improve postnatal depression and weight loss? A systematic review. Arch Womens Ment Health. 2017;20(5):595–611.
18. Nascimento SL, Pudwell J, Surita FG, Adamo KB, Smith GN. The effect of physical exercise strategies on weight loss in postpartum women: a systematic review and meta-analysis. Int J Obes (Lond). 2014;38(5):626–35.
19. Liu N, Wang J, Chen DD, Sun WJ, Li P, Zhang W. Effects of exercise on pregnancy and postpartum fatigue: a systematic review and meta-analysis. Eur J Obstet Gynecol Reprod Biol. 2020;253:285–95.
20. Woodley SJ, Lawrenson P, Boyle R, Cody JD, Mørkved S, Kernohan A, Hay-Smith EJC. Pelvic floor muscle training for preventing and treating urinary and faecal incontinence in antenatal and postnatal women. Cochrane Database Syst Rev. 2020;5(5):CD007471.
21. Wu YM, McInnes N, Leong Y. Pelvic floor muscle training versus watchful waiting and pelvic floor disorders in postpartum women: a systematic review and meta-analysis. Female Pelvic Med Reconstr Surg. 2018;24(2):142–9.
22. Szumilewicz A, Kuchta A, Kranich M, Dornowski M, Jastrzębski Z. Prenatal high-low impact exercise program supported by pelvic floor muscle education and training decreases the life impact of postnatal urinary incontinence: a quasiexperimental trial. Medicine. 2020;99(6):e18874.

23. Moossdorff-Steinhauser HFA, Albers-Heitner P, Weemhoff M, et al. Factors influencing postpartum women's willingness to participate in a preventive pelvic floor muscle training program: a web-based survey. Eur J Obstet Gynecol Reprod Biol. 2015;195:182–7.
24. Lamina S, Agbanusi E. Effect of aerobic exercise training on maternal weight gain in pregnancy: a meta-analysis of randomized controlled trials. Ethiop J Health Sci. 2013;23(1):59–64.
25. American College of Obstetrics and Gynecology (ACOG). Technical bulletin: exercise during pregnancy and the postnatal period. Washington, DC: ACOG; 1985.
26. Bø K, Artal R, Barakat R, Brown WJ, Davies GAL, Dooley M, Evenson KR, Haakstad LAH, Kayser B, Kinnunen TI, Larsén K, Mottola MF, Nygaard I, van Poppel M, Stuge B, Khan KM, IOC medical commission. Exercise and pregnancy in recreational and elite athletes: 2016/17 evidence summary from the IOC expert group meeting, Lausanne. Part 3-exercise in the postpartum period. Br J Sports Med. 2017;51(21):1516–25.
27. World Health Organization (WHO). WHO guidelines on physical activity and sedentary behaviour. Geneva: World Health Organization; 2020.
28. Murray-Davis B, Grenier L, Atkinson SA, Mottola MF, Wahoush O, Thabane L, Xie F, Vickers-Manzin J, Moore C, Hutton EK. Experiences regarding nutrition and exercise among women during early postpartum: a qualitative grounded theory study. BMC Pregnancy Childbirth. 2019;19(1):368.
29. American College of Obstetricians and Gynecologists (ACOG). Physical activity and exercise during pregnancy and the postpartum period. Committee Opinion No. 650. American College of Obstetricians and Gynecologists. Obstet Gynecol. 2015;126:e135–42.
30. Cary GB, Quinn TJ. Exercise and lactation: are they compatible? Can J Appl Physiol. 2001;26(1):55–75. English, French.
31. Bø K, Artal R, Barakat R, Brown WJ, Davies GAL, Dooley M, et al. Exercise and pregnancy in recreational and elite athletes: 2016/2017 evidence summary from the IOC expert group meeting, Lausanne. Part 5. Recommendations for health professionals and active women. Br J Sports Med. 2018;52(17):1080–5.
32. USDHHS—U.S. Department of Health and Human Services. Physical activity guidelines for Americans. 2nd ed. Washington, DC: U.S. Department of Health and Human Services; 2018. https://health.gov/sites/default/files/2019-09/Physical_Activity_Guidelines_2nd_edition.pdf#page=79. Accessed 20 Aug 2021.
33. ACOG—American College of Obstetricians and Gynecologists. Exercise after pregnancy. 2019. https://www.acog.org/womens-health/faqs/exercise-after-pregnancy. Accessed 20 Aug 2021.
34. ACOG—American College of Obstetricians and Gynecologists. ACOG Committee opinion no. 804: physical activity and exercise during pregnancy and the postpartum period. Obstetr Gynecol. 2020;135(4):e178–e88.
35. ACSM—American College of Sport Medicine. ACSM information on Pregnancy Physical Activity. American College of Sports Medicine; 2020. https://www.acsm.org/docs/currentcomments/exerciseduringpregnancy.pdf. Accessed 20 Aug 2021.
36. AGDH—Australian Government. Department of Health. Guidelines for physical activity during pregnancy. Guidelines for physical activity during pregnancy (health.gov.au): Australian Government. Department of Health; 2021.
37. RANZCOG. The First Few Weeks Following Birth, 2021. https://ranzcog.edu.au/womens-health/patient-information-resources/first-few-weeks. Accessed 20 Aug 2021.
38. Campos MDSB, Buglia S, Colombo CSSS, Buchler RDD, Brito ASX, Mizzaci CC, Feitosa RHF, Leite DB, Hossri CAC, Albuquerque LCA, Freitas OGA, Grossman GB, Mastrocola LE. Position statement on exercise during pregnancy and the post-partum period—2021. Arq Bras Cardiol. 2021;117(1):160–80. English, Portuguese.
39. Gaston A, Cramp A. Exercise during pregnancy: a review of patterns and determinants. J Sci Med Sport. 2011;14:299–305.
40. Bauman AE, Sallis JF, Dzewaltowski DA, Owen N. Toward a better understanding of the influences on physical activity: the role of determinants, correlates, causal variables, mediators, moderators, and confounders. Am J Prev Med. 2002;23(2 Suppl):5–14.

41. Bauman AE, Reis RS, Sallis JF, Wells JC, Loos RJ, Martin BW. Correlates of physical activity: why are some people physically active and others not? Lancet. 2012;380(9838):258–71.
42. Gaston A, Vamos CA. Leisure-time physical activity patterns and correlates among pregnant women in Ontario, Canada. Matern Child Health J. 2013;17(3):477–84.
43. Lim S, O'Reilly S, Behrens H, Skinner T, Ellis I, Dunbar JA. Effective strategies for weight loss in post-partum women: a systematic review and meta-analysis. Obes Rev. 2015;16(11):972–87.
44. Santos-Rocha R. Active at home/Active outdoors YouTube Channel. https://www.youtube.com/channel/UCEUWdoBeh5rgfM0kZOn9Xtg/videos.
45. Santos-Rocha R. Active Pregnancy YouTube Channel: https://www.youtube.com/channel/UC0Vyookwc0mcQ5T70imtoNA/playlists.
46. Santos-Rocha R, Corrales-Gutierrez I, Szumilewicz A, Pajaujiene S. Exercise testing and prescription in pregnancy. In: Santos-Rocha R, editor. Exercise and physical activity during pregnancy and postpartum. Evidence-based guidelines. 2nd ed. Cham: Springer International; 2022, Ch. 8.
47. Goom T, Donnelly G, Brockwell E. Returning to running postnatal. Guidelines for medical, health and fitness professionals managing this population. The Association of Chartered Physiotherapists in Sports and Exercise Medicine; 2019.

Strengthening Competencies of Future Healthcare Professionals to Promote Physical Activity During Pregnancy

11

Jennifer Wegrzyk, Mathilde Hyvärinen, Claire De Labrusse, and Franziska Schläppy

Abstract

Pregnancy is an opportune time to adopt healthy behaviors. Healthcare professionals from diverse disciplines play a crucial role in educating pregnant women on an active lifestyle. As a trusted source of information, they can promote physical activity and behavioral change during and beyond pregnancy. Consequently, they can increase well-being, reduce the risk of complications during the perinatal period and lower the rate of noncommunicable diseases in the future. Meaningful learning environments can support students in identifying with their role as future promoters of physical activity, understanding social determinants of health, and providing personalized counseling in physical activity. This chapter focuses on educational strategies (using the examples of women-centered education programs in Switzerland) and digital health to empower future healthcare professionals in the promotion of physical activity during the perinatal period.

Keywords

Physical activity · Pregnancy · Health promotion · Health education

---

J. Wegrzyk (✉) · M. Hyvärinen · C. De Labrusse · F. Schläppy
HESAV—School of Health Sciences, HES-SO—University of Applied Sciences and Arts Western, Lausanne, Switzerland
e-mail: jennifer.masset@hesav.ch; mathilde.hyvaerinen@hesav.ch; clairedelabrusse@hesav.ch; franziska.schlappy@hesav.ch

R. Santos-Rocha (ed.), *Exercise and Physical Activity During Pregnancy and Postpartum*, https://doi.org/10.1007/978-3-031-06137-0_11

11.1 Introduction

Since 2020, the World Health Organization (WHO) guidelines on Physical Activity (PA) and sedentary behavior address for the first-time women during pregnancy and postpartum as a specific target population based on solid evidence on health benefits for mother and child [1]. These guidelines are directed at policymakers with the aim to align local, national, and international strategies and directly concern health practitioners of different disciplines working with women in the perinatal period (e.g., obstetrics, nursing and midwifery, physiotherapy, exercise physiology, adapted physical activity, nutrition). In current practice, barriers to advise PA in perinatal care (and particularly during pregnancy) are mainly a lack of knowledge of existing guidelines and—if knowledge exists—confidence to convey concrete and individually adapted exercise workouts due to mother–child safety concerns [2–4]. Yet, pregnant women are in regular contact with professionals in primary care who are a trusted source of information during a period of life where women are generally more receptive to health behavioral change [5, 6]. This critical teachable period presents an opportunity for health education. Previous studies highlighted promising results of sustained exercise levels among pregnant women after physical activity counseling [7, 8]. Moreover, health practitioners (mainly studied in the field of midwifery) largely identify with their professional responsibility of promoting PA in the perinatal period [9, 10].

As future multipliers in the field of health education, undergraduate students in the healthcare sector are key players to advocate behavioral change in tomorrow's society [11]. Traditionally, pregnant women have been advised to reduce their PA level as harmful effects were assumed [3, 12]. Thus, proactive dissemination and implementation of current guidelines are important as pregnant women may still receive conflicting information. Innovative programs co-designed and realized by all parties (i.e., pregnant women; interprofessional experts, and students in maternity care as well as PA) allow for locally relevant and contextually appropriate interventions to address PA promotion during the perinatal period and beyond.

The Covid-19 pandemic profoundly changed healthcare and health education and reinforced social isolation, depression, anxiety, and physical inactivity in pregnant women [13]. More than ever, healthcare professionals need to be encouraged to adopt more positive and holistic health-oriented approaches (according to the salutogenic understanding [14]) in the perinatal period to strengthen physical, mental, and social well-being while focusing on individuals' capacities and abilities [15].

The purpose of this chapter is to highlight some educational strategies including interprofessional collaboration and community participation allowing students to identify with their role as PA promoters and to experience meaningful learning in a real-life setting. Moreover, the emergence of digital tools presents an opportunity for health education. Students should understand the opportunities and limitations of digital health in future practice and be prepared for learning as a lifelong process.

11.2 Going Beyond Knowledge Acquisition

Knowledge acquisition (concerning pregnancy-related body adaptations, recommendations of PA, and related health benefits) is not sufficient to render students capable of becoming future healthcare "practitioners." Previous studies suggest that health professionals lack important interpersonal skills to guide pregnant women with regard to lifestyle management [16]. Interactive formats of training as a complement to traditional front-of-class teaching can enable students to understand and experience attitudes and reasons why some pregnant women face difficulties in engaging in regular PA, i.e., leisure activities and/or structured exercise programs. As pointed out by a recent systematic review [17], barriers to PA during pregnancy have been mostly studied on an intrapersonal level and comprise lack of time, motivation, confidence, knowledge, and support; fatigue and pregnancy-related discomfort [18]. Longitudinal studies have shown not only interindividual but also intraindividual variability in behavioral constructs depending on the gestational age in a cohort of pregnant women [19–21]. Thus, students cannot apply a one-size-fits-all solution. They should adapt education strategies according to diverse expectations, preferences, and needs depending on pregnant women's personal characteristics and specific stages during the perinatal period.

11.3 Trends and Examples of Existing Programs in Healthcare Education to Promote Physical Activity in Perinatal Care

As a framework to guide educational programs, Kolb's "experiential learning theory" describes learning as a process by which a learner creates knowledge and meaning from direct experience [22]. Experiential learning in undergraduate and graduate curricula of healthcare studies can be provided by an environment that is activity-based and close to real-life experience of the future professional setting to help students identifying with their role as future health promoters. Such an environment encourages students to reflect on their counselling skills to promote PA, to apply critical thinking and experimenting strategies to solve problems in direct exchange with peers and pregnant women. Finally, hands-on experience provides an opportunity to gain transversal knowledge about the concerns and needs of women. This section presents examples of education programs promoting PA in direct exchange with women during pregnancy and postpartum.

11.3.1 Interprofessional and Community-Based Education: Bringing Future Healthcare Professionals and Pregnant Women Together

Many healthcare services provided during pregnancy have the potential to be team-based and training opportunities in interprofessional settings are encouraged by the

WHO [23]. Pregnant women themselves request that future healthcare professionals should work together in group sessions to provide consistent messages and centralized information [24]. Health practitioners should know when, how, and toward whom to refer women in need of complementary support [10, 25, 26]. In particular, (future) midwives are ideally placed for collaborative practice because they occupy a central role in providing regular, health-oriented advice in perinatal care [2]. Several studies addressing lifestyle interventions, such as diet and physical activity in view of weight management during pregnancy and postpartum, highlight the need and efficiency of interprofessional education for both women and professionals [10, 27–29].

Broadening health education from the classroom to the community can make the learning experience more meaningful for students and reinforce motivation and commitment [30, 31]. The direct contact between the woman and the health professional (in this case the student midwife), has the potential to enhance the health education of both parties [32]. Walker et al. (2019) point to the concept of co-design as an interprofessional opportunity between healthcare professionals and pregnant women to develop and conduct woman-centered instead of practitioner-driven programs for healthy maternal lifestyles. Providing woman-centered care is the cornerstone of midwifery education as midwives deliver maternity care tailored to the needs and wishes of every woman and her family [33, 34]. These mutually beneficial engagements aim at improving quality care and adherence to the designed intervention.

Moreover, regular participation in interprofessional, community-based education allows students to gain insight into social determinants of health and to acquire cultural competencies [35]. Students need to be confronted with issues of diversity and inclusion strategies to understand and address health inequities [36] to appropriately encourage at-risk groups of women to engage in PA (e.g., without stigma and use of negative language [37]). Particularly, women with low socioeconomic status demand for professionally guided group training sessions promoting individually tailored and safe PA contextual to diverging expectations, needs, and environmental conditions [38].

To conclude, the implementation of interprofessional and community-based education in health professionals' curricula is both legitimate and needed as the setting reflects the reality of future working conditions. Finally, the exposure to a variety of interprofessional and community-based education programs allow undergraduate students at an early level to identify their interest and skills.

11.3.1.1 "Move Your Baby" as an Example for Interprofessional and Community-Based Education

Since 2018, the School of Health Sciences Lausanne (HESAV), Switzerland, integrated PA promotion into the midwifery BSc program. During the two-year study course, students participate in 8 obligatory hours of theory courses and workshops (basic) and 10 optional hours of theoretical and practical courses (advanced). Practical courses take place within the community-based program *Move Your Baby* (MYB, [39]) designed to create an interactive, "win–win" learning environment for midwifery students and pregnant women. Weekly, free-of-charge sessions are supervised by interprofessional specialists in midwifery and adapted physical activity and correspond to current recommendations (strengthening, balance, endurance, and flexibility exercises). The program is based on the active learning strategies including inquiry or problem-based, group-based learning [40], and interprofessional education guidelines [41]. Students are encouraged to reflect on their understanding, consolidate and apply their theoretical knowledge (e.g., evaluating perceived effort and physiological body responses and detecting potential warning signs), and identify with their future professional role in the field of health promotion.

The preliminary results of the program suggest that free-of-charge sessions favor diversity and inclusion of pregnant women with different socioeconomic backgrounds and that students are incited to individually adapt communication strategies. In terms of fixed objectives (i.e., providing evidence-based counsel, conceiving personalized programs, developing animation skills, understanding the future professional setting, and arguing the professional role of PA promotion), students perceived the pedagogical effectiveness of the program as high whereas pregnant women were very satisfied with the program and stated improved well-being after regular attendance [42].

11.4 Training in Behavioral Change Theory and Interventions for Pregnant Women

Lifestyle advice is often insufficient to elicit sustained change in the health behavior of pregnant women beyond pregnancy and postpartum. Challenges of practicing PA are numerous for pregnant women and include lack of knowledge about PA recommendations, unawareness of how to engage in PA, social norms, and unavailability of PA classes [5, 43, 44]. Students' understanding of principles to overcome barriers to exercise during pregnancy (e.g., through self-efficacy as a predictor for behavioral change and self-care management) may improve future interventions targeting behavioral change during pregnancy [45]. According to Michie et al. 2011, behavior change interventions– based on the Capability-Opportunity-Motivation Behavior (COM-B) framework (cf. Chap. 2)—refer to a coordinated set of activities designed to change specific behavioral patterns [46]. Professionally guided, free-of-charge programs such as MYB allow for active participation and could improve self-efficacy, thus providing a real opportunity for pregnant women to initiate behavioral changes.

As a complement to relevant behavior change theory (as part of knowledge transfer), skill acquisition through behavioral training is an important component to develop students' capability to encourage sustained PA behavior (Fig. 11.1). Next to skill training, interprofessional and community-based education promotes changes in attitudes and beliefs while developing students' professional identity [10] and impacting their motivation. All three components (i.e., Capability, Opportunity, and Motivation) contribute to the targeted students' behavior to encourage pregnant women in becoming agents in the management of their health (Fig. 11.1).

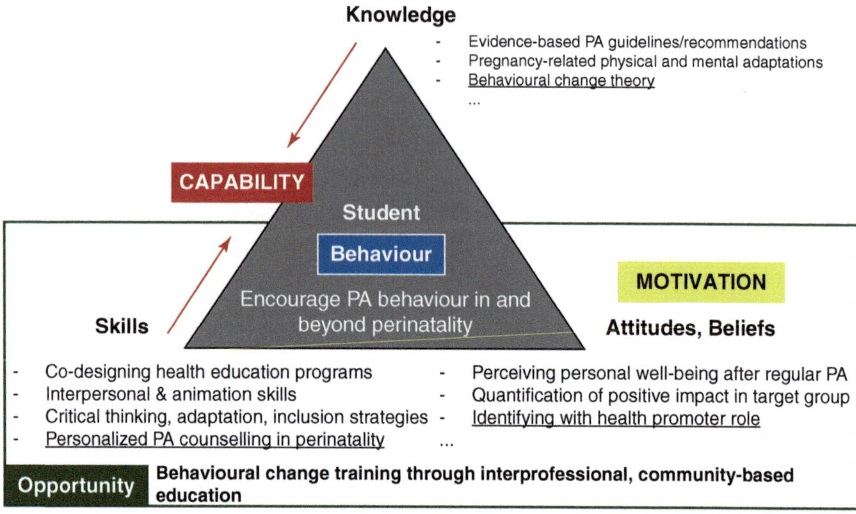

Fig. 11.1 Strengthening students' behavior in encouraging sustainable physical activity (PA) behavior in pregnant women. In color: components of the Capability-Opportunity-Motivation-Behavior (COM-B) framework [46]. An interprofessional, community-based learning environment provides behavioral change training as an opportunity (in green) for students: (1) to apply their knowledge in practice (skills) to develop their capability (in red) in providing personalized PA counseling during pregnancy; (2) to develop attitudes and beliefs to identify with their role as health promoters and to increase motivation (in yellow). All three components of the COM-B framework are interconnected and contribute to the targeted behavior

In terms of motivation, future healthcare professionals should ideally be provided the opportunity to adopt exercise habits themselves to experience health benefits and to become credible role models [47, 48]. Curricula should therefore encourage students to comply with current PA recommendations (for the general adult population) to positively impact attitudes in future practice. Such affective education (i.e., through positive emotional experiences of regular engagement in PA) attributes a personal sense of value to healthy behavior, favors positive reinforcement from peers, and underlines the importance of a healthy lifestyle across pregnancy and postpartum [28]. The commission report by Public Health England and Sport England [49] demonstrates that PA can be successfully integrated into medical school curricula and that students can co-design its implementation to develop self-determined motivation.

For midwifery training in Australia, Kothe et al. (2019) state that students are generally taught the importance of health promotion during pregnancy, risk identification, and lifestyle management. However, they receive insufficient guidance on behavioral change techniques that limit gestational weight gain if needed [27]. Interestingly, those existing curricula focus on pregnancies at high risks thus being disease-centered (pathogenic). In contrast, health promotion programs like MYB focus on lifestyle and health management for the general population thereby presenting a health-centered (salutogenic) approach. Such systematic counseling is of particular importance during pregnancy as reduced PA levels and increased sedentary activities are common throughout pregnancy regardless of prepregnancy PA levels [50] and a contributor to social inequities [1].

11.4.1 Continuation of Health Education Activities into Postpartum

Women need to adjust to their mother's role after giving birth. Coping with postpartum challenges, such as fatigue, sadness or anxiety, and intensive caregiving likely impedes the maintenance of healthy behaviors [51]. During the postpartum period, women are vulnerable to physical inactivity and weight gain, and in need of professional support to maintain or improve their own health behavior [52]. As pointed out by Herval et al. 2019, education programs that start during pregnancy and continue postpartum seem to be more effective in terms of health behavior compared to those programs offered exclusively during pregnancy [53]. This implies that students should be informed about (and ideally participate in) local opportunities, e.g., free-of-charge activities such as "Gym Poussette" [54] existing in Switzerland since 2018. The year-round program focuses on cardiorespiratory and strength capacities and has been successfully extended to ten towns within Western Switzerland. The idea is to promote women's physical fitness while allowing them to spend time with their children (present and often included in the exercises) and to create a social parent network via adapted weekly, exercise sessions. Similar offers exist in the German-speaking part of Switzerland, such as "buggy fit" [55].

11.4.2 Emphasis on Lifelong Learning and Consequences for Students' Evaluation

Students' competencies are usually assessed at given time points during the curriculum to assure and adapt learning progress. Authentic, innovative assessment of attitudes and skills (e.g., critical thinking and adaptability to different contexts) for self-motivated and life-long learning should be included [56]. For instance, the construction of an (electronic) e-portfolio to auto-evaluate learning progress during the studies can serve the transition from undergraduate studies to the future health profession. Portfolios allow students to integrate and consolidate knowledge and experience and have been shown to foster independent learning in graduating midwifery students in the continuum of education [57].

Most importantly, students should be given the opportunity to apply their acquired competencies in future professional settings (e.g., maternity departments and birth centers) to consolidate their experience in view of lifelong learning. Currently, students seem to lack role models during internships because professionals rarely—or not adequately—address health promotion (particularly for PA) during pregnancy [3, 4, 43, 58]. A lack of environmental resources is recurrent barrier cited in the literature [2–4, 58]. A Swedish study highlighted economical cutbacks and organizational changes implying the delegation of additional responsibilities to midwives making it difficult to set aside time for PA counseling [43]. Improved working environments (including career opportunities and professional recognition) would require policy changes on an institutional level towards PA promotion providing sufficient resources for infrastructure and advanced training. These opportunities may include a "mentor"-system for new graduates to assure ongoing professional development in the field of health promotion [10]. Moreover, improved access, availability, and awareness of suitable activities in the local community may support health professionals to promote PA [2]. The WHO Regional Office for Europe cites evidence that healthcare professionals' motivation through positive work environments improves woman-centered care, and health outcomes [59]. Woman-centered care has been for many years the most adequate model of care as it improves maternal and fetal outcomes and maternal satisfaction and reduces healthcare providers' risk of burn-out [60–62].

11.5 Education in Digital Health to Encourage Physical Activity During Pregnancy

Digital Health comprises information and communication technology for the promotion, prevention, and treatment of diseases and has become pivotal in healthcare education for pregnant women, future healthcare professionals and current healthcare practitioners in perinatal care [63]. In terms of PA tracking, digital health is associated with eHealth platforms (internet and mobile apps) and smart devices (including wearable sensor technology) to quantify and encourage PA behavior. These digital interventions can provide more cost-effective promotion of PA than conventional in-person programs as they can reach pregnant women anywhere and anytime. In terms of efficiency, technology-based lifestyle apps can improve motivation and overcome barriers to weight loss and PA during pregnancy and postpartum [64]. However, students need to be sensitized to the limitations of virtual care technologies (e.g., difficult correction via distance, social isolation) which might differently impact pregnant women depending on their socioeconomic status [65].

Pregnancy-related apps are increasingly available—more than in any other medical domain [66]. This popularity could be explained by the fact that childbearing women widely use smartphones and value the use of online resources [67]. User engagement seems to be associated with applications that are interactive (i.e., including feedback systems), supported by educational principles, and visually appealing. Yet, little evidence exists on the quality of eHealth platforms including underlying theoretical bases of behavioral change techniques [67]. Students should therefore become familiar with reliable and validated rating scales to evaluate the quality of existing mobile tools and interventions (e.g., the "mobile application rating scale (MARS)" [68]).

Moreover, a recent systematic review focusing on digital interventions targeting diet, physical activity, and gestational weight gain in pregnancy concluded that—in contrast to interpersonal interventions—poor evidence exists on the effectiveness of the exclusive use of digital delivery to improve health outcomes [69]. Physical encounters between health professionals and the community user will continue even though communication technology and "blended learning approaches" (i.e., a combination of online and face-to-face education) are likely to increase due to their convenience and potential for collaborative and active learning [70]. Immediate messaging applications—providing information and support to pregnant women as a complement to home visits - present a promising communication tool and contribute to the continuity of postpartum women-centered care [71]. However, "whatsapping" practice has not yet been framed as a guideline and should be studied in view of potential unequal access to care.

Moreover, healthcare professionals might increasingly use quality apps to propose and monitor exercises remotely. Guidance of pregnant women at distance implies the understanding of wearable sensor technology in order to continuously and objectively assess PA in everyday life [72]. Undergraduate training in using digital aids would support students in the healthcare sector to successfully integrate these tools into practice [73]. In this context, ethical (such as privacy issues) and social implications (such as built-in biases that might aggravate health disparities) would need to be addressed.

To conclude, digital health education should develop a critical mind and openness to innovation in future health professionals to implement quality tools for the promotion of PA in practice. As a complement to traditional PA counseling, those digital tools might favor a shift towards empowerment of women during pregnancy and alter health-seeking behaviors. Future professionals in maternity care should acquire the expertise to test, identify and recommend effective digital interventions including customizable mobile applications of quality to women that are willing to use e-health tools. Moreover, experts in obstetrics and physical activity should participate in co-designing future technology for telemedicine, mobile medical devices, virtual/augmented reality applications, and privacy and regulatory considerations.

11.6 Future Research

Interprofessional and community-based education have been frequently reported in health education. Interprofessional education is mainly limited to experts in the medical domain/obstetrics (physicians, midwives, nurses specialized in maternal care) and should be enlarged to include experts in other domains (e.g., physical activity, nutrition). Conclusions on the effectiveness of interprofessional and community-based health education intervention yet need to be provided for students and pregnant women. Effectiveness studies are also lacking for online lifestyle interventions for the high number of mobile applications currently available on the market.

Interestingly, most of the existing student-oriented health education interventions in pregnancy concern the promotion of PA only indirectly, for instance, as a component of weight management [10, 28, 52, 74]. Yet, regular PA has the potential to be considered as an independent entity resulting in beneficial physical, mental, and social health outcomes beyond weight gain and obesity prevention. In current literature, to the best of our knowledge, only the pilot design *Move your Baby* (Hyvärinen et al.—unpublished) evaluated the effect of a focused educational intervention on improving undergraduate students' competencies in PA promotion during pregnancy. Randomized controlled and longitudinal study designs including large samples and standardized reporting guidelines are needed to assess the effectiveness of existing programs in terms of (1) students' competencies, (2) behavioral change in pregnant women, and (3) proving causality.

The Covid-19 pandemic highlighted the importance of salutogenic approaches [75] including the domain of obstetrics [76]. All types of health-oriented interventions (individual face-to-face counseling, physical group, and online education) should focus on exploring and promoting PA in culturally diverse populations of pregnant women with different socioeconomic backgrounds, and on comparing opportunities linked to healthcare systems of different countries to discover opportunities for the future [44].

11.7 Conclusion

Students trained in perinatal care and the promotion of PA during pregnancy and postpartum will possess the required competencies to identify and act as future health promoters if curricula contents and practice in community/professional learning environments allow for[1]:

Knowledge Acquisition Concerning pregnancy-related physical and mental adaptations, current guidelines on PA during pregnancy, and behavioral change theory and techniques. Knowledge should also refer to the existence of opportunities for pregnant women concerning digital health and local educational programs offered (examples of Switzerland: *Move your Baby*, *GymPoussette*).

Evidence-Based Practice in Community-Based (Woman-Centered) and Interprofessional Education/Collaboration Experiential learning in real-life settings of future professions promotes competencies, such as the animation of group sessions and personalized counseling skills. With regard to behavioral change theory, students can experience attitudes, facilitators, and barriers of pregnant women as well as social determinants of health. Sufficient hands-on training contributes to a meaningful learning environment in view of the development of self-confidence as an important prerequisite in the promotion of physical activity programs.

[1] Note that listed education strategies are interdependent. For instance, community-based learning and diversity of needs of a heterogenous group of pregnant women favours interprofessional education / collaboration and life-long learning. Adequate use of digital health technologies can promote the entirety of educational aspects.

Acquisition of Attitudes and Skills in View of Self-Motivated, Life-Long Learning Learning is a continuous process grounded in experience to develop critical thinking and adaptability in the field of perinatality (ideally during pregnancy and postpartum). Students can experience and evaluate behavioral change (including own experience of regular PA well-being) through implications in longitudinal intervention designs.

Training in Digital Health for PA Promotion The COVID-19 pandemic accelerated the process of integrating information and communication technologies in the educational system to improve efficiency. Students need to use and understand limitations and opportunities of these technologies for future practice.

Figure 11.2 relies on the components of the COM-B model [46] and illustrates interprofessional and community-based education. Behavioral change training applies to both students and pregnant women and lays the foundation for well-being and meaningful learning.

Finally, institutional policies and practices need to comply with evolving societal needs and the respective healthcare systems and confront students with inclusion strategies to address health improvement and health inequities. Thus, collaborative effort and willingness for experimentation and adaptation of curricular goals are needed to create efficient learning environments.

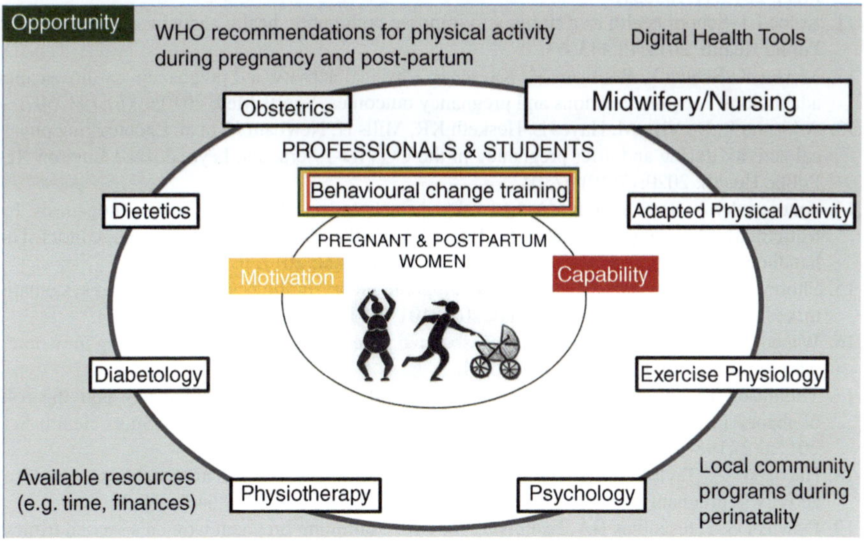

Fig. 11.2 Interprofessional and community-based education in physical activity promotion. Woman-centered approach in perinatal care. Highlighted role of midwives/specialist nurses in maternity care as they are in regular contact with the target group. In color: components of the Capability-Opportunity-Motivation-Behavior (COM-B) framework as mentioned in Chaps. 2 and 4

References

1. Bull FC, Al-Ansari SS, Biddle S, Borodulin K, Buman MP, Cardon G, et al. World Health Organization 2020 guidelines on physical activity and sedentary behaviour. Br J Sports Med. 2020;54(24):1451–62.
2. De Vivo M, Mills H. "They turn to you first for everything": insights into midwives' perspectives of providing physical activity advice and guidance to pregnant women. BMC Pregnancy Childbirth. 2019;19(1):462.
3. Hopkinson Y, Hill DM, Fellows L, Fryer S. Midwives understanding of physical activity guidelines during pregnancy. Midwifery. 2018;59:23–6.
4. Malta MB, Carvalhaes MA, Takito MY, Tonete VL, Barros AJ, Parada CM, et al. Educational intervention regarding diet and physical activity for pregnant women: changes in knowledge and practices among health professionals. BMC Pregnancy Childbirth. 2016;16(1):175.
5. Olander EK, Darwin ZJ, Atkinson L, Smith DM, Gardner B. Beyond the 'teachable moment'—a conceptual analysis of women's perinatal behaviour change. Women Birth. 2016;29(3):e67–71.
6. Phelan S. Pregnancy: a "teachable moment" for weight control and obesity prevention. Am J Obstet Gynecol. 2010;202(2):135 e1–8.
7. Aittasalo M, Pasanen M, Fogelholm M, Kinnunen TI, Ojala K, Luoto R. Physical activity counseling in maternity and child health care—a controlled trial. BMC Womens Health. 2008;8:14.
8. May LE, Suminski RR, Linklater ER, Jahnke S, Glaros AG. Exercise during pregnancy: the role of obstetric providers. J Am Osteopath Assoc. 2013;113(8):612–9.
9. McParlin C, Bell R, Robson SC, Muirhead CR, Araujo-Soares V. What helps or hinders midwives to implement physical activity guidelines for obese pregnant women? A questionnaire survey using the theoretical domains framework. Midwifery. 2017;49:110–6.
10. Walker R, Olander EK, Hill B, Willey S, Skouteris H. Weight management across pregnancy and postpartum care: the need for interprofessional education and collaboration. Nurse Educ Pract. 2019;41:102651.
11. Kolbe LJ. School health as a strategy to improve both public health and education. Annu Rev Public Health. 2019;40:443–63.
12. Melzer K, Schutz Y, Boulvain M, Kayser B. Physical activity and pregnancy: cardiovascular adaptations, recommendations and pregnancy outcomes. Sports Med. 2010;40(6):493–507.
13. Atkinson L, De Vivo M, Hayes L, Hesketh KR, Mills H, Newham JJ, et al. Encouraging physical activity during and after pregnancy in the COVID-19 era, and beyond. Int J Environ Res Public Health. 2020;17(19):e7304.
14. Antonovsky A, Sagy S. Aaron Antonovsky, the scholar and the man behind salutogenesis. In: Mittelmark MB, Sagy S, Eriksson M, Bauer GF, Pelikan JM, Lindstrom B, et al., editors. The handbook of salutogenesis. Cham: Springer International; 2017. p. 15–23.
15. Shorey S, Ng ED. Application of the salutogenic theory in the perinatal period: a systematic mixed studies review. Int J Nurs Stud. 2020;101:103398.
16. Wahedi M. Should midwifes consider associated psychological factors when caring for women who are obese? Br J Midwifery. 2016;24.
17. Thompson EL, Vamos CA, Daley EM. Physical activity during pregnancy and the role of theory in promoting positive behavior change: a systematic review. J Sport Health Sci. 2017;6(2):198–206.
18. Harrison AL, Taylor NF, Shields N, Frawley HC. Attitudes, barriers and enablers to physical activity in pregnant women: a systematic review. J Physiother. 2018;64(1):24–32.
19. Downs DS, Hausenblas HA. Exercising for two: examining pregnant women's second trimester exercise intention and behavior using the framework of the theory of planned behavior. Womens Health Issues. 2003;13(6):222–8.
20. Downs DSH, H.A. Pregnant women's third trimester exercise behaviors, body mass index, and pregnancy outcomes. Psychol Health. 2007;22:545–59.

21. Hausenblas HD, D.S. Prospective examination of the theory of planned behavior applied to exercise behavior during women's first trimester of pregnancy. J Reprod Infant Psychol. 2004;22:199–210.
22. Kolb DA. Experiental learning: experience as a source of leaning and development. Englewood Cliffs, NJ: FT Press; 1984.
23. Organization WH. Framework for action on interprofessional education and collaborative practice. 2010. https://apps.who.int/iris/handle/10665/70185.
24. Aquino M, Olander EK, Bryar RM. A focus group study of women's views and experiences of maternity care as delivered collaboratively by midwives and health visitors in England. BMC Pregnancy Childbirth. 2018;18(1):505.
25. Findley A, Smith DM, Hesketh K, Keyworth C. Exploring womens' experiences and decision making about physical activity during pregnancy and following birth: a qualitative study. BMC Pregnancy Childbirth. 2020;20(1):54.
26. Guthrie TM, de Jersey SJ, New K, Gallegos D. Midwife readiness to provide woman-centred weight gain support: exploring perspectives across models of care. Women Birth. 2020;33(6):e567–e73.
27. Kothe E, Bailey C, Weiner C, Nagle C, Nowson C, Hill B, et al. An investigation of Australian midwifery curricula for obesity management and health behaviour change training. Nurse Educ Pract. 2019;36:54–7.
28. Kothe E, Lamb M, Bruce L, McPhie S, Klas A, Hill B, et al. Student midwives' intention to deliver weight management interventions: a theory of planned behaviour & self-determination theory approach. Nurse Educ Today. 2018;71:10–6.
29. Walker R, Bennett C, Blumfield M, Gwini S, Ma J, Wang F, et al. Attenuating pregnancy weight gain-what works and why: a systematic review and meta-analysis. Nutrients. 2018;10(7):944.
30. Marcus MT, Taylor WC, Hormann MD, Walker T, Carroll D. Linking service-learning with community-based participatory research: an interprofessional course for health professional students. Nurs Outlook. 2011;59(1):47–54.
31. Ramaley J. The changing role of higher education: learning to deal with wicked problems. J High Educ Outreach Engage. 2014;18(3):7–21.
32. Walker R, Morris H, Lang S, Hampton K, Boyle J, Skouteris H. Co-designing preconception and pregnancy care for healthy maternal lifestyles and obesity prevention. Women Birth. 2020;33(5):473–8.
33. de Labrusse C, Ramelet AS, Humphrey T, Maclennan SJ. Patient-centered care in maternity services: a critical appraisal and synthesis of the literature. Womens Health Issues. 2016;26(1):100–9.
34. Leap N. Woman-centred or women-centred care: does it matter? Br J Midwifery. 2013;17(1):12–6.
35. Stubbs C, Schorn MN, Leavell JP, Espiritu EW, Davis G, Gentry CK, et al. Implementing and evaluating a community-based, inter-institutional, interprofessional education pilot programme. J Interprof Care. 2017;31(5):652–5.
36. Mullan F. Social mission in health professions education: beyond Flexner. JAMA. 2017;318(2):122–3.
37. Olander EK, Scamell M. Teaching students about maternal obesity without creating obesity stigma. Nurse Educ Today. 2016;42:59–61.
38. Muzigaba M, Kolbe-Alexander TL, Wong F. The perceived role and influencers of physical activity among pregnant women from low socioeconomic status communities in South Africa. J Phys Act Health. 2014;11(7):1276–83.
39. Move Your Baby. https://moveyourbaby.ch. Accessed Jul 2021.
40. Davidson NM, Major CH. Boundary crossings: cooperative learning, collaborative learning, and problem-based learning. J Excell Coll Teach. 2014;25:7–55.
41. Barr HF, Ford J, Gray R, Helme M, Hutchings M, Low H, Machin A, Reeves S. Interprofessional Education Guidelines Centre for the Advancement of Interprofessional Education. 2017. https://www.caipe.org/resources/publications/caipe-publications/caipe-2017-interprofessional-

education-guidelines-barr-h-ford-j-gray-r-helme-m-hutchings-m-low-h-machin-reeves-s. Accessed Jul 2021.
42. Mathilde Hyvärinen, Franziska Schläppy, Claire de Labrusse, Jennifer Wegrzyk. Pedagogical innovation to promote physical activity in pregnancy: Interprofessional and real-life settings on the example of the educational program Move Your Baby. Eur J Midwifery. 2022;6:32.
43. Lindqvist M, Mogren I, Eurenius E, Edvardsson K, Persson M. "An on-going individual adjustment": a qualitative study of midwives' experiences counselling pregnant women on physical activity in Sweden. BMC Pregnancy Childbirth. 2014;14:343.
44. Zinsser LA, Stoll K, Wieber F, Pehlke-Milde J, Gross MM. Changing behaviour in pregnant women: a scoping review. Midwifery. 2020;85:102680.
45. Cramp AG, Bray SR. A prospective examination of exercise and barrier self-efficacy to engage in leisure-time physical activity during pregnancy. Ann Behav Med. 2009;37(3):325–34.
46. Michie S, Abraham C, Eccles MP, Francis JJ, Hardeman W, Johnston M. Strengthening evaluation and implementation by specifying components of behaviour change interventions: a study protocol. Implement Sci. 2011;6:10.
47. Abramson S, Stein J, Schaufele M, Frates E, Rogan S. Personal exercise habits and counseling practices of primary care physicians: a national survey. Clin J Sport Med. 2000;10(1):40–8.
48. Oberg EB, Frank E. Physicians' health practices strongly influence patient health practices. J R Coll Physicians Edinb. 2009;39(4):290–1.
49. Gates ABR, Ritchie IK. "Embedding physical activity in the undergraduate curriculum"—moving healthcare professionals programme. England: PHEaS; 2018.
50. Fazzi C, Saunders DH, Linton K, Norman JE, Reynolds RM. Sedentary behaviours during pregnancy: a systematic review. Int J Behav Nutr Phys Act. 2017;14(1):32.
51. Behringer J, Reiner I, Spangler G. Maternal representations of past and current attachment relationships, and emotional experience across the transition to motherhood: a longitudinal study. J Fam Psychol. 2011;25(2):210–9.
52. van der Pligt P, Willcox J, Hesketh KD, Ball K, Wilkinson S, Crawford D, et al. Systematic review of lifestyle interventions to limit postpartum weight retention: implications for future opportunities to prevent maternal overweight and obesity following childbirth. Obes Rev. 2013;14(10):792–805.
53. Herval AM, Oliveira DPD, Gomes VE, Vargas AMD. Health education strategies targeting maternal and child health: a scoping review of educational methodologies. Medicine (Baltimore). 2019;98(26):e16174.
54. GymPoussette. https://gympoussettes.ch. Accessed Jul 2021.
55. Buggyfit. https://buggyfit.ch/en/location/zurich/. Accessed Jul 2021.
56. Thibault GE. The importance of an environment conducive to education. J Grad Med Educ. 2016;8(2):134–5.
57. Sidebotham M, Baird K, Walters C, Gamble J. Preparing student midwives for professional practice: evaluation of a student e-portfolio assessment item. Nurse Educ Pract. 2018;32:84–9.
58. Bauer PW, Broman CL, Pivarnik JM. Exercise and pregnancy knowledge among healthcare providers. J Womens Health (Larchmt). 2010;19(2):335–41.
59. UNFPA W, ICM. The state of the world's midwifery 2021. 2021. https://www.unfpa.org/publications/sowmy-2021#:~:text=The%20State%20of%20the%20World%27s%20Midwifery%20(SoWMy)%202021%20builds%20on,a%20particular%20focus%20on%20midwives. Accessed Jul 2021.
60. Donnellan-Fernandez RE, Creedy DK, Callander EJ. Cost-effectiveness of continuity of midwifery care for women with complex pregnancy: a structured review of the literature. Health Econ Rev. 2018;8(1):32.
61. Floris L, Irion O, Bonnet J, Politis Mercier MP, de Labrusse C. Comprehensive maternity support and shared care in Switzerland: comparison of levels of satisfaction. Women Birth. 2018;31(2):124–33.
62. Sandall J, Soltani H, Gates S, Shennan A, Devane D. Midwife-led continuity models versus other models of care for childbearing women. Cochrane Database Syst Rev. 2016;4:CD004667.

63. van den Heuvel JF, Groenhof TK, Veerbeek JH, van Solinge WW, Lely AT, Franx A, et al. eHealth as the next-generation perinatal care: an overview of the literature. J Med Internet Res. 2018;20(6):e202.
64. Sandborg J, Soderstrom E, Henriksson P, Bendtsen M, Henstrom M, Leppanen MH, et al. Effectiveness of a smartphone app to promote healthy weight gain, diet, and physical activity during pregnancy (HealthyMoms): randomized controlled trial. JMIR Mhealth Uhealth. 2021;9(3):e26091.
65. Shaw J, Brewer LC, Veinot T. Recommendations for health equity and virtual care arising from the COVID-19 pandemic: narrative review. JMIR Form Res. 2021;5(4):e23233.
66. Tripp N, Hainey K, Liu A, Poulton A, Peek M, Kim J, et al. An emerging model of maternity care: smartphone, midwife, doctor? Women Birth. 2014;27(1):64–7.
67. Hayman M, Alfrey KL, Cannon S, Alley S, Rebar AL, Williams S, et al. Quality, features, and presence of behavior change techniques in mobile apps designed to improve physical activity in pregnant women: systematic search and content analysis. JMIR Mhealth Uhealth. 2021;9(4):e23649.
68. Stoyanov SR, Hides L, Kavanagh DJ, Wilson H. Development and validation of the user version of the mobile application rating scale (uMARS). JMIR Mhealth Uhealth. 2016;4(2):e72.
69. Rhodes A, Smith AD, Chadwick P, Croker H, Llewellyn CH. Exclusively digital health interventions targeting diet, physical activity, and weight gain in pregnant women: systematic review and meta-analysis. JMIR Mhealth Uhealth. 2020;8(7):e18255.
70. de Jong N, Savin-Baden M, Cunningham AM, Verstegen DM. Blended learning in health education: three case studies. Perspect Med Educ. 2014;3(4):278–88.
71. Perrenoud P, Chautems C, Kaech C. "Whatsapping" the continuity of postpartum care in Switzerland: a socio-anthropological study. Women Birth. 2021;35:e263–74.
72. Runkle J, Sugg M, Boase D, Galvin SL, C CC. Use of wearable sensors for pregnancy health and environmental monitoring: descriptive findings from the perspective of patients and providers. Digit Health. 2019;5:2055207619828220.
73. Poncette AS, Glauert DL, Mosch L, Braune K, Balzer F, Back DA. Undergraduate medical competencies in digital health and curricular module development: mixed methods study. J Med Internet Res. 2020;22(10):e22161.
74. Sandborg J, Henriksson P, Larsen E, Lindqvist AK, Rutberg S, Soderstrom E, et al. Participants' engagement and satisfaction with a smartphone app intended to support healthy weight gain, diet, and physical activity during pregnancy: qualitative study within the HealthyMoms trial. JMIR Mhealth Uhealth. 2021;9(3):e26159.
75. Mana A, Super S, Sardu C, Juvinya Canal D, Moran N, Sagy S. Individual, social and national coping resources and their relationships with mental health and anxiety: a comparative study in Israel, Italy, Spain, and the Netherlands during the coronavirus pandemic. Glob Health Promot. 2021;28(2):17–26.
76. Heinonen K. Strengthening antenatal care towards a salutogenic approach: a meta-ethnography. Int J Environ Res Public Health. 2021;18(10):5168.

Therapeutic Exercise Regarding Musculoskeletal Health of the Pregnant Exerciser and Athlete

12

Augusto Gil Pascoal, Britt Stuge, Patrícia Mota, Gunvor Hilde, and Kari Bø

Abstract

Physical activity during pregnancy is recommended and has been shown to benefit most women. However, some modifications to exercise routines may be necessary due to normal anatomic and physiologic changes and fetal requirements. Therefore, knowledge about the systemic changes of pregnancy should be con-

A. G. Pascoal (✉)
Laboratory of Biomechanics and Functional Morphology, Faculty of Human Kinetics, Interdisciplinary Centre for the Study of Human Performance, University of Lisbon, Cruz Quebrada-Dafundo, Portugal
e-mail: gpascoal@fmh.ulisboa.pt

B. Stuge
Division of Orthopaedic Surgery, Oslo University Hospital, Oslo, Norway
e-mail: britt.stuge@medisin.uio.no

P. Mota
Laboratory of Biomechanics and Functional Morphology, Faculty of Human Kinetics, Interdisciplinary Centre for the Study of Human Performance, University of Lisbon, Cruz Quebrada-Dafundo, Portugal

H&TRC-Health and Technology Research Center, ESTeSL-Lisbon School of Health Technology, Polytechnic Institute of Lisbon, Lisbon, Portugal
e-mail: patricia.mota@estesl.ipl.pt

G. Hilde
Department of Physiotherapy, OsloMet-Oslo Metropolitan University (former: Oslo and Akershus University College of Applied Sciences), Oslo, Norway
e-mail: gunvor.hilde@hioa.no; ghilde@oslomet.no

K. Bø
Department of Sports Medicine, Norwegian School of Sport Sciences, Oslo, Norway

Department of Obstetrics and Gynecology, Akershus University Hospital, Lørenskog, Norway
e-mail: kari.bo@nih.no

R. Santos-Rocha (ed.), *Exercise and Physical Activity During Pregnancy and Postpartum*, https://doi.org/10.1007/978-3-031-06137-0_12

sidered when counseling women who wish to exercise through their pregnancy and should be complemented by the knowledge about the potential effect of exercise (therapeutic exercise) for the prevention and resolution of some common pregnancy-related musculoskeletal conditions. Therapeutic exercise is the systematic and planned performance of exercises that aims to improve and restore physical function.

This chapter presents the scientific evidence foundation on the effect of therapeutic exercises on the prevention and resolution of three commonly pregnancy-related musculoskeletal conditions: pelvic floor dysfunction, diastasis recti abdominis, and low back and pelvic girdle pain. The chapter emphasizes the potential effect of exercise on the prevention and resolution of these musculoskeletal conditions and provides useful information when tailoring therapeutic exercise programs for pregnant women.

Keywords

Pregnancy · Diastasis recti abdominis · Low back pain · Pelvic girdle pain · Pelvic floor muscles · Urinary incontinence

12.1 Introduction

Physical activity during pregnancy is recommended and has been shown to benefit most women. However, some modifications to exercise routines may be necessary due to normal anatomic and physiologic changes and fetal requirements [1]. Pregnant women, therefore, represent a particular gender-based clinical challenge for the therapist and exercise promotor. During pregnancy, the female body undergoes many morphological and physiological changes that affect the musculoskeletal system. The most obvious change in pregnancy is related to the growth of the fetus and the stretching of the abdominal muscles, which may influence the mother's posture and balance. These factors in combination with hormones and weight gain may contribute to a variety of musculoskeletal impairments, trigger the development of musculoskeletal dysfunction, or alter the course of preexisting conditions. The most common pregnancy-related musculoskeletal impairments are pelvic floor dysfunctions, diastasis recti abdominis, and low back and pelvic girdle pain.

Therapeutic exercise is the systematic and planned performance of exercises that aims to improve and restore physical function. Additional goals of therapeutic exercises include pain relief, increased strength, and increased range of motion.

This chapter presents the scientific evidence foundation on the effect of therapeutic exercises on the prevention and resolution of three common pregnancy-related musculoskeletal conditions: pelvic floor dysfunction, diastasis recti abdominis, and low back and pelvic girdle pain. A generic description of each condition is followed by information that could be useful for the development of therapeutic exercise programs for pregnant women.

12.2 Pelvic Floor Muscle Training

In general, it is possible to affirm that all women can benefit from education regarding the role of Pelvic Floor Muscles (PFM) during pregnancy on pelvic floor dysfunctions. The specific treatment of the pelvic floor muscles is critical for the quality of life of women suffering from urinary and anal incontinence, pelvic organ prolapse, and a variety of pelvic pain syndromes. Therapeutic exercises focusing on education and pelvic floor muscle training should be incorporated as a key component for pregnant exercisers and pregnant athlete women.

Several hypotheses have suggested that a trained PFM might reduce the risk of UI during pregnancy and after childbirth [2]. For example, a trained PFM may counteract the hormonally mediated increased laxity of the pelvic floor and the increased intra-abdominal pressure during pregnancy. In addition, it may encompass a greater functional reserve so that childbirth does not cause loss of muscle function to develop urinary leakage. Further, a trained PFM may recover better after childbirth as the appropriate neuromuscular motor patterns have already been learned [2].

PFM Training (PFMT) and the importance of PFMT in restoring function after childbirth were introduced as early as 1948 by Kegel [3]. In an uncontrolled clinical trial from 1952, he reported that 84% of his patients with UI were cured after performing PFMT [4]. According to Bø [5], there are two main rationales for why PFMT works:

- Women learn how to consciously precontract the PFM before and during situations causing increased abdominal pressure (e.g., coughing);
- Increased PFM strength and enhanced hypertrophy take place, building up long-lasting muscle volume to provide structural support, closing the levator hiatus, and lifting the anatomical position of the pelvic floor.

12.2.1 Pre-Contraction

During situations with increased abdominal pressure, the supportive action of the PFM is believed to be important [6–9]. Miller et al. [10] found that older women with SUI could acquire the skill of a well-timed PFM contraction just ahead of and during a cough ("The Knack"), and by this maneuver significantly reduce leakage. The positive effect of the Knack maneuver in reducing leakage during coughing has later been confirmed both among nonpregnant and pregnant women [11]. The rationale to acquire such a skill is to prevent the urethra and bladder base from descending during increased abdominal pressure and thereby prevent leakage. An actual stabilization of the bladder neck by performing pre-contraction just ahead of and during a cough has subsequently been shown in observational studies, using perineal ultrasound, both among both nulliparous continent women [12, 13], and older incontinent parous women [12].

12.2.2 Strength Training

Strength training of the PFM increases PFM strength, provides increased urethral closure pressure, and prevents urethral descent [5, 14]. The PFM, like other skeletal muscles, responds to strength training by improved neuromuscular function, increased cross-sectional area, increased number of activated motor neurons, increased frequency of excitation, and improved muscle "tone" [5, 14, 15]. Specificity and overload are two fundamental principles that carefully must be addressed for effective strength training [14, 16].

To improve a specific skill, that specific skill must be performed. To become a good skier, you need to ski. To effectively improve PFM strength, specific PFM contraction performed in a correct manner needs to be carried out [14]. This means an inward lift and squeezing around the urethra, vagina, and rectum [4, 17, 18]. Avoiding co-contraction of other muscles should be emphasized, as this may mask the actual strength of the PFM contraction being performed [14]. The principle of specificity also draws attention to the fact that a correct PFM contraction may be difficult to perform for some women. Studies on women with UI have shown that >30% were unable to perform a correct PFM contraction [4, 19–21], even after a thorough verbal instruction on how to contract. Assessment of the ability to contract the PFM can easily be performed by visual observation and vaginal palpation [22, 23]. Proper assessment, instruction, and teaching on how to contract correctly are considered crucial to gain benefit from PFMT [24].

To achieve increased cross-sectional area and increased contractile force, the muscles need to be exposed to an overload that is larger than the common load encountered during everyday life [16]. Overload in PFMT can be achieved by performing close to maximal contractions, lengthening the holding periods for each contraction, increasing the number of repetitions and number of sets completed, and reducing the rest intervals [14]. Strength training recommendations for skeletal muscles are 8–12 maximal contractions, 3–4 series, 3–4 times per week [15, 25, 26]. It takes time to achieve increased PFM strength, endurance, and muscle volume [14], and The American College of Sports Medicine recommends the exercise duration period to be at least 15–20 weeks [25]. Strength training with contractions close to maximum and short rest intervals between the contractions usually also increase local muscle endurance [27, 28].

12.2.3 Evidence for Pelvic Floor Muscle Training to Prevent and Treat Urinary Incontinence during Pregnancy

Based on the current evidence presented in a recent Cochrane review by Dumoulin [29], PFMT is better than no treatment, placebo drug, or inactive control treatments for women with UI (any type). The current evidence supports the widespread recommendation (Grade A) for offering supervised PFMT as the first-line treatment for female stress, urgency, or mixed UI [29, 30].

Boyle et al. [31] performed a Cochrane review during pregnancy and 22 trials involving 8485 women (4231 PFMT, 4254 controls) were included in the analysis.

Pregnant women without prior UI (prevention) who were randomized to intensive antenatal PFMT were about 30% less likely to report UI up to 6 months after delivery when compared to women randomized to no PFMT or usual antenatal care (risk ratio (RR) 0.71, 95% CI 0.54–0.95, the combined result of five trials). The results of seven studies showed a statistically significant result favoring PFMT in a mixed population (women with and without incontinence symptoms) in late pregnancy (RR 0.74, 95% CI 0.58–0.94, random-effects model). The fifth International Consultation on Incontinence [30] recommends that pregnant women having their first child should be offered supervised PFMT (Grade A recommendation). To date, there is not enough evidence to conclude on the long-term effect and there are no randomized controlled trials in pregnant recreational or elite athletes.

12.2.4 Can Pelvic Floor Muscle Training Compromise Vaginal Birth?

There has been some concern that a tight and strong pelvic floor might obstruct labor and result in instrumental delivery, perineal trauma and/or injury of peripheral nerves, connective tissue, and muscles [32]. A recent systematic review including 12 RCTs/quasi-RCTs involving 2243 primigravida women concluded that PFM training significantly shortened 1st (mean 28 min) and second stage (mean 10 min) of labor. In addition, antenatal PFM training did not increase the risk of episiotomy, instrumental vaginal delivery, and perineal laceration [33].

12.3 Diastasis Recti Abdominis

Pregnancy and childbirth bring along several changes to a woman's body, especially to the musculoskeletal system [34]. The most obvious change is related to the growth of the fetus and the stretching of the abdominal muscles, which may influence the mother's posture and balance [34].

Today there is a strong focus on the pregnant woman's appearance, especially through social media. Web pages and apps recommend how women should stay thin and get back into shape and regain "a flat tummy" at an early stage of the postpartum period.

Diastasis Recti Abdominis (DRA) or the increased inter-rectus distance is a common condition in women during pregnancy and postpartum [35]. As the fetus grows, the two muscle bellies of the rectus abdominis, connected by the linea alba, elongate, and curve round as the abdominal wall expands, with most separation occurring at the umbilicus [36–38]. The augmented inter-rectus distance is described as a change in the abdominal musculature, specifically in the linea alba and the rectus abdominis sheath, with onset in the last trimester of pregnancy and whose peak of incidence occurs immediately after birth and the first weeks following childbirth [36, 39, 40].

Using the search terms "diastasis recti" and "exercise," 278,000 hits were obtained on Google. In addition, there is easily available advice on how to get rid of what is named "the mum's belly" (e.g., www.mammamage.se; www.

breakingmuscle.com; www.befitmom.com; www.babybellybelt.com; www.tummyzip.com). A systematic review of the scientific literature has found no or very weak evidence behind any of these pieces of advice [41].

12.3.1 Prevention and Treatment

Exercise and surgery are the two available methods to treat diastasis recti abdominis. Akram and Matzen [42] identified 15 studies on surgery and found only one Randomized Controlled Trial (RCT). The RCT compared the results of using two different sutures. The authors concluded that both groups had an adequate correction of DRA 6 months after surgery. This was supported by a recent RCT [43]. However, there are no RCTs comparing surgery with no treatment or exercise, no long-term effect studies, and sparse reports of complications after surgery.

The huge activity in social media recommending a variation of abdominal exercise programs to prevent and treat DRA is in strong contrast to the lack of evidence for any positive effect shown in RCTs. In a systematic review by Benjamin et al. [41], eight studies in the treatment of DRA using abdominal exercises were found: four case studies, two retrospective observational studies, one quasi-experimental posttest study, and one small RCT of a brief training intervention [44]. A new search on Pubmed of August 2017 found only three additional RCTs [43, 45, 46]. These studies score low on the PEDro rating scale of methodological quality (5, 6, and 6 of 10 possible scores of internal validities, respectively), and both exercise protocols, assessment methods, cut-off points for diastasis and results differ (Table 12.1). None of the studies included exercise during pregnancy, and to date, there is, therefore, no knowledge whether the condition can be prevented or reduced with abdominal training or other exercises programs during pregnancy.

It has been suggested that antepartum activity levels may have a protective effect on DRA and exercise may improve post-partum symptoms of DRA [42]. Physiotherapists and exercise instructors prescribe exercises to this population every day, but given the limited research data, there is currently no consensus on which abdominal exercises to recommend narrowing the diastasis [47–50]. Recent research has questioned the use of the commonly used and recommended in-drawing exercises as these appear to widen, rather than narrow the gap measured with ultrasound [35, 51, 52]. Furthermore, one research group recommended contracting the pelvic floor muscles to activate the transverse abdominal muscles to stabilize the linea alba before performing curl-ups [53]. The results of the latter study conferred those contractions of the pelvic floor muscles increased the gap. There are currently no data from RCTs to support the new theory that activation of the transverse abdominal muscles via a pelvic floor muscle contraction can stabilize the linea alba, the validity of the formula used, and what this may mean for the diastasis. Furthermore, the effect of different abdominal exercises to treat low back pain has also recently been questioned. In a systematic review, Smith et al. [54] concluded that stabilization exercise is not more effective than any other form of active exercise in the long term. Based on the current published high-quality RCTs of

Table 12.1 Randomized trials on different exercises on diastasis recti abdominis (DRA)

	Participants	Intervention	Outcome and cut off value for DRA	Results
Mesquita et al. (1999)	50 women (18–40 years) After vaginal delivery Intervention: $N = 25$ Control: $N = 25$	Intervention: 2 supervised sessions with physical therapists 6 h (10 repetitions) and 18 h (20 repetitions) postpartum Abdominal and pelvic floor muscle contractions. Diaphragmatic breathing, pelvic tilt with transverse abdominal and oblique's contraction. Co-contraction of pelvic floor muscles during all exercises Control: no follow-up	IRD measured using a caliper 4.5 cm above the umbilicus 4.5 cm below the umbilicus Diastasis: IRD > 3 cm	0 dropouts Significant larger reduction in IRD in intervention (mean 3.45 cm (SD 0.43) to 2.64 cm (SD 0.45) compared to control (3.16 cm (SD 0.26) to 2.99 cm (SD 0.28)
Walton et al. (2016)	9 women (18–45 years) Cesarean section and vaginal delivery Experimental group: $N = 5$ Control group: $N = 4$	6 weeks intervention (3 times/week of 3 × 10 repetitions). Increasing progression in repetitions. External support by a towel. Both groups: pelvic tilt, pelvic floor muscle exercises, and oblique's contraction Experimental: Plank 10 s with knees on the floor. Control: modified sit-up	IRD measured by ultrasound 4.5 cm above the umbilicus 4.5 cm below the umbilicus Oswestry disability index Pelvic floor distress index Diastasis: Cut-off value not defined	1 drop-out Experimental: IRD: mean 8.75 mm (SD 0.87) to 7.58 mm (SD 2.01) Control: mean 10.97 mm (SD 1.96) to 6.63 mm (SD 1.65) No significant difference between groups, $p = 0.2$ and $p = 0.6$ above and below the umbilicus, respectively
Emanuelsson et al. (2016)	89 participants (27–67 years) 87 women, 2 men Surgery with mesh: $N = 29$ Surgery with Quill: $N = 28$ Abdominal exercise: $N = 32$	3 months (3 times/week with a physical therapist). Exercise for rectus abdominis, obliques, and transversus abdominis	IRD measured by a ruler (halfway between xipoideus and navel and navel and pubic symphysis) SF-36. Ventral hernia pain questionnaire. Abdominal strength: VAS scale and Biodex system 4. Diastasis: IRD: ≥3 cm	3 dropouts No significant improvement on VAS in the exercise group compared to the surgery groups

(continued)

Table 12.1 (continued)

	Participants	Intervention	Outcome and cut off value for DRA	Results
Kamel and Yousif (2017)	60 women (25–35 years) After normal vaginal delivery 2 months postpartum Inclusion: Diastasis >2.5 cm at any point of linea alba	Neuromuscular electrical stimulation + abdominal exercise group: $N = 29$ Abdominal exercise group: $N = 28$ Abdominal exercise: sit up, reverse sit up, trunk twist, U-seat exercise Both groups had a scarf around the abdomen for support. Each exercise has 20 repetitions +4 extra repetitions per week Diaphragmatic breathing	Body mass index. Waist/hip ratio IRD abdominal strength: Isokinetic (Biodex multi-joint system pro, model 850-000; Biodex medical systems Inc.) Peak torque, maximum repetition total work, average power	3 dropouts Inter-rectus distance: Neuromuscular electrical stimulation + abdominal training: 50% reduction Abdominal training: 25.9% reduction, $p < 0.001$ Abdominal strength: Neuromuscular electrical stimulation + abdominals: 75.9%, 95.5%, 76.3% Abdominals: 53.5%, 40.3%, 32.9% increase in peak torque, maximum repetition total work, and average power, respectively. $p < 0.05$ for all comparisons

IRD inter-rectus distance, *VAS* Visual Analog Scale, *SD* standard deviation abdominal training for low back pain, they stated that further research is unlikely to considerably change this conclusion. Nevertheless, abdominal training and especially core training with a focus on the transverse abdominis muscle continues to be highly recommended for both DRA and low back pain [53].

According to the IOC 2016 evidence summary [34, 55], there is no knowledge of the prevalence, risk factors, and prevention and treatment of diastasis in recreational exercisers and elite athletes. However, athletes of most sports are dependent on well-functioning abdominals for sports performance, and therefore may be more vulnerable to the presence of a diastasis than other women. This and the effect of exercise interventions on this specific group of women needs further investigation. Benjamin et al. [41] concluded that there is an urgent need for more studies on the effect of conservative treatment for DRA.

12.4 Low Back and Pelvic Girdle Pain

Although exercise is recommended during pregnancy, some women are inclined to reduce their levels of physical activity [56, 57]. Women with complicated pregnancies or women suffering LBP and/or PGP may have been advised not to participate in exercise activities. The effect of exercise on the prevention of low back and pelvic girdle pain during pregnancy is uncertain. Few trials have been reported to examine the prevention of LBP and/or PGP, and they mainly lacked evidence of a positive effect [58]. Recently, a randomized controlled trial found that group fitness classes for pregnant women, exercising twice a week with a focus on cardiovascular endurance training and strength training, did not affect the prevalence of LBP and PGP during pregnancy or postpartum [59]. Whereas more years of regular physical activity before pregnancy reduced the risk of LBP and/or PGP during pregnancy in one follow-up study [60], a retrospective study comparing athletes who performed plenty of exercise prepregnancy with non-athletic controls found no difference in the prevalence of LBP and/or PGP [61]. In a longitudinal cohort study, a greater loss of physical condition seems to be not a cause but rather a consequence of LBP and/or PGP in pregnancy [62].

12.4.1 Therapeutic Exercise for Pregnancy-Related Low Back and Pelvic Girdle Pain

Several reviews have examined physical therapy interventions for LBP and PGP during pregnancy [63–72]. A recent systematic review showed that exercise reduced the risk of LBP in pregnancy by 9% whereas it had no protective effect on PGP [73]. One systematic review of the Cochrane Collaboration included 26 randomized controlled trials that examined the effects of a variety of interventions for LBP and PGP during pregnancy [58]. Eleven trials examined LBP, four examined PGP and a further 11 trials examined a combination of LBP and PGP (lumbopelvic pain). Evidence of moderate quality suggests that exercise or acupuncture significantly reduced evening PGP or lumbopelvic pain more than normal care alone. A more recent systematic review, including 22 randomized controlled trials, supported the conclusion of the moderate evidence for a positive effect of exercise therapy on pain, disability, and/or sick leave for the treatment of lumbopelvic pain during pregnancy [74]. According to this review, also patient information seems to be a useful intervention, especially when combined with exercises. However, when the authors analyzed LBP and PGP separately, the results were more robust for LBP than for PGP. The European guideline for PGP recommends individualized exercises in pregnancy [72] and a systematic review investigating the effectiveness of complementary and alternative medicine for the management of LBP and/or PGP in pregnancy, found limited evidence to support the use of these interventions [75]. A review of yoga interventions during pregnancy indicates positive outcomes but leads to conclusions that more studies are needed [76].

Whereas individualized exercise and appropriate information to reduce fear and anxiety are recommended for pregnant women, the European guideline for PGP postpartum recommends giving appropriate information and reassuring the patients as part of an individualized multifactorial treatment focusing on specific exercises for motor control and stability [77]. The level of evidence for interventions for PGP postpartum is, however, limited, because few randomized controlled trials have been performed. One systematic review has investigated the effectiveness of physical therapy for the treatment of LBP and PGP related to pregnancy postpartum [78] and included four randomized controlled trials [79–82]. All used exercises for motor control and stability of the lumbopelvic region, but with different interventions. The studies showed high methodological quality. However, only the study by Stuge et al. [79] demonstrated statistically and clinically significant positive and long-lasting effects, where disability was reduced by more than 50% for the exercise group compared to negligible changes in the control group. One more recent randomized study [83], concludes that core stabilization exercises and postural correction are effective in the management of postpartum lumbopelvic pain, however, the methodological quality was low. No studies examining a treatment program for LBP or PGP in elite athletes have been found [34, 55].

The lack of clear evidence supporting the diagnosis, prevention, and treatment of musculoskeletal conditions in the pregnancy and the postpartum period is challenging. Despite the desire of women to stay physically active during pregnancy [84], only a low proportion of pregnant women seem to follow current guidelines for exercise during pregnancy [77]. Even though group exercises during pregnancy have not been shown to influence the prevalence of LBP and/or PGP [59, 85–87], women who exercised seemed to handle their pain disorder better, with reduced need for sick leave [87]. Adhering to an exercise regime is a challenge [59] and it is important that exercises should not provoke pain during or after exercising. It might be that group exercise classes, even supervised, with a focus on cardiovascular endurance training and strength training, are not addressing the pain-provoking factors in individual women. Including heterogeneous samples with and without pain, unspecified LBP, and/or PGP, as well as combining prevention and treatment is likely to be a weak study design and potentially allows for a washout effect caused by the heterogeneity of the patient populations included [88].

The only randomized controlled study showing significant and long-lasting effects included a homogeneous group of patients based on clinical examination and criteria for PGP [79]. The treatment program studied was also individualized and focused on exercises for motor control and stability of the pelvic girdle. The focus of the exercises was to improve force closure with coordination of the local and overall muscle system, especially addressing the dynamic control of a neutral position of the lumbopelvic, subsequently to develop strength and endurance to manage the physical demands facing each individual. Additionally, essential points addressed were sacroiliac joint restrictions, posture, breathing, and cognitive-behavioral perspectives. Cognitive aspects were an important part of the intervention, in addition to the exercises. The women were ordered to perform their 30–60 min exercise program 3 days a week and they adhered closely to this regime. A qualitative study elucidating this treatment program found that by being active agents in managing their PGP the women learned to set themselves proximal goals [89]. Perceived hope and self-efficacy appeared to be essential for developing capacity for self-management and an enhanced ability to benefit from appropriate learning experiences. To improve the quality of treatment, physiotherapists ought to have evidence-based skills, listen attentively, and individualize treatment. The women found the discussion and individualized guidance as positive factors in helping them to cope with their daily lives.

Even though no single exercise therapy has proven to be superior [90], core stabilization exercises have grown in popularity [91] and two different core stabilization strategies exist, with controversy about which is the optimal strategy [92, 93]. The motor control exercise approach emphasizes specific exercises for local muscles, whereas the general exercise approach focuses on exercises on global muscles [94, 95]. A recent review has suggested that therapeutic exercises purporting to restore motor control of specific selected local muscles are unnecessary [92]. However, it has also been emphasized that generic approaches using stabilizing exercises do not address the individual motor control deficits identified in the patients [88]. Increased co-contraction of trunk stabilizing muscles during tasks that provoke pain and an inability to relax muscles are reported in both LBP and PGP [88, 96]. Consequently, interventions should focus less on specific stabilizing muscles and more on daily activities and optimal dynamic control of movements. Inherent underlying maladaptive movements might act as potential ongoing peripheral nociception rather than a strategy to avoid pain [88]. The examination of daily activities can determine whether the movement and pain behaviors are adaptive or maladaptive. With this in mind, individually designed treatment programs of supervised home exercise with regular therapist follow-up sessions to encourage adherence and achieve optimal dosage are recommended for patients with pregnancy-related LBP and/or PGP [79, 97]. Contradictory evidence exists on whether motor control or stabilizing exercises are better than general exercises [98, 99], with one systematic review showing strong evidence that stabilization exercises are not more effective than any other form of active exercise in the long term [54].

Nevertheless, positive changes in motor control have been found to be associated with relief of pain and disability for PGP [79, 100].

In conclusion, pregnant and postpartum women, even those with LBP and/or PGP, should be encouraged to be physically active and health care providers should help the women to find the kind of exercise or physical activity that is optimal for each individual, in her environment.

To assess activity limitations and symptoms there is a need for suitable outcome measures that are reliable and valid for patients with PGP in research and clinical practice [101]. The condition-specific measure, the Pelvic Girdle Questionnaire was developed for pregnant and nonpregnant women [102]. The questionnaire consists of 20 activity items and 5 symptom items on a four-point response scale. The Pelvic Girdle Questionnaire is reliable and valid for both pregnant and postpartum women with PGP; it is simple to administer and feasible for use in research and clinical practice. The Pelvic Girdle Questionnaire has also shown acceptable responsiveness and been shown to discriminate significantly both between pregnant and non-pregnant patients as well as between different locations of pain [103, 104].

12.5 Further Research

This chapter presents the current scientific evidence on the effect of exercise on the prevention and treatment of three commonly pregnancy-related musculoskeletal conditions: pelvic floor dysfunctions, diastasis recti abdominis, and low back and pelvic girdle pain.

To date, there is not enough evidence to conclude the long-term effect of PFMT. To our knowledge, there are no available studies specifically addressing the effect of PFMT among pregnant recreational or elite athletes. These two topics should be explored in further studies.

A lack of evidence exists about the consequences of the diastasis recti abdominis on abdominal wall integrity. Further research should focus on the effect of abdominal strengthening exercises in the reduction of diastasis recti abdominis.

Regarding low back and pelvic girdle pain during pregnancy, high-quality randomized studies are needed to clarify the preventive and/or resolution effect of core stabilization exercises and postural correction. Further, the effect of therapeutic exercise programs for low back or pelvic girdle pain in pregnant elite athletes is unexplored and needs further attention.

12.6 Conclusions

This chapter presents the current evidence on the effect of therapeutic exercise programs in the prevention and resolution of three commonly pregnancy-related musculoskeletal conditions: pelvic floor dysfunction, diastasis recti abdominis, and low back and pelvic girdle pain.

The section on "*Pelvic Floor Muscle Training*" (PFMT) underlines the importance of PFMT during pregnancy. A trained PFM may counteract the hormonally mediated increased laxity of the pelvic floor and the increased intra-abdominal pressure during pregnancy. Further, a trained PFM may encompass a greater functional reserve so that childbirth does not cause the sufficient loss of muscle function to develop urinary leakage. Additionally, a trained PFM may recover better after childbirth as the appropriate neuromuscular motor patterns have already been learned. The current evidence supports the widespread recommendation (Grade A) for offering supervised PFMT as the first-line treatment for female stress, urgency, or mixed UI. The current evidence support PFMT as this is shown to prevent and treat UI during pregnancy and prevent UI postpartum. The fifth International Consultation on Incontinence recommends that pregnant women having their first child should be offered supervised PFMT (Grade A recommendation).

The section on "*Diastasis Recti Abdominis*" explores the effect of exercise on diastasis recti abdominis (DRA) prevention or correction. The potential effect of the abdominal exercise programs on DRA prevention and treatment in pregnant women has been discussed as well as the consequences of this condition on abdominal wall integrity. To date, there is no knowledge whether DRA can be prevented or reduced with abdominal training or other exercise programs during pregnancy.

The topic "*Low Back and Pelvic Girdle Pain*" discuss the existing scientific evidence about the effect of exercise on the prevention and treatment of Low-Back Pain (LBP) and Pelvic Girdle Pain (PGP) during pregnancy. Pregnant women, even those with LBP and/or PGP, should be encouraged to be physically active. Health care providers should help women to find the most appropriate exercise or physical activity for each individual, in her environment. Identification of women's activity limitations and symptoms should be done before engaging in the exercise. For this purpose, there is a need for suitable outcome measures that are reliable and valid for patients with PGP. The condition-specific measure, the Pelvic Girdle Questionnaire was developed for pregnant and nonpregnant women. The questionnaire consists of 20 activity items and 5 symptom items on a four-point response scale. The Pelvic Girdle Questionnaire is reliable and valid for both pregnant and postpartum women with PGP; it is simple to administer and feasible for use in research and clinical practice. The Pelvic Girdle Questionnaire has also shown acceptable responsiveness and been shown to discriminate significantly both between pregnant and non-pregnant patients as well as between different locations of pain.

References

1. American College of Obstetricians and Gynecologists. Physical Activity and Exercise During Pregnancy and the Postpartum Period. ACOG Committee Opinion No. 650. Obstet Gynecol. 2015;126(6):e135–e42.
2. Hay-Smith J, Mørkved S, Fairbrother KA, Herbison GP. Pelvic floor muscle training for prevention and treatment of urinary and fecal incontinence in antenatal and postnatal women. Cochrane Database Syst Rev. 2008;(4):CD007471. https://doi.org/10.1002/14651858.CD007471.
3. Kegel AH. Progressive resistance exercise in the functional restoration of the perineal muscles. Am J Obstet Gynecol. 1948;56(2):238–48.

4. Kegel AH. Stress incontinence and genital relaxation; a nonsurgical method of increasing the tone of sphincters and their supporting structures. Ciba Clin Symp. 1952;4(2):35–51.
5. Bø K. Pelvic floor muscle training is effective in treatment of female stress urinary incontinence, but how does it work? Int Urogynecol J Pelvic Floor Dysfunct. 2004;15(2):76–84. https://doi.org/10.1007/s00192-004-1125-0.
6. Ashton-Miller JA, DeLancey JO. Functional anatomy of the female pelvic floor. Ann N Y Acad Sci. 2007;1101:266–96. https://doi.org/10.1196/annals.1389.034.
7. DeLancey JO. Structural aspects of the extrinsic continence mechanism. Obstet Gynecol. 1988;72(3 Pt 1):296–301.
8. DeLancey JO. Structural support of the urethra as it relates to stress urinary incontinence: the hammock hypothesis. Am J Obstet Gynecol. 1994;170(6):1713–20; discussion 20-3.
9. Ashton-Miller JA, Howard D, DeLancey JO. The functional anatomy of the female pelvic floor and stress continence control system. Scand J Urol Nephrol Suppl. 2001;207:1–7; discussion 106-25.
10. Miller JM, Ashton-Miller JA, DeLancey JOL. A pelvic muscle Precontraction can reduce cough-related urine loss in selected women with mild SUI. J Am Geriatr Soc. 1998;46(7):870–4. https://doi.org/10.1111/j.1532-5415.1998.tb02721.x.
11. Miller JM, Sampselle C, Ashton-Miller J, Hong GR, DeLancey JO. Clarification and confirmation of the knack maneuver: the effect of volitional pelvic floor muscle contraction to preempt expected stress incontinence. Int Urogynecol J Pelvic Floor Dysfunct. 2008;19(6):773–82. https://doi.org/10.1007/s00192-007-0525-3.
12. Miller JM, Perucchini D, Carchidi LT, Delancey JOL, Ashton-Miller J. Pelvic floor muscle contraction during a cough and decreased vesical neck mobility. Obstet Gynecol. 2001;97(2):255–60.
13. Peschers UM, Vodusek DB, Fanger G, Schaer GN, DeLancey JO, Schuessler B. Pelvic muscle activity in nulliparous volunteers. NeurourolUrodyn. 2001;20(3):269–75.
14. Bø K. Pelvic floor muscle exercise for the treatment of stress urinary incontinence: an exercise physiology perspective. Int Urogynecol J. 1995;6(5):282–91. https://doi.org/10.1007/bf01901527.
15. DiNubile NA. Strength training. Clin Sports Med. 1991;10(1):33–62.
16. Åstrand PO. Textbook of work physiology: physiological bases of exercise. In: Human Kinetics; 2003.
17. Bø K, Kvarstein B, Hagen R, Larsen S. Pelvic floor muscle exercise for the treatment of female stress urinary incontinence: I. reliability of vaginal pressure measurements of pelvic floor muscle strength. NeurourolUrodyn. 1990;9(5):471–7. https://doi.org/10.1002/nau.1930090503.
18. Bø K, Kvarstein B, Hagen RR, Larsen S. Pelvic floor muscle exercise for the treatment of female stress urinary incontinence: II. Validity of vaginal pressure measurements of pelvic floor muscle strength and the necessity of supplementary methods for control of correct contraction. NeurourolUrodyn. 1990;9(5):479–87. https://doi.org/10.1002/nau.1930090504.
19. Benvenuti F, Caputo GM, Bandinelli S, Mayer F, Biagini C, Sommavilla A. Reeducative treatment of female genuine stress incontinence. Am J Phys Med. 1987;66(4):155–68.
20. Bø K, Jørgensen J, Larsen S, Oseid S, Kvarstein B, Hagen R. Knowledge about and ability to correct pelvic floor muscle exercises in women with urinary stress incontinence. NeurourolUrodyn. 1988;7:261–2.
21. Bump RC, Hurt WG, Fantl JA, Wyman JF. Assessment of Kegel pelvic muscle exercise performance after brief verbal instruction. Am J Obstet Gynecol. 1991;165(2):322–7. discussion 7-9
22. Messelink B, Benson T, Berghmans B, Bø K, Corcos J, Fowler C, et al. Standardization of terminology of pelvic floor muscle function and dysfunction: report from the pelvic floor clinical assessment group of the international continence society. NeurourolUrodyn. 2005;24(4):374–80. https://doi.org/10.1002/nau.20144.

23. Bø K, Sherburn M. Measurement of pelvic floor muscle function and strength and pelvic organ prolapse. In: Bø K, Berghmans B, Mørkved S, Kampen MV, editors. Evidence-based physical therapy for the pelvic floor. Edinburgh: Churchill Livingstone; 2007. p. 45–112.
24. Bø K, Mørkved S. Pelvic floor and exercise science. In: Bø K, Berghmans B, Mørkved S, Kampen MV, editors. Evidence-based physical therapy for the pelvic floor. Edinburgh: Churchill Livingstone; 2007. p. 113–32.
25. Haskell WL, Lee IM, Pate RR, Powell KE, Blair SN, Franklin BA, et al. Physical activity and public health: updated recommendation for adults from the American College of Sports Medicine and the American Heart Association. Med Sci Sports Exerc. 2007;39(8):1423–34. https://doi.org/10.1249/mss.0b013e3180616b27.
26. Garber CE, Blissmer B, Deschenes MR, Franklin BA, Lamonte MJ, Lee IM, et al. American College of Sports Medicine position stand. Quantity and quality of exercise for developing and maintaining cardiorespiratory, musculoskeletal, and neuromotor fitness in apparently healthy adults: guidance for prescribing exercise. Med Sci Sports Exerc. 2011;43(7):1334–59. https://doi.org/10.1249/MSS.0b013e318213fefb.
27. Bø K, Aschehoug A. Pelvic floor and exercise science: strength training. In: Bø K, Berghmans B, Mørkved S, Kampen MV, editors. Evidence-based physical therapy for the pelvic floor. Edinburgh: Churchill Livingstone; 2007. p. 119–32.
28. Kraemer WJ, Ratamess NA. Fundamentals of resistance training: progression and exercise prescription. Med Sci Sports Exerc. 2004;36(4):674–88.
29. Dumoulin C, Hay-Smith EJC, Mac Habée-Séguin G. Pelvic floor muscle training versus no treatment, or inactive control treatments, for urinary incontinence in women. Cochrane Database Syst Rev. 2014;(5). https://doi.org/10.1002/14651858.CD005654.pub3.
30. Moore K, Dumoulin C, Bradley C, Burgio K, Chambers T, Hagen S, et al. Adult conservative management. In: Abrams P, Cardozo L, Khoury S, Wein A, editors. Incontinence: 5th International Consultation on Incontinence. Paris: SRC—GoogleScholar, ICUD-EAU; 2013. p. 1101–305.
31. Boyle R, Hay-Smith EJC, Cody JD, Mørkved S. Pelvic floor muscle training for prevention and treatment of urinary and faecal incontinence in antenatal and postnatal women. Cochrane Database Syst Rev. 2012;(10). https://doi.org/10.1002/14651858.CD007471.pub2.
32. Kruger JA, Dietz HP, Murphy BA. Pelvic floor function in elite nulliparous athletes. Ultrasound Obstet Gynecol. 2007;30(1):81–5. https://doi.org/10.1002/uog.4027.
33. Du Y, Xu L, Ding L, Wang Y, Wang Z. The effect of antenatal pelvic floor muscle training on labor and delivery outcomes: a systematic review with meta-analysis. Int Urogynecol J. 2015;26(10):1415–27. https://doi.org/10.1007/s00192-015-2654-4.
34. Bø K, Artal R, Barakat R, Brown W, Davies GAL, Dooley M, et al. Exercise and pregnancy in recreational and elite athletes: 2016 evidence summary from the IOC expert group meeting, Lausanne. Part 1—exercise in women planning pregnancy and those who are pregnant. Br J Sports Med. 2016;50(10):571.
35. Mota PG, Pascoal AGBA, Carita AIAD, Bø K. Prevalence and risk factors of diastasis recti abdominis from late pregnancy to 6 months postpartum, and relationship with lumbo-pelvic pain. Man Ther. 2015;20(1):200–5. https://doi.org/10.1016/j.math.2014.09.002.
36. Boissonnault JS, Blaschak MJ. Incidence of diastasis recti abdominis during the childbearing year. Phys Ther. 1988;68(7):1082–6.
37. Fast A, Weiss L, Ducommun EJ, Medina E, Butler JG. Low-back pain in pregnancy. Abdominal muscles, sit-up performance, and back pain. Spine. 1990;15(1):28–30.
38. Gilleard WL, Brown JM. Structure and function of the abdominal muscles in primigravid subjects during pregnancy and the immediate postbirth period. Phys Ther. 1996;76(7):750–62.
39. Coldron Y, Stokes MJ, Newham DJ, Cook K. Postpartum characteristics of rectus abdominis on ultrasound imaging. Man Ther. 2008;13(2):112–21. https://doi.org/10.1016/j.math.2006.10.001.
40. Mota P, Pascoal AG, Carita AI, Bo K. The immediate effects on inter-rectus distance of abdominal crunch and drawing in exercises during pregnancy and the postpartum period. J Orthop Sports Phys Ther. 2015:1–24. https://doi.org/10.2519/jospt.2015.5459.

41. Benjamin DR, van de Water ATM, Peiris CL. Effects of exercise on diastasis of the rectus abdominis muscle in the antenatal and postnatal periods: a systematic review. Physiotherapy. 2014;100(1):1–8. https://doi.org/10.1016/j.physio.2013.08.005.
42. Akram J, Matzen SH. Rectus abdominis diastasis. J Plast Surg Hand Surg. 2014;48(3):163–9. https://doi.org/10.3109/2000656X.2013.859145.
43. Emanuelsson P, Gunnarsson U, Strigard K, Stark B. Early complications, pain, and quality of life after reconstructive surgery for abdominal rectus muscle diastasis: a 3-month follow-up. J Plast Reconstr Aesthet Surg. 2014;67(8):1082–8. https://doi.org/10.1016/j.bjps.2014.04.015.
44. Mesquita LA, Machado AC, Andrade AV. Fisioterapia para Redução da Diástase dos Músculos Retos Abdominais no Pós-Parto. Rev Bras Ginecol Obstet. 1999;21(5):267–72. https://doi.org/10.1590/S0100-72031999000500004.
45. Walton LM, Costa A, LaVanture D, McIlrath S, Stebbins B. The effects of a 6 week dynamic core stability plank exercise program compared to a traditional supine core stability strengthening program on diastasis recti abdominis closure, pain, oswestry disability index (ODI) and pelvic floor disability index scores (PFDI). Phys Ther Rehabil. 2016;3(1):3. https://doi.org/10.7243/2055-2386-3-3.
46. Kamel DM, Yousif AM. Neuromuscular electrical stimulation and strength recovery of postnatal diastasis recti abdominis muscles. Ann Rehabil Med. 2017;41(3):465–74. https://doi.org/10.5535/arm.2017.41.3.465.
47. Carrera Pérez C, Da Cuña CI, González González Y. ¿Cuál es el mejor ejercicio para la rehabilitación de la diástasis abdominal? Rehabilitación. 2019;53(3):198–210. https://doi.org/10.1016/j.rh.2018.12.004.
48. Gluppe SB, Engh ME, Bø K. Immediate effect of abdominal and pelvic floor muscle exercises on Interrecti distance in women with diastasis recti abdominis who were parous. Phys Ther. 2020;100(8):1372–83. https://doi.org/10.1093/ptj/pzaa070.
49. Gluppe SL, Hilde G, Tennfjord MK, Engh ME, Bø K. Effect of a postpartum training program on the prevalence of diastasis recti abdominis in postpartum Primiparous women: a randomized controlled trial. Phys Ther. 2018;98(4):260–8. https://doi.org/10.1093/ptj/pzy008.
50. Theodorsen NM, Strand LI, Bo K. Effect of pelvic floor and transversus abdominis muscle contraction on inter-rectus distance in postpartum women: a cross-sectional experimental study. Physiotherapy. 2019;105(3):315–20. https://doi.org/10.1016/j.physio.2018.08.009.
51. Mota P, Pascoal AG, Sancho MF, Bo K. Test-retest and intra-observer reliability of 2D ultrasound measurements of distance between rectus abdominis in women. J Orthop Sports Phys Ther. 2012;42(11):940–6.
52. Sancho MF, Pascoal AG, Mota P, Bo K. Abdominal exercises affect inter-rectus distance in postpartum women: a two-dimensional ultrasound study. Physiotherapy. 2015;101(3):286–91. https://doi.org/10.1016/j.physio.2015.04.004.
53. Lee D, Hodges PW. Behavior of the Linea Alba during a curl-up task in diastasis rectus abdominis: an observational study. J Orthop Sports Phys Ther. 2016;46(7):580–9. https://doi.org/10.2519/jospt.2016.6536.
54. Smith BE, Littlewood C, May S. An update of stabilisation exercises for low back pain: a systematic review with meta-analysis. BMC Musculoskelet Disord. 2014;15:416. https://doi.org/10.1186/1471-2474-15-416.
55. Bø K, Artal R, Barakat R, Brown WJ, Davies GAL, Dooley M, et al. Exercise and pregnancy in recreational and elite athletes: 2016/17 evidence summary from the IOC Expert Group Meeting, Lausanne. Part 3—exercise in the postpartum period. Br J Sports Med. 2017;50:571.
56. Fell DB, Joseph KS, Armson BA, Dodds L. The impact of pregnancy on physical activity level. Matern Child Health J. 2008;13(5):597. https://doi.org/10.1007/s10995-008-0404-7.
57. Owe KM, Nystad W, Bo K. Correlates of regular exercise during pregnancy: the Norwegian mother and child cohort study. Scand J Med Sci Sports. 2009;19(5):637–45. https://doi.org/10.1111/j.1600-0838.2008.00840.x.
58. Pennick V, Liddle SD. Interventions for preventing and treating pelvic and back pain in pregnancy. Cochrane Database Syst Rev. 2013;(8):CD001139. https://doi.org/10.1002/14651858.CD001139.pub3.

59. Haakstad LA, Bo K. Effect of a regular exercise programme on pelvic girdle and low back pain in previously inactive pregnant women: a randomized controlled trial. J Rehabil Med. 2015;47(3):229–34. https://doi.org/10.2340/16501977-1906.
60. Mogren IM. Previous physical activity decreases the risk of low back pain and pelvic pain during pregnancy. Scand J Public Health. 2005;33(4):300–6.
61. Bø K, Backe-Hansen KL. Do elite athletes experience low back, pelvic girdle and pelvic floor complaints during and after pregnancy? Scand J Med Sci Sports. 2007;17(5):480–7. https://doi.org/10.1111/j.1600-0838.2006.00599.x.
62. Thorell E, Kristiansson P. Pregnancy related back pain, is it related to aerobic fitness? A longitudinal cohort study. BMC Pregnancy Childbirth. 2012;12:30. https://doi.org/10.1186/1471-2393-12-30.
63. Boissonnault JS, Klestinski JU, Pearcy K. The role of exercise in the management of pelvic girdle and low back pain in pregnancy: a systematic review of the literature. J Women Health Phys Ther. 2012;36:69–77.
64. Ho SSM, Yu WWM, Lao TT, Chow DHK, Chung JWY, Li Y. Effectiveness of maternity support belts in reducing low back pain during pregnancy: a review. J Clin Nurs. 2009;18(11):1523–32. https://doi.org/10.1111/j.1365-2702.2008.02749.x.
65. Kanakaris NK, Roberts CS, Giannoudis PV. Pregnancy-related pelvic girdle pain: an update. BMC Med. 2011;9:15. https://doi.org/10.1186/1741-7015-9-15.
66. Katonis P, Kampouroglou A, Aggelopoulos A, Kakavelakis K, Lykoudis S, Makrigiannakis A, et al. Pregnancy-related low back pain. Hippokratia. 2011;15(3):205–10.
67. Lillios S, Young J. The effects of core and lower extremity strengthening on pregnancy_related low back and pelvic girdle pain: a review. J Women Health Phys Ther. 2012;36:116–24.
68. Richards E, Van Kessel G, Virgara R, Harris P. Does antenatal physical therapy for pregnant women with low back pain or pelvic pain improve functional outcomes? A systematic review. Acta Obstet Gynecol Scand. 2012;91(9):1038–45. https://doi.org/10.1111/j.1600-0412.2012.01462.x.
69. Stuge B, Hilde G, Vollestad N. Physical therapy for pregnancy-related low back and pelvic pain: a systematic review. Acta Obstet Gynecol Scand. 2003;82(11):983–90.
70. Vermani E, Mittal R, Weeks A. Pelvic girdle pain and low back pain in pregnancy: a review. Pain Pract. 2010;10(1):60–71. https://doi.org/10.1111/j.1533-2500.2009.00327.x.
71. Verstraete EH, Vanderstraeten G, Parewijck W. Pelvic girdle pain during or after pregnancy: a review of recent evidence and a clinical care path proposal. Facts Views Vis Obgyn. 2013;5(1):33–43.
72. Vleeming A, Albert HB, Östgaard HC, Sturesson B, Stuge B. European guidelines for the diagnosis and treatment of pelvic girdle pain. Eur Spine J. 2008;17(6):794–819. https://doi.org/10.1007/s00586-008-0602-4.
73. Shiri R, Coggon D, Falah-Hassani K. Exercise for the prevention of low back and pelvic girdle pain in pregnancy: a meta-analysis of randomized controlled trials. Eur J Pain. 2018;187:1093–101. https://doi.org/10.1002/ejp.1096.
74. Benten EV, Pool J, Mens J, Pool-Goudzwaard A. Recommendations for physical therapists on the treatment of Lumbopelvic pain during pregnancy: a systematic review. J Orthop Sports Phys Ther. 2014;44(7):464–A15. https://doi.org/10.2519/jospt.2014.5098.
75. Close C, Sinclair M, Liddle SD, Madden E, McCullough JEM, Hughes C. A systematic review investigating the effectiveness of complementary and alternative medicine (CAM) for the management of low back and/or pelvic pain (LBPP) in pregnancy. J Adv Nurs. 2014;70(8):1702–16. https://doi.org/10.1111/jan.12360.
76. Jiang Q, Wu Z, Zhou L, Dunlop J, Chen P. Effects of yoga intervention during pregnancy: a review for current status. Am J Perinatol. 2015;32(6):503–14. https://doi.org/10.1055/s-0034-1396701.
77. Gjestland K, Bø K, Owe KM, Eberhard-Gran M. Do pregnant women follow exercise guidelines? Prevalence data among 3482 women, and prediction of low-back pain, pelvic girdle pain and depression. Br J Sports Med. 2013;47(8):515.

78. Ferreira CWS, Alburquerque-Sendin F. Effectiveness of physical therapy for pregnancy-related low back and/or pelvic pain after delivery: a systematic review. Physiother Theory Pract. 2013;29(6):419–31. https://doi.org/10.3109/09593985.2012.748114.
79. Stuge B, Laerum E, Kirkesola G, Vollestad N. The efficacy of a treatment program focusing on specific stabilizing exercises for pelvic girdle pain after pregnancy: a randomized controlled trial. Spine. 2004;29(4):351–9.
80. Mens JM, Snijders CJ, Stam HJ. Diagonal trunk muscle exercises in peripartum pelvic pain: a randomized clinical trial. Phys Ther. 2000;80(12):1164–73.
81. Bastiaenen CH, de Bie RA, Vlaeyen JW, Goossens ME, Leffers P, Wolters PM, et al. Long-term effectiveness and costs of a brief self-management intervention in women with pregnancy-related low back pain after delivery. BMC Pregnancy Childbirth. 2008;8:19. https://doi.org/10.1186/1471-2393-8-19.
82. Gutke A, Sjödahl J, Öberg B. Specific muscle stabilizing as home exercises for persistent pelvic girdle pain after pregnancy: a randomized, controlled clinical trial. J Rehabil Med. 2010;42(10):929–35. https://doi.org/10.2340/16501977-0615.
83. Chaudry S, Rashid F, Shah S. Effectiveness of core stabilization exercises along with postural correction in postpartum back pain. Rawal Med J. 2013;38:256–9.
84. Backhausen MG, Tabor A, Albert H, Rosthøj S, Damm P, Hegaard HK. The effects of an unsupervised water exercise program on low back pain and sick leave among healthy pregnant women—a randomised controlled trial. PLoS One. 2017;12(9):e0182114. https://doi.org/10.1371/journal.pone.0182114.
85. Eggen MH, Stuge B, Mowinckel P, Jensen KS, Hagen KB. Can supervised group exercises including ergonomic advice reduce the prevalence and severity of low back pain and pelvic girdle pain in pregnancy? A randomized controlled trial. Phys Ther. 2012;92(6):781–90. https://doi.org/10.2522/ptj.20110119.
86. Mørkved SIV, Salvesen KÅ, Schei B, Lydersen S, BØ K. Does group training during pregnancy prevent lumbopelvic pain? A randomized clinical trial. Acta Obstet Gynecol Scand. 2007;86(3):276–82. https://doi.org/10.1080/00016340601089651.
87. Stafne SN, Salvesen KA, Romundstad PR, Stuge B, Morkved S. Does regular exercise during pregnancy influence lumbopelvic pain? A randomized controlled trial. Acta Obstet Gynecol Scand. 2012;91(5):552–9. https://doi.org/10.1111/j.1600-0412.2012.01382.x.
88. Dankaerts W, O'Sullivan P. The validity of O'Sullivan's classification system (CS) for a sub-group of NS-CLBP with motor control impairment (MCI): overview of a series of studies and review of the literature. Man Ther. 2011;16(1):9–14. https://doi.org/10.1016/j.math.2010.10.006.
89. Stuge B, Bergland A. Evidence and individualization: important elements in treatment for women with postpartum pelvic girdle pain. Physiother Theory Pract. 2011;27(8):557–65. https://doi.org/10.3109/09593985.2010.551802.
90. van Tulder M, Koes B. Low back pain (acute). Clin Evid. 2004;12:1643–58.
91. Liddle SD, David Baxter G, Gracey JH. Physiotherapists' use of advice and exercise for the management of chronic low back pain: a national survey. Man Ther. 2009;14(2):189–96. https://doi.org/10.1016/j.math.2008.01.012.
92. Brumitt J, Matheson JW, Meira EP. CCore stabilization exercise prescription, part 2: a systematic review of motor control and general (global) exercise rehabilitation approaches for patients with low back pain. Sports Health. 2013;5(6):510–3. https://doi.org/10.1177/1941738113502634.
93. Bruno P. The use of "stabilization exercises" to affect neuromuscular control in the lumbopelvic region: a narrative review. J Can Chiropr Assoc. 2014;58:119–30.
94. McGill S. Low back disorders: evidence-based prevention and rehabilitation. 2nd ed. Champaign, IL: Human Kinetics; 2007.
95. Richardson C, Hodges P, Hides J. Therapeutic exercise for lumbopelvic stabilization. Edinburgh: Churchill Livingstone; 2004.

96. Stuge B, Saetre K, Ingeborg HB. The automatic pelvic floor muscle response to the active straight leg raise in cases with pelvic girdle pain and matched controls. Man Ther. 2013;18(4):327–32. https://doi.org/10.1016/j.math.2012.12.004.
97. Hayden JA, van Tulder MW, Tomlinson G. Systematic review: strategies for using exercise therapy to improve outcomes in chronic low back pain. Ann Intern Med. 2005;142(9):776–85. https://doi.org/10.7326/0003-4819-142-9-200505030-00014.
98. Gomes-Neto M, Lopes JM, Conceicao CS, Araujo A, Brasileiro A, Sousa C, et al. Stabilization exercise compared to general exercises or manual therapy for the management of low back pain: a systematic review and meta-analysis. Phys Ther Sport. 2017;23:136–42. https://doi.org/10.1016/j.ptsp.2016.08.004.
99. Wang X-Q, Zheng J-J, Yu Z-W, Bi X, Lou S-J, Liu J, et al. A meta-analysis of core stability exercise versus general exercise for chronic low Back pain. PLoS One. 2012;7(12):e52082. https://doi.org/10.1371/journal.pone.0052082.
100. O'Sullivan PB, Beales DJ. Changes in pelvic floor and diaphragm kinematics and respiratory patterns in subjects with sacroiliac joint pain following a motor learning intervention: a case series. Man Ther. 2007;12(3):209–18. https://doi.org/10.1016/j.math.2006.06.006.
101. Boissonnault JS. A review of self-report functional outcome measures in selected obstetric physical therapy interventions. J Women Health Phys Ther. 2009;33(1):7–12.
102. Stuge B, Garratt A, Krogstad Jenssen H, Grotle M. The pelvic girdle questionnaire: a condition-specific instrument for assessing activity limitations and symptoms in people with pelvic girdle pain. Phys Ther. 2011;91(7):1096–108. https://doi.org/10.2522/ptj.20100357.
103. Grotle M, Garratt AM, Krogstad Jenssen H, Stuge B. Reliability and construct validity of self-report questionnaires for patients with pelvic girdle pain. Phys Ther. 2012;92(1):111–23. https://doi.org/10.2522/ptj.20110076.
104. Stuge B, Jenssen HK, Grotle M. The pelvic girdle questionnaire: responsiveness and minimal important change in women with pregnancy-related pelvic girdle pain, low back pain, or both. Phys Ther. 2017;97(11):1103–13. https://doi.org/10.1093/ptj/pzx078.

Nutritional and Energy Requirements of the Pregnant Exerciser and Athlete

13

Maria-Raquel G. Silva and Belén Rodriguez

Abstract

The purpose of this chapter is to identify nutritional requirements for special groups of pregnant exercisers and pregnant athletes such as (1) athletes practicing aesthetic sports, weight competing for sports, and sports of long duration; (2) pregnant exerciser women who restrict or prohibit certain dietary practices or the consumption of important sources of energy and nutrients; (3) adolescent pregnant exercisers; and (4) other pregnant exerciser women in high-risk categories. In addition, risk factors such as low energy availability and eating disorders related to their energy and nutritional requirements are also included. Micronutrients' needs increase much more than macronutrients. Even prior to conception, an increased average intake of folate, iodine, and iron is recommended. However, only at the beginning of the second trimester, a marked increase in vitamins and minerals is observed. A pregnant exerciser or athlete who continues to train during pregnancy may have a total energy expenditure quite high, which depends on the type, intensity, frequency, and duration of the activities performed. Therefore, dietary intakes before, during, and after physical

M.-R. G. Silva (✉)
FP-I3ID, FP-BHS and Faculty of Health Sciences, University Fernando Pessoa, Porto, Portugal

CIAS-Research Centre for Anthropology and Health - Human Biology, Health and Society, University of Coimbra, Coimbra, Portugal

CHRC-Comprehensive Health Research Centre - Sleep, Chronobiology and Sleep Disorders, Nova Medical School, Nova University of Lisbon, Lisbon, Portugal
e-mail: raquel@ufp.edu.pt

B. Rodriguez
Tu Gestor de Salud for Nutrition and Sport, Madrid, Spain

Spanish Paralympic Committee, Madrid, Spain
e-mail: belen.rodriguez@tugestordesalud.com

R. Santos-Rocha (ed.), *Exercise and Physical Activity During Pregnancy and Postpartum*, https://doi.org/10.1007/978-3-031-06137-0_13

exercise are crucial for the maintenance of adequate energy availability. In addition, some unhealthy behaviors such as the consumption of alcohol, smoking, and other stimulant substances, and the lack of sleep should be avoided.

Keywords
Pregnancy · Nutrition · Dietary intakes · Energy · Macronutrients · Micronutrients Exercisers · Athletes · Eating disorders · Sleep

13.1 Introduction

Pregnancy outcomes are related to the previous woman's nutritional status, diet, and household food security as shown in Fig. 13.1.

For those women, who can plan their pregnancies, it is determinant to attain adequate body weight and nutritional profile.

In addition, environmental factors (such as geographic location, daily working hours, among others), genetics, maternal age, socio-demographics, physical activity, and sleep can affect the fetus growth and development and maternal health.

During pregnancy and in the postpartum period, dietary supplementation, breastfeeding, and clinical and nutritional supervision are crucial to promote a healthy and successful post-partum for both (mother and child).

Nowadays, the pandemic caused by the coronavirus disease 2019 (COVID-19) has become a major health problem, including for pregnant women and outcomes; therefore, standard hygiene measures are essential for both mother and child's health.

This chapter will be mainly based on the energy and nutritional requirements of special groups of pregnant exercisers and pregnant athletes such as athletes practicing aesthetic sports, weight competing for sports and sports of long duration; pregnant exerciser women who restrict or prohibit certain dietary practices or the

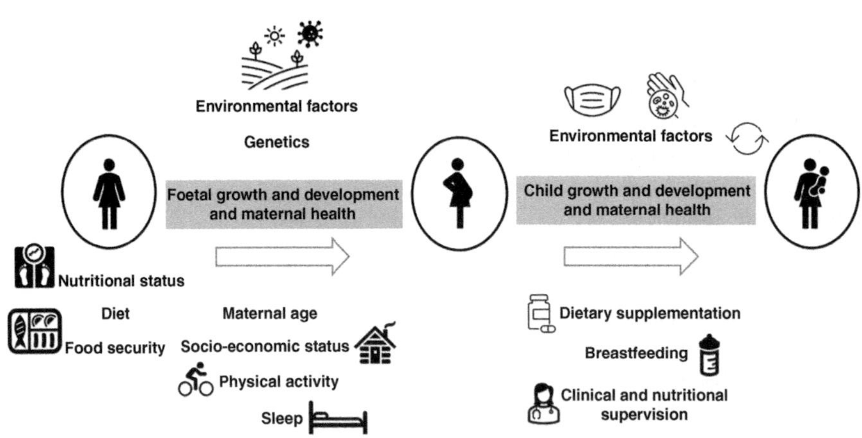

Fig. 13.1 Framework of maternal nutritional status and other variables influencing pregnancy and postpartum, namely child growth and development and maternal health

consumption of important sources of energy and nutrients; adolescent pregnant exercisers; and other pregnant exerciser women in high-risk categories. Also, dietary intakes before, during, and after physical exercise will be analyzed and unhealthy behaviors such as the consumption of alcohol, smoking, stimulant substances, and the lack of sleep will be discussed.

13.2 Nutritional and Clinical Issues During Pregnancy

During pregnancy, the basal metabolism rate rises partly due to the increased mass of active tissue (fetal, placental, and maternal), maternal effort (e.g., cardiovascular and respiratory work), and tissue synthesis; thus, extra energy is needed for the growth of the fetus, placenta, and associated maternal tissues.

Several studies from the 50s and 60s [1, 2] showed that pregnant women with insufficient weight gain presented higher rates of premature birth than those with appropriate weight gain. Therefore, undernutrition was seen as a negative influence factor on the pregnancy outcome.

Nowadays, the opposite significant complication of pregnancy, which is maternal overweight and obesity [3, 4], is preoccupying worldwide medical and scientific communities since the fetus may be exposed to excessive energy availability.

In a recent systematic review and meta-analysis of 90 dietary studies among pregnant women in developed countries (n = 126.242), energy and fiber intakes were generally lower, carbohydrate intake was borderline or lower, and total fat and saturated fat intakes were higher than nutritional recommendations of each specific country [5].

Moreover, it was recently indicated that micronutrient intake during pregnancy is less than optimal [5], which is of great concern since the current consensus lies on the impact of maternal nutrition on both short- and long-term health of the child [6].

Although there are various factors that can negatively affect the maternal nutritional status, such as inadequate energy availability [6], physical inactivity, overweight or obesity [3], and other complications (multiple pregnancies, being an adolescent, alcohol and tobacco consumption, and drugs [7], maternal physiological changes influence nutritional status by increasing energy and nutritional needs [4, 8–10]. These changes can influence not only the mother's health but also fetus growth and development [8].

In well-nourished populations from developed countries, the weight gain during pregnancy is about 12.5 kg and the median infant birth weight is 3.3 kg with a coefficient of variation of 15% [11]. Nevertheless, the average extra energy cost of this typical pregnancy has been calculated to be about 80,000 kcal over the 9-month period, distributed as an extra 150 kcal per day during the first trimester and 350 kcal per day during the second and third trimesters [12].

Therefore, recommendations for energy intakes of pregnant women should be population-specific, because of differences in body size and lifestyles [13].

Anatomical and physiological changes during pregnancy affect the musculoskeletal system at rest and during exercise with weight gain being the most obvious [14].

The characteristics of exercise prescription should be considered in every physical activity framework regardless of its purpose (basic health, recreational pursuits, or competitive activities) [15].

13.3 Special Groups of Pregnant Exercisers and Pregnant Athletes

Some groups of pregnant women should be carefully screened and closely supervised by Sport and Health Professionals as they are more sensitive to an inadequate nutritional status during pregnancy and/or to the development of insufficient or excessive body weight (Table 13.1) [16].

Special groups of pregnant exercisers and athletes are as follows.

13.3.1 Pregnant Athletes Practicing Aesthetic Sports, Weight Competing Sports, and Sports of Long Duration

Athletes practicing aesthetic sports (e.g., any gymnastics discipline, ballet, artistic skating), weight competing sports (e.g., canoeing, judo), and long duration sports (e.g., marathons) normally exhibit lean bodies and reduced body weight, and often present an inadequate energy intake in accordance with their exercise energy expenditure.

Thus, physiological functions, daily activities, and athletic performance can be compromised as these athletes may not achieve adequate amounts of energy available for their daily activities and training demands [17].

Furthermore, they have increased needs for energy and nutrients in prepregnancy, during, and postpregnancy in relation to their pairs (i.e., pregnant women non-athletes) (Fig. 13.2).

Energy availability has been defined as the amount of energy intake minus total energy expenditure normalized to fat-free mass [18, 19], where total energy expenditure is divided into a basal metabolic rate, diet-induced thermogenesis, and activity energy expenditure [20].

Due to the higher metabolic rate and energy expenditure in the synthesis of protein and fat in new tissues in pregnant women, total energy expenditure is higher than in nonpregnant ones (Fig. 13.3).

Table 13.1 Special groups of pregnant exercisers and athletes

Special groups of pregnant exercisers and athletes
Pregnant athletes practicing aesthetic sports, weight competing sports and long duration sports
Pregnant women who restrict or prohibit certain dietary practices
Pregnant adolescents
Pregnant women carrying more than one fetus
Women with multiple pregnancies
Women who are high cigarette smokers, heavy alcohol consumers, and drug abusers (*less frequent*)

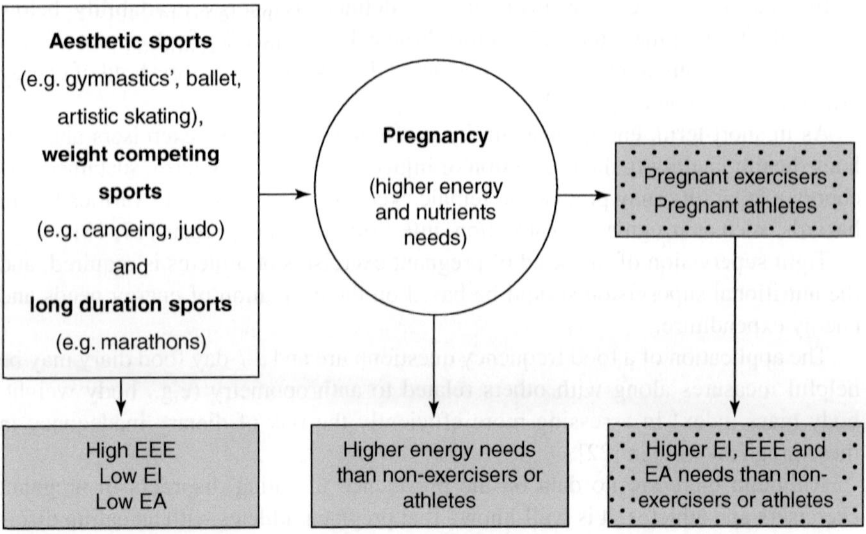

Fig. 13.2 Increased energy needs of pregnant athletes compared to non-athletes (*EEE* exercise energy expenditure, *EI* energy intake, *EA* energy availability)

Fig. 13.3 Partitioning of total energy expenditure in non-pregnancy vs. pregnancy [20]

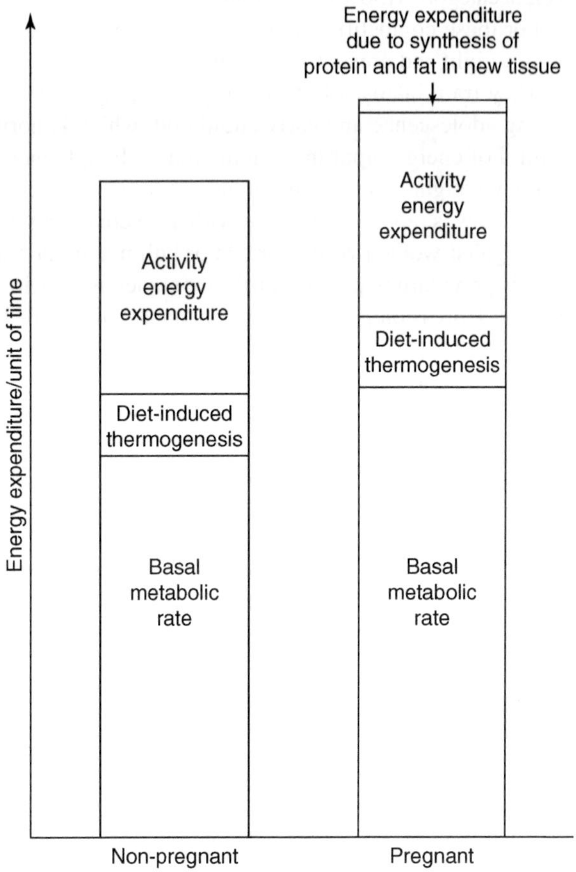

In addition, low energy availability is defined as energy availability below 45 kcal/kg fat-free mass/day [21]. A threshold below 30 kcal/kg fat-free mass/day is associated with amenorrhea and is considered the lowest energy threshold of energy availability for women [17, 19].

As in short-term, energy availability is required to improve exercisers and athletes' health, including the prevention of injury, and in the long term, sustained low energy availability may predispose female exercisers and athletes to various health hazards, such as irregular menstruation, infertility and osteoporosis [17, 18].

Tight supervision of this kind of pregnant exercisers or athletes is required, and the nutritional supervision should be based on the evaluation of energy needs and energy expenditure.

The application of a food frequency questionnaire and a 7-day food diary may be helpful measures along with others related to anthropometry (e.g., body weight, body mass index) in assessing more efficiently the risk of dietary inadequacy in these pregnant women [22].

Although there are no data on the prevalence of eating disorders in pregnant exercisers and athletes, it is well-known that pregnant athletes with an eating disorder, and their offspring, are at particular risk [16, 23].

In fact, the prevalence of eating disorders is higher among athletes (20–22%) than non-athletes (3–9%), with a high frequency in aesthetic sports (42%), sports with weight categories (30%), and weight-sensitive sports such as endurance (24%) [24–29].

For these competitive athletes, energy restriction is common in order to reduce body weight and prevent sports injuries [17].

They train intensively from very young ages and maintain that training regime during adolescence and early adulthood, which is normally characterized by strict control of energy input in combination with high energy output and reduced levels of body weight and body mass index for age. In fact, a mortality rate between 4% and 10% was reported for those with a severe eating disorder [30].

Pregnant women with anorexia or bulimia are at risk to develop anemia, hyperemesis gravidarum, preterm birth, spontaneous abortion, cesarean section, and postpartum depression [31–33]. Their neonates are at for low birth weight, small head [34, 35], and developmental and emotional disturbances [35, 36] such as anxiety, depression, and substance abuse [31, 36].

Additional complications for pregnant women with bulimia involve elevated risk for hypertension, vaginal bleeding, fetal abnormalities, low Apgar scores, breech delivery, and stillbirth [31, 37].

13.3.2 Pregnant Exerciser Women Who Restrict or Prohibit Certain Dietary Practices or the Consumption of Important Sources of Energy and Nutrients

Some pregnant exerciser women restrict or prohibit certain dietary practices or the consumption of energy and nutrients, such as all animal foods (proteins) or milk (calcium, vitamin D); thus, these women are at high risk of inadequate nutrient intake.

In such cases based on a poor diet quality and if a better food selection is not possible, selective supplementation is recommended by the IM [22] in association with clinical (including nutritional) supervision.

13.3.3 Adolescents Pregnant Exercisers

Also, adolescent pregnant exercisers should be carefully supervised, because adolescence is a period of life where diet is likely to be inadequate for dietary intake, especially for energy and some micronutrients intakes, such as calcium, iron, zinc, riboflavin, folic acid, and vitamins A, D, and B-6.

In addition, these young pregnant females are crossing a very demanding period of their own growth and development associated with increased energy needs for the growth and development of the fetus [38]. Therefore, it is recommended for pregnant adolescents to strive for weight gains toward the upper end of the range for women with similar weights for height [22].

13.3.4 Pregnant Exerciser Women in High-Risk Categories

Pregnant exerciser women in high-risk categories, such as exerciser women carrying more than one fetus, with multiple pregnancies, who are high cigarette smokers, heavy alcohol consumers, and drug abusers are normally at high risk of delivering prematurely with low body weight and with new-born's malformations [39].

According to the mentioned subcommittee, special groups of pregnant women should daily take a multivitamin-mineral preparation containing several nutrients beginning in the second trimester as follows: iron = 30 mg/day, vitamin B-6 = 2 mg/day, zinc = 15 mg/day, folate = 300 µg/day, copper = 2 mg/day, vitamin C = 50 mg/day, calcium = 250 mg/day, and vitamin D = 5 µg/day. To improve the absorption of these minerals and vitamins, this supplement should be taken between meals or at bedtime [22].

13.4 Nutritional Status of the Pregnant Exerciser and Athlete

As mentioned before, during pregnancy, energy, and nutrient requirements are normally increased to support maternal metabolism changes, increased blood volume, and red cells expansion, and the delivery of energy and nutrients for the fetus development [6, 16, 40].

The additional energy needs for a pregnant woman with a mean gestational weight gain of 12 kg are estimated to be [13]:

1st trimester	• 325 MJ (77,700 kcal) in total and 375 kJ/day (90 kcal/day)
2nd trimester	• 1200 kJ/day (287 kcal/day)
3rd trimester	• 1950 kJ/day (466 kcal/day)

Table 13.2 Recommendations of the Institute of Medicine and the National Council Research (2009) for total weight gain range in singleton pregnancies by prepregnancy body mass index [22]

Pre-pregnancy BMI (kg/m^2)	Total weight gain (kg)	Total weight gain (lbs)	Weekly weight gain range in the second and thirds trimester, kg (lbs)
Underweight (<18.5 kg/m^2)	12.5–18.0	28–40	0.44–0.58 (1.0–1.3)
Normal weight (18.5–24.9 kg/m^2)	11.5–16.0	25–35	0.35–0.50 (0.8–1.0)
Overweight (25.0–29.9 kg/m^2)	7.0–11.5	15–25	0.23–0.33 (0.5–0.7)
Obese[a] (>30.0 kg/m^2)	5.0–9.0	11–20	0.17–0.27 (0.4–0.6)

[a] Includes obesity class I (30–34.9 kg/m^2), II (35–39.9 kg/m^2) and III (>40 kg/m^2)

However, a pregnant exerciser or athlete who continues to train during pregnancy may have a total energy expenditure quite high, which will depend on the type, intensity, frequency, and duration of the activities performed [23].

Because of the type (high intensity, prolonged, and frequent) of training done by elite athletes, it is likely that weight gain will be less for both mother and fetus than for sedentary women [41].

In accordance with the Institute of Medicine and the National Research Council recommendations [22], an important strategy should be adopted by the pregnant woman that is monitoring her energy intake by comparing her body weight gain and body mass index (Table 13.2).

13.4.1 Energy and Nutritional Requirements for the Pregnant Exerciser and Athlete

The practice of a healthy nutritional intake must be reached by adequate energy availability, including key micronutrients, especially iron, folate, zinc, calcium, vitamin D, and essential fatty acids that promote red blood cell production, enzyme activity, bone development, and brain development [6].

For a reference 17-year-old active woman the estimated average energy requirements, such as 2740 kcal/day and 2852 kcal/day are recommended for the second and the third semester of pregnancy, respectively (Table 13.3), in accordance with the Recommended Dietary Allowances (RDA) from the Food and Nutrition Board/Institute of Medicine (FNB/IM) [42].

An average energy increase of 14%–18% (mean of 16%–Fig. 13.4) is estimated to be the recommended during pregnancy.

However, the German National Consensus Recommendations on Nutrition and Lifestyle in Pregnancy by the 'Healthy Start—Young Family Network considers the increase of only 10% more energy intake in the final months of the pregnancy [43], relying on the slight increases in energy needs, as mentioned before.

Table 13.3 Estimated energy and nutrients requirements for a reference 17-year-old active woman according to the Food and Nutrition Board, Institute of Medicine [16, 42, 44–48]

Dietary reference intakes (DRI's)	Nonpregnant	Pregnant
Energy (kcal/day)	2400	2740–2852[a]
Carbohydrate (g/day)	130	175
Protein (g/day)	46	71
Vitamin A (µg/day)	700	770
Vitamin D (µg/day)	5	5
Vitamin E (mg/day)	15	15
Vitamin K(µg/day)	90	90
Thiamin(mg/day)	1.1	1.4
Riboflavin (mg/day)	1.1	1.4
Niacin (mg/day)	14	18
Pantothenic acid (mg/day)	5	6
Biotin (µg/day)	30	30
Vitamin B-6 (mg/day)	1.3	1.9
Folate (µg/day)	400	600
Vitamin B-12 (µg/day)	2.4	2.6
Vitamin C (mg/day)	75	85
Choline (mg/day)	425	450
Sodium (g/day)	1.5	1.5
Potassium (mg/day)	4.7	4.7
Chloride (g/day)	2.3	2.3
Calcium (mg/day)	1000	1000
Phosphorus (mg/day)	700	700
Magnesium (mg/day)	310	350
Iron (mg/day)	18	27
Zinc (mg/day)	8	11
Selenium (µg/day)	55	60
Iodine (µg/day)	150	220
Copper (µg/day)	900	1000
Manganese (mg/day)	1.8	2
Fluoride (mg/day)	3	3
Chromium (µg/day)	25	30
Molybdenum (µg/day)	45	50
Water (L/day)	2.7	3000

[a]The lower value indicates the second trimester and the highest value indicates the third trimester

Regarding micronutrients, energy needs increase much more than for macronutrients (Fig. 13.4). Even prior to conception, an increased average intake of folate, iodine, and iron is recommended [43]. However, only at the beginning of the second trimester, a marked increase in vitamins and minerals is observed, as can be seen in Table 13.3 and in Fig. 13.4.

Although recommended dietary allowance (RDA) for vitamins D, E and K, biotin, sodium, potassium, chloride, calcium, phosphorus, and fluoride are not increased during pregnancy, estimated energy (as mentioned before), protein, specific

Fig. 13.4 Percentage of increase in DRIs from the non-pregnancy to pregnancy in accordance with the Food and Nutrition Board, Institute of Medicine [42, 44–48]

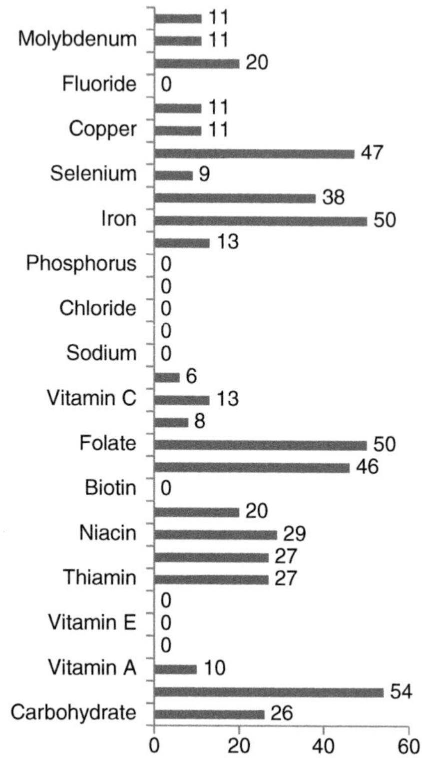

vitamins (vitamin A, thiamin, niacin, pantothenic acid, vitamin B-6, folate, vitamin B-12, vitamin C) and minerals (choline, magnesium, iron, zinc, selenium, iodine, copper, manganese, chromium, and molybdenum) requirements are increased in the second and the third trimesters (Fig. 13.4).

In relation to fiber intake, the FNB/IM recommends an average intake for total fiber of 28 g/day for a pregnant woman (14 g/1.000 kcal × 1.978 kcal/1.000 kcal/ day), slightly higher than the estimated for a nonpregnant woman (25 g/day) [42].

For water intake (from beverages, foods, and drinking water), the FNB/IM recommends an increase from 2.7 L for nonpregnant women to 3.0 L for pregnant women in order to meet hydration needs [48].

13.5 Diet and Physical Exercise

Even though pregnancy adversely affects the performance, most elite athletes prefer to continue to train during pregnancy.

The relatively high intensity, long duration, and frequent workout schedules of most competitive athletes may place them at greater risk of thermoregulatory complications during pregnancy [16].

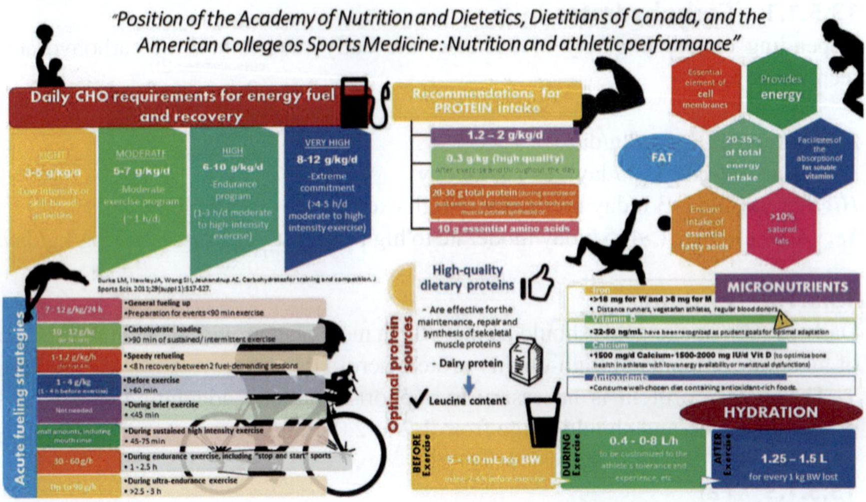

Fig. 13.5 Infographic of the position of the Academy of Nutrition and Dietetics, Dietitians of Canada, and the American College of Sports Medicine about nutrition and athletic performance [51]

Particular attention should be paid to diet and hydration during and between these exercise sessions.

For the pregnant exerciser and athlete, the main ergogenic aid will be the manipulation of diet and hydration.

An ergogenic aid is defined as any training technique, mechanical device, nutritional practice, pharmacological method, or psychological technique that can improve exercise performance capacity and/or enhance training adaptations [49].

Supplementation in pregnancy can be interesting because many women do not comply with the recommendations of some nutrients, namely vitamins or minerals through exclusive feeding.

However, it is important that the food intake and body composition are supervised by an expert and that it is of quality to ensure complete safety for the fetus.

Nutritional needs and manipulation of diet and hydration are like nonpregnant female athletes [50].

In Fig. 13.5, the nutritional needs are explained according to the intensity of the exercise practiced [51].

13.5.1 Daily Requirements by Activity

Daily macronutrients requirements are dependent on the intensity of the physical exercise as follows [51]:

13.5.1.1 Carbohydrates

Depending on the intensity of exercise, the daily requirement of carbohydrates increases:

Light exercise: 3–5 g/kg/day.
Moderate exercise (1 h/day): 5–7 g/kg/day.
High exercise: (1–3 h/day moderate to high exercise): 6–10 g/kg/day.
Very high exercise (>4–5 h/day moderate to high-intensity exercise): 8–12 g/kg/day.

13.5.1.2 Proteins

Daily protein intake goals should be met with a meal plan providing a regular spread of moderate amounts of high-quality protein across the day.

The dietary protein is necessary to support metabolic adaptation, repair and protein turnover, and should range from 1.2 to 2.0 g/kg/day.

13.5.1.3 Fat

Fat intakes that accommodate dietary goals typically range from 20 to 35% of total energy intake.

13.5.2 Dietary Intake Before Physical Exercise

According to the International Society of Sports Nutrition, the daily consumption of high-carbohydrate meals (65%) is recommended to maintain muscle glycogen, while increased ingestion rates are employed (70%) in the 5–7 days leading up to competition as a means of maximizing muscle and liver glycogen stores and to sustain blood glucose during exercise [50].

To get good muscle glycogen stores, it is necessary to follow a carbohydrate-rich diet (600–1000 g or 8–10 g/kg/day) [50].

Carbohydrate and protein levels before doing exercise depends on the duration and the fitness level, but general guidelines recommend the ingestion of 1–2 g/carbohydrates/kg of body weight and 0.15–0.25 g/ protein/kg of body weight 3–4 h before competition [50].

The recommendation to maintain euhydration before exercise is to consume a fluid volume equivalent to 5–10 ml/kg of body weight in the 2 to 4 h before exercise [51].

13.5.3 Dietary Intake During Physical Exercise

As exercise duration increases beyond 60 min, exogenous sources of carbohydrates become important to maintain blood glucose and muscle glycogen stores.

This carbohydrates source should supply 30–60 g/h and can typically be delivered by drinking 1–2 cups of a 6–8% carbohydrates solution (8–16 fluid ounces) every 10–15 min [52].

Because exogenous carbohydrates oxidation rates from single carbohydrates do not exceed 1.0–1.1 g/min, it has been recommended to ensure a carbohydrates intake of 60–70 g/h. A higher carbohydrate intake may result in gastrointestinal problems and a lower intake may result in a suboptimal carbohydrate delivery [52].

The fluid intake should be 0.4–0.8 L/h, although it should be adapted to the tolerance and experience of each athlete [51].

In terms of protein intake, 0.05–0.08 g/kg of body weight in activities or workouts lasting more than 1.5 h is recommended during exercise.

In addition, the relatively high intensity, long duration, and frequent workout schedules of most competitive athletes may place them at greater risk of thermoregulatory complications during pregnancy.

Therefore, particular attention should be paid to maintaining proper hydration during and between these exercise sessions.

Fluid balance during an exercise session can be monitored by weighing before and after the session. Any loss of weight is a fluid loss that should be made up before the next exercise session (1 lb weight loss ≈ 1 pint of fluid).

In addition, the consumption of so-called energy drinks is not recommended, because they normally present high amounts of caffeine [43].

13.5.4 Dietary Intake After Physical Exercise

Following the exercise or training, it is recommended the intake of carbohydrates along with proteins, i.e., 0.8–1–1.2 g/kg of carbohydrates must be ingested together with 0.25–0.4 g/kg of proteins of high quality.

The muscle adaptation to training can be maximized by ingesting 0.3 g/kg of body weight to high quality after key exercise sessions and every 3 to 5 h [53].

Effective rehydration requires the intake of a greater volume of fluid (1.25 to 1.5 L of fluid for every 1 kg of body weight lost).

Again, fluid balance during an exercise session can be monitored by weighing before and after the session. Any loss of weight is a fluid loss that should be made up before the next exercise session (1 lb weight loss ≈ 1 pint of fluid).

13.6 Unhealthy Habits to Avoid

13.6.1 Alcohol, Smoking, and Other Stimulant Substances

Generally, the fetal development is the most susceptible period of exposure to two modifiable lifestyle factors, such as alcohol and tobacco.

The consumption of alcohol during pregnancy promotes a range of effects in exposed children, including hyperactivity and attention problems, learning and memory deficits, and problems with social and emotional development.

The most serious outcome of maternal drinking during pregnancy is fetal alcohol syndrome.

Although it seems clear that heavy alcohol consumption during pregnancy can produce fetal alcohol syndrome, the consequences of drinking at low-to-moderate levels on children's neurodevelopment are much less obvious. Safe levels of alcohol consumption during pregnancy have not yet been established, so it is recommended to avoid alcohol consumption during pregnancy [54].

On the other hand, according to data from epidemiological studies, it is estimated that about 20–30% of women actually smoke during pregnancy and about half of the nonsmoking pregnant women are exposed to passive smoking [54].

Results from a population-based birth cohort (Generation R Study) reflected that children of mothers who continued smoking during pregnancy had a higher risk of behavioral problems at 18 months compared to the children of mothers who never smoke with adjustment for age and gender ($p < 0.05$). According to a recently published analysis, based on the data from prospective Polish Mother and Child Cohort, with an assessment of exposure based on biomarker measurements (3 times in pregnancy and in children at 1 and 2 years of age), cotinine level in saliva collected during pregnancy was significantly associated with decreased motor abilities at 24 months of age ($p = 0.02$) and not with cognitive and language achievements after controlling for a variety of confounders [54]. For these reasons, tobacco consumption should be avoided either actively or passively.

As for caffeine consumption during pregnancy, intake of ≥6 units/day during pregnancy is related to impaired fetal weight and length growth [55].

Pregnant women have slower caffeine metabolism, with 1.5 to 3.5 times longer half-life needed to eliminate caffeine compared to nonpregnant women [56].

The fetal growth characteristics associated with length or skeleton appear to be more affected from the first trimester onwards. Pregnant women should be advised not to consume ≥6 units of caffeine (>540 mg) per day during pregnancy [55].

On the other hand, the American Congress of Obstetricians and Gynecologists states that moderate consumption of caffeine (<200 mg/day) during pregnancy is not a major risk factor for miscarriage or premature birth [57].

As already mentioned, the nutritional environment during embryonic, fetal, and neonatal development plays a very important role in the offspring's risk of developing diseases later in life. Non-nutritive sweeteners furnish the sweet taste without increasing the energy supply.

Animal studies showed that long-term consumption, particularly aspartame, starting during the perigestational period may predispose the offspring to develop obesity and metabolic syndrome later in life [58].

Human extrapolation should be performed very cautiously, as well-designed clinical studies that evaluate the metabolic effects of non-nutritive sweeteners in humans are still lacking.

In turn, adverse effects associated with non-nutritive sweeteners found in animal studies suggest that its use in the human diet as an alternative to nutritive sweeteners during pregnancy should be carefully examined before recommending or not using them [58].

13.6.2 Lack of Sleep

Daily sleep requirements are increased as early as the first trimester of pregnancy, as well as daytime sleepiness in this period of the woman's life cycle [59–65]. In pregnant women, insufficient sleep duration and quality may result from sleep disturbances, such as insomnia, restless legs syndrome, and sleep apnea [66].

Restless legs syndrome is 2 to 3 times more prevalent in pregnant women than in the general population [67], characterized by an unpleasant sensation leading to sudden movement of the legs, often associated with pain, which hinders the onset of sleep.

The scientific literature demonstrates an association between sleep disturbances and negative consequences of pregnancy [68–70], namely a high risk of preeclampsia, cesarean delivery, and depressive symptomatology [71–73].

The peak incidence occurs in the third trimester, and in most cases, the symptoms disappear 1 month after giving birth [67, 74].

These symptoms can be relieved by the movement of the legs, such as walking or kicking. It is probably due to anomalies in the neurotransmitter dopamine [28].

In pregnant women, sleep apnea is associated with overweight and obesity. The breathing is momentarily interrupted and may be accompanied by the typical snoring. Therefore, pregnant women may experience excessive drowsiness during the day, as their sleep may not have been remedial [28].

Since interruption of regular breathing or airway obstruction during sleep may represent serious health complications, symptoms of sleep apnea should be evaluated and monitored during pregnancy [66].

13.7 Conclusion

As pregnancy progresses, several changes occur that will prevent the exerciser or athlete from attaining the same performance levels as before pregnancy.

Weight gain, by itself and in the presence of laxity of joints and ligaments and change in the center of gravity will cause unavoidable limitations in most sporting activities. The ability to stop and start or to change direction will progressively decrease. Any attempts to substitute compensatory movements for finely tuned skill movements result in inefficient movement, a decrease in competitive ability, and an increase in the risk of injury.

Performance in sports in which endurance is important may be adversely affected by the physiological anemia commonly associated with the increased blood volume of pregnancy.

Even though pregnancy adversely affects performance in the competitive athlete, most elite athletes prefer to continue to train during pregnancy.

In fact, pregnant athletes tend to maintain a more strenuous training schedule throughout pregnancy and resume high-intensity postpartum training sooner.

Concerns of the pregnant competitive athlete fall into two general categories: the effects of pregnancy on her competitive ability; and the effects of strenuous training and competition on pregnancy, particularly on her fetus.

Such athletes would certainly require closer obstetric and nutritional supervision than routine prenatal care. Additional testing and intervention should occur as clinically indicated.

References

1. Tompkins WT, Wiehl DG. Nutritional deficiencies as a casual factor in toxemia and premature labor. Am J Obstet Gynecol. 1951;62:898–919.
2. Venkatachalam PS. Maternal nutritional status and its effect on the newborn. Bull World Health Organ. 1962;26:193–201.
3. Dodd JM, Grivell RM, Nguyen AM, et al. Maternal and perinatal health outcomes by body mass index category. Aust N Z J Obstet Gynaecol. 2011;51:136–40.
4. Guelinckx I, Devlieger R, Beckers K, et al. Maternal obesity: pregnancy complications, gestational weight gain and nutrition. Obes Rev. 2008;9:140–50.
5. Blumfield ML, Hure AJ, Macdonald-Wicks L, et al. A systematic review and meta-analysis of micronutrient intakes during pregnancy in developed countries. Nutr Rev. 2013;71:118–32.
6. Grieger JA, Clifton VL. A review of the impact of dietary intakes in human pregnancy on infant birthweight. Nutrients. 2014;7(1):153–78.
7. Perng W, Stuart J, Rifas-Shiman SL, et al. Preterm birth and long-term maternal cardiovascular health. Ann Epidemiol. 2015;25(1):40–5.
8. Gillman MW, Rifas-Shiman SL, Kleinman K, et al. Developmental origins of childhood overweight: potential public health impact. Obesity (Silver Spring). 2008;16:1651–6.
9. Callaway LK, Prins JB, Chang AM, et al. The prevalence and impact of overweight and obesity in an australian obstetric population. Med J Aust. 2006;184:56–9.
10. Ehrenberg HM, Mercer BM, Catalano PM. The influence of obesity and diabetes on the prevalence of macrosomia. Am J Obstet Gynecol. 2004;191:964–8.
11. WHO. Energy and protein requirements. Report of a Joint FAO/WHO/UNU Expert Consultation. Technical Report Series No. 724. Geneva: World Health Organization; 1985.
12. Hytten FE. Nutrition. In: Hytten FE, Chamberlain G, editors. Clinical physiology in obstetrics. Oxford: Blackwell Scientific; 1980. p. 163–92.
13. Butte NF, King JC. Energy requirements during pregnancy and lactation. Public Health Nutr. 2005;8(7a):1010–27.
14. Butte N, Caballero B. Energy needs: assessment and requirements. In: Shils M, Shike M, Ross A, Caballero B, Cousins R, editors. Modern nutrition in health and disease. 10th ed. Baltimore/Philadelphia: Lippincott Williams & Wilkins; 2006. p. 136–48.
15. Artal R, O'toole M. Guidelines of the American College of Obstetricians and Gynecologists for exercise during pregnancy and the postpartum period. Br J Sports Med. 2003;37(1):6–12.
16. Silva M-RG, Bellotto ML. Nutritional requirements for maternal and newborn health. Curr Women Health Rev. 2015;11:41–50.
17. Silva M-RG, Paiva T. Low energy availability and low body fat of female gymnasts before an international competition. Eur J Sport Sci. 2015;15(7):591–9.
18. Loucks AB, Kiens B, Wright HH. Energy availability in athletes. J Sports Sci. 2011;29:S7–15.
19. Rodriguez NR, DiMarco NM, Langley S, et al. Position of the American dietetic association, dietitians of Canada and the American College of Sports Medicine: nutrition and athletic performance. J Am Diet Assoc. 2009;109:509–27.
20. Forsum E, Löf M. Energy metabolism during human pregnancy. Annu Rev Nutr. 2007;27:277–92.
21. Hoch AZ, Pajewski NM, Moraski L, et al. Prevalence of the female athlete triad in high school athletes and sedentary students. Clin J Sport Med. 2009;19(5):421–8.

22. Institute of Medicine and National Research Council of the National Academies. Weight gain during pregnancy: reexamining the guidelines. Washington, DC, USA: Institute of Medicine and National Research Council of the National Academies.; 2009.
23. Bø K, Artal R, Barakat R, et al. Exercise and pregnancy in recreational and elite athletes: 2016 evidence summary from the IOC expert group meeting, Lausanne. Part 1-exercise in women planning pregnancy and those who are pregnant. Br J Sports Med. 2016;50(10):571–89.
24. Sundgot-Borgen J, Torstveit MK. Prevalence of eating disorders in elite athletes is higher than in the general population. Clin J Sport Med. 2004;14:25–32.
25. Sundgot-Borgen J, Torstveit MK. Aspects of disordered eating continuum in elite high-intensity sports. Scand J Med Sci Sports. 2010;20(Suppl 2):112–21.
26. Currie A. Sport and eating disorders—understanding and managing the risks. Asian J Sports Med. 2010;1:63–8.
27. Czech-Szczapa B, Szczapa T, Merritt TA, et al. Disordered eating attitudes during pregnancy in mothers of newborns requiring neonatal intensive care unit admission: a case control study. J Matern Fetal Neonatal Med. 2015;28:1711–5.
28. Silva M-RG, Paiva T. Sleep, nutrition, circadian rhythm, jet lag and athletic performance [in Portuguese]. Lisbon: Portuguese Federation of Gymnastics/Portuguese Institute of Sport and Youthood I.P; 2015.
29. Silva M-RG. Nutritional evaluation and body composition [in Portuguese]. 3rd ed. Porto: University Fernando Pessoa Press; 2015.
30. Nielsen S, Moller-Madsen S, Isager T, et al. Standardized mortality in eating disorders—a quantitative summary of previously published and new evidence. J Psychosom Res. 1998;44:413–34.
31. Cardwell MS. Eating disorders during pregnancy. Obstet Gynecol Surv. 2013;68:312–23.
32. Franko DL, Spurrell EB. Detection and management of eating disorders during pregnancy. Obstet Gynecol. 2000;95(Pt 1):942–6.
33. Mazzeo SE, Slof-Opt Landt MC, Jones I, et al. Associations among postpartum depression, eating disorders, and perfectionism in a population-based sample of adult women. Int J Eat Disord. 2006;39:202–11.
34. Koubaa S, Hallstrom T, Lindholm C, et al. Pregnancy and neonatal outcomes in women with eating disorders. Obstet Gynecol. 2005;105:255–60.
35. Park RJ, Senior R, Stein A. The offspring of mothers with eating disorders. Eur Child Adolesc Psychiatry. 2003;12(Suppl 1):I110–9.
36. Patel P, Wheatcroft R, Park RJ, et al. The children of mothers with eating disorders. Clin Child Fam Psychol Rev. 2002;5:1–19.
37. James DC. Eating disorders, fertility, and pregnancy: relationships and complications. J Perinat Neonatal Nurs. 2001;15:36–48.
38. Brahmbhatt H, Kågesten A, Emerson M, et al. Prevalence and determinants of adolescent pregnancy in urban disadvantaged settings across five cities. J Adolesc Health. 2014;55:6S48–57.
39. van Baaren GJ, Peelen MJ, Schuit E, et al. Preterm birth in singleton and multiple pregnancies: evaluation of costs and perinatal outcomes. Eur J Obstet Gynecol Reprod Biol. 2015;3:34–41.
40. Kaiser LL, Allen L. Position of the American dietetic association: nutrition and lifestyle for a healthy pregnancy outcome. J Am Diet Assoc. 2002;102:1479–90.
41. Artal R, O'Toole M. Guidelines of the American College of Obstetricians and Gynecologists for exercise during pregnancy and the postpartum period. Br J Sports Med. 2003;37:6–12.
42. Food and Nutrition Board/Institute of Medicine. Dietary reference intakes for energy, carbohydrate, fiber, fat, fatty acids, cholesterol, protein and amino acids. Washington, DC: National Academies Press; 2005. http://www.nap.edu/catalog.php?record_id=10490.
43. Koletzko B, Bauer CP, Bung P, et al. German national consensus recommendations on nutrition and lifestyle in pregnancy by the 'Healthy start—young family Network'. Ann Nutr Metab. 2013;63(4):311–22.
44. Food and Nutrition Board/Institute of Medicine. Dietary reference intakes for vitamin a, vitamin K, arsenic, boron, chromium, copper, iodine, iron, manganese, molybdenum, nickel, silicon, vanadium, and zinc. Washington, DC: National Academies Press; 2001. http://www.nap.edu/catalog/10026.html.

45. Food and Nutrition Board/Institute of Medicine. Dietary reference intakes for thiamin, riboflavin, niacin, vitamin B6, folate, vitamin B12, pantothenic acid, biotin, and choline. Washington, DC: National Academies Press; 1999. http://www.nap.edu/catalog.php?record_id=6015.
46. Food and Nutrition Board/Institute of Medicine. Dietary reference intakes for vitamin C, vitamin E, selenium, and carotenoids. Washington, DC: National Academies Press; 2000. http://www.nap.edu/catalog.php?record_id=9810.
47. Food and Nutrition Board/Institute of Medicine. Dietary reference intakes for calcium and vitamin D. Washington, DC: National Academies Press; 2011. http://www.nap.edu/catalog.php?record_id=13050.
48. Food and Nutrition Board/Institute of Medicine. Dietary reference intakes for water, potassium, sodium, chloride, and sulfate. Washington, DC: National Academies Press; 2005. http://www.nap.edu/catalog/10925.html.
49. Buford TW, Kreider RB, Stout JR, et al. International Society of Sports Nutrition position stand: creatine supplementation and exercise. J Int Soc Sports Nutr. 2007;4(1):6.
50. Kerksick C, Harvey T, Stout J, et al. International Society of Sports Nutrition position stand: nutrient timing. J Int Soc Sports Nutr. 2008;3(5):17.
51. Thomas DT, Erdman KA, Burke LM. Position of the academy of nutrition and dietetics, dietitians of Canada, and the American College of Sports Medicine: nutrition and athletic performance. J Acad Nutr Diet. 2016;116(3):501–28.
52. Jeukendrup AE, Jentjens RLPG, Moseley L. Nutritional considerations in triathlon. Sports Med. 2005;35(2):163–81.
53. Jentjens RL, Wagenmakers AJ, Jeukendrup AE. Heat stress increases muscle glycogen use but reduces the oxidation of ingested carbohydrates during exercise. J Appl Physiol. 2002;92(4):1562–72.
54. Polańska K, Jurewicz J, Hanke W. Smoking and alcohol drinking during pregnancy as the risk factors for poor child neurodevelopment—a review of epidemiological studies. Int J Occup Med Environ Health. 2015;28(3):419–43.
55. Bakker R, Steegers EAP, Obradov A, Raat H, Hofman A, Jaddoe VWV. Maternal caffeine intake from coffee and tea, fetal growth, and the risks of adverse birth outcomes: the generation R study. Am J Clin Nutr. 2010;91(6):1691–8.
56. Rhee J, Kim R, Kim Y, et al. Maternal caffeine consumption during pregnancy and risk of low birth weight: a dose-response meta-analysis of observational studies. PLoS One. 2015;10(7):e0132334.
57. American College of Obstetricians and Gynecologists. Committee opinion: moderate caffeine consumption during pregnancy. Obstet Gynecol. 2010;116(462):467–8.
58. Araujo JR, Martel F, Keating E. Exposure to non-nutritive sweeteners during pregnancy and lactation: impact in programming of metabolic diseases in the progeny later in life. Reprod Toxicol. 2014;49:196–201.
59. Hedman C, Pohjasvaara T, Tolonen U, Suhonen-Malm AS, Myllyla VV. Effects of pregnancy on mothers' sleep. Sleep Med. 2002;3(1):37–42.
60. Mindell JA, Jacobson BJ. Sleep disturbances during pregnancy. J Obstet Gynecol Neonatal Nurs. 2000;29(6):590–7.
61. Lee KA, Gay CL. Sleep in late pregnancy predicts length of labor and type of delivery. Am J Obstet Gynecol. 2004;191(6):2041–6.
62. Lee KA, Zaffke ME, McEnany G. Parity and sleep patterns during and after pregnancy. Obstet Gynecol. 2000;95(1):14–8.
63. Le Bon O, Staner L, Hoffmann G, et al. The first-night effect may last more than one night. J Psychiatr Res. 2001;35(3):165–72.
64. Silva M-RG, Paiva T. Poor precompetitive sleep habits, nutrients' deficiencies, inappropriate body composition and athletic performance in elite gymnasts. Eur J Sport Sci. 2016;16(6):726–35.
65. Silva M-RG, Paiva T. Sleep during pregnancy: neurophysiology, disturbances and sleep hygiene [in Portuguese]. In: Santos-Rocha R, Branco M, editors. Active pregnancy—physi-

ological and biomechanical adaptations during pregnancy and postpartum. Lisbon: Foundation for Science and Technology; 2016.

66. Centers for Disease Control and Prevention. National Sleep Awareness Week. MMWR Morb Mortal Wkly Rep. 2011;60(8):233.
67. Picchietti DL, Hensley JG, Bainbridge JL, et al. Consensus clinical practice guidelines for the diagnosis and treatment of restless legs syndrome/Willis-Ekbom disease during pregnancy and lactation. Sleep Med Rev. 2014;22:64–77.
68. Chang JJ, Pien GW, Duntley SP, et al. Sleep deprivation during pregnancy and maternal and fetal outcomes: is there a relationship? Sleep Med Rev. 2010;14:107–14.
69. Nodine PM, Matthews EE. Common sleep disorders: management strategies and pregnancy outcomes. J Midwifery Womens Health. 2013;58:368–77.
70. Okun ML, Schetter CD, Glynn LM. Poor sleep quality is associated with preterm birth. Sleep. 2011;34:1493–8.
71. Ramirez JO, Cabrera SA, Hidalgo H, et al. Is preeclampsia associated with restless legs syndrome? Sleep Med. 2013;14:894–6.
72. Vahdat M, Sariri E, Miri S, et al. Prevalence and associated features of restless legs syndrome in a population of Iranian women during pregnancy. Int J Gynecol Obstet. 2013;123:46–9.
73. Wesstrom J, Skalkidou A, Manconi M, et al. Prepregnancy restless legs syndrome (Willis-Ekbom disease) is associated with perinatal depression. J Clin Sleep Med. 2014;10:527–33.
74. Ismailogullari S, Ozturk A, Mazicioglu MM, et al. Restless legs syndrome and pregnancy in Kayseri, Turkey: a hospital based survey. Sleep Biol Rhythms. 2010;8:137–43.

Diet Recommendations for the Pregnant Exerciser and Athlete

14

Rui Jorge, Diana Teixeira, Inês Ferreira, and Ana-Luisa Alvarez-Falcón

Abstract

Dietary habits play a decisive role during pregnancy and just a well-planned balanced diet can provide all the nutritional needs that this stage of life demands. Frequent exercisers and athletes also have high nutritional requirements and can benefit from a personalized diet either for health or performance purposes. Therefore, a pregnant exerciser and athlete has increased and specific dietary needs which are scarcely explored in the scientific literature.

R. Jorge (✉)
Agrarian School of Santarém - ESAS, Polytechnic Institute of Santarém, Santarém, Portugal

Sport Sciences School of Rio Maior - ESDRM, Polytechnic Institute of Santarém, Rio Maior, Portugal

School of Health Sciences - ESSLei, Polytechnic Institute of Leiria, Leiria, Portugal

Nova Medical School - Nova University of Lisbon, Lisbon, Portugal
e-mail: rui.jorge@esa.ipsantarem.pt

D. Teixeira
NOVA Medical School - FCM, NOVA University of Lisbon, Lisbon, Portugal

Comprehensive Health Research Centre - CHRC, NOVA Medical School - FCM, NOVA University of Lisbon, Lisbon, Portugal
e-mail: diana.teixeira@nms.unl.pt

I. Ferreira
Directorate General of Health, Ministry of Health, Lisbon, Portugal
e-mail: iferreira@dgs.min-saude.pt

A.- L. Alvarez-Falcón
Dietetics Unit, University Hospital of Gran Canaria, Dr. Negrin, Las Palmas de Gran Canaria, Spain
e-mail: aalvfal@gobiernodecanarias.org

R. Santos-Rocha (ed.), *Exercise and Physical Activity During Pregnancy and Postpartum*, https://doi.org/10.1007/978-3-031-06137-0_14

This chapter aims to fill the gap between evidence-based knowledge on the impact of dietary habits during pregnancy and particularly the pregnant exerciser and athlete, bridging the gap between science and practice and help researchers, nutrition and exercise professionals, and even pregnant exercisers and athletes with a summary of the main diet recommendations for pregnant exercisers and athletes.

Keywords
Pregnancy · Nutrition · Diet · Athletes · Exercisers

14.1 Introduction

Undoubtedly, adequate nutrition plays a crucial role prior to and during pregnancy, influencing mother, infant, and pregnancy outcomes. Moreover, the importance of nutrition is very well demonstrated when a substantial body of research suggests that several conditions that are present in adulthood (e.g., obesity, cardiovascular diseases, diabetes, metabolic syndrome) originate in fetal life and are influenced by diet [1, 2].

Dietary aspects assume even higher importance in special populations such as pregnant exercisers and athletes, whose energy and nutritional requirements are higher than their nonpregnant counterparts, prior to, during, and post-pregnancy. Additionally, due to the particularities of the practiced sport, these women could be more prone to having an inadequate nutritional status and weight (e.g., pregnant athletes practicing aesthetic sports [gymnastics, ballet, artistic skating], weight competing sports [canoeing, judo], pregnant women who restrict certain food items) [3].

This chapter aims to provide an overview of evidence-based dietary advice to promote a healthy pregnancy in pregnant exercisers and athletes. The chapter finishes with a set of practical recommendations mainly intended to support all professional groups (e.g., trainers, exercise physiologists, and other sports professionals) that follow and provide counseling to this group of pregnant women.

14.2 Diet Quality During Pregnancy

Pregnant women are recommended to pay particular attention to the quality of their diet [4]. A high-quality diet may be defined as one which is hygienically safe, nutritious, balanced, adapted to individual requirements, and capable of ensuring a good state of health and preventing disease [5].

Compared to the energy requirements, the requirement for individual vitamins and minerals increases much more in pregnancy (namely vitamin A, folate, iodine, and zinc). However, excluding folate and iodine, and other vitamins and minerals in particular dietary patterns (e.g., vegetarian or vegan diets), the higher requirements of vitamins and minerals can be easily achieved by adequate food choices [4]. Due to this, pregnant women are generally encouraged to have a high-quality diet, balanced and varied, characterized by: an abundant consumption of food items with a high nutrient density (high content of essential nutrients relative to their energy content), such as vegetables, fruits, legumes, wholegrain cereals; moderate consumption of animal-based foods (e.g., milk and dairy products, low fat-meat, oily fish, eggs); and a limited consume of sweets, snacks, sugar-containing beverages and oils with a high content of saturated fatty acids (coconut, palm oil) [4]. Despite that, data on dietary quality of pregnant exercisers and athletes is scarce.

14.2.1 Determinants of Dietary Quality

Some researchers had evaluated the association between maternal diet quality during pregnancy and health outcomes in early life and childhood. Tahir et al. observed that a higher maternal diet quality from pregnancy until 3 months postpartum was inversely associated with infant weight-for-length from birth to 6 months, and with infant body fat percent at 6 months [2]. Findings in concordance with other studies [6, 7] suggest the association between maternal diet quality and infant body composition, namely with neonatal and infant adiposity. Dietary intake during pregnancy is also associated with a higher risk of offspring asthma [8]. Therefore, it is important to identify and recognize the determinants of dietary quality in pregnant women.

Various sociodemographic, pregnancy-related, cultural, environmental, and lifestyle factors (such as age, sex, education, parity, body mass index, and physical activity level) seem to influence diet quality [9, 10]. Accessing these determinants is important since they potentially influence and can contribute to target nutritional interventions. For example, Suárez-Martínez et al. have observed that pregnant women with younger age, previous deliveries, lower educational levels, and unhealthy lifestyles, such as lack of physical activity, have a higher risk of having a low adherence to the Mediterranean dietary pattern, which is an example of a dietary pattern generally recognized as a healthy for pregnant women [11]. The lack of studies investigating pregnancy determinants is in contrast with theoretical and empirical literature framing pregnancy as a physiologically and psychologically, but in high- and upper-middle-income countries, evidence consistently points to a social gradient whereby women who are older, more educated, and with higher incomes are more likely to follow a healthy diet [10].

14.2.2 Dietary Sources of Nutrients

Nutritional needs for pregnancy and physical activity can be ensured if the pregnant women's diet follows the principles of healthy eating, recommended by the majority of the food-based dietary guidelines (e.g., food pyramid, healthy eating plate), that is, ensuring a complete, balanced and varied diet [12–14]. Generally, foods from each one of the groups of the food-based dietary guidelines should be consumed daily (complete diet), and foods belonging to the larger groups should be consumed in greater quantities (e.g., cereal products, vegetables, and fruit) compared to foods belonging to smaller groups (e.g., oils and meat) (balanced diet) and different foods should be consumed within each group, varying daily and weekly (varied diet) [12]. Encouraging to drink water and promoting the intake of fish, fruits, and vegetables and on the other hand advising against drinking sugar-sweetened beverages and the intake of sugary foods, red and processed meats are recommendations displayed across most food-based dietary guidelines, alongside with the frequent promotion of legumes intake and olive oil and nuts intake as preferable fat sources [13, 15]. Since during pregnancy and in more physically active individuals, energy and nutritional needs are increased for some nutrients, food-based dietary guidelines usually advise on eating bigger portions of the recommended foods (e.g., if the recommendation presented in the food guide is to intake three to five portions of fruit per day, in more active women five portions of fruit per day would be preferable than three portions of fruit per day), but within the same recommended proportions.

14.2.2.1 Protein Dietary Sources

Protein deficiency during pregnancy has several consequences, including inadequate fetal growth. Furthermore, protein is always crucial to an athlete, so it is especially critical in the pregnant exerciser diet. Note that not only the quantity but also the quality of the protein provided by the diet is an important factor. The protein of animal origin, due to its greater bioavailability and the presence of all essential amino acids, has high nutritional quality; however, the composition of saturated fatty acids and trans fatty acids should be considered when choosing food (animal protein sources usually have more saturated fatty acids than vegetable protein food sources) [16]. Notwithstanding vegetable protein food sources alone can adequately provide all protein needs, when well-balanced or in the presence of a higher total protein intake [17].

A balanced dietary pattern between protein sources of animal origin with a better lipid profile (e.g., fish, lean meat), complemented with good protein sources of vegetable origin such as pulses, whole grains, and nuts, is adequate to meet the protein needs at this stage of the life cycle [16].

To achieve adequate protein intake:

- Include dairy products (e.g., milk, cheese, yogurt) at breakfast and snacks.
- Alternate between eating poultry, fish, pulses (e.g., beans, chickpeas, broad beans, peas, lentils), or eggs.
- Choose to include preferably white meat (i.e., rabbit, chicken, turkey).
- Consume fish 2–3 times a week (fish with low levels of methylmercury—see Sect. 14.6.

14.2.2.2 Carbohydrates and Fiber Dietary Sources

Concerning the choice of food, priority should be given to complex carbohydrates from whole grains, legumes, fruit, and vegetables over free sugars such as added sugar and that naturally present in honey, corn syrup, fruit juices, and fruit juice concentrates, which induce a faster and more accentuated glycemic response [18].

Carbohydrates are the main source of energy for the performance of the body's functions, so their consumption during pregnancy and/or physical activity is of great importance. During pregnancy, blood sugars are more susceptible to moving out of their normal range. With all the extra demands on the body, proper pregnancy nutrition requires to take in an adequate amount of carbohydrates. This will help the body to sustain healthy blood sugar levels throughout your workout. From the carbohydrates that the mother ingests, glucose is obtained, which is the main source of energy and fundamental for the development of the fetus, and fiber, which is important for regulating its intestinal transit. Therefore, it is important to ingest, daily and several times a day, foods rich in carbohydrates, such as wholegrain bread, potatoes, rice, pasta, and oats [12]. Since the size of body carbohydrate stores is relatively limited, the carbohydrate provides a key fuel for the brain and central nervous system and a versatile substrate for muscular work where it can support exercise over a large range of intensities due to its utilization by both anaerobic and oxidative pathway and that there is significant evidence that the performance of prolonged sustained or intermittent high-intensity exercise is enhanced by strategies that maintain high carbohydrate availability (i.e., match glycogen stores and blood glucose to the fuel demands of exercise), while depletion of these stores is associated with fatigue in the form of reduced work rates, impaired skill and concentration, and increased perception of effort, it is important to consider a personalized supply of carbohydrate before, during, and in the recovery between training sessions or events to enhance carbohydrate availability in athletes [19], including pregnant exercisers and athletes.

- Choose the whole-grain versions in at least half of your daily carbohydrate sources (e.g., whole pasta, rice, or bread, and oat flakes).
- Choose wholegrain products with reduced fat, sugar, and salt content.
- Prefer fresh fruits over juices or purees.
- In the main meals serve at least half of the dish with vegetables.
- Reduce consumption of sugary products (e.g., cakes, sweets, pastries, biscuits).

14.2.2.3 Fat and Omega 3 Dietary Sources

Food-based fat has essential functions in the body as a great energy supplier, transport of some vitamins (A, D, E, K), protection against cold, and development of the fetal central nervous system and retina [20]. There are no specific dietary recommendations for pregnant women, however, they have increased needs for essential fatty acids, namely omega-6 and omega-3 [16, 18]. Fat intake in athletes should follow food-based guidelines and be individually adjusted based on training level and body composition goals [21].

To achieve adequate fat intake:

- For cooking and seasoning food, prefer olive oil.
- Include at least a small portion (20 g) of nuts (e.g., walnuts, hazelnuts, peanuts, or almonds), at least 4 times per week.

- Consume 2–3 servings (233–250 g) of fish per week, taking into account the fish species that should be privileged/limited during pregnancy, considering their mercury content.

14.2.2.4 Folate Dietary Sources

Folate supports the growth of the placenta and fetus. Maternal folate deficiency is associated with an increased incidence of congenital malformations, neural tube defects, including anencephaly and spina bifida, and possibly cleft lip and congenital cardiac malformations [20]. Therefore, and despite supplementation being present, it is recommended to increase the consumption of fruit and vegetables rich in this vitamin (e.g., watercress, cabbage, beetroot, brussels sprouts, asparagus), as well as the consumption of whole grains (e.g., whole bread, whole pasta, and rice) and pulses (e.g., lentils, peas, beans, chickpeas, broad beans) [22].

14.2.2.5 Vitamin C Dietary Sources

Vitamin C plays a key role due to its antioxidant activity and promotes iron absorption. During pregnancy, the needs are increased, so citrus fruits, kiwi fruit, strawberry, or vegetables such as green and red peppers, red cabbage, or those with dark green leaves should be included daily in the pregnant women's diet [16].

14.2.2.6 Vitamin D Dietary Sources

Vitamin D is naturally present in a few foods, but it can be produced endogenously through the action of ultraviolet radiation from sunlight on the skin [16, 20, 23]. Thus, moderate daily sun exposure is recommended, taking into account measures to prevent skin cancer, to prevent vitamin D deficiency, and insufficiency [24]. Besides most fish and some foods fortified with vitamin D, the majority of foods do not have vitamin D or are a relatively small vitamin D source (e.g., eggs and dairy products). Athletes who live at higher latitudes (i.e., > 35th parallel), that mainly train indoors, with darker skin, with higher body fat content, mostly train in the early morning and evening periods, that have most of their skin covered (e.g., clothing, equipment, and screening/blocking lotions) during the exercise sessions, are at increased risk for Vitamin D insufficiency and deficiency [25].

14.2.2.7 Calcium Dietary Sources

Inadequate calcium intake contributes to the development of osteopenia, paresthesias, muscle cramps, and increases the risk of preeclampsia, and intrauterine growth restriction [16, 20]. Calcium is transported in the placenta by active transport, and to meet fetal needs, maternal calcium absorption at the intestinal level is doubled during pregnancy [16, 20, 26].

Dairy products such as milk, cheese, and yogurt are a great source of calcium, so they should be included in the mother's diet. Low-fat products should be favored when possible. If the consumption of dairy products is contraindicated, calcium can also be found in other foods, such as calcium-fortified soy vegetable drinks (check the label for calcium content); calcium-fortified breakfast cereals (check the label);

canned fish (such as canned sardines); some dark green leafy vegetables (e.g., kale, arugula, and watercress); nuts including almonds, hazelnuts, and seeds [22].

14.2.2.8 Iron Dietary Sources

Insufficient iron intake during pregnancy can compromise oxygen transport to the fetus, and consequently its development, and is associated with increased cardiovascular risk in adulthood. Maternal iron deficiency should be avoided as it is associated with an increased risk of low birth weight, prematurity, perinatal mortality, and neurodevelopmental disorders [27].

The absorption of heme iron, present in animal products, is considerably superior to the absorption of non-heme iron, found in plant foods, in which phytates and phenolic compounds inhibit iron absorption, which can also be increased by the consumption of vitamin C.

Canned sardines, lean meat (e.g., rabbit, chicken, turkey), red meat (e.g., beef), and eggs are good sources of animal-derived iron. Pulses (e.g., white beans, butter and red beans, lentils, and chickpeas), and some vegetables (e.g., spinach, lettuce, arugula, broccoli) are considerable important plant-based iron sources.

To improve iron absorption:

- Include a source of vitamin C (e.g., orange, mandarin, kiwi, strawberry) at lunch and dinner.
- Avoid drinking tea or coffee with main meals (consume 1–2 h before or after).
- Include different sources of iron (meat or fish with pulses or vegetables).

14.2.2.9 Magnesium Dietary Sources

Magnesium is a cofactor and activator of several enzymatic reactions (>300), being essential for the metabolism of macro and micronutrients, cell growth, and for ensuring the structure and permeability of cell membranes, the response of the immune system, and prevention of inflammation. At the end of pregnancy, the fetus accumulates 1 g of magnesium and its maternal deficit can interfere with fetal growth and development [28].

Whole grains are one of the main dietary sources of magnesium, so they must be included in at least half of the cereals and derivatives consumed throughout the day.

14.2.2.10 Iodine Dietary Sources

Iodine is part of the thyroxine molecule, which plays a key role in metabolism, fetal neuronal myelination, and gene expression. During pregnancy, the synthesis of thyroid hormones increases by 50% which also explains the increase in iodine requirements at this stage [16]. Severe deficiency in this mineral is associated with postpartum hypothyroidism, perinatal mortality, congenital malformations, neonatal hypothyroidism, and impaired fetal neurocognitive development [16]. Inadequate iodine intake is associated with the development of attention deficit or hyperactivity disorders, decreased intelligence quotient, and in more severe cases cretinism [16, 29]. However, high levels of iodine should also be taken into account because they potentially induce the same effects as deficiency [16].

In order to contribute to the proper intake of iodine, a varied diet should be ensured, including foods that are usually sources of iodine, in particular: fish, milk, other dairy products, and eggs.

14.2.2.11 Zinc Dietary Sources

Zinc is an important component of more than 200 enzymes, nucleotides, proteins, and hormones, participating in protein synthesis, nucleic acid metabolism, cell division, gene expression, antioxidant defense, immune, neurological, and vision function [16, 20]. Severe zinc deficiency induces congenital malformations, including anencephaly, and if moderate can compromise fetal growth, brain development, and immune function [16, 20, 23]. Women with untreated zinc deficiency are at increased risk of miscarriage, intrauterine growth restriction, preeclampsia, preterm birth, and intrapartum hemorrhage [23].

Good sources of zinc are meat, cheese, nuts and seeds (e.g., pine nuts and pumpkin seeds), whole grains, and whole-grain bread.

14.2.2.12 Selenium Dietary Sources

Selenium plays an important role in antioxidant activity, with a relevant role in fertility [16]. Decreased selenium levels are associated with recurrent miscarriages, preeclampsia, intrauterine growth restriction, glucose intolerance, changes in lipid profile, and impairment of cognitive and psychomotor development [16, 30]. Selenium food sources vary depending on the soils and water used in food production. Among the foods with the highest content are oat seeds and oat bran.

14.2.3 Dietary Patterns

14.2.3.1 Mediterranean Diet

If initially the Mediterranean Diet was just used to describe the traditional dietary patterns of countries around the Mediterranean Sea, nowadays, it is the most widely studied dietary approach to healthy eating and disease prevention, being strongly associated with cardiovascular, metabolic, cognitive, and possibility antineoplastic benefits [31]. The Mediterranean dietary pattern is characterized by a high intake of extra virgin (cold pressed) olive oil, vegetables, fruits, cereals, nuts, and pulses; moderate intake of fish, meat, dairy products, and red wine; and a low intake of eggs and sweets [32]. Usually, Mediterranean Diet is graphically represented through the use of a pyramid. At the bottom of the pyramid, are represented food items that are the base of this diet, plant-based foods (fruits, vegetables, cereals, bread, pasta, rice, couscous, olive oil, olives, nuts, seeds, herbs), which should be consumed in higher proportions and frequency due to their richness in key nutrients and protective substances (vitamins, micronutrients, fiber, omega-3 fatty acids, polyphenols, flavonoids). At the upper levels, we found foods of animal origin, which should be eaten in moderation [33]. Besides considerations regarding the proportion and frequency of food consumption, the Mediterranean Diet pyramid highlights concepts, such as moderation/frugality, socialization, physical activity, adequate rest, and seasonality [33].

Prior to and during pregnancy, a higher adherence to the Mediterranean dietary pattern has been associated with a lower gestational weight gain and with a reduced risk of developing gestational diabetes [34–37]. Therefore, as will be hereafter addressed, in Sect. 14.5.2, Mediterranean Diet could be used as a preventive tool against gestational diabetes.

Although more randomized controlled trials are necessary, a growing body of evidence shows the benefits of following a Mediterranean dietary pattern during pregnancy on children's health, namely regarding the reduction of the risk of early preterm birth, birth defects (e.g., anencephaly), asthma, and allergy [8, 38]. Based on the Mediterranean dietary pattern, pregnant women can adapt the total portions in terms of their daily physical activity.

14.2.3.2 Vegetarian Diets

Worldwide, the adoption of vegetarian and vegan diets has become more popular and common. Although vegetarian diets could be associated with a higher risk of having macro and micronutrient deficiencies, the evidence demonstrates that these dietary patterns could provide an adequate nutrient intake and be considered safe, if

Table 14.1 Potential nutritional deficits associated with the type of vegetarian diet

	Iron	Zinc	Calcium	Iodine	Vitamin B12	Vitamin D	EPA/DHA	Protein
Lacto-ovo-vegetarian (eliminates meat and fish, but includes dairy products and eggs)	X	X				X	X	X
Lacto-vegetarian (eliminates meat, fish, and eggs, but includes dairy products)	X	X				X	X	X
Ovo-vegetarian (eliminates meat, fish, and dairy products, but includes eggs)	X	X	X	X	X	X	X	X
Vegan (exclude consumption of any animal products, even honey, gelatin, or other animal-derived ingredient)	X	X	X	X	X	X	X	X

EPA eicosapentaenoic acid, *DHA* docosahexaenoic acid

very well-planned [39–41]. The risk of nutritional deficiencies and dietary inadequacy is greater as the diet becomes more restrictive, as shown in Table 14.1.

A well-planned and balanced intake of key nutrients (proteins, iron, vitamin D, calcium, iodine, n-3 fatty acids, zinc, vitamin B12) is very important during pregnancy. Particular care is required for pregnant exercisers and athletes, whose nutrient requirements are increased.

A study conducted in the United States has shown that vegetarian diets during pregnancy were not associated with gestational diabetes, anemia, or preeclampsia [42]. However, if the diet is unbalanced, with nutritional deficiencies in the key nutrients previously mentioned, a higher risk of fetal impairment (low birth weight, neurological disabilities, and fetal malformations) could emerge [39].

The adoption of vegetarian diets during pregnancy should include a wide variety of plant foods and adequate supplementation. Specially attention should be given to the intake of foods rich in the following nutrients:

Proteins:

Although protein needs are particularly high during pregnancy, could be easily achieved, if energy requirements are met [39]. Beans, grains, nuts, seeds, pseudocereals (e.g., buckwheat, quinoa), soy-based food products (e.g., "soy milk," "soy yogurt," tofu, tempeh), and meat analogs based on wheat or soy are good sources of proteins in vegetarian diets. Dairy products and eggs are also important sources of protein for lacto-ovo-vegetarians. In strength athletes' protein needs are even higher, but, as mentioned before, vegetable protein food sources alone can adequately provide all protein needs, when well-balanced or in the presence of a higher total protein intake [17].

Vitamin B12:

Vitamin B12 is a water-soluble vitamin found in substantial quantities only in animal sources, a fact that justifies the utilization of supplements and fortified foods in vegetarian and vegan diets. Vitamin B12 supplementation is mandatory for all vegans [40].

Zinc:

Nuts, seeds, pulses, soy, grains, nutritional yeast, zinc fortified products (e.g., breakfast cereals), are examples of good sources of zinc. In vegetarian and lacto-ovo-vegetarian diets zinc's intestinal absorption is reduced when compared with an omnivore diet. This impairment in zinc absorption could be explained by the phytate content of vegetarian diets. For this reason, vegetarians should be encouraged to increase the consumption of the foods mentioned. Food preparation techniques like soaking beans and pulses, sprouting, and sourdough leavening of bread, increase zinc bioavailability. Zinc absorption is also increased, if zinc-rich foods are consumed with foods that contain organic acids (e.g., citric acid), such as fruits and vegetables of the Brassicaceae family (e.g., broccoli, cabbage, cauliflower, kale, collards, turnip, Chinese cabbage, common radish, horseradish) [39, 40, 43].

Iron:

Vegetarian diets have been associated with iron deficiency, so vegetarian pregnant women should enrich their diets with beans, lentils, and other iron-fortified foods, such as bread and breakfast cereals. Non-heme iron from plants is worst absorbed than heme iron from animal food sources, like meat, eggs, and dairy products, for this reason, pregnant women are advised to eat vitamin C-rich foods (e.g., citrus fruits or tomatoes) together with iron-rich foods [39]. Considering that physical training may increase the Estimated Average Requirement in female athletes by 30 to 70% [44], that iron requirement are progressively increased during pregnancy and that vegetarian diets have been associated with iron deficiency [39], concerns regarding iron deficiency could easily arise regarding the pregnant exerciser and athlete who follow a vegetarian diet, being essential to prevent iron deficiency in the fetus by preventing iron deficiency in the pregnant woman.

Calcium:

As highlighted in the table above ovo-vegetarian and vegan diets are associated with calcium intakes below the recommended. The requirements for this mineral can be met in a vegetarian diet, by choosing plant food rich in calcium [40]. Calcium can be found in low-oxalate foods (high bioavailability), such as Chinese cabbage, broccoli, kale, turnip greens, and soy products. With lower calcium availability, we could name "soy milk" (if fortified with calcium), sesame seeds, almonds, and beans [39].

Close support by health professionals capable of providing nutritional counseling, planning the pregnant woman's diet, and monitoring nutrient intake in the different phases of pregnancy is strongly encouraged to avoid a compromise of maternal health and ensure the adequate fetus's physiological development.

14.2.4 Other Relevant Dietary Aspects

14.2.4.1 Hydration

Since water is profusely present in the components of maternal weight gain (e.g., fetus, placenta, amniotic fluid, blood), by the end of pregnancy water represents about two-thirds of the increase in maternal weight [45]. There are physiological changes in the hydrodynamics, increasing the water content in the body and in how it is regulated, for instance, the exchange of water from the mother to the fetus increases as the pregnancy progresses and as an example, the volume of amniotic fluid is recognized as a predictor of fetal well-being [46].

Pregnant women who experience frequent nausea and vomiting during pregnancy and who perform prolonged exercise should pay even more attention to proper hydration because they can be at greater risk for dehydration) due to the higher chances of negative fluid balance [47, 48].

Hydration status is of paramount importance during pregnancy. Usually, it is recommended that pregnant women should have a total water intake of around 3 L (total water includes all water contained in food, beverages, and drinking water)

[49], but since factors such as temperature, humidity, clothing, and sweating (highly influenced by exercise) influence dehydration this recommendation should be individualized considering the previous factors. Usual dietary intake should also be considered while defining the amount of fluids that a pregnant women should have, since almost every food has relevant amounts of water in its constitution [50].

A fluid intake equivalent to 5–10 mL/kg of body weight for 2–4 h before exercise is a standard guideline of an adequate fluid intake before exercise [19]. During an exercise session fluid intake should be customized to avoid dehydration or hyperhydration, since multiple factors (e.g., exercise intensity, duration, fitness, heat acclimatization, altitude) play a role in the variability of fluid loss between individuals [19]. In the course of an exercise session fluid balance can be estimated by weighing before and after the exercise session, and the fluid loss should be compensated before the next exercise session with a fluid intake of around 1.25–1.5 times the estimated fluid loss during the previous session [19]. It is important to emphasize that effective rehydration requires a greater intake of fluids than the total fluid loss during the exercise session [19].

Hydration is also a key factor in attenuation, a condition that is estimated to affect more than a quarter of pregnant women: constipation. Constipation is also aggravated if there is a need to use iron supplements because constipation is one of the common adverse effects of iron supplementation that is both prevalent in pregnant women as well in female athletes [51, 52]. On the other hand, if diarrhea is present, hydration and electrolyte need increase enormously in order to compensate for the acute water and electrolyte losses [49].

14.2.4.2 Caffeine

Caffeine is an alkaloid (1,3,7-trimethylxanthine) that stimulates the central nervous system due to its nonselective antagonistic action of adenosine receptors. It is naturally present in tea leaves, guarana berries, kola nuts, coffee, and cocoa beans, as well as in more than 60 plant species. It is an ingredient in a wide variety of foods, such as cakes, ice cream, cola drinks, energy drinks, and dietary supplements for weight loss and to increase sports performance. Coffee is the natural drink with the highest and most varied caffeine content. The concentrations will depend on the genetic differences of the grain, the degree of roasting, as well as the time and way of preparing it [53].

Caffeine has been shown to acutely enhance cognitive function (including attention and vigilance) and to improve exercise performance when consumed in doses of 3–6 mg/kg body mass, but high doses of caffeine (e.g., 9 mg/kg body mass) are associated with a high incidence of side-effects and do not seem to be required to elicit an ergogenic effect [54].

About 80% of pregnant women consume caffeine on a daily basis [55] and 74% of athletes use caffeine as an ergogenic aid, mostly endurance sports athletes [54] which raises the importance to access the safety of caffeine consumption during pregnancy.

Caffeine reaches and increases in the fetoplacental compartment, as the maternal plasma caffeine levels increase, and the caffeine maternal blood levels increase with pregnancy due to progressive reductions in its metabolism. Higher caffeine

Table 14.2 Mean caffein content of common beverages and foods

Foods and beverages	Caffeine
Mug of filter coffee	140 mg
Mug of instant coffee	100 mg
Mug of regular tea, or green tea	75 mg
Can of energy drink, 250 mL	80 mg
Can of cola	40 mg
Bar of plain dark chocolate, 50 g	Less than 25 mg
Bar of plain milk chocolate, 50 g	Less than 10 mg

British Nutrition Foundation [61]

consumption during pregnancy can reduce the blood flow to the placenta causing complications and in the worst-case scenario miscarriage [55].

Observational data associates caffeine intake with increased risk for negative pregnancy outcomes, such as miscarriage, stillbirth, and lower birth weight [56, 57], and even prepregnancy caffeine consumption at levels >400 mg/day was associated with increased risk of spontaneous abortion particularly at weeks 8–19 of gestation [58].

The maximum daily caffeine intake recommended for pregnant women is 200 mg [59], and the American College of Obstetricians and Gynecologists states that "Moderate caffeine consumption (less than 200 mg per day) does not appear to be a major contributing factor in miscarriage or preterm birth [60]. The relationship of caffeine to growth restriction remains undetermined. A final conclusion cannot be made at this time as to whether there is a correlation between high caffeine intake and miscarriage" [60].

In Table 14.2 the mean caffein content of common beverages and foods is presented.

Even though most of the evidence available on this topic is observational, several authors of recent research conducted on the impact of caffeine intake on pregnancy outcomes suggest that pregnant women should minimize caffeine intake during pregnancy [55–57].

14.2.4.3 Low- and Non-Calorie Sweeteners

Low- and non-calorie sweeteners are food additives that are added to a variety of foods and beverages in place of sugars either during the manufacturing process or as table-top sweeteners. They can be added to a wide range of sugar-reduced or sugar-free products, such as soft drinks, chewing gum, confectionery, frozen desserts, dessert mixes, yogurts, and puddings depending on the approved conditions of use [62].

Based on the current scientific evidence and recent World Health Organization recommendations as well as guidance from other scientific bodies, it is recommended the reduction of free sugar intake to less than 10% of total energy intake [63]. The consumption of foods and beverages with low- and non-calorie sweeteners to replace those with added sugars can be an option to reduce sugar and energy intake, provided that the use of such products does not induce a compensation for energy intake. Low- and non-calorie sweeteners range in sweetness from 30 (cyclamate) to 650 (sucralose) times sweeter than sugar [62].

Absorption of low- and non-calorie sweeteners into the bloodstream occurs in the small intestine and can be transferred to a fetus through the placenta and to an infant through breast milk. Although some low- and non-calorie sweeteners are fully degraded (e.g., aspartame), most of them (e.g., sucralose, acesulfame K, saccharin) circulate in the body unmetabolized and are found in the blood, urine, and feces [64]. Currently, an acceptable daily intake for each substance is established. The acceptable daily intake is the amount of a substance that people can consume daily throughout their lives, without any appreciable risk to health. Various international regulatory organizations, such as the Food and Agriculture Organization, the World Health Organization, the European Food Safety Authority, and the Food and Drug Administration, have endorsed the safety of low- and non-calorie sweeteners, within the limits of the acceptable daily intake established for each compound, in terms of carcinogenicity, mutagenicity, teratogenicity, and reproductive and developmental toxicity [62].

According to regulatory agencies such as the European Food Safety Authority and the Food and Drug Administration, low- and non-calorie sweeteners intake is safe in pregnant women when the intake does not exceed the recommended limits (Table 14.3). At the postpartum, the advice for lactating women is similar to that for pregnant women [62, 65]. However, foods and drinks containing artificial sweeteners should not replace more nutritious options (e.g., the consumption of more processed drinks in replacement of dairy-based drinks or water), as can happen in

Table 14.3 Acceptable daily intakes of common low- and non-calorie sweeteners [66]

Low- and non-calorie sweeteners	Acceptable daily intake expressed as mg/kg of body mass/day	Recommendations during pregnancy mg/kg of body mass/day
Acesulfame-K (E-950)	15	15
Aspartame (E-951)	40	40
Cyclamate (E-952)	11	Not recommended
Saccharin (E-954)	5	Not recommended
Sucralose (E-955)	15	15
Steviol glycoside (E-960)	4	Accepted for steviol glycoside Dried or raw stevia leaf infusions are not recommended

specific foods and food supplements commonly used by athletes (e.g., meal substitutes, sports bars, pre-and postexercise shakes, gainers).

Pregnancy is not an optimal period to lose weight and low-calorie diets are not recommended, but moderate consumption of low- and non-calorie sweeteners in pregnant or lactating women can be justified by the need to replace sugary foods or drinks in those women with type I or gestational diabetes, or those who for any other reason need to pay special attention to weight management and therefore control their weight gain [62, 67].

14.3 Impact of Maternal Diet on Offspring Health

As mentioned by Koletzko [68], the hypothesis that early life nutrition and growth influence the subsequent risk of disease and the term "programming" was proposed in 1974 by Dörner. In 1977, Forsdahl correlated higher infant mortality in Norway with a subsequent increased risk of cardiovascular mortality, suggesting that poverty during childhood and adolescence, followed by prosperity, are risk factors for cardiovascular disease and that nutritional deficit could cause permanent damage [69]. Later, Barker et al. argued that the fetus exposed to malnutrition decreases its growth rate to reduce nutritional needs. This period of malnutrition could also decrease the function of key organs, altering negative feedback metabolic mechanisms, and increase vulnerability to adverse environmental factors in the future [70].

Over time, these assumptions were consolidated in the concept of the origins of the development of health and disease [71], which proposes that the environment to which we are exposed in critical periods of development has an effect permanent effect on tissue structure and metabolism and, consequently, on long-term health. Thus, the concept of "metabolic programming" is based on the evidence that environmental exposures early in life program the individual's development, metabolism, and health in the future. Currently, we are aware of several environmental factors with this programming effect, including smoking, maternal exposure to endocrine disruptors, maternal nutrition, and maternal physical activity. Of these exposures, nutrition is a determinant, so the concept of "metabolic nutritional programming" refers to early nutritional exposures in critical or sensitive periods of development that, through programming effects, have a long-term impact [72].

A healthy woman at the time of conception is more likely to have a successful pregnancy and a healthy child. In turn, maternal malnutrition (nutritional changes such as pre-obesity, obesity, and malnutrition/low weight) during pregnancy has been associated with an increased risk of complications in different maternal-fetal outcomes, namely preeclampsia, gestational diabetes, macrosomia (more than 4000 g at birth), congenital malformations, fetal death, low birth weight, breastfeeding failure, and maternal mortality, as well as metabolic programming for the disease in adulthood of the newborn [73].

Furthermore, evidence suggests that the optimization of nutritional status and proper weight management during pregnancy and lactation can be cost-effective strategies for preventing chronic noncommunicable diseases caused by inadequate eating habits [74]. All of this imposes the need to conceptualize an intervention that promotes women's health and its surveillance, from a preconceptional perspective.

Due to the excessive focus on weight control, weight-class restrictions, and aesthetic requirements for sport, many female athletes sometimes choose to adopt specific and restrictive dietary patterns, which may predispose the development of eating disorders, in fact, the prevalence of eating disorders is higher in female athletes (6–45%) when compared to male athletes (0–19%) [75].

Considering that the pregnant exerciser and athlete have higher nutritional requirements, it could be hypothesized that the adoption of restrictive diets could be associated with adverse consequences for the mother and the baby (such as spontaneous abortion, preterm delivery, and fetal growth restriction). Therefore, everyone in the sports system should be aware and has a role to play in the recognition of situations of disorder eating or eating disorders [76]. In addition, we would like to highlight, once again, the importance of the personalized evaluation of the adequacy of the dietary intake and dietary pattern in a pre-natal phase.

Evidence also suggests that interventions that improve maternal nutritional status are effective and sustainable means to achieve health gains and reduce health inequalities for future generations [77]. Dietary interventions during pregnancy are safe and cost-effective to limit excessive weight gain during pregnancy, improve maternal and child health, and reduce the risk of gestational diabetes, gestational hypertension, preeclampsia, premature birth, abortion. and metabolic disorders [78–80].

14.4 Food Safety for Pregnant Women

Food safety is important for everyone and in any phase of the life cycle, but in pregnant women, its importance is even higher, since pregnant women are at particularly high risk for foodborne infections [81], and the potential consequences of higher exposure to food contaminants can harm not just the women but mostly the fetus [82] and during pregnancy dietary supplements are often consumed [83] which may increase the risk of exposure to unwanted adulterants [84]. In addition, pregnant exercisers and athletes usually eat more than their sedentary counterparts and therefore have a higher risk of contact with bacteria, parasites, and viruses, and higher exposure to contaminants through food and drinks. Besides that, beyond the common "pregnancy supplements," the use of ergogenic supplements by pregnant exercisers and athletes can be of concern.

14.4.1 Food-Borne Infections

Among the most common causes of foodborne infections are bacteria (e.g., Salmonella), parasites (e.g., *Toxoplasma gondii*), and viruses (e.g., Norovirus) [85].

Pregnancy is an exceptional immune tolerant condition [86] which may lead to increased susceptibility of pregnant women to foodborne infections from pathogens such as *Listeria monocytogenes*, and *Toxoplasma gondii* which have a predilection for the maternal-fetal unit and may induce severe illness in the mother and/or fetus increasing the risk of premature labor, abortion, intrauterine death, or early perinatal death [87].

Since pregnant exercisers and athletes often have augmented energy and protein needs than their sedentary counterparts, it is probable that pregnant exercisers and athletes have to eat larger daily amounts of food, eventually larger amounts of animal food sources (which are more likely to contain harmful pathogens) [88] and

Table 14.4 List of common foods with higher and lower risk for food-borne infections during pregnancy (adapted from [88])

Type of food	Higher Risk	Lower Risk
Meat and poultry	Raw or undercooked meat and poultry	Meat and poultry cooked until a minimum internal temperature of around 74 °C/165 °F
Seafood	– Raw and undercooked fish, shellfish, and food containing raw or undercooked seafood (e.g., sushi or ceviche) – Refrigerated smoked fish Partially cooked seafood (e.g., shrimp and crab)	– Previously cooked seafood heated to 74 °C/165 °F – Canned fish and seafood – Seafood cooked until 63 °C/145 °F
Milk and cheese	– Unpasteurized (raw) milk – Soft cheeses made from unpasteurized (raw) milk (e.g., feta, brie, camembert)	– Pasteurized milk – Hard cheeses – Processed cheeses – Cream cheese – Mozzarella – Soft cheeses that are labeled “made from pasteurized milk”
Eggs	Foods that contain raw or uncooked eggs	– At home: recipes that call for raw or undercooked eggs are made with pasteurized eggs – When eating out: Ask if pasteurized eggs were used
Vegetables and sprouts	Unwashed fresh vegetables, including lettuce/salads, and raw sprouts	– Washed fresh vegetables, including salads – Cooked vegetables and sprouts
Deli meats and deli salads	– Deli, and luncheon meats that have not been reheated – Deli salads prepared without preservatives in a deli-type store or restaurant	– Deli, and luncheon meats reheated to steaming hot or 74 °C/165 °F – Deli salads freshly prepared at home
Pâtés	Unpasteurized, refrigerated pâtés or meat spreads	Canned or shelf-stable pâtés or meat spreads

perhaps have a higher probability to contact with dangerous microscopic pathogens. Therefore is even more important for pregnant exercisers and athletes to be aware of what they can do to reduce the risk of food-borne infections.

In Table 14.4 a list of common foods is displayed and categorized as being of higher or lower risk option among different types of foods.

Besides avoiding high-risk foods, to avoid foodborne infections during pregnancy is also fundamental to comply with some basic food safety rules, such as wash hands and surfaces often, separate, and avoid cross-contaminate (e.g., keep raw foods separate from ready-to-eat foods), cook to proper temperatures (use a meat thermometer if need be) and refrigerate promptly.

14.4.2 Dietary Contaminants Exposure

Contaminants in food can be very diverse, but we can classify them into three levels: (1) formed during culinary processing, generally associated with frying, grilling, and barbecuing; (2) present in different packaging materials (e.g., bisphenol A and phthalates), which under certain conditions, such as heat, migrate to the food; (3) present in an unanticipated, unintentional way in the food matrix (e.g., mycotoxins, heavy metals, dioxins, pollutants that persist in the environment and accumulate in food such as organochlorine pesticides) [89].

The main concern arising from exposure to food contaminants is related to acute toxic, carcinogenic, mutagenic, and reproductive effects. Currently, exposure to these compounds, mainly due to the consumption of contaminated food, is associated with impacts on health, such as metabolic disease, cancer, neurodevelopmental deficiency, and neurodegenerative disease, among others.

However, a significant part of these contaminants has endocrine disruptor activity—substances in our environment, food, and consumer products that interfere with hormone biosynthesis, metabolism, or action resulting in a deviation from normal homeostatic control or reproduction and causing harmful effects on living organisms, including humans, even in small concentrations. In 2012, the World Health Organization warned that "the risk of illness from exposure to endocrine disrupting chemicals may be significantly underestimated" [90].

The risk associated with exposure to endocrine disruptors is especially relevant at times of the life cycle with greater susceptibility, such as the preconception and intrauterine development phase. Maternal, but also paternal, exposure to toxic chemicals before, close to conception, and during pregnancy can adversely affect the quality of eggs, sperm, and embryos, with consequences on fertility, child health, adulthood, and offspring through fetal programming [91–95].

However, eating habits are not only determinants of exposure to contaminants, but there is also an interaction between them [96]. Optimizing nutritional intake and adequate nutritional status during preconception and pregnancy, namely vitamins and minerals, are important not only to help promote normal fetal development but also as a protective influence on the mechanisms of toxicity of environmental contaminants and risk of diseases [97]. In this context, it is still important to deepen the knowledge about the risk-benefit of ingesting certain foods during pregnancy, as is the case of fish with higher mercury content. Contradictory epidemiological findings regarding the health effects of fish consumption can also be explained by the mixed effects of beneficial nutrients and harmful chemicals contained in fish. Recently, increasing evidence is beginning to emerge implying not only the importance of nutritional status but also the use of protective bioactive food components, specifically from the Mediterranean diet, to decrease the general toxicity of environmental pollutants [96].

Additionally, food is the main route of exposure to microplastics, namely through the ingestion of contaminated water, seafood, and salt. Microplastics can contain two types of harmful chemical co-contaminants, often with endocrine-altering effects, not only including plastic additives, such as phthalates, bisphenol A, and brominated flame retardants, but also chemicals absorbed from the surrounding environment (e.g., heavy metals, persistent organic pollutants, polycyclic aromatic hydrocarbons, polychlorinated biphenyls) [98]. Food safety authorities, notably the European Food Safety Authority, are concerned about the implications of microplastics for food safety, food accessibility, and hence human health [98]. In this context, it is not surprising that the evidence of the adverse consequences of microplastics has been increasing, however, having been recently detected in human placentas, it is even more pertinent and necessary to develop more studies to evaluate the effects of microplastics on the development of the fetus.

Since food packaging can be of concern and considering that athletes tend to consume more often sports foods, sports drinks, and sports supplements (e.g., protein bars, gainers, energy gels), among other potential risks, packaging should also be criteria to be taken in account for the decision of which products to purchase and consume.

14.4.3 Food Supplements

As mentioned before pregnant active women have increased nutritional needs of several micronutrients, such as folate, iodine, iron, and magnesium when compared to their non-pregnant counterparts. Despite the fact that ideally, the intake of most nutrients should come from food, and that, in general, no vitamin and mineral supplements are required if an athlete is consuming adequate energy from a variety of foods to maintain body weight [19], pregnant women and pregnant exercisers and athletes are often recommended to supplement their diet with key micronutrients like folic acid, iodine, and iron.

The advantages of micronutrient supplementation during pregnancy are well-established for some micronutrients, as folate (usually supplemented as folic acid) [99–102] but on the other hand, there is a relative paucity of data concerning the use of multivitamins and multimineral supplements during pregnancy, which does not allow the generalization of advising micronutrient and multimineral supplements to most pregnant women [103, 104], moreover, there are even some micronutrients that its supplementations should be carefully evaluated (e.g., vitamin A), since can cause hypervitaminosis [105].

Regardless of the above, one of the main issues regarding nutrient supplementation during pregnancy is the regulation of the supplements (food supplements vs. drugs with nutrients). While in most countries drugs are extensively studied for safety and efficacy before being commercialized, food supplements are often considered safe until proven unsafe and are not systematically and mandatorily tested and monitored prior to and after being commercialized, being common the existence of adulterated or contaminated food supplements available in the market (around 20%) [106]. Food supplement adulteration is an emerging food safety problem and that effective control by food regulatory authorities is needed to safeguard consumers [107] and while this issue is not adequately addressed, a conservative approach and the advice to just take well-regulated supplements (i.e., drugs with nutrients) probably is the approach with less risk for pregnant women. Despite the fact that specific food supplements for pregnant women are scarcely studied regarding contaminants, some evidence raises concerns about the potentially harmful levels of heavy metals (e.g., lead, mercury, and arsenic) found in food supplements (not in well-regulated drugs with nutrients) throughout the world [108].

Notwithstanding, national-level guidelines and personalized doctor advice should prevail on the decisions about who, when and with what to supplement in each specific case.

14.5 Diet in Special Conditions

All women, including pregnant exercisers or even athletes, can experience a higher weight gain than expected during pregnancy and/or develop gestational diabetes [109], and both for weight management and for gestational diabetes management, diet is a major tool to effectively control these conditions [110–112].

14.5.1 Excessive Weight Gain During Pregnancy

Pregnancy is a period of rapid physiologic weight gain [113], and complying with the weight gain recommendations during pregnancy seems to help achieve better pregnancy outcomes, however, women often find it difficult to do not exceed the weight gain recommendations [114]. Curiously, the evidence available on the increased odds of excessive prenatal weight gain in elite athletes versus active and sedentary controls is very weak [109], which stresses the relevance of a careful weight management in pregnant athletes. Even in a sample of Olympics, European, and World Championships medalists, these elite athletes decrease training volume throughout pregnancy and had a statistically similar average weight gain during pregnancy from controls (mean (SD): 12.3 kg (4.1 kg) vs. 13.3 kg (3.4 kg), $p = 0.28$) [115].

Providing adequate energy intake through the diet considering the pregnant woman's energy needs is fundamental to control the weight gain during pregnancy and therefore avoiding excessive weight gain throughout pregnancy [113]. To respond to the physiologic weight gain during pregnancy, which among others also includes fetus growth and development, is usually recommended an increase in pregnant women's energy intake [116], conversely, women report little or no change in energy intake during pregnancy, what can imply that current recommendations to increase energy intake may, therefore, encourage excessive weight gain and eventually adverse pregnancy outcomes [113]. In light of the above, maintaining the pre-pregnancy energy intake during pregnancy eventually can allow a normal weight gain as a consequence of the previously reported common decrease in physical activity during pregnancy.

Regardless of the aforementioned, diet as a whole, and not just energy intake, has a relevant role in reducing the risk of excessive gestational weight gain [111], for instance, a Mediterranean-style diet intervention on physically active pregnant women showed the capacity to reduce gestational weight gain [110]. Inclusively, evidence suggests that the complexity of interactions with advice sources, body dissatisfaction, feelings of control, as well as perceived risks of weight gain may lead to ineffective weight management interventions during pregnancy while focusing on a healthy diet and physical activity levels may be more useful and less stigmatizing than focusing on weight [117], since controlling body weight during pregnancy is not a behavior, but performing a concrete dietary choice is.

Additionally, pregnancy is often considered a period of great motivation for behavior change and seems that the perceived benefits for the mother and the baby enhances the intentions to change eating behaviors, such as eating more fruits and vegetables and eating less high-fat and sugary foods [57], which can be seen as a good opportunity to improve long-lasting dietary habits.

14.5.2 Gestational Diabetes

Worldwide, gestational diabetes prevalence varies hugely between countries, mostly due to socioeconomic determinants and the mean age of childbirth [118]. Diet may play a role in the onset of gestational diabetes [118, 119], but is in the managing of diabetes that diet has a key role [112].

Dietary factor's relevance to gestational diabetes is immediately stamped on weight management since body mass index and gestational weight gain are modifiable risk factors for the onset of gestational diabetes [120]. Pregnancy is associated with increased insulin resistance as a metabolic adaptation to the nutritional demands of the placenta and fetus, but in pregnant women with obesity, this mechanism is exacerbated [121]. Insulin resistance is normally compensated by an adaptive increase in pancreatic β-cell mass together with enhanced glucose-stimulated insulin release, but eventually, the excessive fat during pregnancy can create a pro-inflammatory environment that can disrupt the response of the β-cells to the endocrine signals of pregnancy and limit the adaptive changes in β-cell mass and function, resulting in an increased risk of gestational diabetes [121].

Dietary counseling focus on the type, amount, and distribution of carbohydrates during the day, regarding the nutritional status, physical activity level, and pharmacotherapy of the pregnant woman is the bedrock for successful management of gestational diabetes and reducing both short-term and long-term complications in both mother and offspring [112]. A number of different kinds of dietary approaches are used worldwide, and there is no agreement among specialists as to what constitutes an ideal approach [122]. Limiting carbohydrates and increasing fat intake seem counterproductive, in fact, instead of restricting, it is beneficial to focus on the quality of carbohydrates and promote vegetables and fruits consumption and on allowing the intake of higher levels of complex, low-to-medium glycemic index carbohydrates and adequate fiber, again through higher consumption of vegetables and fruits [122]. In fact, active pregnant women who followed a Mediterranean diet decreased by 35% the risk of gestational diabetes in comparison with usual care controls, being the main dietary changes of the intervention protocol the incentive to include in their diet a high intake of nuts, extra virgin olive oil, fruit, vegetables, unrefined grains, and legumes; moderate to high consumption of fish; low to moderate intake of poultry and dairy products, such as yogurt and cheese; low consumption of red meat and processed meat; and avoidance of sugary drinks, fast food, and food rich in animal fat [110].

Regardless of the aforementioned, no particular diet or dietary protocol appears to be superior to another, nonetheless, more intensive diet counseling and more frequent visits to the Registered Dietitian during pregnancy are associated with better management of gestational diabetes and with favorable changes toward a healthy eating pattern [122].

14.6 Practice-Oriented Dietary Guide for an Active Pregnancy

Based on the compilation of all the references used as an information source for the elaboration of this chapter, we present this practice-oriented dietary guide as a summary of the main dietary advice during pregnancy and particularly for pregnant exercisers and athletes.

14.6.1 General Dietary Advice

- Restrictive diets should be avoided during pregnancy.
- Consider the energy content of the diet alongside overall nutritional quality, following the most consensual dietary guidelines for healthy eating (e.g., food guides), which are generally in line with the adequate dietary principles for good pregnancy management in terms of both weight control and gestational diabetes prevention and management.

- Healthy dietary patterns such as Mediterranean Diet fit all the recommendations for pregnant women, and sportswomen, and should be promoted as a good diet for pregnant exercisers.
- Vegetarian diets can be appropriate and nutritional adequate during pregnancy and in athletes, although must be very well-planned to provide all the energy and nutritional needs. Special attention should be given to nutrients, such as protein, vitamins (vitamin D, vitamin B12), minerals (zinc, iron, calcium, iodine), and omega-3 fatty acids. The nutritional adequacy of a vegetarian diet must be assessed individually.
- Pregnant women should be aware of the expected weight gain during pregnancy (e.g., 11 to 16 kg in normal-weight women).
- Appropriate nutritional supplementation, namely folic acid, iodine, and iron supplementation should be initiated after an assessment and prescription by a Medical Doctor and preferably using well-regulated supplements (i.e., drugs with nutrients) instead of "regular" food supplements, always taking into consideration national-level guidelines and personalized doctor advice about when and with which nutrients to supplement.
- In the case of a pregnant exerciser an example of a simple hydration plan can be the intake of about 0.5 L (5–10 mL per kg of body weight) of liquids about 2–4 h before starting to exercise, the intake of 0.4–0.8 L per hour of exercise and a reposition of 1.25–1.5 L per each 1 L of the fluid deficit during the exercise session. Sweat loss during an exercise session can be estimated by weighing without clothing before exercising and weighing again without clothing after exercise (after drying with a towel). The weight difference will be mainly due to sweat loss. If liquids were intake during the exercise session, the amount of liquids intake should be deducted from the final result (e.g., if a woman was 60 kg before exercise and drank 0.5 L of water during the exercise session, and at the end of the exercise session was 59.5 kg, it means that the sweat loss was about 1 L, i.e., 60–59.5 + 0.5 of water ≈ 1 L of sweat loss).
- In case of constipation, the triad: drinking sufficient fluids, sufficient intake of dietary fiber (e.g., through foods such as whole grains and derivatives, vegetables, seeds, fresh and dried fruits such as kiwi, orange, fig, and plum) and regular and sufficient physical activity seem to be the most efficient lifestyle approach.
- If needed (e.g., gestational diabetes or weight management), consume foods with low- and non-caloric sweeteners (acesulfame potassium, aspartame, sucralose) in moderate amounts, adhering to the acceptable daily intake standards set by regulatory agencies. Avoid foods with cyclamate, saccharin, and raw stevia leaf, as well as their infusions and extract.
- Pregnant women should minimize caffeine intake during pregnancy up to a daily maximum of 200 mg per day, which is equivalent to about two espresso coffees. Opting for decaffeinated versions is a good way to reduce caffeine intake. We advise against using caffeine supplementation as an ergogenic aid in case of pregnancy.

14.6.2 Food Safety Advice

Simple advices as the following will reduce the risk of contact with microorganisms that can be especially dangerous during pregnancy [88]:

- Properly wash and disinfect hands always before and after handling food, after going to the toilet, after being in contact with animals, or after being in contact with places where animals may have been (e.g., if you are gardening, handling earth, or sand).
- Wash and properly disinfect the vegetables and fruits you eat.
- Separate raw food from cooked or previously washed and disinfected food, in order to avoid cross-contamination (e.g., never place cooked food in a container where raw food was previously, without properly washing and disinfecting the container).
- If you leave food to defrost in the refrigerator (e.g., meat or fish) always place them in closed containers to prevent the liquid resulting from the defrosting from spilling and potentially contaminating other foods.
- Ensure that the food is properly defrosted before cooking it.
- Properly cook food (i.e., get to an adequate cooking temperature during the appropriate time), especially foods such as meat, fish, or eggs (always opt for the "well-done" options).
- If you reheat the food (leftovers), make sure it gets to boiling temperature, or if you use the microwave assure, they are well cooked internally.
- Always check and respect the expiration date of food.
- Recommendations for decreasing exposure to endocrine disruptors [123, 124]:
- Use of natural and minimally processed, fresh, seasonal, and local foods, as well as the consumption of moderate amounts of meat.
- Respect seasonality and prefer locally sourced food.
- Reduce the consumption of ultra-processed foods, which are usually packaged and rich in fat (where most of the contaminants are present), in addition to also containing salt, sugar, and industrial formulations typically with five or more ingredients, with additives and substances, such as oils, salt, antioxidants, stabilizers, and preservatives.
- Avoid packing hot food/meals in plastic containers.
- Use packaging and materials (plastic boxes, utensils, cling film, etc.) always following the instructions.
- Respect the temperature conditions, that is, do not use packaging or other materials to heat or prepare food, unless this is expressly indicated.
- Do not use returnable packaging or recyclable packaging for other products, especially for nonfood or hazardous products, such as bleach, detergents, thinners, etc.
- Read labels carefully: many of the compounds are already described on food labels/cosmetics (e.g., bisphenol A, phthalates).
- Do not store food in metal containers after opening; prefer a nonmetallic container with a lid.

- Consume 2–3 servings weekly (equivalent to 233–350 g) of fish with low levels of methylmercury (anchovies, herring, canned tuna, cod, horse mackerel, golden bream, pollock, sole, hake, sardine, plaice, rainbow trout, shrimp, squid, crab, crayfish, octopus) and varying species as consumed. The consumption of fish in a larger quantity (> 3 servings per week) can entail risks in terms of exposure to methylmercury, but its consumption in an amount of less than two servings can compromise the benefits associated with the consumption of fish, specifically at fetal neurodevelopment level.
- Limit the consumption of fish/mollusks species with a high content of methylmercury, namely eel, marlin, sturgeon, pouting, grouper, sea bream, halibut, pike, moray eel, snapper, catfish, goldfish, perch, ray, sea bass, salmon, redfish, monkfish, trout; halibut, fresh or frozen tuna, beetle, sandpaper, dye maker).
- Avoid the consumption of shark (dogfish), blue shark, swordfish, mackerel, potato fish, crab (dark meat), lobster, and similar large crustaceans (head and chest), and oysters.

Any of the advices present in this practice-oriented guide excludes the need for a personalized evaluation, prescription, monitoring, and adaptation of dietary intake, made by health professionals during the different phases of pregnancy.

References

1. Dunford AR, Sangster JM. Maternal and paternal periconceptional nutrition as an indicator of offspring metabolic syndrome risk in later life through epigenetic imprinting: a systematic review. Diab Metab Syndrome. 2017;11(Suppl 2):S655–62.
2. Pullar J, Wickramasinghe K, Demaio AR, Roberts N, Perez-Blanco KM, Noonan K, Townsend N. The impact of maternal nutrition on offspring's risk of non-communicable diseases in adulthood: a systematic review. J Glob Health. 2019;9(2):020405.
3. Silva M-R, Doñate B, Carballo K. Nutritional requirements for the pregnant exerciser and athlete: evidence-based guidelines. In: Santos-Rocha R, editor. Exercise and sporting activity during pregnancy. Berlin: Springer; 2019. p. 327–45.
4. Koletzko B, Cremer M, Flothkötter M, Graf C, Hauner H, Hellmers C, Kersting M, Krawinkel M, Przyrembel H, Röbl-Mathieu M, et al. Diet and lifestyle before and during pregnancy—practical recommendations of the Germany-wide healthy start—young family network. Geburtshilfe Frauenheilkd. 2018;78(12):1262–82.
5. Guerrero M, Pérez-Rodríguez F. Diet quality indices for nutrition assessment: types and applications (chapter 14). In: Functional food—improve health through adequate food. London: IntechOpen; 2017.
6. Shapiro ALB, Kaar JL, Crume TL, Starling AP, Siega-Riz AM, Ringham BM, Glueck DH, Norris JM, Barbour LA, Friedman JE, et al. Maternal diet quality in pregnancy and neonatal adiposity: the healthy start study. Int J Obes (Lond). 2016;40(7):1056–62.
7. Chen L-W, Aubert AM, Shivappa N, Bernard JY, Mensink-Bout SM, Geraghty AA, Mehegan J, Suderman M, Polanska K, Hanke W, et al. Maternal dietary quality, inflammatory potential and childhood adiposity: an individual participant data pooled analysis of seven European cohorts in the ALPHABET consortium. BMC Med. 2021;19(1):33.
8. Chen LW, Lyons B, Navarro P, Shivappa N, Mehegan J, Murrin CM, Hébert JR, Kelleher CC, Phillips CM. Maternal dietary inflammatory potential and quality are associated with

offspring asthma risk over 10-year follow-up: the lifeways cross-generation cohort study. Am J Clin Nutr. 2020;111(2):440–7.
9. Pestoni G, Krieger J-P, Sych JM, Faeh D, Rohrmann S. Cultural differences in diet and determinants of diet quality in Switzerland: results from the National Nutrition Survey menuCH. Nutrients. 2019;11(1):126.
10. Doyle IM, Borrmann B, Grosser A, Razum O, Spallek J. Determinants of dietary patterns and diet quality during pregnancy: a systematic review with narrative synthesis. Public Health Nutr. 2017;20(6):1009–28.
11. Suárez-Martínez C, Yagüe-Guirao G, Santaella-Pascual M, Peso-Echarri P, Vioque J, Morales E, García-Marcos L, Martínez-Graciá C. Nela Study Group T: adherence to the Mediterranean diet and determinants among pregnant women: the NELA cohort. Nutrients. 2021;13(4):1248.
12. Rodrigues SS, Franchini B, Graça P, de Almeida MD. A new food guide for the Portuguese population: development and technical considerations. J Nutr Educ Behav. 2006;38(3):189–95.
13. Food-based dietary guidelines. http://www.fao.org/nutrition/education/food-dietary-guidelines/regions/en/.
14. Herforth A, Arimond M, Álvarez-Sánchez C, Coates J, Christianson K, Muehlhoff E. A global review of food-based dietary guidelines. Adv Nutr. 2019;10(4):590–605.
15. Quarta S, Massaro M, Chervenkov M, Ivanova T, Dimitrova D, Jorge R, Andrade V, Philippou E, Zisimou C, Maksimova V, et al. Persistent moderate-to-weak mediterranean diet adherence and low scoring for plant-based foods across several Southern European countries: are we overlooking the mediterranean diet recommendations? Nutrients. 2021;13(5):1432.
16. Raymond J, Morrow K. Krause and Mahan's food & the nutrition care process. 15th ed. Amsterdam: Elsevier Health Sciences; 2020.
17. Rogerson D. Vegan diets: practical advice for athletes and exercisers. J Int Soc Sports Nutr. 2017;14:36.
18. European Food Safety Authority. Dietary reference values for nutrients. Summary report, vol. 14; 2017. p. e15121E.
19. Thomas DT, Erdman KA, Burke LM. American College of Sports Medicine joint position statement. Nutrition and athletic performance. Med Sci Sports Exerc. 2016;48(3):543–68.
20. Mousa A, Naqash A, Lim S. Macronutrient and micronutrient intake during pregnancy: an overview of recent evidence. Nutrients. 2019;11(2):443.
21. Rosenbloom CA, Coleman EJ. Sports nutrition: a practice manual for professionals. 5th ed. Chicago, IL: Academy of Nutrition and Dietetics; 2012.
22. Tabela da Composição de Alimentos. http://portfir.insa.pt.
23. World Health Organization. WHO guidelines approved by the guidelines review committee. In: WHO recommendations on antenatal care for a positive pregnancy experience. Geneva: World Health Organization; 2016.
24. Direção-Geral da Saúde. Norma no 004/2019: Prevenção e Tratamento da Deficiência de Vitamina D. Lisboa: Saúde DaoGd; 2019.
25. Larson-Meyer DE, Willis KS. Vitamin D and athletes. Curr Sports Med Rep. 2010;9(4):220–6.
26. Hyde NK, Brennan-Olsen SL, Bennett K, Moloney DJ, Pasco JA. Maternal nutrition during pregnancy: intake of nutrients important for bone health. Matern Child Health J. 2017;21(4):845–51.
27. Georgieff MK. Iron deficiency in pregnancy. Am J Obstet Gynecol. 2020;223(4):516–24.
28. Dalton LM, Fhloinn DMN, Gaydadzhieva GT, Mazurkiewicz OM, Leeson H, Wright CP. Magnesium in pregnancy. Nutr Rev. 2016;74(9):549–57.
29. Abel MH, Ystrom E, Caspersen IH, Meltzer HM, Aase H, Torheim LE, Askeland RB, Reichborn-Kjennerud T, Brantsæter AL. Maternal iodine intake and offspring attention-deficit/hyperactivity disorder: results from a large prospective cohort study. Nutrients. 2017;9(11):1239.
30. Farias PM, Marcelino G, Santana LF, de Almeida EB, Guimarães RCA, Pott A, Hiane PA, Freitas KC. Minerals in pregnancy and their impact on child growth and development. Molecules. 2020;25(23):5630.

31. Lăcătuşu C-M, Grigorescu E-D, Floria M, Onofriescu A, Mihai B-M. The Mediterranean diet: from an environment-driven food culture to an emerging medical prescription. Int J Environ Res Public Health. 2019;16(6):942.
32. Davis C, Bryan J, Hodgson J, Murphy K. Definition of the Mediterranean diet; a literature review. Nutrients. 2015;7(11):9139–53.
33. Bach-Faig A, Berry EM, Lairon D, Reguant J, Trichopoulou A, Dernini S, Medina FX, Battino M, Belahsen R, Miranda G, et al. Mediterranean diet pyramid today. Science and cultural updates. Public Health Nutr. 2011;14(12a):2274–84.
34. Slomski A. Mediterranean diet during pregnancy. JAMA. 2019;322(12):1134.
35. Olmedo-Requena R, Gómez-Fernández J, Amezcua-Prieto C, Mozas-Moreno J, Khan KS, Jiménez-Moleón JJ. Pre-pregnancy adherence to the Mediterranean diet and gestational diabetes mellitus: a case-control study. Nutrients. 2019;11(5):1003.
36. Koutelidakis AE, Alexatou O, Kousaiti S, Gkretsi E, Vasios G, Sampani A, Tolia M, Kiortsis DN, Giaginis C. Higher adherence to Mediterranean diet prior to pregnancy is associated with decreased risk for deviation from the maternal recommended gestational weight gain. Int J Food Sci Nutr. 2018;69(1):84–92.
37. Amati F, Hassounah S, Swaka A. The impact of Mediterranean dietary patterns during pregnancy on maternal and offspring health. Nutrients. 2019;11(5):1098.
38. Biagi C, Nunzio MD, Bordoni A, Gori D, Lanari M. Effect of adherence to Mediterranean diet during pregnancy on children's health: a systematic review. Nutrients. 2019;11(5):997.
39. Sebastiani G, Herranz Barbero A, Borrás-Novell C, Alsina Casanova M, Aldecoa-Bilbao V, Andreu-Fernández V, Pascual Tutusaus M, Ferrero Martínez S, Gómez Roig MD, García-Algar O. The effects of vegetarian and vegan diet during pregnancy on the health of mothers and offspring. Nutrients. 2019;11(3):557.
40. Baroni L, Goggi S, Battaglino R, Berveglieri M, Fasan I, Filippin D, Griffith P, Rizzo G, Tomasini C, Tosatti MA, et al. Vegan nutrition for mothers and children: practical tools for healthcare providers. Nutrients. 2018;11(1):5.
41. Melina V, Craig W, Levin S. Position of the academy of nutrition and dietetics: vegetarian diets. J Acad Nutr Diet. 2016;116(12):1970–80.
42. Yisahak SF, Hinkle SN, Mumford SL, Li M, Andriessen VC, Grantz KL, Zhang C, Grewal J. Vegetarian diets during pregnancy, and maternal and neonatal outcomes. Int J Epidemiol. 2021;50(1):165–78.
43. Agnoli C, Baroni L, Bertini I, Ciappellano S, Fabbri A, Papa M, Pellegrini N, Sbarbati R, Scarino ML, Siani V, et al. Position paper on vegetarian diets from the working group of the Italian Society of Human Nutrition. Nutr Metab Cardiovasc Dis. 2017;27(12):1037–52.
44. DellaValle DM. Iron supplementation for female athletes: effects on iron status and performance outcomes. Curr Sports Med Rep. 2013;12(4):234–9.
45. Hytten FE. Weight gain in pregnancy. In: Clinical physiology in obstetrics. Oxford: Blackwell Scientific; 1980. p. 193–230.
46. Beall MH, van den Wijngaard JP, van Gemert MJ, Ross MG. Amniotic fluid water dynamics. Placenta. 2007;28(8–9):816–23.
47. ACOG Committee Opinion No. 650. Physical activity and exercise during pregnancy and the postpartum period. Obstet Gynecol. 2015;126(6):e135–42.
48. Tulmaç ÖB, Kılıç R, Yaman S, Aktulum F, Şimşek G, Erdinç S. Evaluation of the vestibular system with video head impulse test in pregnant women with hyperemesis gravidarum. J Obstet Gynaecol Res. 2021;47(1):96–102.
49. Institute of Medicine. Dietary reference intakes for water, potassium, sodium, chloride, and sulfate. Washington, DC: The National Academies Press; 2005. https://doi.org/10.17226/10925.
50. Malisova O, Bountziouka V, Panagiotakos DB, Zampelas A, Kapsokefalou M. The water balance questionnaire: design, reliability and validity of a questionnaire to evaluate water balance in the general population. Int J Food Sci Nutr. 2012;63(2):138–44.
51. Bradley CS, Kennedy CM, Turcea AM, Rao SS, Nygaard IE. Constipation in pregnancy: prevalence, symptoms, and risk factors. Obstet Gynecol. 2007;110(6):1351–7.

52. Goodrich JA, Frisco DJ, Kim S, Holliday M, Rueda M, Poddar S, Byrnes WC. The importance of lean mass and iron deficiency when comparing hemoglobin mass in male and female athletic groups. J Appl Physiol. 2020;129(4):855–63.
53. Jung S, Kim MH, Park JH, Jeong Y, Ko KS. Cellular antioxidant and anti-inflammatory effects of coffee extracts with different roasting levels. J Med Food. 2017;20(6):626–35.
54. Guest NS, VanDusseldorp TA, Nelson MT, Grgic J, Schoenfeld BJ, Jenkins NDM, Arent SM, Antonio J, Stout JR, Trexler ET, et al. International society of sports nutrition position stand: caffeine and exercise performance. J Int Soc Sports Nutr. 2021;18(1):1.
55. Darakjian LI, Kaddoumi A. Physiologically based pharmacokinetic/pharmacodynamic model for caffeine disposition in pregnancy. Mol Pharm. 2019;16(3):1340–9.
56. James JE. Maternal caffeine consumption and pregnancy outcomes: a narrative review with implications for advice to mothers and mothers-to-be. BMJ Evid Based Med. 2021;26(3):114–5.
57. Poole R, Kennedy OJ, Roderick P, Fallowfield JA, Hayes PC, Parkes J. Coffee consumption and health: umbrella review of meta-analyses of multiple health outcomes. BMJ. 2017;359:j5024.
58. Gaskins AJ, Rich-Edwards JW, Williams PL, Toth TL, Missmer SA, Chavarro JE. Pre-pregnancy caffeine and caffeinated beverage intake and risk of spontaneous abortion. Eur J Nutr. 2018;57(1):107–17.
59. European Food Safety Authority. Panel of dietetic products, nutrition and allergies. Scientific opinion on the safety of caffeine. EFSA J. 2015;13:4102.
60. ACOG CommitteeOpinion No. 462. Moderate caffeine consumption during pregnancy. Obstet Gynecol. 2010;116(2 Pt 1):467–8.
61. British Nutrition Foundation. What not to eat when pregnant. Scotland: British Nutrition Foundation; 2018. p. 2.
62. Serra-Majem L, Raposo A, Aranceta-Bartrina J, Varela-Moreiras G, Logue C, Laviada H, Socolovsky S, Pérez-Rodrigo C, Aldrete-Velasco JA, Meneses Sierra E, et al. Ibero-American consensus on low- and no-calorie sweeteners: safety, nutritional aspects and benefits in food and beverages. Nutrients. 2018;10(7):818.
63. WHO. WHO guidelines approved by the guidelines review committee. In: Guideline: sugars intake for adults and children. Geneva: World Health Organization; 2015.
64. Palatnik A, Moosreiner A, Olivier-Van Stichelen S. Consumption of non-nutritive sweeteners during pregnancy. Am J Obstet Gynecol. 2020;223(2):211–8.
65. Fitch C, Keim KS. Position of the academy of nutrition and dietetics: use of nutritive and nonnutritive sweeteners. J Acad Nutr Diet. 2012;112(5):739–58.
66. Evaluations of the Joint FAO/WHO Expert Committee on Food Additives (JECFA) list of chemicals in functional class sweetener. http://apps.who.int/food-additives-contaminants-jecfa-database/search.aspx?fc=66#.
67. Cavagnari BM. Non-caloric sweeteners in pregnancy and lactation. Revista espanola de salud publica. 2019:93.
68. Koletzko B. Developmental origins of adult disease: Barker's or Dorner's hypothesis? Am J Hum Biol. 2005;17(3):381–2.
69. Forsdahl A. Are poor living conditions in childhood and adolescence an important risk factor for arteriosclerotic heart disease? Br J Prev Soc Med. 1977;31(2):91–5.
70. Barker DJ, Osmond C. Infant mortality, childhood nutrition, and ischaemic heart disease in England and Wales. Lancet (London, England). 1986;1(8489):1077–81.
71. Barker DJ, Thornburg KL. The obstetric origins of health for a lifetime. Clin Obstet Gynecol. 2013;56(3):511–9.
72. Koletzko B, Brands B, Grote V, Kirchberg FF, Prell C, Rzehak P, Uhl O, Weber M. Long-term health impact of early nutrition: the power of programming. Ann Nutr Metab. 2017;70(3):161–9.
73. Lowensohn RI, Stadler DD, Naze C. Current concepts of maternal nutrition. Obstet Gynecol Surv. 2016;71(7):413–26.

74. Poston L, Harthoorn LF, Van Der Beek EM. Obesity in pregnancy: implications for the mother and lifelong health of the child. A consensus statement. Pediatr Res. 2011;69(2):175–80.
75. de Borja C, Holtzman B, McCall LM, Carson TL, Moretti LJ, Farnsworth N, Ackerman KE. Specific dietary practices in female athletes and their association with positive screening for disordered eating. J Eat Disord. 2021;9(1):50.
76. Wells KR, Jeacocke NA, Appaneal R, Smith HD, Vlahovich N, Burke LM, Hughes D. The Australian Institute of Sport (AIS) and National Eating Disorders Collaboration (NEDC) position statement on disordered eating in high performance sport. Br J Sports Med. 2020;54(21):1247–58.
77. World Health Organization. Good maternal nutrition—the best start in life. Copenhagen; 2016.
78. Thangaratinam S, Rogozinska E, Jolly K, Glinkowski S, Roseboom T, Tomlinson JW, Kunz R, Mol BW, Coomarasamy A, Khan KS. Effects of interventions in pregnancy on maternal weight and obstetric outcomes: meta-analysis of randomised evidence. BMJ (Clin Res Ed). 2012;344:e2088.
79. Englund-Ögge L, Brantsæter AL, Sengpiel V, Haugen M, Birgisdottir BE, Myhre R, Meltzer HM, Jacobsson B. Maternal dietary patterns and preterm delivery: results from large prospective cohort study. BMJ (Clin Res Ed). 2014;348:g1446.
80. Aaltonen J, Ojala T, Laitinen K, Poussa T, Ozanne S, Isolauri E. Impact of maternal diet during pregnancy and breastfeeding on infant metabolic programming: a prospective randomized controlled study. Eur J Clin Nutr. 2011;65(1):10–9.
81. O'Brien SJ, Larose TL, Adak GK, Evans MR, Tam CC. Modelling study to estimate the health burden of foodborne diseases: cases, general practice consultations and hospitalisations in the UK, 2009. BMJ Open. 2016;6(9):e011119.
82. Gómez-Roig MD, Pascal R, Cahuana MJ, García-Algar O, Sebastiani G, Andreu-Fernández V, Martínez L, Rodríguez G, Iglesia I, Ortiz-Arrabal O, et al. Environmental exposure during pregnancy: influence on prenatal development and early life: a comprehensive review. Fetal Diagn Ther. 2021;48(4):245–57.
83. Blumberg JB, Cena H, Barr SI, Biesalski HK, Dagach RU, Delaney B, Frei B, Moreno González MI, Hwalla N, Lategan-Potgieter R, et al. The use of multivitamin/multimineral supplements: a modified Delphi consensus panel report. Clin Ther. 2018;40(4):640–57.
84. Denham BE. Dietary supplements in the USA: problematic trends. Public Health Nutr. 2021;24(9):2771–5.
85. Canadian Paediatric Society. Foodborne infections. Paediatr Child Health. 2008;13(9):779–88.
86. Adar T, Grisaru-Granovsky S, Ben Ya'acov A, Goldin E, Bar-Gil Shitrit A. Pregnancy and the immune system: general overview and the gastroenterological perspective. Dig Dis Sci. 2015;60(9):2581–9.
87. Smith JL. Foodborne infections during pregnancy. J Food Prot. 1999;62(7):818–29.
88. Food and Drug Administration. Food safety: for pregnant women, their unborn babies, and children under five. Nutrition CfFSaA: Center for Food Safety and Applied Nutrition; 2020.
89. Teixeira D, Pestana D, Calhau C, Graça P. Linhas de Orientação sobre Contaminantes de Alimentos, Direção-Geral da Saúde. Lisboa: Direção-Geral da Saúde; 2015.
90. World Health Organization, United Nations Environment Programme, Inter-Organization Programme for the Sound Management of Chemicals, Bergman A, Heindel J, Jobling S, Kidd K, Zoeller T. State of the science of endocrine disrupting chemicals 2012: summary for decision-makers. Geneva: World Health Organization; 2013.
91. Wigle DT, Arbuckle TE, Turner MC, Bérubé A, Yang Q, Liu S, Krewski D. Epidemiologic evidence of relationships between reproductive and child health outcomes and environmental chemical contaminants. J Toxicol Environ Health B Crit Rev. 2008;11(5–6):373–517.
92. Yazbeck C, Thiebaugeorges O, Moreau T, Goua V, Debotte G, Sahuquillo J, Forhan A, Foliguet B, Magnin G, Slama R, et al. Maternal blood lead levels and the risk of pregnancy-induced hypertension: the EDEN cohort study. Environ Health Perspect. 2009;117(10):1526–30.
93. Miranda ML, Edwards S, Maxson PJ. Mercury levels in an urban pregnant population in Durham County, North Carolina. Int J Environ Res Public Health. 2011;8(3):698–712.

94. Kalloo G, Wellenius GA, McCandless L, Calafat AM, Sjodin A, Romano ME, Karagas MR, Chen A, Yolton K, Lanphear BP, et al. Exposures to chemical mixtures during pregnancy and neonatal outcomes: the HOME study. Environ Int. 2020;134:105219.
95. Kalloo G, Wellenius GA, McCandless L, Calafat AM, Sjodin A, Karagas M, Chen A, Yolton K, Lanphear BP, Braun JM. Profiles and predictors of environmental chemical mixture exposure among pregnant women: the health outcomes and measures of the environment study. Environ Sci Technol. 2018;52(17):10104–13.
96. Chan-Hon-Tong A, Charles MA, Forhan A, Heude B, Sirot V. Exposure to food contaminants during pregnancy. Sci Total Environ. 2013;458-460:27–35.
97. Koletzko B, Brands B, Poston L, Godfrey K, Demmelmair H. Early nutrition programming of long-term health. Proc Nutr Soc. 2012;71(3):371–8.
98. EFSA Panel on Contaminants in the Food Chain (CONTAM). Presence of microplastics and nanoplastics in food, with particular focus on seafood. EFSA J. 2016;14(6):e04501.
99. Bulloch RE, Lovell AL, Jordan VMB, McCowan LME, Thompson JMD, Wall CR. Maternal folic acid supplementation for the prevention of preeclampsia: a systematic review and meta-analysis. Paediatr Perinat Epidemiol. 2018;32(4):346–57.
100. Haider BA, Bhutta ZA. Multiple-micronutrient supplementation for women during pregnancy. Cochrane Database Syst Rev. 2017;4(4):CD004905.
101. Lassi ZS, Kedzior SG, Tariq W, Jadoon Y, Das JK, Bhutta ZA. Effects of preconception care and periconception interventions on maternal nutritional status and birth outcomes in low- and middle-income countries: a systematic review. Nutrients. 2020;12(3):606.
102. Viswanathan M, Treiman KA, Kish-Doto J, Middleton JC, Coker-Schwimmer EJ, Nicholson WK. Folic acid supplementation for the prevention of neural tube defects: an updated evidence report and systematic review for the US preventive services task force. JAMA. 2017;317(2):190–203.
103. Biesalski HK, Tinz J. Multivitamin/mineral supplements: rationale and safety—a systematic review. Nutrition. 2017;33:76–82.
104. Zeisel SH. Is maternal diet supplementation beneficial? Optimal development of infant depends on mother's diet. Am J Clin Nutr. 2009;89(2):685s–7s.
105. Bastos Maia S, Rolland Souza AS, Costa Caminha MF, Lins da Silva S, Callou Cruz R, Carvalho dos Santos C, Batista Filho M. Vitamin a and pregnancy: a narrative review. Nutrients. 2019;11(3):681.
106. Tucker J, Fischer T, Upjohn L, Mazzera D, Kumar M. Unapproved pharmaceutical ingredients included in dietary supplements associated with US Food and Drug Administration warnings. JAMA Netw Open. 2018;1(6):e183337.
107. Rocha T, Amaral JS, Oliveira M. Adulteration of dietary supplements by the illegal addition of synthetic drugs: a review. Compr Rev Food Sci Food Saf. 2016;15(1):43–62.
108. Costa JG, Vidovic B, Saraiva N, Do Céu Costa M, Del Favero G, Marko D, Oliveira NG, Fernandes AS. Contaminants: a dark side of food supplements? Free Radic Res. 2019;53(sup1):1113–35.
109. Wowdzia JB, McHugh TL, Thornton J, Sivak A, Mottola MF, Davenport MH. Elite athletes and pregnancy outcomes: a systematic review and meta-analysis. Med Sci Sports Exerc. 2021;53(3):534–42.
110. Al Wattar B, Dodds J, Placzek A, Beresford L, Spyreli E, Moore A, Gonzalez Carreras F, Austin F, Murugesu N, Roseboom TJ, et al. Mediterranean-style diet in pregnant women with metabolic risk factors (ESTEEM): a pragmatic multicentre randomised trial. PLoS Med. 2019;16(7):e1002857.
111. Muktabhant B, Lawrie TA, Lumbiganon P, Laopaiboon M. Diet or exercise, or both, for preventing excessive weight gain in pregnancy. Cochrane Database Syst Rev. 2015;(6):CD007145.
112. Rasmussen L, Poulsen C, Kampmann U, Smedegaard S, Ovesen P, Fuglsang J. Diet and healthy lifestyle in the management of gestational diabetes mellitus. Nutrients. 2020;12(10):3050.
113. Jebeile H, Mijatovic J, Louie JCY, Prvan T, Brand-Miller JC. A systematic review and metaanalysis of energy intake and weight gain in pregnancy. Am J Obstet Gynecol. 2016;214(4):465–83.

114. Rogozińska E, Zamora J, Marlin N, Betrán AP, Astrup A, Bogaerts A, Cecatti JG, Dodd JM, Facchinetti F, Geiker NRW, et al. Gestational weight gain outside the Institute of Medicine recommendations and adverse pregnancy outcomes: analysis using individual participant data from randomised trials. BMC Pregnancy Childbirth. 2019;19(1):322.
115. Sundgot-Borgen J, Sundgot-Borgen C, Myklebust G, Sølvberg N, Torstveit MK. Elite athletes get pregnant, have healthy babies and return to sport early postpartum. BMJ Open Sport Exerc Med. 2019;5(1):e000652.
116. Butte N, King J. Energy requirements during pregnancy and lactation. Public Health Nutr. 2005;8(7a):1010–27.
117. Johnson M, Campbell F, Messina J, Preston L, Buckley Woods H, Goyder E. Weight management during pregnancy: a systematic review of qualitative evidence. Midwifery. 2013;29(12):1287–96.
118. Zhu Y, Zhang C. Prevalence of gestational diabetes and risk of progression to type 2 diabetes: a global perspective. Curr Diab Rep. 2016;16(1):7.
119. Zhang GH, Chen ML, Liu SS, Zhan YH, Quan Y, Qin YM, Deng SP. Effects of mother's dietary exposure to acesulfame-K in pregnancy or lactation on the adult offspring's sweet preference. Chem Senses. 2011;36(9):763–70.
120. Weschenfelder F, Hein F, Lehmann T, Schleußner E, Groten T. Contributing factors to perinatal outcome in pregnancies with gestational diabetes-what matters most? A retrospective analysis. J Clin Med. 2021;10(2):348.
121. Szlapinski SK, Hill DJ. Metabolic adaptations to pregnancy in healthy and gestational diabetic pregnancies: the pancreas—placenta axis. Curr Vasc Pharmacol. 2021;19(2):141–53.
122. Kapur K, Kapur A, Hod M. Nutrition management of gestational diabetes mellitus. Ann Nutr Metab. 2021:1–13.
123. EFSA Panel on Contaminants in the Food Chain (CONTAM). Scientific opinion on the risk for public health related to the presence of mercury and methylmercury in food. EFSA J. 2012;10(12):2985.
124. UN Committee recommends new dietary intake limits for mercury. https://apps.who.int/mediacentre/news/notes/2003/np20/en/index.html.

GPSR Compliance

The European Union's (EU) General Product Safety Regulation (GPSR) is a set of rules that requires consumer products to be safe and our obligations to ensure this.

If you have any concerns about our products, you can contact us on ProductSafety@springernature.com

In case Publisher is established outside the EU, the EU authorized representative is:

Springer Nature Customer Service Center GmbH
Europaplatz 3
69115 Heidelberg, Germany

Batch number: 10732031

Printed by Printforce, the Netherlands